Gut and Physiology Syndrome

Natural treatment for

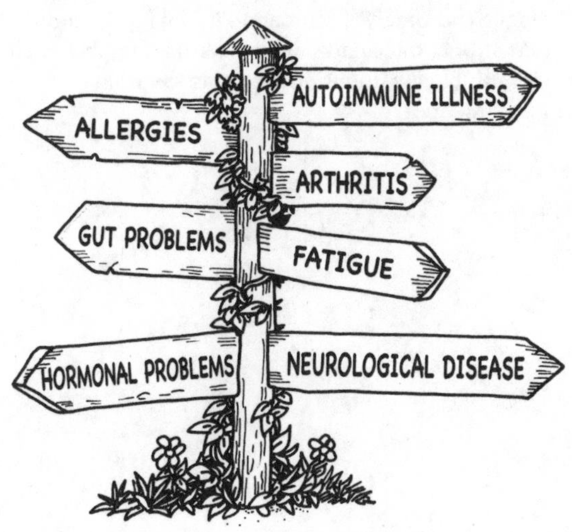

Dr. Natasha Campbell-McBride

MD, MMedSci (neurology), MMedSci (nutrition)

Gut and Physiology Syndrome

ISBN: 978–0–9548520–7–8

Medinform Publishing

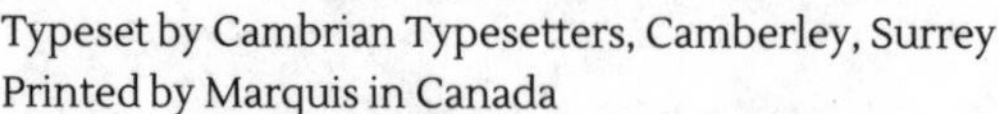
Typeset by Cambrian Typesetters, Camberley, Surrey
Printed by Marquis in Canada

*To GAPS people all over the world,
who have the courage to take control of their
health and go on a journey of personal growth
and transformation through overcoming a
chronic illness.*

Reviews

Dr Natasha Campbell-McBride has written a very important book!

Not only she has demonstrated the vital role of microbiome in all chronic disease, but has given us a practical healing protocol on how to deal with the problem. Her views on autoimmune disease are deep and based in clinical experience.

This book should be read by every person with a chronic degenerative disease, and by every medical professional, who works with these patients.

I warmly recommend it !

Professor Yehuda Shoenfeld, MD
Zabludowicz Center for Autoimmune Diseases
Chaim Sheba Medical Center, Israel

Dr. Natasha has done it again! *Gut and Physiology Syndrome* takes an in-depth look at the underlying causes of today's health crisis—environmental and dietary poisons—and then provides a comprehensive plan for detoxification and nourishment to achieve the good health and clear mind, that is the birth right of every adult and every child. Especially appreciated are suggestions for reviving our natural instincts for knowing what to eat for our own particular metabolism. *Gut and Physiology Syndrome* is an important contribution to our collective search for good health.

Sally Fallon Morell, President
The Weston A. Price Foundation

I recently had the opportunity to review Natasha Campbell-McBride's new book *Gut And Physiology Syndrome.* Natasha has been a valued colleague and friend of mine for many years. In fact, there are few other medical people who have had such a positive influence on my thinking and my practice of medicine as Natasha. Natasha is a creative thinker and a deep seeker for the truth wherever it may lie. Natasha revolutionized the world of medicine with her original GAPS concepts and books. She showed us in clear and practical terms, that microbes are not our enemies and that learning to work with our internal microbiome is one of the keys to not only our own health, but the health and survival of our planet.

The beauty of Natasha's work is that, unlike most, she takes this new understanding of our crucial relationship with the microbial world and put it into a doable, effective, action plan. Natasha's GAPS Diet has been a cornerstone of my medical work for the greater part of a decade.

With her new book, Natasha expands on her vision of the role of our microbiome in our entire physiology. She continues to break new ground as she gently pushes us into a new more honest, realistic and ecological understanding of life. This work is a tremendous contribution towards remediating our current medical situation: one, in which our current medicine is largely another source of sickness and disease, to one, where we can begin to heal the tremendous suffering we are experiencing all around us. Please buy this book, think about what is being said and, if possible, put these ideas into action. Our world depends on it!

Dr Thomas Cowan, MD

This book is a gem! A wealth of information about the central role of the gut microbiome in maintaining the health of all the organs of our body. A central theme is that infectious disease only happens when our tissues are unhealthy, due to nutritional deficiencies and toxic chemical exposures, and infection is part of a repair mechanism to restore health. For example, fungi release nanoparticles that can absorb toxic metals and facilitate their removal from the body. This book will change your perspective on health and disease and teach you how to heal your body naturally.

Dr Stephanie Seneff, PhD

This book is a tour de force! A revelation! With chronic illness affecting over half the US population, with a new generation of children sicker and dying younger than their parents' generation – if this continues we are facing the deterioration of our civilization and humanity. Dr Campbell-McBride reveals the damage is mostly self-inflicted!

Dr Campbell-McBride does more than show us the causes of illnesses, she gives us practical ways of reversing (and preventing) the deterioration of health and offering us hope for true healing. This book should be required reading in every medical school.

Established ways are slow to adapt and change. Therefore, it is up to the individual healthcare practitioner, the parent with a chronically ill child, or adult (seeking to reverse conditions they were told were incurable), the health-conscious consumer (wishing to optimize and preserve their well-being and that of their family) to read this book. Lives are at stake.

Tedd Koren, DC, Developer of Koren Specific Technique, and author of *Cancer is Natural, So is the Cure* and *Childhood Vaccination: Questions All Parents Should Ask.*

Well, Dr Natasha has done it again! This book abounds rational information and wisdom. Her explanation of the body's physiology is brilliant, yet easy to comprehend.

Gut and Psychology Syndrome was a revelation to the world of autism and mental illness. Gut and Physiology Syndrome restores hope to all people suffering from chronic diseases and unexplained symptoms.
I can't thank her enough!

Beatrice Levinson, Traditional Naturopath, Certified GAPS Practitioner

Contents

Introduction

Modern medicine has divided the human body into different systems and compartments. We have a cardio-vascular system, a nervous system, a digestive system, a respiratory system, a muscular-skeletal system and many more. To treat problems in those systems we have cardiologists, neurologists, psychiatrists, gastroenterologists and other specialists. The reason for this division is that medical science has accumulated a huge amount of information which is impossible for one person to know in its entirety. A specialist can learn in depth about one aspect of human physiology.

However, from the beginning it became clear that there is a problem with specialisation. The human body is one entity; it functions as a whole. Every system, every organ, every cell communicates, affecting each other and working together. Unfortunately, specialists in different disciplines often do not communicate with each other, avoid affecting each other and do not work together. Cardiology may focus on the heart function without considering what is going on in the rest of the body. Gastroenterology often thinks that the digestive system has no relation to other organs and systems, while psychiatry usually behaves as if the brain functions completely separately from the body. Is it a surprise then that some diseases have long been pronounced 'incurable'?

Many medics are uncomfortable with this situation and are trying to work in a more holistic way.

The more I worked with children and adults with learning disabilities and mental illness in my clinic, the more I realised that what caused their mental problems was also causing a plethora of their physical problems. What kind of physical problems? Painful and stiff joints, hay fever and asthma, allergies and food intolerances, bed-wetting and cystitis, painful muscles and bones, lack of energy and debilitating fatigue, headaches, chronically blocked and runny nose, various skin rashes and eczema, hair loss and alopecia, poor muscle density and strength, bad breath and mouth ulcers, body odour, poor blood sugar control, hormonal abnormalities, neurological symptoms, diarrhoea, constipation, abdominal pain and bloating, and many other physical symptoms.

The body works as a whole: whatever affects the brain and causes mental symptoms is at the same time affecting other organs in the body, which in turn respond with their own uncomfortable symptoms. My first book *Gut and Psychology Syndrome (GAPS). Natural treatment for autism,*

ADD/ADHD, dyspraxia, dyslexia, depression, schizophrenia and more focussed on the brain function of the person. So, it was logical to call the physical part of the problem *Gut and Physiology Syndrome,* which also abbreviates to *GAPS* in the English language.

What is GAPS?

All diseases begin in the gut! This is what Hippocrates, the father of modern medicine, concluded more than two thousand years ago. And the more we learn with our modern scientific tools the more we realise just how correct he was. Indeed, every chronic disease begins in the gut. *GAPS,* which stands for *Gut and Psychology Syndrome* and *Gut and Physiology Syndrome,* establishes a connection between the state of a person's digestive system and the health of the rest of the body.

Our digestive system holds the roots of our health; GAPS conditions stem from the unhealthy gut.

The list of GAPS conditions is long; I divided them into two groups:

1. Gut and Psychology Syndrome

2. Gut and Physiology Syndrome

Gut and Psychology Syndrome or GAPS includes learning disabilities and mental disorders, such as autism, ADHD/ADD, dyslexia, dyspraxia, addictions, depression, obsessive-compulsive disorder, bipolar disorder, schizophrenia, epilepsy, eating disorders and many other conditions which affect the function of the brain. Many of these conditions have no established diagnostic labels and present themselves as a mixture of various symptoms: mood alterations, memory and cognitive problems, behavioural and social problems, panic attacks, anxiety, involuntary movements, various tics and fits, sensory problems, etc. When the brain is in trouble it can produce any mixture of symptoms. You may find it useful to read my first book, which covers Gut and Psychology Syndrome, even if your individual health problem is not listed on its cover.

Gut and Physiology Syndrome or GAPS includes various chronic physical conditions which stem from an unhealthy gut, such as all autoimmune conditions (celiac disease, rheumatoid arthritis, type one diabetes, multiple sclerosis, amyotrophic lateral sclerosis, systemic lupus erythematosus, osteoarthritis, Crohn's disease, ulcerative colitis, autoimmune skin problems, etc.), asthma, eczema, various allergies, food allergy and intolerance, chronic fatigue syndrome, fibromyalgia, myalgic encephalomyelitis, multiple chemical sensitivity, arthritis, menstrual problems, endocrine disorders (thyroid, adrenal and other), neurological diseases and all chronic digestive disorders (such as irritable bowel syndrome, gastritis, colitis, oesophagitis, etc). Many conditions do not fit into any diagnostic box and can present as a mixture of symptoms: digestive problems, fatigue, muscular weakness, cramps and abnormal muscle tone, pains and aches in joints and muscles, skin problems, hormonal abnormalities, etc.

In every person the symptoms from both GAP Syndromes overlap: people with mental problems suffer physical symptoms (painful joints and muscles, fatigue, skin problems, allergies, asthma, hormonal problems, autoimmunity), while people with physical conditions have mental symptoms (such as depression, 'brain fog', inability to concentrate, mood swings, sleep abnormalities, memory problems, anxiety, panic attacks, tremors, tics, fits, etc.). When the digestive system is unwell, so instead of being a source of nourishment it becomes a major source of toxicity in the body, nothing in the body can function well. Any organ, any system, any cell can show symptoms of distress – usually many of them respond with some symptoms. As a result, GAPS patients are often the most difficult (if not impossible) for mainstream medicine to fathom and to help.

Indeed, you may have been told by your medical practitioner that your disease is 'incurable', and that all you can do for the rest of your life is 'manage the symptoms' with various medications, while your body progressively deteriorates. This is happening with an ever-increasing number of adults and children in our modern world. More than that: diseases are becoming 'younger' – disorders which used to be found largely in adults are now found in children, and children succumb to them at a younger and younger age.

Here is an approximate list of symptoms and conditions which may belong to the *Gut and Physiology Syndrome.*

Addictions
Alcoholism
Allergy, various forms
Alopecia
Amyotrophic lateral sclerosis (*Lou Gehrig's disease*)
Anaemia
Arthritis, various forms
Atopic conditions
Autoimmunity
Asthma
Back pain, chronic
Bed-wetting
Blood sugar instability

Celiac disease
Chronic fatigue syndrome
Colitis
Constipation, chronic
Crohn's disease
Cyclical vomiting syndrome
Cystitis
Diabetes, type one and type two
Diarrhoea, chronic
Digestive illness
Ear infections, chronic
Eczema
Failure to thrive
Fatigue
Fibromyalgia
Food allergy and food intolerance
FPIES (*Food Protein Induced Enterocolitis Syndrome)* and its variations
Fussy eating
Gastritis
Gastroesophageal Reflux Disease (*GERD*)
Glue ear (*chronic otitis media with effusion*)
Gluten sensitivity
Hay fever
Hair loss
Headaches
Hormonal problems
IBS (*Irritable Bowel Syndrome*)
Immune system insufficiency
Infertility
Lupus
Lyme disease
Malabsorption and malnourishment
ME (*Myalgic Encephalomyelitis*)
Menstrual problems
Migraine
Milk allergy
Mould sensitivity / allergy
Multiple chemical sensitivity
Multiple sclerosis
Neurological illness
Neuropathy, various forms
Nephropathy
Oesophagitis

Osteoarthritis
Osteoporosis
PANDAS (*Paediatric Autoimmune Neuropsychiatric Disorders Associated with Streptococcus*)
Parasites
PCOS (*Polycystic Ovaries Syndrome*)
PMS (*Peri-Menstrual Syndrome*)
Psoriasis, psoriatic arthritis
Reflux
Restless Leg Syndrome
Rosacea
Rheumatoid arthritis
Sinusitis, chronic
Thyroid problems
Ulcerative colitis
Urinary problems
Vaginal thrush, other vaginal problems

This list is not complete; many other chronic health problems begin in the gut. No doctor can have an extensive clinical experience with all of these conditions. However, from the way these disorders develop and the way they respond to treatment, I have no doubt that, at their root, they are GAPS disorders. That is why I recommend implementing the *GAPS Nutritional Protocol* as baseline treatment for all of these conditions. This protocol has been designed to heal your gut, to make the very roots of your health robust and functioning as they should.

Every human being is unique and will have a unique response to the treatment. Some will recover fully just with the *GAPS Nutritional Protocol*. Some will require other health treatments added to the GAPS Programme, such as homeopathy, acupuncture, medicinal herbs, removing toxic metals, psychotherapy, bioresonance, light, sound, massage, physiotherapy, spiritual treatment, natural spa treatment, hypobaric oxygenation, sauna, detox programmes, etc. No matter what your individual situation is, *GAPS Nutritional Protocol* will lay a solid foundation for your full recovery; it will give the roots of your health the best chance to heal. Once you have built this solid foundation, you will find that all those other healing methods work much better for you, starting to make a real difference, because the root of the problem has been addressed. And the root of every chronic disease is to be found in the digestive system! This book will explain why.

In the next chapter we will be talking about what lives inside your digestive system and who takes care of it. We will be talking about gut flora. There is a growing epidemic of abnormalities in gut flora in modern humans and this epidemic is getting deeper with every generation. This epidemic is the basis for all chronic disease epidemics in the world. Make no mistake: the state of your gut flora is the cause of your disease, no matter how far from the gut your symptoms may be located! Whether you are suffering from rheumatoid arthritis, multiple sclerosis, allergies, asthma, neuropathy or a skin disorder, the cause of your disease is in the gut. By the time you have finished reading this book you will have no doubt about it.

The human body is a wonderful creation: it has a full ability to heal and maintain itself programmed into it! You have to allow your body to use this divine programme. Healing begins from understanding what is going on in your body. Knowledge is the key: no matter how chronic and severe your health problem may be, you must know why you are developing it and where it came from. Without this knowledge fear takes hold, and fear can only destroy. This book will give you an understanding of where your chronic disease came from and how to find your way to good health.

Let us begin!

Good health begins in the soil inside us!

If you don't like bacteria, you're on the wrong planet.

Stewart Brand

Did you know that your body is populated by a myriad of microscopic creatures? Your skin, your mucous membranes, your heart, your lungs, your blood vessels, your abdominal cavity and all your other organs and tissues are teeming with life. The variety and diversity of microbes we all carry on and in ourselves are staggering; it is a world just as amazing and complex as life on Earth itself! The fact is: we are never alone! The human body is an ecosystem of life forms, inseparable from each other and dependent upon each other.

The majority of these microbes live inside our digestive systems. They are called gut flora and, more recently, gut microbiota or gut microbiome.[1] In this book we focus on the gut flora, because it is the headquarters of our body's microbial flora. What happens in the gut flora has a profound effect on every other microbial community in the body (in the blood, on mucous membranes, inside organs and tissues). It is also the easiest part of our microbiome for us for influence. So, by working on our gut flora and keeping it healthy and well, we can keep the body's microbiome healthy, so it behaves as a good friend to us rather than a powerful foe.

Our gut flora is a mixture of uncountable species of bacteria, fungi, viruses, protozoa, worms and all sorts of other creatures. Different life forms inside the human digestive system live together in harmony controlling each other, planting each other, harvesting each other, eating each other, assisting each other and competing with each other. Recent research has discovered that about 90% of all cells in the human body are in our gut flora![2] So, our bodies make-up just 10% of us, a shell, a habitat for that mass of microbes living inside our digestive systems! This microbial community is an organ in its own right! The more we learn about this microbial world the more we realise what an important part of us it is. Our health very much depends on the health of our gut flora. No matter how far from the gut an organ in your body is, it is greatly affected by the gut flora's composition, state and functions.[3]

We have all seen a picture of a plant with its roots in the soil. But if we look at the image of our gut wall under the microscope, we see a very similar picture. The absorptive surface of the human gut has tiny finger-like protrusions, called villi. The surface of these villi is covered by thin, long, stringy hair called microvilli, which under the microscope look very much like the hair roots of a plant. Then we see that this hairy surface inside us is not clean and shiny at all, it is covered by a sticky 'dirty-looking' substance; the spaces between villi are full to the brim with it, so only the tips of the villi are visible. In different places this substance is brown or lighter coloured, and under the microscope it looks very much like soil in its structure. What is this substance? Let us examine it.

All microbes in this world build little homes for themselves. Most creatures on our planet build some sort of shelter for themselves, including us humans! The microbes in our gut do the same; they secrete various substances (polypeptides, gluelike adhesins, glycoproteins, proteoglycans and many more) to surround themselves with and create perfect cosy homes to live in. This sticky substance has a name – biofilm.[4] As we have a myriad of different microbes in the gut, living together in a complex mixture, their biofilms are mixed together, creating that 'dirty-looking' sticky cover on the gut wall, filling up all the deep crevices and crypts between villi and other structures. This is our own soil and the 'roots' of our health are sitting in that soil.

Western science started researching gut flora only recently. However, we have been researching soils on our planet for much longer and know a little about them. In order for us to understand our gut flora, I think, it is a good idea to look at the structure of the soil under our feet.

A complex mixture of different life forms lives in healthy soil: fungi, bacteria, viruses, protozoa, nematodes, arthropods, worms, insects. Larger creatures, such as moles, voles, mice and other animals visit frequently to feed on the microbes, worms and insects, contributing to the overall fertility of the soil. All these life forms, great and small, form one ecosystem, diverse and balanced, where every creature plays an important part.[5] The same picture can be seen in the human gut. A healthy gut flora has a large diversity of different life forms: bacteria, viruses, fungi, protozoa, flukes, worms and all sorts of other creatures living together in harmony in their own soil, which they create for themselves. Your gut wall is imbedded in this 'soil', coated and protected by it, fed and nourished by it, rooted in it with its many protrusions, villi and microvilli. The bigger the diversity of different life forms in your gut flora – the healthier you are!

Let us have a look at the life forms in our gut, based on what we have studied so far. I am sure there are many other creatures there which we have not yet discovered. And those that we have discovered, we have not yet researched to any great degree.

Fungi

The most active place in the soil is an area around plant roots, because the roots secrete sugars.[6] A myriad of microbes lives in this area feeding on these secretions, none so important as fungi, called mycorrhiza.[7] These fungi create an extension of the root system of the plant; they attach themselves to the roots and grow a fine network of long filaments with many branches, spreading to a large area around the root. Through mycorrhiza all plants growing in an area are connected to each other underground: two trees may be many metres away from each other, but they are connected through this fungal network, sharing information, nutrition and water. Grasses and bushes between these trees participate in this network through the mycorrhiza on their roots. In fact, researchers now talk about the whole planet being wrapped in a fungal 'blanket' of fine filaments – a network probably much more sophisticated than our World Wide Web.[8] Just as the arteries and capillaries in our bodies bring nutrients to our cells, this fungal network brings nutrients to the plant roots. Thanks to mycorrhiza, the root system of the plant becomes many times bigger and more efficient at feeding the plant. Apart from feeding it, mycorrhizal network protects the plant from toxic metals and other poisons which may exist in the soil.[9] In the human body the blood transports hormones, neurotransmitters, enzymes and many other information-carrying substances. Mycorrhiza does the same underground: it carries information from one plant to the next. The flow of information, nutrients, water and more can go any way, back and forth through the mycorrhizal network. This network is dynamic: new filaments grow all the time and connect to the whole network, while other filaments disappear. This fungal network provides soil with a fine structure, a road system of a sort, and a myriad of small creatures (bacteria, viruses, archaea, protozoa and other) live on this structure. Just as we – humans – build our homes along streets, lanes and roads that deliver goods back and forth for us, the microbes build their 'homes' along the mycorrhizal 'road system'.

Recent research into human gut flora has discovered some 60-70 species of different fungi living in the gut of healthy people.[10] No doubt future research will discover that their numbers are much greater than that. The fact that these fungi thrive in the gut of a healthy person means that they are there for a purpose. Do they create mycorrhiza inside us to participate in digestion and absorption of food? There is no doubt about it! These fungi provide our microbial community with a structure; their network of thin filaments makes a 'road network' in the gut flora. Along this network smaller creatures can build their homes (their 'houses, villages and towns') and thrive. Nutrients, information and water are delivered to their 'homes' via this 'road network' and wastes are taken away. These long filaments would transport nutrients and water through the gut flora and to our gut wall for us to absorb. So, our ability to benefit from the food, we eat, would depend greatly on the fungal population inside our gut flora!

Let us look further. The absorptive surface of the human gut has finger-like protrusions (called villi), which are covered by thin long stringy hair (called microvilli). When we look at microvilli under the microscope, we see that they are covered by a thick 'forest' of long thin filaments with many branches. It is called glycocalyx.[11] What is it made from? From molecules similar to that fine network of fungal filaments in the soil (the mycorrhiza) – glycoproteins, proteoglycans and others. Glycocalyx is present not only in the gut wall but on all our mucous membranes, inside our blood vessels and in other places in the body.[11] Is glycocalyx in our bodies an equivalent of mycorrhiza in the soil? Is it of fungal origin? Hopefully future research will find that out.

When it comes to fungi, so far we have largely focused on a ubiquitous yeast, called candida, which lives in the human body. Hundreds of candida species have been discovered so far. In a healthy person candida produces no symptoms, but in a person with compromised gut flora it can overgrow and become a dangerous parasite. Candida is a normal part of our human microbiome, and in a balanced gut flora with a large diversity of microbes it is beneficial for us.[12] From clinical experience we already know that candida protects us from mercury and other toxic metals, [13] just as mycorrhiza in the soil protects plants from mercury and other toxic metals. This fungus absorbs and retrains mercury, thus protecting us. For example, from clinical experience, we know that people who have amalgam fillings in their teeth can never get rid of candida overgrowth in their gut, because the body uses it to protect itself from mercury and other toxic substances leaching from the amalgams.[14] I am sure that future research will discover other beneficial functions of candida in the body. We may also discover that, what we thought was candida, is actually a large community of many other species of fungi, fulfilling complex services for us.

When we try to attack candida with antifungal drugs, we attack many other species of fungi in the body, which are likely to be beneficial for us. I have patients in my clinic who have developed severe illness after a course of an antifungal drug. Experienced health practitioners will tell you how difficult it is to 'eliminate' candida from the body; in fact, it is impossible. When we attack candida, it releases mercury and other toxins back into the system, making us very ill. As soon as we stop attacking candida, it re-grows quite quickly. The only way to deal with candida is to restore diversity in the gut flora, so other microbes take the fungi under control. It is also necessary to remove the toxins which these fungi are protecting us from. As long as these toxins remain in the system, the fungi will grow because they are Nature's universal decomposers. If there is anything dead or damaged that needs to be broken down and re-cycled fungi will be there, active and thriving, and the human body is no exception! When the body is polluted, damaged and full of decaying material, we will have an overgrowth of fungi inside, causing unpleasant symptoms.

Fungal overgrowth is an unbalanced situation. We, human beings, are good at creating unbalanced situations in Nature, including in our own bodies. As soon as we find a microbe, we want to kill it, whether it is in the soil, in the water, in the air or inside us. Research has shown that the best and most efficient policy against candida overgrowth is having a healthy population of beneficial bacteria in the body, *Lactobacilli* in particular.[15] They eat fungi, controlling their growth and proliferation.[16] Antibiotics destroy these beneficial bacteria in the gut leaving candida uncontrolled.[17] That is why most cases of fungal overgrowth in humans happen after courses of antibiotics. When you kill some part of the balanced microbial community in the gut flora, it becomes unbalanced and disease always follows. Did you know that approximately three-quarters of all antibiotics produced in the Western world are fed to poultry, cows and pigs in our industrial agriculture?[18] These antibiotics remain in the eggs, milk and meat we get from these animals.[19] Add to that the fact that most pesticides, fungicides, herbicides and other agricultural chemicals, used extensively in the production of plants for humans, are antibiotics in their nature.[20] Every time we eat bread, vegetables, fruit or any other commercially produced plants we consume antibiotics.[21] In the West, people have been eating these contaminated foods for several decades now, damaging their gut flora and promoting fungal overgrowth in their bodies.

Let us come back to the soil where plants grow. The microbes in the soil produce gluelike substances, which give the soil its crumbly texture and ability to hold water. For example, mycorrhiza produces a 'glue' called glomalin.[22] Candida also produces a 'glue' (agglutinin-like adhesins, fibrinogen, fibronectin and other), which creates complexes with bacteria, viruses and other microbes in the gut, and their gluelike secretions and biofilms![23] These complexes absorb large amounts of water, keeping the gut wall moist, well-lubricated and protected. The same happens in the soil: gluelike microbial products are important reasons why healthy soils absorb and hold large amounts of water. Modern agriculture uses chemicals and practices which destroy these gluelike substances in the soil, and the microbes which produce them. As a result, the soil cannot hold water, so arable lands become prone to drought, while every rain runs off these fields, creating floods in villages and towns downstream. The same situation happens in the gut when we destroy our gut flora with antibiotics and other chemicals: the gut wall loses its protection, lubrication and moisture.

It may turn out that fungi are some of the most important inhabitants of a healthy human gut! They provide the very basis and structure for our gut flora; we need to cultivate them and take care of them.

Bacteria

Bacteria are the most researched part of our gut flora; thousands of species have been discovered and the list is growing. According to current research, they comprise some 60% of the dry mass of the stool (human faeces), that is why they are considered to be the most numerous inhabitants of the human gut.[24]

Most research into gut flora is done by studying human stools. However, our gut flora does not live in the stool; it lives on the wall of the gut. What we have in the stool is spent microbes and other dead matter that is being discarded by the body. The fact that bacteria finish up in the stool in large numbers does not necessarily mean that they are the most numerous and most important members of our gut flora. All it means is that the body discards them in large numbers for some reason. In order to see the real gut flora, we need to study biopsy samples of the gut wall.[25] Millions of routine biopsies are carried out by mainstream gastroenterologists all over the world, but these samples are hardly ever sent for microbiological examination. Hopefully, mainstream practices will change in the future, but at the moment it is stool that is being tested. So, the research we have so far is not very reliable. But that is what we have, so let us have a look at it.

The bacterial composition of your stool very much depends on what kind of meal has come out of you. If it included some animal foods (meat, fish, eggs and dairy) then your stool is likely to be dominated by *bacteroides*.[26] But if it largely contained plant matter then your stool will be dominated by *prevotella* species.[27] None of these bacteria are 'good' or 'bad' necessarily, but it shows that food has a powerful effect on the composition of microbial flora. This confirms our knowledge that to heal the gut in people with abnormal gut flora we need to change the person's diet.

Recent research in bacteria has discovered that they have 'flexible' genetics.[28] Their genes are free-floating, enabling them to discard some genes into their environment and pick up other genes: there is some sort of 'free gene market' for these microbes. Based on this discovery researchers now propose that there are no isolated species of bacteria in

Nature, but a continuum where genetics are constantly exchanged and changed.[29] One species of bacterium can become another by choosing genetics based on their environment and needs. This process is active inside our bodies: in our gut, on our mucous membranes and in every other tissue and organ. The gene exchange can happen not only between bacteria, but between microbes and our own cells.[30]

Different parts of the human digestive system have been found to have different bacteria living there.

The mouth and oesophagus are richly populated by microbes. Some 600–800 different species of bacteria have been identified in the oral cavity alone.[31] Different structures in the mouth have different flora on them (the teeth, the gums, the tongue, mucosa of the cheeks, tonsils, etc). When this flora is balanced and there is appropriate diversity of microbes, those areas stay healthy. It is very interesting that all the groups of bacteria, present in the human stool, are also present in our saliva! It appears that ancient traditional cultures around the world knew something about this. Apparently, in rural China there was a tradition for the grandparents to put some of their saliva into the mouth of a new-born baby in the family.

The stomach produces hydrochloric acid, which creates a very hostile environment for microbes. As a result, the human stomach is considered to be the least populated area of our digestive system (0–10^3 colonies per millilitre of stomach content).[32] However, some microbes like living in an acidic environment and are found in the stomach: *yeasts (including candida), helicobacter pylori, some streptococci, staphylococci and lactobacilli.*[33] No doubt this list is incomplete. Pathologists (who do post-mortem examinations) sometimes find worms in the stomachs of people, plus we have not yet studied viruses, archaea and other microbes, many of which live happily in very acidic environments in nature. These are normal inhabitants of a healthy stomach, they live in the top layers of the mucosa of the stomach lining, and in every person their number is individual. All of these microbes are capable of causing disease, but as long as the stomach's mucosa is healthy and produces normal amounts of acid they do us no harm and, very likely, do a lot of good services for us too.[34]

The trouble is, in our modern world, people take painkillers, anti-inflammatory drugs and antibiotics regularly, which damage the protective mucous layers of the stomach.[34] This allows resident bacteria and yeasts to get deeper into the wall of the stomach and impair acid production.[35] Once the stomach acidity becomes low, all sorts of other microbes come in and settle on the walls of the stomach, and our resident microbes overgrow and become a problem. The person develops indigestion, heart-burn, belching, reflux and other symptoms. People take antacid drugs for heart-burn and indigestion, which reduce stomach acid production even further, making the whole situation worse long term. If this situation continues, more severe problems can develop, such as stomach ulcers and cancer.[36] *Helicobacter pylori* is considered to be responsible for ulcers and cancer in the stomach. However, the majority of people, who have this microbe living in their stomachs, are perfectly healthy, because healthy stomach mucosa does not allow microbes to get deep into the stomach wall and cause trouble. The stomach mucosa has to be damaged first by drugs or something else in order for *H. pylori* to become a problem.

Helicobacter pylori is now considered to be a normal inhabitant of the human digestive system; babies are supposed to acquire it fairly soon after birth. Research shows that in countries with traditional ways of life the majority of small children have this microbe in their stomachs, while in Western countries only about 5% of children have it.[37] The absence of this microbe in the gut of children and adults is linked to high rates of asthma, allergies and obesity.[38] Our appetite and food consumption are controlled by hormones produced in the stomach and duodenum: ghrelin, leptin and other. *Helicobacter pylori* appears to be involved in the normal production of these hormones.[39] In the absence of *H.pylori,* the production of these hormones becomes unbalanced, leading to poor appetite control, abnormal metabolism and weight gain. Remember that our industrial agriculture deliberately feeds antibiotics to poultry and livestock to fatten them up more quickly, because antibiotics damage their gut flora and normal appetite regulation, and encourage growth of particular microbes associated with obesity. So, if your doctor has found *H.pylori* in your stomach, don't rush to take antibiotics to eliminate it. This microbe should only be attacked in cases of stomach ulcers, stomach cancer or another serious stomach problem, and only as part of a holistic protocol, which includes appropriate diet.

Many people with low stomach acid production and an overgrowth of microbes in the stomach suffer from belching and bloating, because yeasts, archaea and other microbes in their stomachs produce too much gas. Your stomach is positioned underneath your heart (separated by the diaphragm). When the stomach fills with gas, it can push the heart up into an unnatural position, which can cause a heart problem: heart racing, abnormal rhythm and palpitations. This usually happens when you are driving or sitting in a way that doesn't give your abdomen much room to expand. Releasing the gas though belching can stop the heart symptoms. But, long term, we have to address the stomach problem in order to help the heart.

The small intestine has more bacteria living in it than the stomach, and the further from the stomach we get, the richer that flora becomes. In the duodenum (the highest part of the small intestine) very few microbes are found (0–10^5 colonies per millilitre of intestinal content) and the species are very similar to the stomach population (*yeasts, streptococci, staphylococci and lactobacilli*). In the ileum (the last third of the small intestine) the flora is the richest (10^3–10^6 colonies per millilitre of content), and the lowest end becomes very similar to the flora of the bowel, dominated by *Bacteroides, Clostridia* and *coliforms*.[40] The numbers of bacteria in the small intestine very much depend on the level of stomach acid production, particularly in the first two-thirds of the intestines. If the stomach produces normal amounts of acid, then the small intestine is sparsely populated. But, if the person has low acidity in the stomach, then the small intestine will have a much bigger population of microbes in it. People who have an overgrowth of microbes in their small intestine may be diagnosed with IBS (Irritable Bowel Syndrome) or SIBO (Small Intestinal Bacterial Overgrowth). Studying the gut flora of the small intestine is quite difficult, which is why we don't have much knowledge in this area yet. And what is largely being researched is only the content of the intestine, not the samples of the intestinal wall (where our real gut flora lives). There is no doubt that intestinal permeability (or 'leaky gut') is caused by abnormal microbial flora on the wall of the small intestine.[41] The bulk of food absorption happens in this part of our digestive system. So, when it is damaged and not working well, we cannot digest and absorb food properly, and as a result develop multiple nutritional deficiencies.

The bowel (colon or large intestine) has the richest population of microbes living in it; this is where the bulk of our gut flora resides.[42] An ever-growing number of different species of bacteria is being identified in human stools; the more we study this mixture of microbes the more we realise just how complex it is and how little we know about it. The predominant groups of bacteria in the stool of healthy people are *Bacteroides, Fusobacteria, Bifidobacteria, Eubacteria, Peptostreptococci* and *Clostridia*.[43] Researchers are concerned that we are not able to culture or identify large numbers of species, which gives us a very incomplete picture.

Our human bowel can be seen as an equivalent of the rumen of herbivorous animals. Herbivorous animals (grazing animals which eat only grass and other plants) have a very special digestive system with several stomachs full of microbes, called rumen.[44] It is not the cows (sheep, deer, horses, goats or other ruminants) that digest the grass and other plants, they eat, but their microbial flora in the rumen. Some 70% of all carbohydrates (sugars) in the grass are converted by the rumen microbes into saturated fat (short-chain fatty acids); these sugars absorb in that form.[45] The same thing happens in our bowel: complex carbohydrates, which did not get digested higher up, are converted into short-chain fatty acids and absorbed. They play many useful roles in the body. The difference between humans and herbivorous animals is that their rumen is at the beginning of their digestive systems, while our 'rumen' – the bowel – is at the end. Humans and herbivorous animals have very different digestive systems, which handle food differently.

A large part of the research into bacteria in the stool has focussed on so-called prebiotics – carbohydrates which feed bacteria. Prebiotics, starch and fibre are considered to be good food for bacteria in the gut, and we have many supplements on the market with these substances: FOS (fructooligosaccharides), inulin and others. The problem is that prebiotics, starch and fibre feed equally the 'good' and the 'bad' microbes in the gut. If your gut is largely populated by the beneficial microbes, they will feast on the starch, fibre and prebiotics, grow larger colonies and make you healthier as a result. But, if your gut is dominated by pathogenic microbes, then they will feed on these carbohydrates and grow bigger and stronger, and make you very sick as a result.[46] GAPS people have pathogens dominating their gut flora, so prebiotics, starch and fibre are not good for them: they cause bloating, flatulence, abdominal pain and abnormal stools. These patients have to work on changing their gut flora first, removing pathogens and re-establishing beneficial microbes, before they can try foods containing those complex carbohydrates.

Archaea

Archaea are generally similar in size and shape to bacteria, but are considered to be a different group of microbes. They are some of the most ancient and most numerous microbes on the planet, and they are able to use all sorts of things as food and for producing energy: sugars, metals, gases, ammonia and even sunlight. *Methanobrevibacter smithii* – an archaea found in the human gut – is thought to complete the process of fermentation in the bowel.[47] Archaea produce gases, methane in particular. So, people with excessive gas production and symptoms of bloating, belching and flatulence are likely to have an overgrowth of this group of microbes. Archaea are very efficient at extracting energy and calories out of food. For example, a study in anorexic patients has discovered an overgrowth of archaea in their digestive systems.[48] Anorexic patients eat very little, so their gut flora grows archaea to extract as much energy and calories as possible from food, so the person can survive on their meagre ration. We know very little about this group of microbes, but it is a fact that they are very numerous in healthy soil and in the healthy gut flora of animals and humans.[49] I am sure that future research will discover that they fulfil many beneficial functions for us.

Viruses

Did you know that the food industry uses viruses for killing bacteria on ready-to-eat meat products, cheese and many other foods?[50] And that our hospitals use viruses for cleaning catheters and other medical equipment?[51] These viruses are called bacteriophages (bacteria-eaters). They were first discovered in 1896 by a British microbiologist E. H. Hankin in the Ganges and Yamuna rivers in India. Bacteriophages in these rivers provided protection from cholera, dysentery and other infections by eating microbes which cause them. These viruses invade bacteria and destroy them. When they are introduced into the human body, they don't touch our cells but find their specific bacteria and kill them. Bacteriophages were developed as medicine in the former Soviet Union for dealing with antibiotic-resistant bacterial infections.[52] But we don't have to introduce them into our bodies! Recent research is discovering that our gut wall is covered by them![53] The biggest populations of bacteriophages are found in the gut of healthy animals (including humans) and in healthy soil. Sea-water is rich in these viruses (about 9×10^8 per ml of sea-water) and so are all other natural unpolluted waters of rivers, lakes and oceans. Undoubtedly, this is one of the reasons why swimming in natural waters has been prized for centuries as a healing procedure. Wherever there are bacteria, we find viruses – bacteriophages – and our gut flora is rich in both. All other mucous membranes and many other tissues in the body are rich in viruses, which probably protect us not only from bacteria, but from fungi, archaea and other microbes.

So, the human body is full of viruses! Among them there are many that can cause disease; yet they are normal inhabitants of the human body. For example, the *herpes* family of viruses can live in the skin, mucous membranes, immune cells and the nervous system.[54] There are some 130 species of herpes virus discovered so far and at least eight of them were found in humans. These include herpes viruses 1, 2, 6 and 7, varicella-zoster virus, EBV (Epstein-Barr virus), cytomegalovirus and Kaposi-associated herpesvirus. Animal research shows that resident herpes viruses protect their host from bacterial infections and help our immune system to deal with cancer cells and pathogenic viruses.[55] They live in our organs silently without causing any problems until we compromise our immune system and the internal environment of the body. Then they can become active and cause a transient disease: shingles, cold sores, chicken pox, infectious mononucleosis and other. These illnesses are necessary for the body to be cleansed and the immune system rebalanced. Having done their jobs, these viruses go back to their little 'homes' and become dormant again.

Another well-known resident virus in the human body is *papilloma virus*, which lives in the skin and all our mucous membranes, including the gut. There are some 170 species of this virus found so far and they normally do us no harm. I am sure that future research will show that they are beneficial for us in some way. But, when the microbial balance in the body is damaged by antibiotics and other man-made chemicals, these viruses can participate in active disease (warts and cancers on the skin and mucous membranes in the mouth, throat, lungs, digestive system and genital organs). There is no need to fear this virus and vaccinate against it! It is a normal and an essential inhabitant of the human body.[56] Instead, we need to protect our mucous membranes with a healthy diverse community of microbes – our body flora. This flora will protect you not only from viruses, but from anything else that can damage your mucous membranes and skin.[57]

Another virus called *norovirus* is common in humans. Every winter many people in the northern hemisphere get this 'tummy bug', leading to a few days of vomiting and diarrhoea. Animal experiments have shown that norovirus can restore normal gut flora, which has been damaged by antibiotics.[57] Not only gut flora is restored, but the immune function and normal physical state of the gut wall as well. Norovirus infection only lasts a few days, causing transient vomiting and diarrhoea; not a big price to pay for restoring your gut flora! Vomiting and diarrhoea are major cleansing functions of the digestive system. They are not pleasant, but they flush toxins, parasites and other disease-causing things out of your gut, leaving it cleaner and healthier as a result.

From clinical experience we know that some of the most severe cases of gut dysbiosis happen after a long course of antiviral drugs. We do not yet know what damage these drugs do to our resident viral population, let alone how to correct that damage. Healthy soils on our planet are teeming with viruses, but our industrial agriculture is destroying them together with all other life forms. We, humans, are doing the same to our resident viruses when we use antiviral drugs.

Protozoa

Protozoa are one-cell organisms with animal-like behaviour. In the soil protozoa eat bacteria and fungi, releasing their nutrients to feed the roots of the plants.[58] They are important members of the microbial community of the rumen in herbivorous animals, where they help to break down plant matter and release nutrients from it. I am sure that something similar happens in the human gut. Amoeba, giardia, cryptosporidium and other protozoa, commonly found in the human stool, can cause diarrhoea, abdominal pain and other digestive symptoms. Yet the majority of people who test positive for these microbes are perfectly healthy. When the gut flora is well-balanced, protozoa live there in small numbers and are controlled by other members of the community. But, if the balance has been upset, just like with any other microbe, they can get out of control and cause problems.

Worms

Let us start with earth-worms. These modest creatures are irreplaceable for the health of the soil. They swallow organic matter and other particles in the soil and digest them. What comes out of the other end is the best compost in existence, called worm castings, rich in humus and ready-made pre-digested nutrients for plants.[59] Moving through the soil earth-worms create channels for air and water, making the soil softer, richer and healthier, supporting microbial life and re-cycling organic matter. The more earth-worms a patch of soil contains, the more fertile and productive it is.[60]

Let us now have a look at the worms inside our digestive systems. Make no mistake – we all have them! From tiny threadworms to several-feet-long tapeworms, they are a part of normal human gut flora, an essential part. In the last ten years the interest and research into intestinal worms has intensified. Two varieties are receiving particular attention: porcine whipworm (*Trichuris suis*) and hookworm (*Necator americanus*). Taking live eggs of these worms as medicine (helminth therapy) has been demonstrated to re-balance the immune system and reduce inflammation, allergies and autoimmunity.[61] A number of published clinical trials have shown that deliberate introduction of worms into the digestive system can alleviate symptoms of Crohn's disease, ulcerative colitis, asthma, hay fever, multiple sclerosis, type one diabetes and other chronic diseases.[62] Do these worms play the same role for us as earth-worms for the planet? Do they aerate and enrich the 'soil' inside our digestive systems? I have no doubt that they do all that and more.

If we think about it, the presence of worms in our digestive systems is inevitable. The larvae of hookworms live in the soil. They burrow through the skin of your feet into the lymphatic system, travel to the digestive system, mature and lay eggs, which are then excreted in faeces and returned into the soil. For millennia we, human beings, walked barefoot. So, we all had hookworms for most of our existence on this planet.[63] Other worms are acquired the same way, or by drinking water from streams, rivers and lakes and eating food contaminated with soil. For most of our existence on this planet that is exactly what we, humans, did! Humans have always had worms and there is no need to fear them. As long as there is diversity in the gut flora, where no particular species can get out of control, these worms cause us no trouble; in fact, they bring us many benefits.

Industrial agriculture destroys worm populations in the soil. Most arable fields in the Western world have no worms left at all. The same is happening in the gut flora of humans: chemicals in our food and pharmaceutical drugs destroys many life forms in our gut, including worms. As a result, people suffer from digestive problems, allergies, autoimmunity and other chronic illnesses. On the other hand, overgrowth of various worms in the body can also cause disease. Like all other creatures inside us, worms have to be in balance and in harmony with the rest of the microbial community of the body.

The life cycle of common worms indicates that there can be no microbe-free tissues or organs inside us. Common worms lay eggs in the gut. The larva that hatches from those eggs, burrows through the gut lining and travels through the body to complete different stages in its development. Some larvae mature in the lungs and liver, some in the brain and eyes, some in the heart and spleen – no organ can be free of them. These creatures have their own gut flora and many microbes living on their surface, which they carry and seed throughout your body.[64] And that is only one way for various microbes to populate your body; there are other ways. Bacteria are often infected with viruses, protozoa are infected with bacteria, archaea and viruses and they seed these infections wherever they are in our bodies. Indeed, recent research is finding resident microbes living in our blood vessels, our brain, lungs, heart and other organs. So, the human body is not 'clean' inside! It is a diverse eco-system full of all sorts of life forms living together in every organ and tissue, not only in the gut, skin or a mucous membrane. This is a fascinating area of study where we may discover the real causes of many illnesses and the real sources of good health!

The subject of the human microbiome becomes even more interesting when we look at another aspect of microbes – a natural phenomenon, called pleomorphism.

Pleomorphism

Pleomorphism is the amazing ability of microbes to change shape and form to the point of looking and behaving like something completely different. As mentioned above, bacteria have been found to exchange their genetics between one another, other microbes and even our human cells.[65] Depending on the environment, food supply and the stage in their life cycle, microbes can become unrecognisable. In many cases microbiology has been studying different forms of one creature, thinking that they were entirely different microbes. A good example of this is L-forms of bacteria, which are attracting a lot of interest in microbiology today.[66] These bacteria lack a substance called peptidoglycan and, as a result, have no rigid cell wall. They are difficult to study and can look like chlamydia, mycoplasma, nano-microbes, fungal spores, cists, fungus, viruses, archaea, parasites or anything else. They can multiply by all sorts of unusual methods and can take many different shapes, forms and sizes. In the blood, they can attach themselves to blood cells and even live inside them while still being perfectly active.[67] They are found in the blood of healthy and sick people and are 'stealth' microbes. They can stay inactive for long periods of time inside our cells waiting for the right disease-causing environment in the body, when they can change and take part in the disease process. They are involved in all chronic degenerative conditions in humans and animals, so it is important for us to know about them.

Cell-wall deficient (L- forms) bacteria were first described in 1935 at the Lister Institute. In a healthy situation they do not trigger any immune response and do not appear to cause any harm. But, when the environment in the body changes, they can proliferate, grow out of proportion, change shape and size and become pathogenic.[66] They are thought to be involved in chronic and relapsing infections, autoimmunity, autism, chronic inflammation and cancer.[68] For example, they have been found in tumours and the blood of cancer patients, where they transform from single cell creatures to complex structures that look like fungal mycelia.[69] They can live very comfortably inside white blood cells (the very cells that are supposed to be killing microbes!) and even multiply there.

Cell-wall-deficient microbes can pass from mother to foetus.[70] We get them during our foetal development and our immune system does not react to them. They are resistant to antibiotics; in fact, a course of antibiotics stimulates their growth.[71] Antibiotics don't allow bacteria to form a proper cell membrane, and it was believed for a long time that this kills the bacteria. Now we know that many of them don't die; they just adapt to life without a tough cell membrane as L- forms and can become even more dangerous, creating chronic non-specific symptoms in the body. It is believed by researchers that ubiquitous use of antibiotics in the modern world is responsible for the existence of a large variety of cell-wall-deficient microbes in modern humans and animals.[66,72] They are impossible to destroy by established antibacterial methods (antibiotics, chlorination and other chemicals, pasteurisation, boiling and other). As a result, they are found in foods and water, pharmaceutical medicines and vaccines, as well as in all the body fluids of animals and humans.[66,72] There are many chronic illnesses which show the presence of large numbers of these cell-wall-deficient microbes (including Lyme disease, autoimmune disease, mental illnesses and cancer). A good example is PANDAS (*Paediatric Autoimmune Neuropsychiatric Disorders Associated with Streptococcal*

Infections): some researchers are now convinced that this disease is caused by a cell-wall-deficient form of streptococcus created by penicillin-type antibiotics.[73] Cell-wall-deficient microbes often hide inside our cells and are very difficult for the body to deal with; that is why they are perfectly designed to participate in chronic degenerative diseases.[67,68,70]

A number of L-forms of fungi (cell-wall-deficient or without cell walls at all) have been recently found in the blood of autistic children and their mothers: *Aspergillus fumigatus*, *Candida parapsilosis*, *Cryptococcus albidus* and *Rhodotorula mucilaginosa*.[70] It was demonstrated that these fungi are very active and capable of pleomorphing (changing) into invasive forms and that they produce powerful toxins. For example, *Aspergillus fumigatus* releases gliotoxin, which is a strong immune system suppressant.[70,74] When the immune system is suppressed, the body can get inhabited by all sorts of other microbes. On top of that, gliotoxin and other fungal metabolites are known to damage the nervous system, particularly in a developing child. Researchers are now posing a question: is silent infection with *Aspergillus fumigatus* (aspergillosis) and other filamentous fungi the cause of autism and the other neurodevelopmental disorders, that have gained epidemic proportions in Western children?[70,75] It has been shown that these fungi move from the mother's body into the body of the developing foetus during pregnancy, so these children are already born with this infection.[70,74] Antibiotics have been shown to cause fungal dysbiosis in humans and animals for decades. The presence of antibiotics in our food, water and environment is ever growing and, undoubtedly, plays an important role in this epidemic. Testing for fungi has always been a challenge for mainstream medicine and, since we could not test for them, for a long time fungal dysbiosis has been dismissed as non-existent. New scientific data allows us to see the fungal colonisation of our bodies by cell-wall-deficient fungi (L-forms), which can be far more invasive than the fully evolved forms.[70,77] In addition, these fungal L-forms produce nanoparticles – the tiniest possible particles we can detect.[77,78] Nanoparticles are so small that there is no barrier in the body that they cannot cross; they can get anywhere. The mothers of autistic children pass these nanoparticles to their unborn children.[70] Perhaps, we are all born with these nanoparticles.

I don't believe that Nature does anything without good reason! Why would a child acquire fungal nanoparticles from the mother before being born? Perhaps there is a useful purpose for them. Research provides us with a clue: fungal nanoparticles absorb toxic metals such as Al, Sb, Ba, Hg, Pb, Cd, and Tl.[70,76] GAPS patients routinely test positive for toxic metals. Perhaps the nanoparticles of fungi collect these poisons and help the body to remove them? Being so small, fungal nanoparticles can be an efficient mechanism in cleaning toxic metals out of every cell and every tissue in the body. The association of fungal overgrowth in the body with metal toxicity is well known; fungi absorb toxic metals and play a role in protecting us from them.[82] Unfortunately, it is not a perfect way for us to deal with metal toxicity, as fungi produce many toxins of their own, causing unpleasant symptoms.

L-forms of various bacterial species have also been found in the blood of autistic children recently: *Enterococcus agglomerans, Rhizobium radiobacter, Enterococcus faecalis, Pseudomonas aeruginosa, Morganella morganii, Chryseobacterium indologenes, Brevibacterium casei* and *Aeromonas sobria.*[70] The blood of their mothers has demonstrated the presence of L-forms of *Serratia marcescens, Enterococcus faecalis, Pseudomonas aeruginosa, Providencia rettgeri, Brevibacterium casei* and *Morganella morganii.* These bacteria are also passed to the foetus from the mother during pregnancy and all of them are capable of inflicting their own damage on the human body. As these bacterial L-forms pleomorph into other forms, their ability to damage us and to cause disease can change. For decades our main weapon against bacteria has been antibiotics. The problem is that antibiotics are only capable of influencing a bacterium in a particular form.[78,79] We are now learning that bacteria can change their forms many times, and our ubiquitous use of antibiotics has been stimulating that process. The new forms can be resistant to all existing antibiotics. Growing antibiotic resistance in bacteria is causing increasing worry among the mainstream medical community.[80,81]

The good news is that many natural interventions can force cell-wall-deficient microbes to go back to their original form, so the body can deal with them effectively. These natural interventions are the GAPS-type diet, high fever, sauna, probiotics, fermented foods, sunbathing, removing man-made toxins, electromedicine, oxygen therapy and other.[74,75,77]

Although the Western mainstream medical establishment largely ignores the concept of pleomorphism, many brilliant scientists and medics have confirmed its existence and continue to do so. Let us look at the history of how pleomorphism was discovered and what we have learned about it.

It is thought that the phenomenon of pleomorphism was first described by a brilliant French biologist Antoine Bechamp (1816–1908), who identified microscopic entities in all healthy creatures.[83] He named these structures *microzymas* and observed that they took part in building normal healthy tissues; they were harmless while the body was healthy and well. However, when the environment in the body changed, due to poor nutrition, toxicity or trauma, these *microzymas* transform into viruses, bacteria, protozoa or fungi and start destroying the body. Based on his research, Bechamp came to the conclusion that microbes do not cause disease. Instead, their function is to dismantle a body with an unhealthy metabolism (abnormal terrain). He wrote: 'Bacteria found in man and animals do not cause disease, ... they will not or cannot attack healthy tissues.[83,84] First the body has to become diseased through poor nutrition, pollution or trauma in order for the harmless *microzymas* to transform into pathogenic microbes. This very important discovery goes completely against the *germ theory* that has dominated our thinking for more than a hundred years. The germ theory states that microbes come to us from outside and attack us without any reason. Instead, Bechamp found that most microbes do not come into the human body from outside; they live inside our bodies all of our lives in a harmless state fulfilling useful functions for us. As long as the body is properly nourished, not polluted with man-made chemicals, and is looked after with kindness and care, these microbes will never attack it. Once the body is diseased or damaged, pathogenic microbes arise from within the body and destroy it.

A highly respected German physician, pathologist and scientist Rudolf Virchow (1821–1902) agreed with Bechamp. He stated that microbes were using infected organs as a habitat, but were not the cause of disease. He wrote: 'If I could live my life over again, I would devote it to proving that germs seek their natural habitat: diseased tissue, rather than being the cause of diseased tissue'.[84]

A famous British nurse Florence Nightingale (1820–1910) concluded that diseases are 'reactions of a kindly Nature against the conditions into which we have placed ourselves'. She stated that she had seen cases of smallpox which 'could not by any possibility have been caught from anybody', but arose anew from within her patients' bodies.[84]

The concept of pleomorphism was further developed by a brilliant German scientist Guenther Enderlein (1872–1968). He coined the word *pleomorphic* from the Greek 'many forms'. He observed how microbes can change into many different forms, depending on changes in their environment, and how harmless microbes can transform into pathogenic ones.[85,86] Through his research he confirmed Bechamp's theory that infections arise from within the body through wrong living and thinking. He called Bechamp's *microzymas 'protits'* and stated that they are a normal part of every cell and tissue in a human body, that they are indestructible and outlive the body (continue living after the body dies). As long as the body retains a healthy metabolism, they are harmless. But when the body becomes diseased, they evolve into viruses, bacteria and, ultimately, fungi and destroy the body. He concluded that fungi are the culmination of the evolution of *protits* into pathogenic microbes and described this evolution in the following fungi: *Mucor racemosus, Aspergillus niger, Penicillium chrysogenum, Penicillium roque-fortii, Aspergillus ruber, Mucor mucedo, Candida para-psilosis* and *Candida albicans*.[86] He created a complex protocol with natural remedies (called SANUM remedies), aimed at changing the inner environment of the body in order to force pathogenic microbes to evolve back to their harmless state of '*protits*' and go back to harmonious symbiosis with the body. He stated that using antibiotics does not kill the bacterium; instead it forces this bacterium to mutate into other forms, which can be much more pathogenic and cause a long-term degenerative disease (the cell-wall-deficient forms or L-forms that we know today). According to Enderlain's research microbes cannot be killed. All our antimicrobial inventions only force them to mutate into other forms, which may be difficult or impossible to detect.

Another renowned German doctor and researcher Wilhelm Reich (1897–1957) has looked at pleomorphism from another angle.[87] He discovered '*bions*', which appear to be Bechamp's *microzymas* or Enderlein's *protits*. He observed how, with changes in the environment, these bions turn into bacteria and amoeba. The bions can form from organic or inorganic material as microscopic clumps of molecules (like crystals do), but then they become 'alive' and continue evolving into living microbes. His research led him to the conclusion that life on Earth is being created all the time, every second, every minute. Based on his research Wilhelm Reich wrote *The Bion Experiments on the Origin of Life* in 1938 (translated into English in 1979).[87]

Standard science tells us that life on Earth evolved eons ago. But research into pleomorphism shows us that living creatures appear on our beautiful planet all the time, evolving into microbes of different sizes and complexity, which eventually become fungi. Fungi are very special, because they belong in both plant and animal kingdoms and can continue evolving further in both directions.[87,88] This process of life creation is going on everywhere, including inside our own bodies. The catalyst of this process appears to be the environment! Changes in the environment, both inside and outside our bodies, command these microscopic entities to evolve into something beneficial or pathogenic, or to return to their original harmless form.

Many other scientists and doctors have confirmed what Bechamp, Enderlein and Reich discovered. Amongst them are Bruno Haefeli, Royal Raymond Rife, Virginia Livingston-Wheeler, Eleanor Alexander-Jackson, Lida Mattman, Irene Corey Diller, Ludwik Gross, Gaston Naessens, Kurt Olbrich, Bernhard Muschlien and others.[89] Most of these researchers used microscopes which allowed them to view microbes in their *living* state, active, moving and propagating. Unfortunately, the standard microscopes widely used today kill the microbes, which gives a very limited and altered information.

Emerging research into microbial pleomorphism shows us again how little we know about microbes, how immensely adaptable and clever they are, and how misguided it is to think that we can defeat them with our modern inventions. But let us go deeper! New research into human and animal bodies now talks about holobiome and hologenome: the full collection of human and microbial cells, making one ecosystem with mixed genetics.[88] A large percentage of human genetics is now considered to be of microbial origin.[90] For example, more than a third of human genes are thought to be of bacterial origin and some 10% come from viruses.[91] On top of that, microbes living in our bodies exchange genetics with our cells and allow us to adapt genetically to changes in the environment. The whole holobiome and hologenome are now thought to be passed from parents to their babies during pregnancy and birth. This leads us to theories of evolutionary biology, which are coming to the conclusion that human and animal bodies evolved from communities of microbes.[92] At some point in the evolution of life on Earth single-cell microbes have come together and formed communities, where gradually different cells specialised to be different organs to do different functions. But, despite the fact that they have changed and specialised, these cells have never forgotten who their predecessors were – microbes! We are not only co-existing with a plethora of microbes inside us, but our human bodies are likely to have a microbial origin. So, when we attack microbes, who are we attacking? It is a known fact that antibiotics kill our immune cells.[93] Many human immune cells (and other blood cells) are likely to have a microbial origin, possibly descending from protozoa, because their shape and behaviour are very similar to the shape and behaviour of this group of microbes.

We humans have co-existed with all kinds of creatures on our beautiful planet for eons, and a human body is a complex and magnificent ecosystem, full of microbes and descending from microbes. If we take care of this ecosystem, it will maintain its diversity and serve us well. But, when the body gets polluted and poisoned with processed foods, chemicals, drugs, electromagnetic radiation and other man-made inventions, pathogenic microbes can arise from within our bodies and become our most powerful enemies. It is possible that these pathogens arise not only from our microbiome, but from our own cells, because they themselves may have originated from microbes sometime in the evolution of life on Earth.

To conclude this chapter, let us return to the soil inside us – our gut flora – because it is the biggest community of microbes in the human body. This community is the one we can affect most directly through the food we eat. As this community gets healthier, in my clinical experience, it takes care of the rest of the human microbiome – the microbes which live in other organs and tissues. As we heal the gut, the whole metabolism and the environment of the body changes, which in turn will make the whole microbial community and the whole human body healthier.

Healthy soil is Nature's co-operative, where every little thing is contributing and benefitting from the whole. Remove one of these elements and the balance is gone. Suddenly species, that used to be perfectly benign as part of the whole, start overgrowing and causing trouble. Our industrial agriculture has been creating this imbalance with impunity for decades. Agricultural chemicals destroy many life forms in the topsoil. As a result, the soil stops supporting plants well and they become malnourished and sick, so more chemicals are needed. If you speak to farmers in the Western world, many will tell you that, without chemicals, nothing would grow on their soils at all.

We have been doing the same to the soil inside us, to our gut flora, for decades. Antibiotics damage and change many species of bacteria in the gut creating an imbalance and reducing biodiversity. After every course of antibiotic your gut flora becomes more and more unbalanced and impoverished, unable to feed you or look after you. Add to that antifungal, antiprotozoal and antiviral drugs. And what about the agricultural chemicals which we consume daily with our food? They will do the same to the 'soil' inside your gut as they do to the soil on the fields, where your food is grown. Having damaged your gut flora, pharmaceutical drugs and agricultural chemicals then absorb into your bloodstream and damage microbial diversity everywhere else in your body.

'A nation that destroys its soil destroys itself', proclaimed American president Franklin Roosevelt in 1937. All life on Earth depends on that thin layer of topsoil that covers our planet, without it there will be no life and no food! According to environmental sciences, every desert in the world is man-made, including the Sahara, Gobi, Middle Eastern and Australian deserts.[94] Many fertile soils in the Western world are turning into deserts thanks to modern industrial agriculture. The same is happening to the digestive systems of people in our world. Many patients in my clinic are so malnourished, so deficient in essential nutrients that, no matter how good the quality of their food may be, their gut simply cannot digest or absorb it. The 'soil' inside them is damaged and has turned into a 'desert' which cannot support life. Like a plant which is trying to grow in a sick soil, the human body cannot thrive if its roots are in sick gut flora!

Many people don't know that one of the main causes of global warming on our planet is industrial arable agriculture. Its practices release phenomenal amounts of carbon and other elements from the soil into the air. It has been calculated that, if we converted even a proportion of our arable fields to pasture and forest where diverse microbial communities in the soil thrive, the soils would absorb large amounts of carbon from the atmosphere and convert it into humus – a very stable carbon compound. These fields can eliminate global warming and save our planet! Can we do the same with our gut flora? Can we reverse the damage in our 'soil' and turn the 'deserts' in our digestive systems and elsewhere in the body back into lush 'forests' and 'grasslands' with a diverse community of life forms? The answer is – yes, we can! That is what this book is about.

What does gut flora do for us?

All great things have their origin in that which is small.

Lao Tzu

Protection from invaders and toxins

If you flattened the absorptive surface of the human digestive system it would cover a very large area (some researchers say a tennis court, some say even larger). Mother Nature has protected this 'tennis court' by covering every square millimetre with a thick layer of 'soil' – our gut flora – a complex community of life forms living in their own biofilm.

Remember, biofilm is a sticky substance microbes produce to make a home for themselves.[1] A very important part of that biofilm is mucus produced by the gut wall.[2] This mucus is both a barrier between the gut wall and the microbes and, at the same time, a major habitat for our gut flora. In fact, the mucus forms the basis for the soil inside us. Mucus looks quite magical under the microscope; it contains large molecules shaped like bottlebrushes, each made out of a central protein backbone with strings of sugars coming from it. These molecules are called mucins; they give mucus its gel-like consistency.[3] Between these 'bottlebrushes' there is a whole 'soup' of nutrients for microbes to live on – a rich table full of food laid for them – but only in the outer layers of the mucus cover. As we go deeper into the mucus, it contains chemicals and immune factors which do not allow microbes close; by the time we penetrate to the gut wall it looks almost sterile. Every mucous membrane in the body produces this magical cover, providing a perfect ground for our body flora to live on, whether it is in our nose, throat, sinuses, lungs, digestive system, urinary tract or elsewhere.

Healthy gut flora is an immensely complex and diverse community of creatures great and small, which produce every antibacterial known to man, antiviral, antifungal and many other substances, most of which we haven't yet fully researched.[4] Using these molecules different species control each other, not allowing any one to overgrow and cause trouble. At the same time, they protect the gut from any microbes and parasites which come in from the outside.

Our gut flora protects us from any damaging chemicals we may swallow with food and drink, or which may have been produced as by-products of digestion.[5] It has been known for a few decades now that microbes can remove toxins from soils contaminated by industry.[6] Bacilli, yeasts and fungi, protozoa and other microbes have been used in a procedure called bioremediation, when microbes are used to neutralise industrial chemicals. Our gut flora can do the same – it neutralises dangerous chemicals. If the gut flora cannot destroy the chemicals, it will chelate them (from the Greek word *chēlē* meaning 'a claw'). Like the claw of a crab, chelators in your gut flora grab hold of toxins until they are taken out of your body in your stool. This happens to toxic metals (such as mercury, lead, cadmium, arsenic and aluminium), carcinogens and many other chemicals. In fact, our resident gut bacteria are some of the strongest chelating agents we know, protecting us from some of the most harmful chemicals in existence.[7] The most researched species are *Lactobacilli, Bifidobacteria, Propionibacteria, E. coli, Enterococci* and *Bacillus subtilis*. These bacteria can neutralise and chelate chemicals even when they are dead; they have substances in their cell walls which do these jobs for us. Animal research shows that, when the gut flora is damaged and cannot neutralise and chelate toxins, our digestive systems absorb large amounts of toxic metals and other damaging chemicals. Once they are inside the body, they can cause a lot of damage in many organs and systems.[8]

A major source of mercury (and other toxins) for people all over the world is amalgam fillings in teeth; they release mercury into our saliva, which goes into our digestive system.[9] We all know people who have several amalgam fillings in their teeth, and yet they seem to be healthy, and their digestive systems are functioning well. Why are they not affected? These people are blessed with a healthy gut flora, which is dealing with this mercury onslaught all the time and protecting the body from it. But when these people have a course of antibiotics, very often they start developing symptoms of mercury toxicity.[10] The antibiotics damage their gut flora, reducing its protection, and mercury starts absorbing into the bloodstream.

A major source of mercury in our food is fish, shellfish and seaweed. Humanity has polluted the oceans with many chemicals, including toxic metals. As a result, Western governments recommend that their populations reduce seafood consumption. People with healthy gut flora are protected, but people with damaged gut flora have to be careful. Seafood is an excellent source of high-quality nutrition; it is very sad to lose it! This is just one example of what we humans are doing to our planet and, ultimately, to ourselves.

Gut flora determines your response to pharmaceutical drugs.[11] Every human being has a unique gut flora. Microbes in your gut can inactivate the drug, make it more potent or alter its action in an unpredictable way. The pharmaceutical industry knows this, but because research into gut flora composition is very new, nothing can be done about it at the moment.

Appropriate digestion and absorption of food

Your gut wall is covered by very special epithelial cells, called enterocytes. These cells complete the digestion of food and then absorb it. They work very hard and soon wear out, so they live a very short life (just a few days), die and are replaced by newly born enterocytes. This process is called *Cell Regeneration* and it is a wonderful gift to us from Nature. It allows our bodies to heal any damage, regenerating and rejuvenating itself.[12] This process is active all our lives and it goes on in every organ and tissue in the body. For example, every three to four months you have a 'new' liver, because most of your liver cells have been shed and replaced by newly born young cells.[13] Cell regeneration is particularly active in the gut wall; it renews our gut lining all the time and allows us to heal the gut, no matter how damaged it may be.

From animal research we know that the whole process of cell renewal is run and orchestrated by our gut flora.[14] When we damage the gut flora this process goes wrong, the enterocytes degenerate, many of them mutate (some even turn cancerous) and are unable to digest and absorb food for us. The health and well-being of our gut wall is predetermined by the state of our gut flora! Not only does it protect enterocytes from anything damaging, but the microbes in our 'soil' produce substances which nourish these cells and provide them with energy.[15] In other words, our gut flora is the 'housekeeper' of our digestive system. You cannot develop any digestive disorder, whether it is as mild as IBS or as severe as cancer, without damaging the gut flora first. If your gut flora is strong, diverse and healthy, it will protect you. People who are blessed with such healthy 'soil' have a strong constitution, able to withstand many assaults from the environment: poor diet, starvation, stress and overwork. But as soon as their gut flora is damaged, even mild influences can damage their health.

As the 'housekeeper' of your digestive system, the gut flora makes sure that your gut is in a fit state to digest and absorb food properly. Digestion and absorption of food relies very heavily on the activity of our gut flora. Microbes in our 'soil' produce enzymes, acids and other substances to assist in breaking down proteins, fats and carbohydrates, cleave off minerals and vitamins, and ensure that they all absorb in the right shape and form. Every nutrient has to come into the body 'holding hands' with other nutrients; no vitamin or protein is supposed to be alone, isolated. And every nutrient has to be in a certain biochemical shape. The only way to accomplish this is though properly digested food; no supplement in the world can do that for you. When your gut flora is damaged you cannot digest food well. No matter how good the quality of food you may be eating, your body will not benefit fully from it and so will not be nourished well.

Production of vitamins and hormones

Your gut flora makes sure that your digestive system is able to feed you properly, and not all of that nourishment comes from food alone. There are many nutrients that are provided for us by our gut flora; the microbes in the gut actively synthesize them. They come from food as well, but the gut flora is the main source of these substances for us: the whole B-vitamins group (thiamine, riboflavin, niacin, pyridoxine, cyanocobalamin, folate, pantothenic acid, biotin, etc), vitamin K2 (menaquinone), many amino acids and other molecules.[16] These are some of the most essential nutrients without which we cannot live or function well. That is why Mother Nature has provided us with our own little factory inside our digestive system to produce these substances for us all the time. There is a very complex 'conversation' going on between the body and the gut flora, where the body asks for so much vitamin B12, for example, and the gut flora releases it in the right amount and the right biochemical shape for the body to use. We can never replicate this with supplements! Supplements generally do not provide the correct biochemical form of these nutrients; as a result, the body very often cannot use vitamins from supplements.

People who damage their gut flora typically look pale and have low stamina and ability to cope with stress – they develop *anaemia*. In order for us, humans, to have healthy blood we need a good supply of the whole spectrum of B vitamins coming from our gut flora. So, in order to deal with anaemia long term, we need to focus on restoring the 'soil' inside us. As an immediate remedy for anaemia the person needs to eat liver, which is one of the richest sources of B vitamins and iron, on a daily basis. Red meats (lamb, beef and game) and organ meats (liver, kidneys, tongue, tripe, etc) provide iron in the right biochemical form for human physiology. Taking iron supplements does not remedy anaemia; this has been proven conclusively in many international studies.[17] Iron supplements provide a perfect food for many iron-loving microbes in the gut, allowing them to grow and proliferate, which causes unpleasant digestive symptoms and a deeper imbalance in the gut flora.

Recent research has shown that eating liver will not only provide all the B vitamins and iron necessary for us (and a plethora of other essential nutrients), but is also a good source of vitamin C.[17] For a long time we believed that vitamin C could only come from plant foods. However,

I have a growing group of patients who have to follow the No-Plant variation of the GAPS Diet for many months, sometimes years. These people cannot eat any food from the plant kingdom at all (no vegetables, no fruit, no greens, no nuts, no beans), and yet they thrive and look very healthy. There are no signs of any nutritional deficiencies in these people, and so I am often asked 'Where do these patients get their vitamin C from?' Clearly, we don't know everything about vitamin C yet! Recent research has indicated that various microbes in our gut flora can produce vitamin C for us.[18] These patients eat liver and other organ meats on a daily basis, so obviously these foods provide them with plenty of vitamin C.

Vitamin K2 (menaquinone) is a very interesting substance that plays many roles in the body.[19] Our gut flora is the main and sometimes the only source of this vital vitamin. Without it, our bodies cannot use minerals appropriately, calcium in particular. If you have a K2 deficiency, calcium does not go to your bones and teeth, so you develop osteoporosis and tooth decay. Instead calcium settles in soft tissues: in your blood vessels (causing high blood pressure and heart disease), in your brain (calcifying important structures), in your joints and ligaments (causing arthritis), and in your liver and kidneys (forming stones). Fermented foods can provide good amounts of this vitamin. Good examples are well-aged traditional high-fat cheeses in Europe and fermented soya products in Asia (natto in particular). These foods can be used as an immediate remedy by people with abnormal gut flora, but long term we need to work on restoring the 'soil' inside us, so it can start producing vitamin K2.[19]

Our gut produces some 40 hormones, and it is becoming more and more apparent that our gut flora takes part in this process. In addition, the gut flora produces many hormones of its own and takes part in the metabolism of our hormones. For example, many of our steroid hormones are excreted from the body in bile, which carries them into the gut. Recent research has discovered that a common bacterium in the gut flora, called *Clostridium scindens,* can convert our steroid hormones into androgens – male hormones, such as testosterone.[20] From androgens our gut flora can produce oestrogens and other steroid hormones. The researchers in this area now consider the gut microbiome to be an endocrine organ.[21] To confirm that, another group of researchers have discovered a so-called 'estrobolome' (bacterial genes which take part in oestrogen metabolism in the gut).[22] When the gut flora is damaged these hormones are not processed properly and can lay the ground for estrogen-dependent illnesses in the body, including cancer (endometriosis, menstrual abnormalities, breast cancer, uterine and ovarian cancers, prostate cancer, colorectal cancer, malignant melanoma, etc).[23] Hormones are very powerful molecules; they have many functions in the body and affect many tissues and cells at the same time. Production and processing of hormones makes our gut flora even more powerful in its ability to affect our lives.

Production of neurotransmitters

Production of neurotransmitters is a major function of our gut.[24] Neurotransmitters are chemicals used by our nervous system; they act as messengers between the nerve cells and play many other important roles. The more we research neurotransmitters the more we discover that many of them are manufactured in the gut, and then transported to the brain. Good examples are serotonin and dopamine: about 95% of serotonin and about 50% of dopamine are produced in the gut.[25] Serotonin is our 'happy' neurotransmitter; it makes us feel content, relaxed and joyful. People whose gut is unable to produce enough serotonin become depressed and negative. They are often diagnosed with depression and treated with drugs that increase levels of serotonin in the brain. Another neurotransmitter missing in depression is dopamine. This is our 'motivational' neurotransmitter: it makes us get out of bed in the morning, brush our hair, wash our face, dress and get on with our lives. People whose gut is unable to produce enough dopamine don't want to get out of bed in the morning, they often don't brush their hair or wash their faces for days; they have no motivation to do anything in life – a major symptom of depression. A group of researchers in Norway examined faeces from 55 people and found certain bacteria in depressive patients which were not present in healthy people.[25] Depression is a GAPS condition and should be treated with the GAPS Nutritional Protocol. Once the gut is healed, it starts producing normal amounts of serotonin and dopamine, and depression melts away. Many GAPS people may not be diagnosed with depression, but looking at their personalities it is clear that their gut is not supplying them with enough serotonin and dopamine. Another very important neurotransmitter produced by our gut flora is *gamma-amino butyric acid* (GABA). People whose gut does not produce enough of this substance suffer from anxiety, panic, insomnia and depression, and are prone to drug and alcohol abuse.[26] As I have mentioned elsewhere in this book, many of these people do not have digestive symptoms (pain, abnormal stool, gas or reflux)! They do not believe that their depression, obsessions, anxiety or any other mental symptoms may possibly be connected to the gut. However, when we test their gut flora, we find it to be abnormal and, when we treat their gut, these mental symptoms disappear. The human body has a wonderful ability to compensate for abnormalities, to work around them. The digestive system in these people may compensate for abnormalities for many years, while their abnormal flora is causing mental and physical illness.

Our gut has been called 'the second brain'. Some researchers even call it 'the first brain' because of the complexity of its nervous system, production of hormones, neurotransmitters and many other active substances. Recent research in microbiome has discovered that our gut flora is a major part of that 'brain'. Through producing various active substances our gut microbes can dictate our behaviour and mood, and even our thoughts! Many of our desires, food preferences and mood changes are not our own; they are imposed upon us by the microbes in our gut. And it is not surprising: the genetic composition of our gut flora outnumbers our own by 100-200, while their cell composition outnumbers ours by ten. Every food addiction you have is likely to be imposed on you by your gut flora; the microbes in your gut are addicted to that particular food and are demanding it by giving you an irresistible urge to eat it.[27] This is particularly the case in people with obesity, diabetes, autoimmunity and mental illness, and the typical addictions are to processed carbohydrates (sugar, chocolate, bread, pasta, snacks, etc).

Microbes in our gut have their own circadian rhythms: they produce various chemicals and do different things in a rhythmic daily fashion, according to the movement of the sun.[28] Worms, flukes and other intestinal inhabitants are a good example: during the day the majority of them live outside our digestive system (in the abdominal cavity, around the liver, in the mesentery and its fat, sometimes in the lungs and chest cavity), but at night they travel into the digestive system to feed.[29] Many people with worm infestations have poor sleep because the worms are most active at night, causing symptoms of abdominal pain, belching, gas production and active peristalsis. Recent research has discovered that microbial circadian rhythms inside us affect the rhythms of our own biological clock. The ability of our liver to detoxify and clean the blood, our pancreatic function, digestive function, blood and lymph circulation, functions of our nervous system and the rest of the body are strongly affected by the circadian rhythms of microbes in the gut.[28] Modern lifestyles of staying up late, eating late in the evening and international travel disrupt the circadian rhythms of microbes in the gut, which can change your metabolism and predisposition to disease. For example, it is a well-known fact that obesity and diabetes are more common amongst people whose circadian rhythms are disrupted by shift work or jet lag. Research has shown that these people have different gut flora compared to people without those health problems.[30] Our bodies are an ecosystem; they do not belong to us alone! They are a community of many life forms, living in the same space and working in co-operation. Our lifestyle choices can change the whole ecosystem, with many consequences.

Where does the gut flora come from?

In 2016 it was discovered that the uterus is not sterile but has a rich microbial flora of its own![31] In healthy women it is dominated by *Lactobacilli*, and this flora plays a vital role in conception and pregnancy. A placental microbiome has been identified, and the interesting thing is that its microbial population resembles oral flora (the flora in the mouth) more than the flora in the groin of the woman. Women with abnormal uterine flora often cannot conceive or sustain pregnancy, making it a major reason for infertility.[32] During pregnancy the baby swallows liquids in the uterus which transfer uterine and placental flora into the baby's gut. Recent analysis of the first stool from newborn babies (meconium) shows that it already contains a community of microbes, largely dominated by *Lactobacilli* and *physiological E. coli*.[33] So, the gut flora starts forming in the baby during pregnancy. Then, during the time of birth, the baby's body flora receives a large boost from the bodily flora of the parents. When the baby goes through the birth canal of the mother it swallows mouthfuls of microbes which live in the mother's vagina. Vaginal flora is quite rich and largely comes from the bowel of the woman. So, if the mother has abnormal gut flora, the flora in her vagina will also be abnormal and she will pass it to her baby at birth. The father also has a rich microbial flora in the groin, which comes out of his bowel, and he shares that flora with the mother on a regular basis. So, both parents pass their gut flora to the child at the moment of natural birth through the microbial flora in the mother's birth canal.

If the child has been born through a caesarean section then this important step is missing. Studies have found that the gut flora of babies delivered by caesarean section has lower microbial diversity and an absence of *Bifidobacteria* species, which are very important for the normal development of the baby's immune system and gut.[34] Babies born naturally have richer gut flora dominated by *Bifidobacteria*. So, the way the baby is delivered has a deep impact on the composition of the baby's gut flora. A child starting life with abnormal gut flora will have a compromised immune system and a compromised constitution.

We have an epidemic of abnormalities in gut flora in the world, particularly in industrialised countries. As gut flora passes down the generations, this epidemic worsens. Before talking about the health of any child in my clinic I always talk about the health of the parents and grandparents; and a typical scenario has emerged. After the Second World War the grandparents, who generally received healthy gut flora from their parents, may have had a few courses of antibiotics, which slightly damaged their gut flora. They passed this partially damaged flora to their children. Their children were born at a time when breastfeeding was going out of fashion (replaced by artificial formulas), when antibiotics were given to children for every cough and sneeze, and when junk food was increasingly becoming a large part of children's diet. All these factors created generations of people with far more damaged gut flora than in their parents. The gut flora of women, on average, is more damaged than that of men because many of them took contraceptive pills for quite a few years before having children. The Pill has a very damaging effect on the gut flora and the immune system of a woman. So, by the time the younger generations decide to have children, their gut flora is far more seriously damaged than in their parents' generation, and that is what they pass to their babies. The situation is worsening with each generation. The epidemic of GAPS or abnormal gut flora increases every year.

A child starting life with abnormal gut flora will have compromised immune system and compromised constitution. On top of that, there is another very damaging factor passed to our babies from the mothers – a toxic load the child is born with. Women in our modern world are storing increasing amounts of toxic chemicals in their bodies starting from early childhood (from food and water, personal care products, make-up, hair dyes, other vanity chemicals and the environment). The mother's body unloads toxins into the child during pregnancy, so our babies are born with an ever-growing toxic load, undermining their constitution further. Testing of umbilical blood of new-borns has found some 287 toxins, including mercury, pesticides and fire retardants.[35] The US National Academy of Sciences (NAS) estimated in 2006 that over 60,000 US children are born each year at risk for life-long problems because of dangerous blood levels of mercury in their mothers. It is the first born that usually gets the majority of that toxicity. Any further children usually benefit from a cleaner pregnancy, unless the mother has exposed herself to large amounts of toxins between pregnancies.

But let us come back to the gut flora. The mother's breast and breast milk are a rich source of microbes for the child's gut flora; the nipples of the breastfeeding mother and the milk ducts in her breasts add their own microbes to the milk. So, the breast milk is a probiotic food! It can contain up to 10^9 microbes/L in healthy mothers and the most frequently found bacteria are *staphylococci, streptococci, corynebacteria, lactobacilli, micrococci, propionibacteria, bifidobacteria* and *ruminococci*.[36] In addition, breast milk provides the right food for the right composition of microbes in the baby's digestive system. That is why breastfed babies develop healthier gut flora than bottle-fed babies. The milk of a breastfeeding mother is very similar in its composition to her blood; it has alive and active immune cells, immunoglobulins, enzymes, growth factors, hormones, neurotransmitters and many other components. All of these vital elements take part in the proper maturation of the gut wall, gut flora, immune system, nervous system and all other organs and systems of the child's body. No formula in the world can ever imitate that. Bottle-fed babies develop deficient gut flora, which predisposes them to allergies, autoimmunity, learning disability and other health problems.[37] Research shows that giving even some formula as a supplement to a breastfed baby will have a damaging effect on the baby's gut flora: it is not as healthy as the gut flora in exclusively breastfed babies. Unfortunately, the majority of parents in the Western world give their babies formula even if the child is breastfed.

In our modern world many women have polluted bodies and unhealthy gut flora, generating a stream of toxicity. All these toxins finish up in the woman's blood and milk. I have a large number of families in my clinic where the mother had to stop breastfeeding because her milk was making her child ill. Babies with type one diabetes, FPIES (*Food Protein Induced Enterocolitis Syndrome*), severe allergies, severe eczema, severe digestive problems, epilepsy and severe problems with mental and physical development are often in this category. When the mother cannot breastfeed her baby, the best solution is *not* formula! The best solution is a healthy wet nurse – another breastfeeding woman who would share her milk with your baby. For more on the subject of wet nursing, turn to the chapter *A–Z*.

Introducing solids is another important stage in the gut flora development of the child. Children who are weaned onto processed grains and processed milk – the most common weaning foods in the Western world – develop more damage in their gut flora, gut wall and immune system. In *Part Four* of the first GAPS book (*Gut and Psychology Syndrome*) I have described how a baby should be weaned, particularly a GAPS baby. This is the way people in traditional societies used to introduce solids to their babies. Continuing to breastfeed while slowly introducing homemade foods to your child will ensure that your child develops a healthy gut, a healthy immune system and robust health overall. Unfortunately, a large percentage of babies in the Western world are GAPS babies and their proportion is growing every year. So, I recommend introducing solids to all babies in a traditional way.

Fully weaned babies and toddlers are considered to have a similar gut flora to adults. Research into gut flora so far has focused largely on bacteria. I am sure future research will find out that many other microbes are involved in the development of the baby's gut flora.

What happens to the gut flora after weaning? Unfortunately, in our modern world it is under threat from every side. In the first GAPS book in the chapter *What can damage gut flora?* I described in detail all the risk factors. Here, we will just summarise them. Antibiotics, by far, are the most damaging influence; not only from prescription medications but also from food. Many chemicals used by our agriculture and food industry are antibiotic in their nature (though they may not be labelled as such). Pharmaceutical drugs, prescribed for long periods of time, damage gut flora: steroids, the contraceptive pill, sleeping pills, statins, painkillers, etc.[38] Modern food, full of processed and chemical ingredients, changes the composition of the gut flora very unfavorably. Pollution, exposure to industrial chemicals, electromagnetic pollution, ionizing radiation and many other factors in our environment have a very detrimental effect on the composition of our gut flora. Long-term stress, dental treatments, physical exertion, alcohol and drug abuse, smoking and other lifestyle choices can damage gut flora too. Every human being carries a unique mixture of microbes in the body. All the damaging factors listed above will change that bodily flora in an unpredictable way, predisposing us to different health problems. Science has only just started studying gut flora; we don't have reliable methods of testing our microbiome, let alone correcting any abnormalities. In the meantime, the state of our gut flora predetermines the state of the rest of our bodies. And the more we study our bodily flora the more we realise that nothing in the human body is sterile! Microbes are everywhere – in our body cavities, blood vessels and organs. I would like to repeat this: our bodies are highly evolved ecosystems, communities of various microbes, life forms and cells living together in harmony, supporting each other and using each other. When we attack microbes with antibiotics or other chemicals, we attack the very essence of our bodies.

Friend or foe?

When the 'soil' in your digestive system gets damaged, instead of being your friend, it becomes a major enemy. Every microbe in the gut, even those deemed 'beneficial', can start producing a plethora of toxic substances. These toxins absorb through the damaged gut wall and get distributed around the body. For example, a family of bacteria called *Clostridia* are normal inhabitants of the human gut, but they are capable of producing very powerful toxins that affect the brain and the rest of the nervous system. When the gut flora has a normal healthy diversity of different microbes, clostridia are controlled and do us no harm. But when the gut flora is damaged, they can take part in disease process (from digestive problems and abnormal muscle function to neurological symptoms). Overgrowth of clostridia in the gut has been found in autistic children and people with mental illness, autoimmune disease and digestive disorders.[39]

Yeast overgrowth is very common and typically develops after antibiotic treatments. The most researched yeast is the family of *Candida*, which can produce many toxins in the gut. Candida, when out of control, grows long filaments through the gut wall making it porous and leaky.[40] Having spread from the gut, candida can grow in any organ or tissue in the body, which can lead to many health problems (from inflammation to cancer). For example, it is now recognized that the majority of asthma cases have a fungal origin.[41] All chronic illnesses, from mental to physical, have some fungal involvement.

Many other microbes in the gut can cause problems when out of control. We know that a common soil microbe found in the gut flora, *Streptomyces achromogenes*, can produce a toxin (streptozotocin) which gets into the bloodstream and destroys beta cells in the pancreas, causing type one diabetes.[42] *Coxsackievirus B* is also strongly associated with type one diabetes; this virus lives in the gut flora of humans. There is a strong association between a common microbe, which lives in the human gut, called *Klebsiella pneumonie,* and ankylosing spondylitis – a severe autoimmune disease.[43] People with another autoimmune disease – rheumatoid arthritis – were found to have an overgrowth of *Prevotella copri* in the gut, a particular bacterium that is not found in such numbers in healthy people.[44] Migraine sufferers have an overgrowth of nitrate-reducing microbes, while people with Parkinson's disease have microbes which undermine production of neurotransmitters in the gut and the brain. In addition to various toxic chemicals these microbes can produce so-called super-antigens – substances which can trigger autoimmune disease in the body.[45] Attempts to destroy these microbes using antibiotics are not the way to deal with the situation. We need to work on restoring diversity in the gut flora, so other microbes can bring down and control the disease-causing ones naturally.

There is no end to the microbes that can overgrow when the diversity of our gut flora is gone, and we have only just started researching them. Microbes take part in disease in the digestive system and anywhere else in the body, including mental and neurological illness, diabetes, obesity, cancer, allergies and autoimmunity. They interact with prescription drugs and contribute to toxic side effects. It is beyond the scope of this book to look at all the toxins produced by abnormal gut flora; in my first GAPS book I described some well-researched toxins. All we need to know is that unhealthy, unbalanced gut flora creates a river of toxicity, flowing from the gut into your body, and that the mixture of toxins is likely to be very individual.

Good health begins in the gut! A person with damaged gut flora is malnourished, because food is not digested and absorbed properly, and the gut flora is not providing B vitamins, vitamin K2 and other vital substances. The person develops allergies and intolerances to foods, because the gut wall is damaged and leaky and so absorbs food undigested. The digestive system deteriorates, because its housekeeper – the healthy gut flora – is not there to look after it. So, the person develops digestive symptoms: abnormal stool (diarrhoea, constipation or a mixture), abdominal pain, overproduction of gas, reflux, indigestion, etc. People with these symptoms are usually diagnosed with IBS (Irritable Bowel Syndrome), which should be renamed 'gut dysbiosis' in my opinion. The protective function of the gut is diminished, so the person is absorbing toxins from the environment (toxic metals, petrochemicals, agrochemicals, by-products of the digestive process and other damaging substances). The unbalanced mixture of microbes in the gut creates their own plethora of toxic chemicals, absorbing through the damaged gut wall. And alive active microbes and the larva of parasites escape the gut and travel around the body.

In short, instead of being a source of nourishment, which our digestive system is supposed to be, it becomes a major source of toxicity in the body, causing disease. Hippocrates, the father of modern medicine, stated almost two thousand years ago: 'All diseases begin in the gut!' No matter whether the disease is a chronic physical or mental disorder, he was absolutely right! Your digestive system holds the roots of your health! So, no matter what chronic illness we may suffer from, we have to start treating it from the roots – the digestive system with its gut flora. It doesn't matter if you have digestive symptoms or not, the roots of your chronic illness are likely to be found in your gut. I have had many patients who didn't think that their gut was a problem, because they didn't have diarrhoea, constipation, bloating, gas or any other digestive symptoms. But when we started treating the gut with the GAPS Nutritional Protocol, their chronic illnesses started disappearing: from rheumatoid arthritis to multiple sclerosis, from chronic fatigue syndrome to asthma, from fibromyalgia to mental illness and from diabetes to obesity.

Our immune system is closely connected to our gut flora. Every change in the gut flora has a profound effect on our immune function. Let us have a look at how that happens.

Immune system

"Give me a medicine to produce a fever, and I can cure any disease."

Hippocrates

We know that our bodies are equipped with a system to protect us from invaders – microbes, parasites and toxins – called the immune system. What many people don't know is that about 80–85% of our immune system is located in the gut wall.[1] So, our digestive system can be seen as the biggest and one of the most important immune organs in the body! The immune system can be compared to an army with most of the commanding echelons located in the gut wall: the 'generals', the 'admirals' and the 'officers'. And this is not surprising considering that some 90% of all cells in the human bodies are in the gut flora.[2] The immune system located in the gut wall has a very complex and close relationship with the gut flora.[3] The gut flora feeds it, informs it, balances it and keeps it healthy and well. Any army commander has to have information about the enemy in order to make decisions. It appears that a very large percentage of the information, your immune system is acting upon, comes from the gut. When the gut flora is healthy and normal, the data coming from it keeps the immune system well-balanced and functioning normally. But, when the gut flora gets damaged, the immune system has to act upon a very different data – a data that brings disease and disorder.[4]

A very important part of our immune system is THE LYMPHOID TISSUE. It is a fine mesh of fibres inhabited by immune cells, and it is spread all over the body through all our tissues and organs.[5] In various parts of this mesh lymph nodes are positioned where the lymphoid tissue becomes dense and well organised to trap and neutralise dangerous microbes and toxins. Lymphoid tissue is present in every mucous membrane of the body: in the mouth, nose and throat, digestive system, sinuses, eyes, lungs, urinary system and genital organs. It plays a very important role there, because that is where the human body comes in contact with the outside. Food, microbes, toxins and chemicals from the environment are met by the lymphoid tissue; it is the first barrier they have to face in the body. Infectious microbes from the environment normally enter your body through the mucous membranes, where they come into contact with the lymphoid tissue. There the microbe is properly dealt with and information about it is memorised, leading to temporary or permanent immunity against that particular infection. It doesn't matter where the infection entered the body (the nose, mouth, throat or elsewhere), the information about it will be known by the whole lymphoid tissue everywhere in the body. And, of course, every mucous membrane is richly populated by microbial flora, which interacts with the lymphoid tissue.[6] Depending on the composition of this flora the lymphoid tissue can be very healthy and efficient or it can malfunction.

Normally an infection is not supposed to get directly into the body, because it cannot get past the lymphoid tissue. Unfortunately, what do we do with vaccinations? We inject microbes and their toxins directly into the body! We breach the barrier of the lymphoid tissue, which is supposed to deal with the infection first in order to develop proper immunity against it. That is one of the reasons why, in many instances, vaccinations fail to develop lasting immunity against microbes.

Your immune system is a hungry organ, it needs feeding all the time. A person with abnormal gut flora does not digest or absorb food properly and so develops multiple nutritional deficiencies.[7] As a result, the immune system becomes malnourished and unable to function well and to respond to infections; this person has developed *immune deficiency*. I have seen many children with physical and mental disabilities whose parents state that their child has never had a fever or a common cold. Colds are thought to be caused by viruses, but it is not the virus that creates the fever, the runny nose, the headache, the cough and all the other symptoms of a common cold. It is your immune system who creates all these symptoms; the immune system that is responding to the virus and dealing with it. In a person with abnormal gut flora the immune system can be malnourished and unable to respond to the virus. That is why the child gets no fever or any other symptoms of the cold, while the viruses come into the body of the child without being opposed. When we test these children, we find chronic viral infections active in their bodies.[8] The same happens to many adults with damaged gut flora: their immune systems are in no fit state to mount a response to viruses or any other microbes and toxins in the environment. Often, when we start treating the person with the GAPS Nutritional Protocol, they develop a fever and all the symptoms of their first common cold. This is a cause for celebration; it means that the immune system has started working!

The challenges coming from abnormal gut flora and an unhealthy gut are often too overwhelming for the immune system. In a GAPS person, instead of being a source of nourishment, the gut becomes a major source of toxicity; a river of toxins flows through the gut wall into the body and, of course, the immune system reacts to that. Alive and active microbes pass through the gut wall, and the immune system has to react to them as well. On top of that, in a person with abnormal gut flora the gut wall gets damaged; it becomes porous and leaky. Undigested food absorbs through this damaged gut wall and the person develops symptoms of food allergies and intolerances, because the immune system is trying to deal with these undigested foods.[9]

The responses of our immune system have been divided into two groups: non-specific and specific. The *non-specific* part of the immune system reacts the same way to different kinds of attack and reacts quickly. Examples of these responses are fever, inflammation, production of liquids (tears, mucus, saliva, etc), sneezing, coughing, vomiting and diarrhoea. *Specific* immunity takes time to develop and can lead to autoimmune disease. Let us have a look at these two branches of our immune system in more detail as GAPS people have a problem with both of them.

Non-specific responses of the immune system.

If you get exposed to a common microbe or a toxin for a short period of time and your *non-specific immunity* is strong, it will deal with the situation fully and completely. The process can be quite dramatic though and quite uncomfortable: you can develop a high temperature, headache, aching body, drop in energy, vomiting, diarrhoea, pain, coughing, runny nose, sneezing, increased tear production, increased mucus production, etc. All of these symptoms are caused by your immune system; these are the 'weapons' it uses to fight the infection and expel it. It is very important to allow your body to do this work! Yes, while this work is being done you may feel miserable. But if you allow this process to complete without using painkillers, anti-fever drugs, anti-coughing drugs, antihistamines or any other medications, then you will recover fully and come out of this illness stronger than before.[10] It is important to respect your body while it is doing the work: stay in bed, rest, sleep, keep warm and eat correctly. But, if you fight the *symptoms* of the problem, which are the tools your immune system is using, then the disease will not be dealt with correctly. It will linger in the body laying the ground for *the specific response*, which may lead to a far more serious situation – a chronic autoimmune disease.

Specific responses. All autoimmunity is born in the gut!

The specific response develops when your exposure to the toxins, undigested foods and microbes has become chronic. This allows your immune system the time to develop antibodies (immunoglobulins). The activity of specific antibodies is called autoimmunity and it is thought to lead to autoimmune disease. A person with abnormal gut flora has a constant flow of toxins, undigested foods and microbes coming into the body from the gut. That is why GAPS people almost always have autoimmunity.

What is autoimmunity?

The mainstream explanation for autoimmunity is that your immune system 'mistakenly' attacks your healthy organs and tissues, so powerful drugs are being used to beat the immune system down 'to stop it attacking the body'.[11] Since it is the immune system that causes the *symptoms* of the disease (pain, inflammation and abnormal function), the drugs reduce the symptoms, giving an illusion that the person is 'getting better'. But the disease inevitably progresses and gets worse over time. The drugs, which used to 'help', gradually stop working. New, more powerful drugs have to be used to supress the immune system and hence reduce the symptoms, while the disease continues to destroy the body of the person. Our mainstream medicine has been doing this for decades. The complete failure of this approach has led to autoimmune diseases being pronounced 'incurable'. Patients are told that there can be no recovery and only symptoms can be controlled somewhat, while the body progressively deteriorates.

If a disease is 'caused' by the immune system, then suppressing it should cure the disease, shouldn't it? The fact that it doesn't work should suggest that, perhaps, the theory is wrong. The real question is: why would your immune system attack your own body? Is our immune system misguided or badly designed? Or is it doing exactly what it is supposed to do under the circumstances?

The textbook mechanism of autoimmunity, taught to students in medical schools, is a so-called *molecular mimicry phenomenon*. This theory states that, once your immune system develops antibodies – specific weapons – against a specific protein of a microbe, for example, it finds similar proteins in your own body and attacks them as well. Why would your immune system make such a mistake? Doesn't the immune system know proteins in its own body, is it blind or not-clever-enough to see the difference between its own protein and a microbial one? This theory presumes that human immune system doesn't really know what it is doing, and the mainstream drug treatments are based on this presumption.[12]

The idea of a molecular mimicry phenomenon was first developed in studying rheumatic fever. The real cause of this disease is still debated, but commonly accepted opinion is that the immune system creates antibodies against a protein in a bacterium (*group A beta-haemolytic streptococcus*), which causes *strep* throat infections.[13] It is thought that this protein is similar to a protein in our heart valves. The theory states that, once the immune system has this 'weapon' against the streptococcus, it uses it to destroy the heart valves, leading to heart failure. Rheumatic fever used to be a common disease in the West in the pre-antibiotic era. Since antibiotics have been invented, every strep throat infection is treated to kill the streptococcus, so rheumatic fever has become uncommon in the West. Antibiotics are life-saving medications. Unfortunately, today many prescriptions do not fall into that category but, when it comes to strep throat, it is one example when antibiotics may be necessary. But, shouldn't the fact that antibiotics work so well in this situation, lead us to a thought that rheumatic fever may be caused by an infection in the heart, rather than a 'misguided' immune system? If the infection is elsewhere, *Streptococci* produce powerful toxins, which go into the bloodstream and may damage the heart valves. Perhaps, the immune system does not attack perfectly normal tissues 'by mistake', but tries to deal with damaged tissues? What if streptococci produce something that changes the structure of proteins in the heart valves, making them abnormal and diseased? After all, it is the job of the immune system to find abnormal proteins and try to clear them out of the body.

Recent research is confirming that microbes can indeed change the structure of proteins. Microbes produce various enzymes, one of which is being researched extensively as a potential mechanism for autoimmunity and allergy. This enzyme is called *microbial transglutaminase (mTg)*. It has an ability to bind proteins into a form of glue by cross-linking them together, and our commercially sold processed foods are full of this 'glue'.[14] Since its discovery in 1989 *microbial mTg* has been used extensively by the food industry in the production of processed meats, fish, dairy, baked products (including breads, buns, cakes and desserts), sweets, gelatine and other concoctions. These proteins, cross-linked by *mTg*, have been found to damage the gut lining and trigger autoimmunity in the body, amongst many other destructive influences on human health.[15] It is estimated that the average Western person now consumes approximately 15 mg of microbial transglutaminases in processed foods daily, and these damaging molecules are now also being used by industry in the manufacture of probiotic foods and nutritional supplements.[16]

Microbial *mTg* in the gut is known to bind with proteins in our food (gluten, for example). When these complexes of *mTg* connected with gluten absorb, the immune system produces antibodies against them.[17] On top of that, these complexes damage the gut lining making it porous and leaky. In a GAPS person abnormal gut flora produces plenty of *mTg*, which can absorb and bind to proteins, turning them into abnormal molecular formations.[18] Our immune system has to clear this debris, using inflammation, allergy and autoimmunity.

The human body produces transglutaminases too, which accomplish a multitude of functions in our organs and tissues (*tTg or tissue transglutaminase*). In its biochemical structure our *tTg* is quite different from the one produced by microbes, and our immune system knows the difference. It is microbial *mTg* that triggers autoimmunity and allergy when it gets where it is not supposed to be.[16]

Our immune system does not only deal with microbes and their biproducts. In modern humans the immune system is very busy dealing with man-made toxicity, and this work load is getting bigger by the day. Toxic chemicals, radiation, electro-magnetic pollution and other man-made influences, just like microbial enzymes, can also damage proteins in the human body. Our immune system surveys the body all the time. When it finds these contaminated and damaged proteins, it recognises them as abnormal and deals with them, employing all sorts of mechanisms and tools it has in its toolkit, including antibodies. Unfortunately, when your doctor finds antibodies in your blood, you are likely to be diagnosed with an 'autoimmune disease' and given mainstream immune-suppressing treatments. Is this label 'autoimmune disease' appropriate? Perhaps, we should rename this situation a *CONTAMINATION DISEASE*? Such a term would lead us away from attacking our own immune system, which is working hard to clean out disease-causing debris. Instead, we could think about how we can reduce our exposure to toxicity and assist our immune system in removing it. I have no doubt that all autoimmune diseases are born in the gut, and some leading immunologists are starting to come to the same conclusion.[19]

The contamination mechanism is common in GAPS patients and a good example is *GAPS Collagen Disorder*.

Collagen is one of the most ubiquitous proteins in the human body; in fact, it is estimated that about a third of all protein in your body is collagen.[20] It forms a strong and flexible network of fibres and, in a way, 'holds the body together'. Your joints, ligaments, fascia, skin, blood vessels, bones, teeth, muscles, gut wall and many other tissues and organs have a large amount of collagen fibres in their structure. They form a so-called *connective tissue* in the body. Unfortunately, due to its amino acid composition, collagen is a magnet for toxicity: toxins attach themselves to collagen molecules, contaminating and damaging them.[21] The immune system uses various tools to clean the contaminated collagen fibres or, if it cannot clean and save them, to dismantle and remove them (your immune system knows what is appropriate under the circumstances). As a result, the very structure of the body suffers. People with this problem usually have 'loose' joints and muscles, low muscle density and tone, low density in their skin and tissues.[22] They are often 'double-jointed' or have hyper-mobile joints. When they stand straight, their knee joints often over-bend backwards; when they straighten their arms, the elbow joints over-bend. Many of them can bend their fingers back all the way to their forearm. They often trip over their own feet and get a reputation for being 'clumsy'. They fall over easily and hurt themselves, twist their ankles and wrists and can even dislocate their joints. They often have flat feet, because the ligaments in the foot are not strong enough to hold all the bones in the right position. As their fascia are also loose, these people are prone to developing hernias in their abdominal wall or groin and can even have organ prolapse. Their spine is often painful, because the spinal column is made out of many small joints, which become loose and do not provide good support. These people bruise very easily, because our blood vessels are made out of collagen to a large degree; the walls of the blood vessels become weak and break easily, leading to bruising. Collagen is a structural element of all the capsules, sheaths and other supporting structures of our nervous system, particularly its peripheral part. Damage to the collagen can manifest itself as a neurological disorder, such as carpal tunnel syndrome, peripheral neuropathy and other. All these problems happen because the major structural protein in the body – collagen – is being contaminated. In my experience, GAPS collagen disorder is the background of many so-called autoimmune diseases.

What kind of toxins can contaminate our collagen and other proteins? Unhealthy gut flora is by far the main source of toxicity in our bodies, which includes improperly digested foods absorbing through the damaged gut wall. But many toxins can also come in from the environment. A good example is *glyphosate* – a common herbicide (sold under many names, one of which is *Roundup*). Glyphosate is a synthetic amino acid, and it is an analogue of glycine – the most abundant amino acid in collagen. Recent research shows that glyphosate is capable of replacing glycine in the structure of proteins in the body.[23,24] When this happens to collagen, the very essence of your body is under threat. Your immune system will find this changed collagen and try to clean it or remove it, using inflammation, antibodies and other mechanisms. In the last decade glyphosate has become one of the most widely used agricultural chemicals. It is poisonous and it is everywhere – in our food and water, even in organically produced food. The increase in its use goes in parallel with the increase in modern degenerative diseases.[23,24] Other agricultural chemicals, such as herbicide glufosinate, insecticide l-canavanine and many other are being implicated in the development of autoimmune disease. Many vaccines are contaminated with these chemicals, because they are manufactured with the use of collagen and other proteins from animals, which were fed commercially produced foods full of glyphosate and other agricultural poisons. The MMR vaccine (measles, mumps and rubella) has been recently verified to have this contamination.[25] Commercially produced gelatine (collagen from animals), foods containing gelatine and gelatine capsules for packaging nutritional supplements and medications are often contaminated in this way as well. There is no doubt that the increasing use of glyphosate and other agricultural chemicals is responsible for a growing epidemic of collagen disorders and autoimmune illnesses in the world.

Pharmaceutical drugs can cause autoimmunity and inflammation in the body. A good example is *Drug-Induced Lupus Erythematosus (DIL)*. Some 38 common drugs, prescribed for long periods of time, are known to cause this severe autoimmune disease.[26] Amongst them are some antibiotics, anti-epileptic drugs, anti-arrhythmic drugs, blood pressure medication, anti-inflammatory and anti-psychotic drugs. When the drug is stopped, the symptoms of *DIL* disappear. Drugs are toxins and, as with any toxin, they can attach themselves to proteins in your body (collagen in particular) and start a disease. Another example of chemically induced disease is rheumatoid arthritis: it has a strong association with the toxic chemicals in cigarette smoke, cosmetics, insecticides and other man-made chemicals.[27]

One group of toxins, which we humans have filled our modern environment with, are fat-soluble chemicals used by agriculture, the food industry, the personal care industry, modern building materials, clothes, furniture, etc. Abnormal gut flora will also provide a plethora of these toxins. Some toxic metals belong to this group: mercury, lead, arsenic, nickel, cadmium, copper and aluminium. Fat-soluble toxins have a strong ability to cause disease when they accumulate in the body, particularly in high-fat tissues. Just like in the case with collagen, toxic metals attach themselves to proteins in high-fat tissues and change their three-dimensional structure, attracting the attention of the immune system.[28] Our brain and the rest of the nervous system are high-fat tissues and can become a dumping ground for toxic metals and other fat-soluble toxins. Most chronic degenerative neurological conditions have this mechanism as part of the cause of the disease: multiple sclerosis, amyotrophic lateral sclerosis, neuropathies, Parkinson's disease, dementia, etc.

The bone marrow is a high-fat tissue and can also become a target for toxic metals and other fat-soluble toxins. Our immune cells and blood cells are born in the bone marrow; it is their 'maternity unit'. As this maternity unit gets contaminated by man-made chemicals, the very structure of the immune system and the blood is under threat. The person may develop different forms of autoimmune anaemia, low levels of different blood cells and immune cells (neutropenia, thrombocytopenia, Evan's syndrome), autoimmune lymphoproliferative syndrome and other. There is an epidemic of leukaemia in the Western world; today it is the most common cancer in children.[29] There is no doubt that the child's exposure to fat-soluble toxins from the mother during pregnancy, from vaccinations and the environment is an important cause of this epidemic.[30]

Our endocrine organs have a high proportion of fats in their structure: thyroid gland, adrenals, sex glands, pancreas and other. They also have a high proportion of collagen in their structure (the stroma and the capsule of the gland). Toxic metals and other poisons can accumulate in these organs, disrupting the hormonal balance in the body, causing a plethora of symptoms and problems. A person with this situation may develop autoimmune polyendocrine syndrome, autoimmune pancreatitis, type one diabetes, Hashimoto's thyroiditis, Graves' disease, endometriosis, autoimmune oophoritis and other disorders.

Autoimmune disease is becoming more common. Science has identified close to 200 autoimmune conditions so far, and the list keeps growing. The most commonly known autoimmune illnesses are celiac disease, type one diabetes, systemic lupus erythematosus, Sjogren's syndrome, Hashimoto's thyroiditis, Graves' disease, rheumatoid arthritis, ankylosing spondylitis, multiple sclerosis, myasthenia gravis, pernicious anaemia, Addison disease, dermatomyositis, reactive arthritis and psoriasis. But there are dozens of diagnoses that are less common. The more we study autoimmunity, the more we realise that all chronic diseases have an autoimmune component, because (quite rightly) the immune system uses all its tools (including antibodies) to deal with contamination of our tissues and organs. We also need to remember, that every contaminated place in the body becomes a breeding ground for microbes (fungi in particular). These creatures will add their own toxicity to the mix and attract the attention of the immune system in their own unique way. We will talk about this in further chapters.

In so-called autoimmune disease the exposure to contamination is chronic and long-term, but it is within our power to stop this exposure! The first thing that must be done is healing and sealing the gut wall, and the GAPS Nutritional Protocol will do that effectively. This will stop the toxicity flowing from the damaged gut into the body. The GAPS Diet will feed the immune system properly making it strong and up to the job, while providing plenty of nutrients for re-building and restoring damaged organs and tissues. The recovering gut flora will rebalance the immune system, making it well-informed and efficient. We can also take active steps to remove toxicity from the body using natural methods. And we can change our life-style, reducing exposure to environmental toxins. When all this is achieved, suddenly an 'incurable' disease becomes perfectly curable! Thousands of people around the world, who have recovered from autoimmune diseases through natural methods, will testify to this effect.

The word *autoimmunity* comes from a Greek prefix '*auto*', meaning '*self*', and *immunity* – the immune system. The mainstream concept of autoimmunity means that your immune system attacks self – normal healthy tissues in your body, causing a disease. My clinical experience has led me to the conclusion that this concept is a mistake. I am convinced that our immune system is never misguided! The immune system is not our enemy, it is a magnificent and powerful ally given to us by Mother Nature. It has not been designed to cause disease, but to free us from disease! We must respect its work and do everything in our power to assist it, if we want to recover from any chronic illness or lead a healthy life.

Food allergies and intolerances

Our gut flora is the housekeeper of the gut wall: it protects it, feeds it and orchestrates the cell regeneration process – the wonderful process, which renews the gut wall's structure all the time. When gut flora is abnormal, something terrible happens: your gut wall gets damaged. Let us see what that means.

Enterocytes, which cover your gut wall, stick to each other at their sides, forming so-called tight junctions between them. Food is not supposed to absorb between those cells: the tight junctions will not allow that. Instead food is supposed to be taken inside the enterocytes, which analyse it, improve it and then allow it through into your blood and lymph. But when the gut flora is abnormal, pathogenic microbes produce toxins which damage tight junctions and open the gut wall to invasion.[31] As a result, your gut wall becomes porous and leaky; the food, you eat, doesn't get a chance to be digested properly before it absorbs through this damaged gut wall and finishes up in your bloodstream. Your immune system finds these undigested food particles and responds to them. The reaction of the immune system to undigested food clinically manifests as *food allergy or intolerance* and can present as an asthma attack or a panic attack, a skin rash or migraine, a bout of cystitis or a drop in energy, lapses of memory or heart palpitations, emotional instability or arthritis, etc.[32] The reactions can be immediate or delayed. For example, at the same moment you could be reacting to bread you have just eaten, plus ham you ate yesterday, plus eggs you ate a few days ago and plus tomatoes you ate two weeks ago. So, on any given day you have no idea what you are reacting to, as all these reactions overlap. People do laboratory tests for food allergy and intolerance and start removing foods out of their diet. They remove and remove until there is virtually nothing left to eat, but they are still reacting! As long as your gut wall is like a sieve, you are absorbing most foods undigested and are reacting to everything you eat. Instead of focusing on food, we must focus on healing and sealing the gut wall. Once those holes in the gut are sealed, the food will start digesting properly before it absorbs. And, as a result, your food allergies and intolerances will disappear. Thousands of people around the world have done this by following the GAPS Introduction Diet. It takes time to heal and seal your gut wall. But, as this process gets under way, your allergies will start disappearing one by one.

How do allergies develop?

Our immune system is immensely complex and has many branches and departments. One of the most researched and important branches is called Th1. This branch is responsible for normal reactions to anything in the environment. For example, when your Th1 is working properly, you don't need to know how much pollen is in the air (from grasses and flowers). Your Th1 will deal with the pollen and you will never develop hay fever. Thanks to well-functioning Th1 you don't need to know how many dust mites live in your pillow, or how many chemicals you are breathing in daily, or what effect different foods can have on your body. With healthy Th1 you can look after animals (cats, dogs, horses) and have no allergic reactions to them. What keeps our Th1 healthy and well? Our gut flora! When the gut flora is well-balanced and diverse, we have a strong fully-functional Th1.[33] But when the gut flora is damaged, your Th1 can become disabled. As a result, the immune system has to use other branches to deal with the environment, mainly a branch called Th2 (as far as we know at the moment). This branch has not been designed to deal with pollen, dust mites, chemicals, foods and animals, so it uses inappropriate tools for the job. As a result, you start developing hay fever, asthma, eczema, chronic rhinitis, allergic conjunctivitis, allergies to animals, foods and chemicals, all the way to anaphylactic reactions. This immune imbalance between Th1 and Th2 is called *atopy*.[34] An atopic person is primed for reacting to anything in an allergic, hypersensitive way. This situation is a GAPS condition; it develops due to abnormal gut flora. It is becoming more and more common in the world, and our medicine is creating an ever-increasing list of diagnostic labels for this group of patients. Let us have a look at some of them.

Mast Cell Activation Disorder and eosinophilia

Mast cells are white blood cells (immune cells) which are found everywhere in the body. Their main home is our connective tissue – the tissue that holds our bodies together and is present everywhere. They concentrate in very large numbers in all our mucous membranes, because that is where the body comes in contact with the outside. They are present in the brain and the rest of the nervous system, and they are in your blood. Mast cells play many important roles in the body participating in inflammation, autoimmunity, healing wounds, dealing with chemicals, microbes and parasites and developing long-term immunity against various infections.[35]

Remember the last time you were bitten by a mosquito? What happened after that quite quickly? You developed an itchy red lump on your skin, which stayed itchy for a few days. This is caused by the activity of your mast cells: they release powerful molecules (histamine, serotonin, heparin, proteases, eicosanoids, thromboxane, prostaglandins, platelet-activating factors, eosinophil-attracting factors, cytokines, etc) causing inflammation. These active molecules are contained in granules – special 'bags' inside the mast cells. Histamine is one of the most researched molecules amongst them. It plays an important role in inflammation and allergy: it dilates the blood vessels in the area and makes them leaky, leading to swelling of the tissues. At the same time, it activates the nerve endings leading to the feelings of pain and itch. As a result, that mosquito bite turns into a swollen, red and itchy lump. In a person with a normal balanced immune system the lump is no more than 0.5–0.6 cm in diameter and disappears in a few days. But in an atopic person the lump is large, red, very itchy and lingers for much longer.

Mast cells are involved in allergic reactions mediated by immunoglobulins (IgM, IgG, IgE, etc). Immunoglobulins are antibodies – special molecules which learn about an invader and then recognise it at any time. The invader may be a particular microbe, chemical or improperly digested food. As soon as immunoglobulins detect the presence of an invader, they bind to the mast cells and make them release chemicals into your system, causing the symptoms of an allergic reaction. The reaction can be local (such as eczema or allergic rhinitis) or it can be systemic and very powerful, such as anaphylactic shock.

Mast cells can respond to many different stimuli, releasing chemicals from their 'bags' and starting a powerful cascade of symptoms in your body. When your gut wall is damaged and leaky, all sorts of things absorb into your blood and lymph and get distributed around the body: undigested foods, toxins and antigens from the activity of your abnormal gut flora, alive microbes, and toxins from the environment. All of these things can activate your mast cells. In some people all their mast cells in the body become activated, leading to a disorder called *MCAD (Mast Cell Activation Disorder*) or *MCAS (Mast Cell Activation Syndrome*).[36]

In MCAD/MCAS the mast cells produce their powerful mix of chemicals chronically (all the time) or recurrently, which leads to a plethora of unpleasant symptoms in many organs and tissues. The symptoms can range from easy bruising, flushing and itchy skin, feeling cold, dizziness, low blood pressure, diarrhoea, abdominal pain, nausea and vomiting to brain fog, headaches, poor memory, coughing, wheezing, inflammation in the eyes, general fatigue and musculoskeletal problems. Periodically people with this disorder may have anaphylaxis with difficulty breathing, rapid pulse, nausea, vomiting, dizziness and fainting. The reactions depend on what mixture of toxins and undigested foods are entering the body through the damaged gut wall on any particular day. In order to deal with this disorder, we need to focus on healing and sealing the gut wall. Once the gut is healed, the flow of toxins and undigested foods will stop, and the mast cells will have a chance to 'calm down' and stop releasing their powerful chemicals.

Mast cells do not work alone. They work together with other immune cells such as eosinophils. Eosinophils are known to be involved in fighting parasites and in allergy. They accumulate in any tissue which is responding to allergy: in the skin of eczema patches, in the lungs in asthma, in the mucous membranes of the nose and sinuses in allergic rhinitis. Just like mast cells, they also have 'bags full of chemicals', which are released during an allergic reaction. When the gut wall is damaged and leaky, undigested foods and toxins penetrate the gut wall and it attracts large numbers of eosinophils. They accumulate in the gut wall leading to a diagnosis of an eosinophilic gut disorder. Depending on where the main symptoms are the person may be diagnosed with *eosinophilic oesophagitis, eosinophilic gastritis, eosinophilic gastroenteritis* or *eosinophilic enterocolitis*. In all of these disorders the wall of the gut is infiltrated with large numbers of eosinophils, releasing their powerful chemicals and contributing to the digestive symptoms (pain, reflux, gas production, abnormal stool and malabsorption). In parallel the person usually has high levels of eosinophils in the blood (eosinophilia). There is no point fighting eosinophils and mast cells themselves, they are only a response of your immune system to the unhealthy situation in your gut. We need to deal with the real cause of your illness: abnormal gut flora and damaged gut wall.

There are many new diagnostic labels being created all the time for atopic people. These disorders (MCAD/MCAS and eosinophilic gut disorders) are becoming quite common in the Western world. They are due to the fact that the gut flora is abnormal. As a result, the immune system loses its balance and the person becomes atopic – primed for developing allergies. Another disorder in this group is *histamine intolerance (HIT)*. This is another new diagnostic label. There are a few studies already published about this disorder and the numbers of people affected are growing. Let us have a look at it.

Histamine and other biogenic amines

Biogenic amines are powerful molecules produced from amino acids. Many microbes in our gut and in the environment can convert amino acids into biogenic amines, such as histamine (made from an amino acid histidine), serotonin and tryptamine (made from an amino acid tryptophan), tyramine (made from an amino acid tyrosine), phenylethylamine (made from an amino acid phenylalanine) and many others.[37] These amines can act in the body as powerful neurotransmitters and hormones affecting many functions in many organs. Our gut flora is a very important source of biogenic amines in the body. Production of biogenic amines is complex and, in a healthy situation, is tightly controlled. One of the mechanisms of controlling them is enzymes which destroy excesses of these molecules: *Diamine Oxidase (DAO), Monoamine Oxidase (MAO)* and others. A healthy gut wall produces these enzymes to deal with any excess of biogenic amines in food. On top of that enterocytes – the cells that line the gut wall – produce their own enzymes for dealing with these molecules. The trouble is, in a person with abnormal gut flora the gut wall is damaged and often unable to produce enough of these enzymes. In addition, the damaged leaky gut wall allows biogenic amines to absorb between enterocytes, without being properly controlled by these cells.[38]

The clinical picture of *HIT* (*histamine intolerance*) includes the activity of many biogenic amines, not only histamine. The symptoms of excess biogenic amines in the body are numerous and involve many organs. A person may develop headaches, vertigo, nausea, vomiting, diarrhoea, abdominal pain, low blood pressure, fast heart rate, abnormal heart rhythm, itchy skin rash, eczema, wheezing and breathlessness, runny nose and sneezing, menstrual problems, etc. Histamine and other biogenic amines increase the permeability of our blood vessels, which can lead to rapid swelling of tissues and anaphylactic reactions.

Histamine and other biogenic amines are produced not only by microbes, but also by many cells in the human body: immune cells (such as mast cells and eosinophils), gut cells, neurones, smooth muscle cells, endothelium in our blood vessels, etc. It is normal for our bodies to produce these substances. At present we have little knowledge about their functions and how they are balanced, but the fact that our bodies produce them should tell us not to fear these molecules.

Most microbes in our environment and the microbes, which ferment our food, produce biogenic amines.[39] That is why foods, which have been fermented or stored for some time (even leftovers of yesterday's meal) can contain large amounts of biogenic amines. Many fresh foods have these substances too plus they may have other substances, which liberate histamine or impair the enzymes DAO and MAO, creating an excess of biogenic amines in the body. So, it is not possible to avoid histamine and other biogenic amines in our food completely.

The foods which can increase histamine level in the body are: fermented, pickled, preserved, salted, smoked or canned foods, mature cheeses, food leftovers, shellfish, vinegar, acidic fruit (kiwi, lemon, lime, pineapple, plums, etc), most berries (strawberries in particular), papaya, nuts, chocolate, tomatoes, all varieties of tea and coffee, beans and pulses, wheat germ, alcohol, raw egg white and yeast-containing foods. Many chemicals added to processed foods can make histamine intolerance worse (benzoate, sulphites, nitrites, MSG and glutamate, food dyes, etc).

These are foods which are generally considered to have low histamine level: fresh meats, fresh fish, fresh eggs, fresh vegetables, fresh milk and freshly fermented yogurt, some fruit (choose by trial and error), butter, herbal teas and fresh herbs.

These lists of foods are approximate as reactions are very individual. Histamine is only a small part of the whole picture. The real reason for being ill is the fact that the gut flora is abnormal, the gut wall is damaged and porous, and the immune system is out of balance, making the person atopic. Humanity has been eating fermented and less-than-perfectly-fresh foods for all of its existence – foods full of biogenic amines. Only very recently have humans suddenly become sensitive to these molecules. Why? Because of what we are doing to our gut flora. HIT is part and parcel of food allergy and intolerance caused by the damaged leaky gut. In order to deal with any food allergy, including HIT, we need to focus on healing and sealing the gut wall; we must restore its proper integrity. Then foods will digest properly before absorbing into your body, and the reactions will disappear. And most importantly, as your gut heals, your immune system will re-balance itself and you will stop being an atopic person – a person prone to allergies.

As with any food allergy and intolerance, it is necessary to go through the *GAPS Introduction Diet* slowly and patiently. The first stages of this diet have virtually no histamine-rich foods, and fermented foods are introduced very gradually starting with tiny amounts. Every human being is unique and has a unique gut flora, so adjust the diet for yourself. If you are very sensitive to biogenic amines, start without fermented foods, but soon start trying to have a tiny amount of homemade whey, yogurt, kefir, sour cream or sauerkraut juice. At some point you will find that you can tolerate them. Fermented foods will help to normalise your gut flora, improve its balance and increase its diversity.[40] All fermented foods have probiotic microbes in them, which cause a 'die-off' reaction. In most people biogenic amines play a part in that 'die-off'. In fact, symptoms of histamine intolerance are part and parcel of the die-off reaction in many people. This reaction should be controlled at a manageable level, but it cannot be avoided completely.

A person with histamine intolerance has to be careful what probiotic bacteria they choose to take. The most common lactobacilli, used in probiotics and in fermentation of food (*Lactobacillus casei* and *Lactobacillus bulgaricus*), can produce histamine and probably should be avoided by a histamine-sensitive person.[41] Some species, such as *Lactobacillus rhamnosus, Bifidobacterium infantis, Bifidobacterium longum, Lactobacillus plantarum*, and possibly *Lactobacillus reuteri* are thought to reduce the production of biogenic amines. However, this is based on some limited research which we cannot fully rely upon yet. And in the clinical experience different people can have very different reactions to probiotic bacteria.

Atopic people have a lot going on in their bodies; histamine is only one small facet of the whole picture. So, I recommend not being too focused on histamine (and other biogenic amines). The real cause of the disorder is GAPS. Work on changing your gut flora and healing and sealing your gut wall using the GAPS Nutritional Protocol. In my experience, following the GAPS Introduction Diet is important for this group of patients. Once your gut wall is sealed, food will be digested properly before it absorbs. As a result, your body will no longer need to activate your mast cells, eosinophils and other immune cells. These cells will 'calm down' and stop releasing histamine and other powerful molecules, which cause the symptoms of allergy, HIT, MCAD and eosinophilic gut disorders. Recovering gut flora will re-balance your immune system; the Th1 branch will start functioning again. Once that has happened, you can say good-bye to allergies! Whatever your main diagnosis may be (hay fever, asthma, eczema, allergies, MCAD, HIT, eosinophilia or even anaphylaxis), you can recover from it!

The following letter from a mother demonstrates this point well.

'At the age of 18 months testing found that our son was allergic to all food, anaphylactic to at least ten foods. He was put on a hypoallergenic formula, which he lived on for some 3.5 years. The only food he was given was a mixture of rice, pears, tinned sweet corn and sugar. He was having many anaphylactic reactions that were out of control, he broke his arm twice, and he was taking up to seven medications including steroids. He was intolerant to all food. I found an online group called GAPS Kids which helped me to realise that my son had FPIES (Food Protein Induced Enterocolitis Syndrome) and, most importantly, that it was resolvable. This group helped me to start a boy, who was allergic to all food, on a protocol where food was the healer!

We had to start by putting drops of lamb broth into his formula. It took us three months to build his tolerance, so that he was now having half a bottle of broth mixed with his formula every day. Just from adding broth, he had now garnered three safe GAPS foods: zucchini, butternut pumpkin and carrot, as well as one safe broth: lamb. With this we could begin the GAPS Introduction Diet. We

stopped the formula and his morning sneezing and congestion cleared up immediately. He had been intolerant to the formula all this time! Within four days of starting the GAPS Introduction Diet my son could tolerate a portion of his most allergenic food: egg yolk. Within 11 days he could tolerate his second most allergenic food: almonds. We went through the Introduction Diet in six weeks. My son now had an incredible number of safe foods and he was putting on so much solid weight. He had this beautiful colour to replace the pale white ghostly look. For the first time in his life he was able to join the family for Christmas lunch, and he closed his eyes the entire meal for the joy of tasting delicious nourishing food. He was devouring meat, organ meats, egg yolks, broth, soup, almond bread and a huge array of vegetables by the time we reached the Full GAPS Diet.

My son healed fast, but then we hit a wall when he slowed down to a crawl. Over the next three years we found the following 'cherries-on-the-top' massively increased his healing: clearing parasites (he had Dienthamoeba Fragilis and Blastocystis Hominis), taking the issue of water quality seriously and filtering out fluoride and chlorine, cranio-sacral therapy and resolving his tongue tie.

The whole family has been on the GAPS Protocol. Last Christmas we decided to order a pizza and ate it with no reactions at all! We had all healed enough. GAPS has completely transformed our future, not just our health, but our lifestyle. We purchased five acres of land and now are living on our dream farm. We are going to grow our own biodynamic food; we have our own spring-fed water supply and we are going to raise organic free-range chickens.' Mary K.

Bless the fever!

Fever is good for us! It is a major tool our immune system uses for killing disease-causing microbes, destroying toxins and removing cancer cells. If you have a fever for a few days and do not interfere with it, but allow your body to run high temperature for as long as it needs to, you clean your body, remove chronic infections, prevent cancer formation and rejuvenate yourself.[42] Researchers are experimenting with inducing fever in patients with incurable cancers, chronic fatigue syndrome and other severe illnesses, and are finding that fever can be very effective in the treatment of these disorders. During fever your immune system re-sets itself, re-balances its various branches, re-groups and becomes more effective at dealing with the environment.

Traditional societies around the world have known this for centuries, where increasing the body temperature on a regular basis was done as a prophylactic measure.[43] Russian banja, Scandinavian sauna, Turkish baths, Roman baths, sweat lodges of the Native Americans, bathing in hot springs in Japan, Iceland and other places around the world have long been prized as heath-giving activities. Whole families in those cultures consider them to be a very important part of their weekly routine. Studies have been conducted showing that regular use of sauna and Russian Banya prevents many chronic illnesses from developing in the first place and can be very helpful in healing from those illnesses.

If you allow your immune system to use fever to the full, you can prevent autoimmunity from developing in your body. The trouble is, people are afraid of fever and, as soon as their temperature starts rising, they start taking medications to bring it down. If your immune system is not allowed to use fever properly, the ground will be laid for developing autoimmunity, chronic inflammation, allergies, chronic infections, parasites and cancer in the future.

It is particularly vital to allow fever to run in our babies and small children.[44] Children are born with immature immune systems, which require education. The first fever your child develops is a major educational experience for the child's immune system. If the fever is not allowed to run, the child's immune system has missed an important lesson. Instead it has received a wrong lesson, which may lay the ground for allergies and autoimmunity in the future. Of course, it can be quite frightening for parents to see their baby or toddler 'on fire' and feeling ill. So, it is natural for them to want to stop the fever and to see their child well again. This is the time to focus on what is best for the child: let the fever run! Just keep your child warm and well hydrated. In most cases the fever will only last for 12–24 hours; and when your child has come out of it, he or she will have a stronger and healthier immune system! Majority of fevers are caused by common colds, which generally do not need a doctor's attention. But, obviously, it is important to make sure that the fever is not caused by a serious infection, such as meningitis, which requires medical treatment.

What do we need to do when we develop a fever? Follow the same recommendations for your babies and children as well as for yourself.

Stay in bed, keep warm and keep sweating. Sweating is very healing; toxins leave your body and your temperature comes down naturally. Keep a few sets of pyjamas or night shirts, which you can change regularly as they absorb your sweat. Put a large cotton towel underneath yourself; cover yourself with another large cotton towel and put a warm blanket on top of it. When we have fever we feel cold and may even shiver. To keep warm, we must wear only natural fibres – cotton and wool, no synthetics!

While running fever it is important to stay well-hydrated. Keep drinking hot water with a large piece of fresh lemon in it (the lemon will provide minerals and vitamin C). Make a butter–honey mixture and eat a few teaspoons of this mixture with every cup of hot water. To make butter–honey mixture mix 200g (7 oz) of organic raw butter (or organic ghee) with 1–6 teaspoons of honey to your taste. (Start with one teaspoon of honey and keep tasting the mixture and adding honey until your taste buds are happy). Keep this mixture at a room temperature next to your bed. If butter is not tolerated for some reason use coconut oil, homemade tallow or any other animal fat (please look in the recipe section for how to make tallow). Add a pinch of natural salt to the butter–honey mixture. When we sweat, we lose a lot of salt from the body; replenishing it is important.

There is an old proverb: starve the fever, feed the cold! When we have a high temperature we don't want to eat; food becomes a burden for the body to deal with when it needs to spend all its resources on fighting the disease. Just drinking plenty of hot water with lemon and eating the butter–honey–salt mixture is quite enough. When your temperature starts coming down, you can start eating food. What food is best to start from? It is very important to start with food that is easy to digest and which will feed your immune system. The best food in this situation is homemade meat stock, and chicken stock is very pleasant to start from (chicken should be organic and soy-free). To make chicken stock put a whole chicken and giblets into a 4–5 l (7–8¾ pt.) pan, fill it with water, add a tablespoon of natural salt and cook for 2–3 hours. The resulting stock will be clear and delicious. Keep drinking as much of this stock as you want all day. When you become hungry, eat the chicken, which you made the stock with, focussing on the skin, the fat, the brown meat on the bones and the soft parts of the bones (not the breast!). I strongly recommend eating the chicken with your hands, without using cutlery! If you eat with your hands, your body will instinctively lead you to the bits of the chicken that are best for your health at that moment; using cutlery will not allow this instinct to express itself. By taking a portion of the chicken stock, adding a few non-starch vegetables to it and cooking for 20 minutes you can make a good soup. Keep eating this soup and the chicken, drinking the chicken stock, and drinking hot water with lemon and the butter–honey mixture. If chicken is not tolerated for some reason, use other meats on the bone for making the stock (lamb, beef, goose, duck, game, etc). It is good to add a few teaspoons of homemade kefir, sour cream, whey or yogurt to your soups. They will add probiotic bacteria and enzymes to your meals, which will stimulate immunity and heal your gut lining. Do not eat anything else! Following these simple recommendations, you will come out of your fever stronger and healthier than you were before.

A small proportion of babies and small children can develop *febrile seizures* during high temperature (usually higher than 39°C/ 102.2°F). When this happens, the child may twitch or have other involuntary movements and lose consciousness for a few seconds. Febrile seizures are not epilepsy and generally require no treatment. Don't try to restrain the child, just keep him or her safe and remove blankets and clothing to reduce the child's temperature a little. Generally, there is no need to be overly concerned about febrile seizures, they pass on their own and leave no lasting damage. Seizures are a cleansing procedure for the brain; fever initiates powerful cleansing in the body, which may involve the nervous system. Keeping your child well-hydrated and giving him or her the butter–honey–salt mixture will ensure that the child's body goes through the fever safely without any complications. To prevent febrile seizures, keep the temperature below 39°C/102.2°F while allowing the fever to run. The best way to do this is to undress the child and apply a moist cloth over the skin. If this measure doesn't work, then dissolve a small tablet of aspirin (75 mg) in a cup of warm water and give the child a few teaspoons of this water. Instead of aspirin you can use a natural willow tea. It is important not to bring the temperature down too much, but just reduce it below the critical level of 39°C/102.2°F. If the seizure lasts longer than 10–15 minutes or the child has recurrent seizures, then it is important to seek medical assistance.

Bless the common cold!

Nature doesn't do anything without good reason! Common viruses associated with common colds have a very important mission in Nature: they provide regular cleaning for our bodies. Nobody catches a virus by accident! When you 'catch a virus' it means your body needs this virus to remove accumulated toxins. If a group of people is exposed to the same virus on the same occasion, only some will develop the cold, while others will not. Why do you think that happens? The people who 'got the virus' needed some cleansing done. We live in a polluted world: every day we breath in plethora of chemicals from car exhausts, indoor pollution, aeroplane travel, agricultural and industrial pollution. These chemicals accumulate in the mucous membranes of your nose, sinuses and breathing passages. When you catch a cold, you get a runny nose, sneezing, coughing – the functions designed to clean up the mucous membranes of your nose, sinuses and breathing passages. If those areas of your body are clean, your body will not use the virus, and you will be one of the 'lucky ones' who did not get the common cold. The cold often raises your body temperature, which means that your body has to do some deeper cleansing in other organs and systems, not just in your breathing passages. The body will use the fever to get rid of cancer cells and stored toxins and chemicals. So, by the time you have recovered from a common cold, you have a body which is cleaner and healthier overall.

The common cold is not a haphazard situation that develops in your body by accident. It is a finely orchestrated event where the virus and your body work together as partners, for your good. So, when you catch a common virus, it is not a time to start taking anti-inflammatory drugs, antibiotics and anti-fever medications. It is time to feel blessed: your body is giving you a chance to clean up and prevent a whole host of terrible chronic illnesses from ever developing, such as cancer and autoimmune disease.

Science keeps confirming this fact. A good example is *norovirus* – a common 'tummy bug' in humans. Every winter many people in the northern hemisphere get this virus leading to a day or two of vomiting and diarrhoea. Animal experiments have shown, that norovirus can restore and normalise gut flora which has been damaged by antibiotics.[45] Not only is gut flora restored, but also the immune function and the normal physical state of the gut wall. Vomiting and diarrhoea are major cleansing functions of the digestive system. They are uncomfortable, but they flush out toxins and parasites from your gut, leaving it cleaner and healthier as a result. Some people also develop a high temperature when they get norovirus, which means their bodies need deeper cleansing.

The same applies to common childhood infections: measles, mumps, rubella, chicken pox and scarlet fever. These infections are designed by Mother Nature to 'educate' the immune system of the child and train it to deal properly with the environment.[46] These infections come with a fever, which makes them powerful cleansers. People who have these infections in early childhood typically never develop allergies, autoimmunity or any other immune problems, because their immune system has had a chance to mature properly. In our modern world there is a fear of childhood infections because they may cause complications. The decisive factor in whether a child will sail through the infection or get complications from it, is the child's nutritional status. Children who have nutritional deficiencies in animal protein, animal fat and fat-soluble vitamins (A, D, K and E) are prone to developing complications from infections.[47] All of these nutrients come from animal foods prepared at home:

meats and organ meats, meat stock, animal fat, fish, eggs and high-fat dairy. Children who grow up largely on breakfast cereals, skimmed milk, bread, pasta and sugar will have deficiencies in all those vital nutrients necessary for the immune system to function well. The diet of these children makes them prone to developing complications from *any* infection, not just the ones mentioned.

According to recent research, the presence of uncleared viral infections in the body is an important cause of autoimmune disease, such as inflammatory bowel disease, autoimmune thrombocytopenia, autoimmune thyroid disease, type one diabetes, mental illness and others.[48] The drugs, which people take when they get a common cold, will not do anything to the virus. All they do is stop your immune system from dealing with this virus properly, allowing the virus to settle in your body as a chronic infection. So, taking drugs for common colds is not a good idea but, unfortunately, the majority of people do exactly that. No doubt this practice is a major contributing factor to our epidemic of autoimmune disease, allergy and other immune problems.

So, what should we do when we get a common cold? The important thing is to trust your body and work with it. Avoid all medications and do not reduce the fever or any other symptoms of your cold. They are the tools your immune system is using! Allow your body to do the work unimpeded. While you have a fever, only hot water with the lemon and butter–honey–salt mixture should be consumed. Once the fever subsides, you need to eat foods which nourish the immune system: homemade meat stock, organ meats (liver in particular), fatty meats, vegetable soup made with the homemade meat stock, oily fish with well-cooked vegetables, eggs, butter, sour cream, full-fat yogurt and kefir. Avoid anything made from flour and sugar, as these foods will undermine your immune system.

When you have a cold, it is important to keep warm and well hydrated, sleep as much as you can and avoid any stress or exertion. This means that you should not work when you have a common cold! There is nothing heroic or respectable in going to work with a fever and a cold. Your body is under great strain, it is doing very important work removing toxins and future chronic illnesses from your organs. If you organise your time to allow your body to do that work fully, it will reward you with good health for many years to come. The same applies to your children. Don't send your child to school with a cold and a fever! It is important for your child to rest and sleep as much as possible, and eat nourishing homemade food. Your child's cold may give you a chance to spend some quality time together: talking, playing and cooking good food.

Feed your immune system well!

What kind of foods does our immune system require to be healthy and strong? There is no avoiding the fact that most of these foods are of animal origin: meat, animal fat, organ meats, fish, eggs and high-fat dairy (particularly fermented). These foods will provide protein, fats and fat-soluble vitamins, so necessary for your immune system to be healthy.[49] Vegetables combine with all of these foods very well and will provide some extra nutrients and cleansing substances.

When we have a cold, we need to focus on hot soups and stews, made with homemade meat stock, fatty meats and well-cooked vegetables. Homemade sour cream, butter and ghee should be on the menu every day (unless dairy is not tolerated). Organ meats are very important to eat regularly, liver in particular. Liver is a powerhouse of nutrition; it provides all the nutrients necessary to have a strong and robust immune system. Other organ meats (kidney, heart, tongue, tripe, glands and brain) will provide their own mix of essential nutrients, such as large amounts of cholesterol.

Cholesterol is one of the most vital molecules necessary for our immune system! Animal experiments and human studies have demonstrated that immune cells rely on cholesterol in fighting infections and repairing themselves after the fight.[50] On top of that, LDL (low-density lipoprotein) cholesterol directly binds and inactivates dangerous bacterial toxins, preventing them from doing any damage in the body. One of the most lethal toxins is produced by a widely spread bacterium, *Staphylococcus aureus*, which is the cause of MRSA, a common hospital infection. This toxin can literally dissolve red blood cells. However, it does not work in the presence of LDL cholesterol.[50] People who fall prey to this toxin have *low* blood cholesterol. Considering that today almost all adult patients (and even some children) in our hospitals are prescribed statins to reduce their blood cholesterol, it is no wonder that MRSA has become such a problem as a hospital infection. In order to deal with it effectively we need to take steps *to increase* the cholesterol level in our hospital patients, and feeding them organ meats, animal fat and eggs with bacon daily will be a great help for their immune systems. It has been recorded that people with high levels of cholesterol are protected from infections: they are four times less likely to contract AIDS, they rarely get common colds, and they recover from infections more quickly than people with 'normal' or low blood cholesterol.[51] On the other side of the spectrum, people with low blood cholesterol are prone to various infections, suffer from them longer and are more likely to die from an infection.[52] A diet rich in cholesterol has been demonstrated to improve these people's ability to recover from infections. So, any person suffering from an acute or chronic infection needs to eat high-cholesterol foods to recover. Cod liver oil, rich in cholesterol, has long been prized as a remedy for the immune system. Those familiar with old medical literature will tell you that, until the discovery of antibiotics, a common cure for tuberculosis was a daily mixture of raw egg yolks and fresh cream, very high in cholesterol.[53]

Fermented foods are a great help for our immune system.[54] They provide active probiotic microbes and pre-digested, easy-to-absorb nutrients. Homemade yogurt, kefir, sour cream, cottage cheese and whey are soothing and healing for the digestive system and for the immune system, located in its walls.

Herbs and spices are good for immunity. Curcuma, ginger, garlic, onion, cloves, cumin, caraway, dill, coriander (cilantro) and other herbs and spices in small amounts should be a regular part of our diet. When we don't have an infection, freshly pressed vegetable and fruit juices can also help to keep our immune system and the rest of the body healthy. But it is not a good idea to have them during an active infection!

There are foods which alter the immune balance in the body and make us vulnerable to viruses; they can activate our resident viruses (such as herpes family or papilloma) and they will make it easier for viruses from the outside to come in. These foods are chocolate, fruit and nuts.[55] Many raw vegetables can do that as well, if eaten in excess. When we have a cold or another active infection, we need to avoid these foods. Vegetables need to be cooked in meat stock as a soup or stew, or roasted with a large amount of animal fat. Cooked vegetables have a different effect on the body; they are easier to digest and are more nourishing than raw vegetables. When you have an infection, eat your cooked vegetables hot, not cold, as part of soup, stew or a meal with fatty meat.

People who decide to avoid all animal foods are called vegans. A vegan regimen is not a diet; it is a form of fasting. Fasting is a powerful cleansing procedure, which can be beneficial for a body with a large toxic burden. But we cannot fast forever! Any fast has to be fairly short. When the body finished cleansing it will require feeding, and that is when animal foods must be introduced. Vegetarians who keep themselves healthy eat plenty of eggs and dairy products (animal foods, which sustain them) and, at least occasionally, they eat meat and fish. Misguided veganism has become an important cause of mental and physical illness in the Western world.[56] In all the vegans, I have seen in my clinic, the immune system is in a state of collapse; it is unable to mount a response to the environment. Vegans often say that they never have colds. In reality they get all the viruses that we all get, but their immune system is in no fit state to respond to them, so there is no fever, coughing, sneezing or any other symptoms of a common cold. Please read more on this subject in my book *Vegetarianism Explained. Making an Informed Decision.*

Some nutritional supplements can be helpful for the immune system. Good quality cod liver oil is one of the traditional, time-proven remedies. It provides cholesterol and fat-soluble vitamins (A, D and K_2 if the oil is fermented). Taking it on a regular basis is known to prevent common colds and other infections. An amino acid L-lysine can be very helpful when our resident viruses activate (for example, a herpes virus causing a cold sore). Taking a supplement of L-lysine for a few days right at the beginning of a cold sore developing can arrest the infection. An adult should take 3–6 grams per day; a child can take from 500 mg to 3 grams. Mushroom supplements, such as cordyceps, reishi, coriolus, maitake, shiitake and others have been demonstrated to boost our immunity and assist it in the fight against cancer and chronic infections.[57] Raw bee pollen, dried green juices, colostrum, some herbs, natural vitamin C with zinc and many other natural substances have been shown to be beneficial for our immune system. Apart from L-lysine, most of these supplements need to be taken on a long-term basis, so it is a good idea to consult a health practitioner to get quality supplements.

What else does our immune system need?

The *hygiene hypothesis*, which is finally being accepted by our mainstream, has demonstrated that it is essential for us, humans, to be exposed to microbes in the environment in order to have healthy fully-functional immune systems.[58] It has been demonstrated in a number of studies that people who grew up in close contact with animals, soil, animal manure and other sources of microbes, have healthier immune systems than people who grew up in a 'clean' environment. It is now a known fact that people who have intestinal worms are better protected from autoimmunity and allergy than people who don't have them. The Westerners are obsessed with sterilising their environment, fighting microbes and, as a result, creating immune problems in the population. It is particularly vital for small children to be exposed to microbes in the environment, so keeping things too clean around them is doing them a disservice.

We are children of Nature; it is vital for us to be in close contact with it to keep our bodies healthy. It is important for us to walk bare-foot on the soil and grass and to swim in the natural waters of lakes, rivers and sea. It is important for us to be physically active in the fresh air in natural environments. It is essential for us to be in contact with animals and other forms of life on our beautiful planet. It is essential for us to sunbathe regularly. All of these activities help us build a robust immune system and a healthy beautiful body.

Babies are born with immature immune systems. Mother Nature has created various tools to mature that immune system and prepare it for a long healthy life. These tools are various microbes in the environment, including those that cause childhood infections and common colds. These are our friends; we need to allow our bodies to meet them fully in order to develop healthy strong immune systems. We just need to feed our bodies properly to make the whole process healthy (which, unfortunately, often doesn't happen in modern families). We live in a world teeming with microbes, and our bodies are full of microbes that are essential for our very survival! Their constant interaction with our immune system is part and parcel of good health. The vast majority of microbes on our planet are not only harmless for us, but beneficial. And it is quite possible that our immune cells have evolved from microbes in the first place. Some immune cells look and behave like microbes and it is known that antibiotics kill immune cells.[59] Nature works on co-operation! Everything in Nature supports each other, balances each other out and creates an environment for each other. We must stop fearing Nature and its creatures, instead we must respect them and try to live in harmony with them. Our human body is one of those creatures!

Modern humans have changed their environment substantially removing themselves from Nature. This is the reason for the chronic diseases becoming more and more rampant. The only real answers are to be found in Nature! We must nourish our bodies properly, keep ourselves and our environment unpolluted and allow our immune systems to do their work unimpeded.

I would like to share with the reader a case study of a little girl called Mary (the name has been changed to protect her privacy).

Mary was a healthy baby at birth, but she was given dried formula milk from day one as well as breast milk. She was a restless baby not sleeping for more than 30 minutes at a time and constantly crying. She was diagnosed with colic and the mother was advised to stop breastfeeding and move to formula. As soon as that was done, Mary developed severe eczema all over her body and became even more miserable. Steroid cream was used for eczema, which provided partial relief for a couple of months and then stopped working. She had severe explosive diarrhoea alternating with constipation and her stools were slimy. She reacted to dust, animals and vaccinations with flu-like symptoms, worsening of eczema and swollen face. By 12 months she could tolerate a very limited number of foods and reacted even to those. Testing revealed severe allergies to most foods, including her milk formula so Mary was put onto hydrolysed milk formula, which brought no improvements. After blood tests Mary was diagnosed with

THI – Transient Hypogammaglobulinemia – which is a condition of immunodeficiency (when the immune system does not work properly). The parents were advised to keep Mary away from people, animals, travelling and other environments where she could pick up any infection. The parents were told, that this condition could last for the rest of her life and that there was no treatment for it.

The parents tried elimination diets, fish oils and probiotics, which brought some improvements. Yet, by the age of three Mary was diagnosed with failure to thrive, as she has not put on any weight for two years and was not growing.

Then the parents heard about the GAPS Diet and started it immediately. During the first two months on the GAPS Introduction Diet Mary lost some weight and looked even worse than before. She went through die-off reactions with painful stomach cramps. But, despite the weight loss and stomach cramps, the parents were encouraged by the fact that Mary's stools had become normal and regular and she had started getting some colour in her face (she had been very pale all her life). When the initial difficult period was over, Mary started improving and, by the end of one year on the diet, she was tolerating all foods allowed on the GAPS Nutritional Protocol without any reactions. But, most importantly, her blood tests showed no signs of THI; for the first time in her life Mary had a normally functioning immune system! She was growing, putting on weight and the diagnosis of failure to thrive was removed. Mary stayed on the strict GAPS Diet for two years, after which she was well enough to introduce other foods. Today she is a beautiful thriving young girl who has a pet dog and no health problems of any description.

In conclusion: Mother Nature has equipped us with an amazing protector, called the immune system. Its complexity and power are staggering. All of our lives it is busy maintaining our good health, stamina and well-being. It is never misguided and it always uses the right tools for the job. We must respect its work, because without the involvement of our immune system we cannot survive in this world, let alone recover from any illness! A large percentage of our immune system is located in the gut wall and has a close relationship with the gut flora. When the gut flora is abnormal, the immune system responds to the flow of toxicity coming through the damaged gut wall by using many different tools, including inflammation, allergy and autoimmunity. Every GAPS person has immune activation as part of their individual clinical picture. Their immune system is working very hard trying to deal with a dangerous situation, when the biggest frontier in the body – the gut – is breached and the whole organism is in danger! We must do all we can to assist our immune system by feeding it well and reducing its work-load. In order to help, we must focus on healing and sealing the gut wall, normalising the gut flora, reducing our exposure to environmental toxicity and using natural healing methods for restoring the physical structure and functions of the whole body.

In the next chapter we are going to look at another vital system in the human body – our endocrine organs. All systems and organs in our bodies are affected by the state of the gut flora, including our endocrine glands.

Hormones

Life is like riding a bicycle. To keep your balance you must keep moving.

Albert Einstein

Our endocrine system works as a team: all our hormone-producing organs communicate with each other and balance each other. Parts of the brain (pituitary gland, pineal gland and hypothalamus), our thyroid gland, pancreas, adrenal glands, sex glands, parathyroid glands, thymus and other endocrine organs work together as a magnificent orchestra, playing a very complex symphony of hormone production and regulation.

Our gut flora plays a very important part in this 'symphony'. Microbes in the gut produce their own hormones, enzymes, neurotransmitters and many other active molecules, releasing them into the circulation.[1] The more we research the human microbiome, the more we find that it is involved in our hormonal balance. Its capacity to produce a plethora of different hormone-like substances makes it more powerful than any endocrine gland we have. In fact, our gut flora can be considered to be an active endocrine organ in its own right! And this organ has a strong influence on the rest of our endocrine system. To start with, our gut flora is involved in food digestion and absorption, making sure that all our endocrine glands receive proper nutrients to function. Secondly, it protects the whole body from toxicity, including the endocrine glands, which are very sensitive to toxins.[2] On top of that, it produces active substances to communicate with the brain and the glands. The interaction of our gut flora with the endocrine system is immensely complex and dynamic, giving it great power to affect everything in the body.

Hormones are the rulers of our metabolism! They affect every organ and every cell in the body in a unique and very complicated way. Our hormonal balance is a finely tuned system, very delicate and sensitive, constantly adjusting itself to what is going on in the body and to changes in our environment. If even one hormone changes its function, the rest of the system has to change to keep a balance.

We humans have changed our environment quite dramatically in the last few decades, inside our bodies and outside. Some very important changes are happening in our gut flora. When the composition of the gut flora gets damaged, everything changes in the body! The flow of nutrients, hormones, enzymes and many other powerful substances, coming from the gut to our endocrine organs, becomes different. Instead of supporting our endocrine system, these substances interfere in its work. As a result, a new unhealthy hormonal balance gets established in the body, which brings a multitude of health problems.

In addition to affecting our endocrine system through the gut flora, our modern environment is becoming more and more directly damaging to this vital system.[3] We, humans, have filled our lives with endocrine-disrupting chemicals, which are found in thousands of everyday products. Plastics (in food packaging, household products and other applications), fire retardants in our furniture and clothes (including baby clothes and nappies), the contraceptive pill, HRT (hormone replacement therapy), many other pharmaceutical drugs, dental materials, baby formula and its packaging, personal care products, hair dyes, make-up, paper, cleaning chemicals and laundry detergents, agricultural chemicals and processed food all contain endocrine-disrupting substances. Our bodies get contaminated with these chemicals and they accumulate in our tissues.[4] The most common chemicals found in human bodies are PCBs (polychlorinated biphenyls), BPA (bisphenol A), BPS (bisphenol S), PBDEs (polybrominated diphenyl ethers), phthalates, phenols (alkylphenols, nonylphenols, etc) and DDT.[5] Many chemicals are classified as xenoestrogens, because they mimic natural female hormones – oestrogens. Xenoestrogens disrupt sex hormone balance in women and men, causing abnormal sexual development in children, endometriosis, polycystic ovaries, obesity, neurological and mental problems, breast cancer, prostate cancer and other cancers of reproductive organs in men and women. Babies and children are particularly vulnerable to these poisons.[6]

Endocrine-disrupting substances are also produced in Nature by some plants and fungi.[7] For example, cereals and legumes are known sources of these chemicals.[8] It is essential to prepare these foods properly in order to destroy xenoestrogens and other antinutrients in these plants by soaking, sprouting and fermentation before cooking.[9] Western soya products are a major source of endocrine-disrupting substances in the industrialised world, because soya beans are not properly prepared.[10] In traditional cultures soya has always been fermented prior to using it as food. The same applies to the majority of baked products in the Western world. Grains, and the flour made from grains, have not been properly prepared. In traditional cultures, grains have always been fermented prior to making any food from them.

Plant-based and many industrial endocrine-disrupting chemicals come into the body with food and drink, interacting with our gut flora. A healthy gut flora is able to neutralise many toxins in our digestive system, protecting us. Unfortunately, a growing proportion of humanity has damaged gut flora, populated by an unhealthy mixture of living creatures.

Not only will they not protect us from environmental toxins, but overgrowth of pathogenic fungi, bacteria, protozoa and worms in the human gut can produce many endocrine-disrupting chemicals of their own. These chemicals absorb through the gut lining and interfere in our hormonal balance. This situation is present in all GAPS people to a different degree. Let us talk about the most common scenarios.

Abnormal thyroid function

Our thyroid gland has a powerful effect on our metabolism: our temperature control, metabolic rate, energy production, growth and maturation, food digestion and assimilation, appetite, blood pressure and heart rate, body weight, bone density, mental function, mood, sleep and many other functions. The toxicity produced in the unhealthy gut usually causes low thyroid function.[11] It is possible that, for a short period of time, the person's thyroid gland may become hyperactive, but fairly soon the thyroid function gets impaired. As a result, the person has low metabolic rate and low body temperature, feeling cold all the time regardless of the season and weather. These people are typically overweight and find it difficult to lose weight, though some can be underweight. Their appetite is typically low. They have dry skin and coarse hair, because their sebaceous glands and sweat glands don't work very well. Their heart rate and blood pressure are low. Their muscles are weak and flabby, and their movements are sluggish. They are typically constipated. They are often depressed, apathetic and feel sleepy all the time. The old name for hypothyroidism was myxoedema – swelling of the face and body, because people with this problem accumulate certain proteins (mucopolysaccharides) under their skin and behind their eyes, which attract water and cause swelling.[12] As a result, the person has a typical hypothyroid face – swollen and expressionless with puffy eyes. Swollen ankles are common as is swelling in the limbs and other parts of the body.

Testing for thyroid function very often finds that the thyroid gland of the person produces normal or even high amounts of thyroid hormones. This finding is very common in GAPS people, and it causes confusion amongst doctors and their patients. How can a person with a full clinical picture of low thyroid function have normal (or even high) blood levels of thyroid hormones? The reason for this is *functional deficiency* of the hormones.

What is a functional deficiency?

Hormones are released by our endocrine glands into the bloodstream, which takes them all over the body to do their jobs. In order for any hormone to do its job, it has to find its receptors on the organs and tissues and attach itself to those receptors. The receptors are very specific for every hormone; the hormone fits into the receptor like a key into a keyhole. The trouble is that many toxins, produced by the abnormal gut flora and absorbed into the bloodstream, can also fit into those 'keyholes'.[13] When the toxins occupy the receptors of the thyroid hormone in the body, the hormone has nowhere to attach itself. So it floats around idly and just gets excreted or recycled, while the person develops symptoms of low thyroid function.

Functional deficiency can happen with any hormone in the body, with any nutrient, enzyme, neurotransmitter and any other active molecule, which has to attach itself to a receptor in order to accomplish its mission. GAPS people have a river of toxins, flowing from the gut into the blood and lymph and attaching themselves to receptors of important substances in the body. That is why GAPS people always have functional deficiency of some or many nutrients, hormones, neurotransmitters, enzymes and other molecules. This situation can produce a plethora of symptoms, seemingly unconnected with each other, because the most fundamental functions of the body get impaired. Attaching to receptors is just one mechanism of toxins interfering with hormones; there are other mechanisms. The result is the same: the hormone cannot do its work in the body. In order to deal with this situation we need to remove toxins; and in order to do that we have to start from healing the gut, because the gut is the major source of toxicity.

Another major source of damage for our thyroid function comes from halogens.

What are halogens?

Halogens are a group of elements in the periodic table, which include iodine, chlorine, bromine, fluorine and astatine. Molecules of thyroid hormones contain iodine in their structure. The trouble is that other halogens, such as fluorine, chlorine and bromine have an ability to push iodine out of those molecules, making them dysfunctional and causing hypothyroidism.[14] Where do these halogens come from? In our modern environment they are everywhere and are increasingly difficult to avoid. Chlorine is in our drinking water and processed food. It is toxic and absorbs through our digestive system very well. When we swim in a chlorinated swimming pool we absorb large amounts of chlorine through our skin. We also absorb it through the lungs, because a thick layer of chlorine gas floats above the pool water, and we breathe it in while swimming. Bromides are in all our plastic food wrapping and plastic bottles. It is a major ingredient in pesticides (used in large amounts on strawberries, for example) and food additives (potassium bromide in bread and other baked products, and brominated vegetable oils).[15] Bromides are major ingredients in fire retardants in our clothes, furniture upholstery and carpeting. Fluoride is extremely toxic, it is in our drinking water (in areas where water is fluoridated), in our toothpaste (and other dental products) and non-stick cooking pans, where Teflon and other such materials are used.[16] These environmental halogens (chlorine, bromine and fluorine) are chemically stronger than iodine; they displace it in the body, causing iodine deficiency.

All cells in our bodies use iodine. Apart from the thyroid gland, iodine is used extensively by our brain and the rest of the nervous system, our skin, our digestive system, other endocrine glands (pancreas, thymus, testes and ovaries) and many other organs in the body. Salivary glands absorb iodine in large amounts; that is why saliva is used to test for iodine levels in the body. Our brain absorbs iodine very effectively, and it has a stimulating effect on the brain activity, making us more alert and mentally able. All of our organs suffer when we are exposed to environmental halogens, because they cause iodine deficiency in the body, despite the fact that we may be consuming plenty of this essential element in food. Iodine deficiency creates a background in the body for cancer development, particularly cancers of the stomach, oesophagus, breast, ovaries, endometrium and the thyroid gland.[17] Female hormones (oestrogens) appear to inhibit absorption of iodine. This fact is used as an explanation for why low thyroid function is more common in women than men, with the ratio of 9 to 1.[18] Xenoestrogens, which we discussed earlier, can inhibit absorption of iodine as well.

It is interesting that, apart from our thyroid gland, thyroid hormones can be produced in the body by other organs. Ovaries concentrate iodine and produce a thyroid hormone, called T2 (diiodothyronine), which can be used by the body to make T3 (triiodothyronine) and T4 (levothyroxine). Our white blood cells also can make thyroid hormones for us.[19] We have known for a long time that our brain produces a thyroid-stimulating hormone (TSH), which regulates production of thyroid hormones in the body. Recent research has discovered that, apart from the brain, TSH can be produced by epithelial cells in the gut wall and different immune cells (T cells, B cells, splenic dendritic cells, bone marrow hematopoietic cells and lymphocytes). This means that our gut and our immune system regulate our thyroid function! Considering that some 85% of immunity is located in the gut wall, most of these regulating elements are to be found in the gut. No wonder that the majority of GAPS people have thyroid problems!

The easiest way to test for iodine deficiency and to supplement iodine is to paint a patch the size of your hand somewhere on your skin, using Lugols iodine solution. Lugols iodine solution comes in several different concentrations (from 2% to 15%) and can be easily purchased. The Lugols solution will colour your skin brown and your body will absorb iodine from that patch. If you have no iodine deficiency, the body will take, on average, 24 hours to absorb the solution. (The brown colour stays on your skin for 24 hours and then disappears.) If the brown colour disappears in 12 hours or less, then you have a deficiency in iodine. Painting Lugols iodine solution on your skin not only works as a test, but also as a very safe way to supplement iodine. We call it *the iodine paint* in the GAPS Protocol and use it for children and adults.

Paint a patch of iodine on your skin every bedtime. Check your skin next morning: if the brown colour has gone completely, your body needs more iodine. Keep painting it every bedtime, making the patch no smaller than your hand. Make sure to paint on different areas of skin, because Lugols solution can cause skin irritation if you paint on the same place many times. If, after some weeks of painting iodine on your skin, you still test deficient it may be time to consider supplementing iodine orally. The easiest way is to take an old remedy, called *Iodoral* (iodine/potassium iodide supplement). It comes in tablets of two strengths: 12.5 mg and 50 mg. It is prudent to start from a smaller dose. Take it for a few weeks, while using the iodine paint to test if you need more. Adjust the dose gradually. Some people try to supplement iodine by taking Lugols solution in drops in water, and many different doses are used. This is when iodine supplementation can become quite complicated, and it is beyond the scope of this book to go into this subject in depth. If you want to use higher doses of iodine, please research the subject and consult with an experienced practitioner. It is possible to overdose on iodine, so supplementing higher doses should be undertaken very carefully and under professional supervision.

Low thyroid function is routinely recorded in people with many chronic illnesses: rheumatoid arthritis, fibromyalgia, chronic fatigue syndrome, multiple sclerosis and many other autoimmune and neurological conditions, asthma, allergies, mental illness, migraines, chronic cystitis and nephropathy, psoriasis, etc. – all the conditions which belong to the *Gut and Physiology/Gut and Psychology Syndrome*. The symptoms can be as mild as swollen ankles and puffy eyes, feeling cold all the time and having cold hands and feet, or as severe as a full-blown hypothyroidism.

Toxins coming from the gut, particularly if fat-soluble, can accumulate in the thyroid glands.[20] This attracts the attention of the immune system, and the person can develop inflammation (thyroiditis) of the gland or an autoimmune thyroid disease, such as Hashimoto's thyroiditis, Ord's thyroiditis (with low thyroid function) or Grave's disease (with a hyperactive thyroid). Toxicity accumulation in the thyroid gland can lay the ground for other problems, such as goitre and cancer.

The mainstream treatment for low thyroid function is synthetic hormone replacement. Many patients don't feel well with this approach and use natural thyroid supplements instead, made from freeze-dried animal thyroid glands. These natural supplements supply all the hormones and substances the thyroid gland produces, and in the natural balance. This measure can bring relief. However, in order to deal with the situation fully, addressing the root of the problem, we need to reduce the toxic load in the body. And in order to do that we need to address all the sources of toxicity in the body: halogens in our food, water and environment, iodine deficiency and xenoestrogens. But most importantly we must stop that river of toxicity coming from the digestive system; we need to change the gut flora and heal the gut wall.

Abnormal adrenal function

Our adrenal glands fulfil many functions for us. But the word that is most associated with the adrenals is – stress. These small glands, which sit on top of our kidneys, are responsible for handling stressful situations. They produce adrenaline, noradrenalin and steroids, which change everything in the body to prepare it for the fight-or-flight response. Steroids make sure that fats get broken down to provide the body with plenty of energy, and glucose and glycogen are being produced from proteins to do the same. They shut down the immune and digestive systems, so they don't interfere in your fight and flight. The steroid hormone aldosterone makes sure that the volume of blood and blood pressure are at the right level, to provide your brain and muscles with good circulation (so you can be alert and run away from danger). Androgens, produced by the adrenal cortex, put you in the right mental and physical state for making quick and, possibly, aggressive decisions. Everything in the body prepares for handling a stressful situation: the brain and senses are sharp and in focus, the muscles are ready to contract, and there is plenty of energy from both glucose and fats to fuel the response.

Our adrenal glands are very efficient and have served humanity well for a very long time. Unfortunately, in our modern world they have to deal with a very different stress – toxins and stimulants. Toxins from the environment and the activity of unhealthy gut flora can undermine adrenal function.[21] In a GAPS person there is ongoing stress in the body from food allergies and intolerances, and toxicity coming from the gut. Our adrenal glands can work under pressure for quite a long time, but at a certain point they get 'exhausted' and the person develops low adrenal function.

The first symptom of low adrenal function is fatigue, particularly in the afternoon. This is when people start drinking coffee. Coffee is addictive; the first few cups seem to help with the fatigue, but soon they stop working, and you start increasing the amount of coffee per day. Coffee, sugar, chocolate, smoking and tea are stimulants; they give your adrenals a 'slap to wake-up'. Our adrenals can tolerate these stimulants for a while, but eventually they can get exhausted. These are the most common symptoms of adrenal exhaustion.

- Fatigue most of the day, but then in the evening you may get an unusual boost of energy.
- Difficulty in relaxing and falling asleep, despite being tired.
- Difficulty waking up and then not feeling refreshed in the morning.
- Inability to handle stress, getting 'wound up' easily.
- Tendency to tremble when under pressure.
- Craving for salty and fatty foods.
- Weak immune system and susceptibility to infections.
- Reduced sex drive.
- Lightheaded when rising from a horizontal position.
- Extreme tiredness after exercise.
- Physical problems, such as allergies, asthma, joint pains, low blood pressure, low blood sugar, low muscle tone, poor circulation, weight gain, pain in lower back and numbness in fingers and toes.

The first advice given to people with adrenal fatigue is to rest. Yes, resting is important, but we must address the root of the problem in order to remove it permanently. We must provide proper support for our adrenals and reduce the toxic load in the body. Since the majority of toxicity in our bodies comes from the gut, we must heal and seal the gut wall. In order to do that, we need to address the state of the gut flora. And we must change our diet to make sure that we nourish our adrenals properly.

Our adrenal glands are hungry organs; they need to be fed with high quality nutrition. This is particularly important for people with adrenal problems. It may sound surprising, but the most nourishing foods for our adrenals are animal foods: fresh meats, fish, eggs and fermented dairy, particularly high fat. Homemade meat stock, gelatinous meats, fresh eggs and other foods rich in collagen and phospholipids will nourish and restore the structure of your adrenal glands.

Many adrenal hormones are steroids. All steroid hormones in your body are made from cholesterol. This essential molecule is produced in the glands themselves and also comes from the bloodstream. The blood cholesterol is maintained by our liver; it has a 'factory' inside it manufacturing cholesterol, packaging it into LDL (low-density lipoprotein) and sending it into the bloodstream, to be delivered to the adrenals and other organs. The adrenals convert cholesterol into steroid hormones. So, in order for us to have a healthy adrenal function we need plenty of cholesterol.[22] Unfortunately, increasing numbers of people in the world are unable to produce enough cholesterol, because their bodies are too toxic or have nutritional deficiencies which interfere in the production of cholesterol in the liver and in the adrenals. As a result, they are not able to produce enough steroid hormones! Why is this important?

Hormone adrenalin, produced by our adrenal glands, is called the stress hormone. However, in order for us to cope with daily stress we need the *full* spectrum of adrenal hormones, not only adrenaline. In a person with low blood cholesterol the adrenals may produce plenty of adrenaline, but not enough steroid hormones! Unopposed adrenaline makes the person unable to handle stress in a calm and balanced way. These people can be short-tempered, argumentative, defensive and aggressive; they cannot handle pressure and are prone to tantrums, uncontrollable anger and nervous breakdown. Many GAPS people are in that category. Cholesterol-reducing medications (statins) can cause this situation as well, because they damage the cholesterol-producing 'factory' inside the liver, depriving the body of this essential-to-life substance.[23] As a result, blood cholesterol becomes low, and the person's body cannot produce enough steroid hormones.

Low blood cholesterol is a very serious situation in a human body and must be remedied as soon as possible! Since many GAPS people are unable to produce enough cholesterol, they must obtain it from food. That is one of the reasons why eating foods rich in cholesterol on a daily basis is very important for GAPS people! It can provide vital help for their adrenals and other cholesterol-dependent organs. I have seen many people with poor self-control and aggressive behaviour whose personality changes dramatically as soon as they start eating plenty of cholesterol-rich foods. These people become calm, pleasant and able to handle daily stress in a balanced way. You will find more information on cholesterol in other chapters of this book and in my book *Put your heart in your mouth. What really is heart disease and what can we do to prevent and even reverse it.*

Thyroid gland and adrenals work together. When one gets 'exhausted' the other usually goes the same way, and so many symptoms of low thyroid function and adrenal exhaustion overlap. There are supplements of freeze-dried animal adrenal glands and thyroid glands on the market. It is a good idea to take them together for a while to provide support for your glands. There are some herbs used for adrenal support (liquorice root, ashwagandha, maca root, Siberian ginseng, rhodiola rosea and other). But the most important treatment is changing the diet of the person. To get long-term recovery we need to work on normalising the gut flora, healing the gut and reducing the toxic load in the body.

To understand how stress affects your body, please read the chapter *Healing*.

Sex glands

Apart from adrenals, steroid hormones are produced in our gonads (ovaries in women and testes in men). Oestrogens, progesterone, testosterone, androgens and other sex hormones are produced from cholesterol. Male and female bodies both produce the full range of sex hormones. However, the balance differs in men and women and is extremely complex and finely tuned. It changes constantly in response to changes in the environment and bodily activity.

Gut flora has a very important influence on our sex hormones and current research in this area is discussed in previous chapters.[24] Toxicity coming from the gut and nutritional deficiencies interfere in the balance of sex hormones in the body and can create many symptoms. I see many GAPS children in my clinic with premature or delayed sexual development. Many GAPS youngsters have abnormal 'confused' sexual development, where they may have some male and some female characteristics in their appearance and behaviour. Many women have abnormal menstrual cycles, suffer from PMS (peri-menstrual syndrome), endometriosis, polycystic ovaries, infertility and other problems. Men can suffer from infertility, gynaecomastia (large breasts), problems with libido and various forms of sexual dysfunction. Abnormal bodily shape and confused sexual behaviour can be common in both genders.

I have no doubt that hot flushes are caused by the activity of our gut flora! Hot flushes are a major symptom of menopause in women and men. However, in my clinical experience children, young women (far too young for menopause) and men (young and old) can suffer from hot flushes. These people have abnormal gut flora, where microbes in the gut produce hormone-like substances and other chemicals which cause hot flushes and many other unpleasant hormonal symptoms (mood swings, fatigue, depression, aggressiveness and other).[25] Menopause (in women and men) is supposed to be easy and comfortable; that is how Mother Nature designed it. It is not a disease; it is a natural stage in human life. There should be no major symptoms or problems. People with damaged gut flora usually have a very uncomfortable menopause. *HRT* (*Hormone Replacement Therapy*) has been developed to help with menopausal symptoms. However, in many people it does not help, but instead causes hormone-dependent cancers (of the breast, uterus, prostate and other hormone-sensitive organs).[26] It is foolhardy to interfere with the body's hormonal balance using synthetic hormones (contraceptive pill and HRT)! Our hormonal balance is infinitely complex; we do not understand it fully yet, let alone have the knowledge to interfere in it safely. Only natural methods of correcting your gut flora and metabolism will make your menopause comfortable and symptom-free. GAPS Nutritional Protocol will do that for you.

Women are cyclical creatures: every month they go through a hormonal cycle. In the first half of the menstrual cycle oestrogens are in charge, keeping immunity strong and not allowing any opportunistic microbes to get out of hand.[27] However, in the second half of the month another hormone rules – progesterone; this hormone prepares the woman's body for pregnancy. Every month, during childbearing years, a woman's body gets ready for pregnancy, organising a soft nourishing bed in the uterus for a fertilised egg to plant itself into, and that is progesterone's job. In order not to reject the egg, progesterone suppresses immunity. As a result, opportunistic microbes in the body become active in the second half of the menstrual cycle, and the closer to menstruation the more active they become. They produce toxins and interfere in many functions of the body. PMS (peri-menstrual syndrome) is the result of their activity. These toxins cause migraine headaches and emotional instability (when a woman can be angry or aggressive one minute and then tearful and depressed), sleep problems, blood sugar and blood pressure abnormalities, muscle cramps and other symptoms.[28] It is not you 'going mad'; it is your resident microbes playing with your body.

One of these opportunistic microbes is yeast (candida). Many men and women in the modern world suffer from an overgrowth of yeast due to regular use of antibiotics and contraceptives. In women the second half of the menstrual cycle is the time when yeast activates, causing thrush in any moist and warm place. In men the thrush can be constant or recurrent. The most common places are in the groin and vagina, under breasts and in the armpits, in the mouth and throat, behind the ears and in the ear canals, on the mucous membranes of the digestive system, breathing passages and sinuses. In order to control the yeast, it is important to keep those areas of your body populated by beneficial microbes. In order to do that I recommend an old traditional procedure people used for millennia: keep a glass jar of homemade kefir in your bathroom and apply a small amount daily to all the problem areas. Kefir is the best 'cream' for the nappy area of an infant, and it is essential for children with yeast overgrowth anywhere on their bodies.[29] Kefir has a very diverse and balanced microbial community. When we apply it to our skin and mucous membranes, the microbes in kefir boost the normal flora in the area and reduce pathogenic yeast. It is best to make kefir with raw organic milk or cream. The nourishing substances in it will sooth and heal any damage on the skin or mucous membranes. In order to control the yeast in the digestive system keep eating homemade fermented foods regularly. Following the GAPS Nutritional Protocol will reduce the yeast and other opportunists long term. It is impossible to be free of them (they are normal inhabitants of our bodies), but we can bring them to proper balance with the rest of the microbial community.

A person with abnormal gut flora is primed for developing all sorts of illnesses of the reproductive organs, because these organs are very sensitive to any hormonal change in the body. Our gut flora is a very large source of hormones! The more damaged the gut flora is, the more severe are hormonal abnormalities. I have met young women in their twenties and early thirties, who had such painful and disabling menstruations that they were considering surgical removal of their womb and ovaries. I have met GAPS people with all sorts of confused sexual development and behaviour, having a profound effect on their quality of life. And I have seen recoveries from such 'incurable' illnesses as endometriosis, polycystic ovaries, infertility and sexual disfunction.

In conclusion

Our gut flora is a very important player in our hormonal balance. Various microbes in the gut flora produce nutrients, hormones, neurotransmitters, enzymes and other active substances, which interact with our endocrine system and affect its many functions. When the gut flora is abnormal this interaction goes wrong. On top of that, a plethora of industrial man-made toxicity pollutes the body of a modern human. Many of these toxins act as endocrine disrupters, interfering in the functions of our endocrine glands and the hormones they produce. Hormones are the rulers of our metabolism; they work as a team affecting every cell and every organ in the body. When their balance is upset the person develops a multitude of health problems. GAPS Nutritional Protocol will provide the foundation for healing the endocrine system and bringing our hormones back to normal balance. It is important for the person to be aware of the fact that healing their endocrine system is an important part of their recovery.

The liver and the lungs

The doctor of the future will give no medicine, but will interest his patients in the care of the human body, in diet, and in the cause and prevention of disease.

Thomas Edison

What happens to the flow of nutrients and toxins coming from our digestive system into the rest of the body? This flow separates roughly into two streams: one goes into the blood and another into the lymph.

Our blood is a water-based medium, so water-soluble nutrients and toxins get absorbed into the blood. The blood from the gut gets collected into a system of veins (called *the portal system*), which opens up into the liver. So, *your liver is the first port of call for the water-soluble substances* absorbing through your gut wall.

Lymph is a fat-based medium, so fat-soluble nutrients and toxins from the gut generally absorb into the lymph. The lymph is collected into a long duct (called the *thoracic duct*) going up along the spine and opening into the left subclavian vein. This vein takes the blood-lymph mixture into the right heart, which promptly pumps it directly into the lungs. So, *our lungs are the first port of call for the fat-soluble nutrients and toxins* coming from the digestive system.

Let us talk about these two vital organs – the liver and the lungs – in detail.

The liver

This amazing organ fulfils a myriad of functions for us: processing nutrients from the gut, manufacturing vital nutrients and active substances (such as cholesterol, enzymes, antioxidants and many more), recycling millions of active molecules (enzymes, hormones and neurotransmitters) and doing other important jobs. The liver is our major detoxification organ; it handles toxins from the gut and toxins brought in from the rest of the body, destroying them and recycling them.[1] Because of its detoxifying function many people ask if it is safe to eat the liver of animals. Liver does not accumulate toxins; not only is it safe to eat, but making it a regular part of your menu will help your body to process toxins more effectively.[2] Toxins which the liver cannot destroy are unloaded into the bile, which flushes them out into the digestive system to be removed from the body in stool. Bile is a very important substance produced by the liver. It moves slowly through bile ducts to the gall bladder, which accumulates bile and releases it into the duodenum to digest fats.

Without bile we would not be able to digest dietary fats and would develop deficiencies in fats, fat-soluble vitamins (vitamins A, D, K and E) and essential fatty acids (omega 3, 6, 7, 9). Without these substances your body cannot function well, your cell regeneration is impaired (which means that your body cannot heal or rebuild its tissues) and your immune system collapses. About 50% of the dry weight of a human body is fat and it is essential for a myriad of functions in our organs.[3] A person who lacks bile cannot digest fats, which finish up in the stool, making the stool greasy and pale in colour. At the same time the deficiency in fats creates many problems and symptoms in the body: poor immunity and susceptibility to infections, lack of energy, poor memory and cognitive ability (your brain is a very fatty organ!), endocrine problems, osteoporosis, dry skin and hair, etc. The deficiency in fat-soluble vitamins and essential fatty acids will create another list of debilitating problems. Nothing in the body can function without these substances!

Many GAPS people are in this category; they find it difficult to digest fats. As a result, they have to limit their fat consumption, otherwise they feel bilious, nauseous and unwell after a meal. People who have lost their gall bladder through surgery can also find it difficult to digest fats, because their bile has nowhere to accumulate. And people who follow the anti-fat and low-fat mainstream advice often finish up with this problem as well.[4] In order for the liver to maintain the bile flow we must consume natural fats with every meal. The fat in the food makes the capsule of the liver contract, while the bile ducts relax their walls and become wider; as a result, the bile flows easily out of the liver and the gall bladder into the duodenum. When this stimulation does not happen for a long time, the bile ducts can get blocked with bile stones.

How do we get bile stones?

Formation of bile stones is perfectly normal and goes on in all of us all the time.[4,5] If we cut a bile stone in half and look at it under the microscope, inside it we would find a clump of microbes, mineral crystals with toxic metals or other toxins, fragments of parasites and anything else the body tries to remove. When your liver is unable to destroy something dangerous (a toxin, a group of microbes or a parasite), the liver 'imprisons' it by coating it with bile and making a bile stone. Once formed, these stones are tiny and soft and pass easily through the bile ducts. When we eat a meal with a good fat content, these tiny stones get flushed into your gut and removed from the body in the stool. If a person is on a low-fat diet, there is no stimulation for the liver to contract and the stones stay too long in the bile ducts.[4,5] As a result, calcium salts accumulate in the outer parts of the stone and it becomes bigger with a rough, hard surface. This kind of stone is difficult to pass; it gets stuck in the bile ducts of the liver and blocks them. GAPS people have abnormal gut flora and a high parasitic load in the body. As a result, they can form too many stones; the liver may be unable to flush them out fast enough and the stones can grow large and hard. When enough biliary ducts are blocked with stones the bile stops flowing, so fat digestion becomes impossible.

Apart from the bile, another major digestive juice may not flow into the duodenum – pancreatic juice. In the majority of people the pancreatic duct connects with the biliary duct (forming one shared channel) before opening into the duodenum. If the biliary duct is full of stones, they can block this shared channel, impairing the flow of pancreatic juice. The pancreas in the majority of people has another duct opening into the duodenum (independently from the bile duct) called the duct of Santorini, so the pancreas has another chance to drain itself of its juice. This is a wonderful insurance Nature gave our pancreas because, if its ducts are blocked, enzymes in its own juices can damage the pancreas and cause acute or chronic pancreatitis. Pancreatic juices are essential for digestion of fats, as well as protein, carbohydrates and other elements of food. Despite having the second duct, blockage of the main pancreatic duct will reduce the flow of pancreatic juice and can cause a condition called *pancreatic insufficiency*,[6] which we will talk about later (please, see chapter *A–Z*). It is very difficult to digest food when pancreatic juices are not available!

Do you know how soap is made? Traditionally it was made by cooking fat, ash, lye or another alkaline salt together. When a person has lots of bile stones, the bile does not come into the duodenum to digest fats. As a result, undigested fats combine with alkali (produced by the pancreas) in the gut and form a kind of soap. This 'soap' is a major cause of chronic constipation; it sticks to the walls of the gut and food particles causing problems with the proper transit of food.[7] The vast majority of chronically constipated people have this problem.

Another group of people with this problem are those whose gall bladder has been removed surgically. The usual reason for this very common operation is pain caused by passing a bile stone. The pain can be severe, but by the time it starts the stone has already left the gall bladder and started its journey into the duodenum. So, in most cases there is no point in removing the gall bladder, as the stone has already gone.[8] And indeed, the majority of these operations, called cholecystectomy, find only 'sludge' in the removed gall bladder, no stones. Unfortunately, in our mainstream medicine, removal of the gall bladder has become a standard procedure for any person with pain in the 'gall bladder spot'. The gall bladder is not surplus to requirement, it is an important organ! Without it fat digestion is impaired with many serious consequences. It is best to avoid its removal by dealing with bile stones naturally. For those whose gall bladder has already been removed, I recommend the following procedure to restore normal fat digestion. Many people without gall bladders have restored their fat digestion through the GAPS Nutritional Protocol and are able to eat large amounts of fat with every meal without any problems.

What do we do to remove bile stones and restore fat digestion?

Long-term we take ***GAPS shakes*** twice a day.

> ***GAPS shake recipe:*** *Make a juice from 1 carrot + 2–3 apples (or an equal amount of pineapple) + 1 stick of celery + a small wedge of beetroot + a small piece of white or red cabbage. You can also add a little lemon and some greens. To this juice add 1–2 raw eggs (the yolk and the white) and 4–5 tablespoons of homemade raw sour cream. If sour cream has not been introduced yet, add a similar amount of raw butter or ghee, softened at room temperature, or raw coconut oil. You can also try any animal fat, such as tallow, pork fat, lamb fat, goose fat; olive oil can also be used. Blend in a blender or whisk with a handheld tool. This 'shake' is delicious and will provide you with wonderful raw nutrients, including raw fat and cholesterol. You can add your cod liver oil to this smoothie: it will disguise its taste for you very effectively. Start with small amounts of GAPS shakes, such as 1–2 tablespoons per day (1–2 teaspoons for a child). When one glass is well tolerated, gradually increase to 2 glasses per day, between meals. Drink slowly, 'chewing' every mouthful. The shakes need to be taken on an empty stomach, so first thing in the morning and the middle of the afternoon are good times. GAPS shakes have an ability to slowly soften and dissolve the hard shell of the gall stones, while providing gentle stimulation for the liver capsule to contract and push the stones out.*

While increasing the daily amount of the GAPS shakes, I recommend working slowly on introducing animal fats into your diet. Start from the amount you *can* tolerate and gradually keep increasing it. To assist in digesting fats, I recommend taking supplements of ox bile, which is usually combined with some herbs. Taking 1–2 capsules of these supplements with every meal will help you to digest fat. Once you are able to have a good amount of animal fat with every meal, you can gradually stop taking the supplement. After that I recommend continuing to drink the GAPS shakes for longer. Apart from helping to remove your gall stones and cleansing your liver, they are very tasty and make an enjoyable part of the diet.

For adults I recommend regular coffee enemas. This simple procedure has a powerful cleansing effect on the liver, removing many gall stones. Please read in detail about enemas in the chapter *Bowel Management*.

Passing a gall stone

Passing a gall stone is not pleasant; it causes pain in the gall bladder area, nausea and vomiting. However, when your body has decided to remove a gall stone it will prepare for it. Trust the process and avoid rushing to the hospital, unless you are prepared to lose your gall bladder. When the pain starts, the chances are that the stone has already left the gall bladder, so you may lose this important organ for no good reason. Not only will the liver and gall bladder be prepared properly by the body for removing a stone, but also the pancreas. Remember, that the biliary duct joins with the pancreatic duct before opening into the duodenum. Your body knows how to remove a stone without getting it stuck in the pancreatic duct (which can cause acute pancreatitis). This complication is more likely to happen during man-made interventions, such as *endoscopic retrograde cholangiopancreatography*,[9] or an alternative procedure, called 'liver flush' (when a person consumes a large amount of olive oil in a mixture with grapefruit or lemon juice). I do not recommend liver flush to GAPS people at the beginning of the protocol. A few years later, when your digestive function is much better and you really would like to try this procedure, it will be much safer for you to do so.

Here is what we need to do in order to help the stone pass quickly and with less pain. Keep warm and put a hot water bottle on your liver area. Make a hot bath with 2–3 cups of Epsom salt in it, stay in the bath for as long as it is comfortable. Try to sip on a warm solution of Epsom salt (1 tablespoon dissolved in a glass of warm water; you can sweeten it with some honey). Epsom salt relaxes the smooth muscles in the bile ducts, allowing the stone to pass more easily.[10] You can take some medication which will have the same effect (*drotaverine* or *papaverine*). Obviously, the medication has to be obtained in advance, but if you have some magnesium supplements at home you can take a double dose. Peppermint oil and peppermint tea can also be helpful. To use peppermint essential oil you can add 1–5 drops to your tea or rub the oil on the painful area of your tummy.[11]

Nausea and vomiting are common when passing a gall stone, which can make it very difficult to drink anything. In this case you can dissolve the medication or magnesium supplement under your tongue, and you can hold small mouthfuls of Epsom salt solution in your mouth for a few minutes and then spit them out. The rich capillary network in your mouth will absorb a fair amount of muscle-relaxing substances. Magnesium oil can be quite helpful, because it is applied to the skin. A coffee enema can be very helpful in this situation (if you feel strong enough to do it), as it makes the liver flush the bile out and remove the stone quicker (please read more about coffee enemas in the chapter *Bowel Management*).[12] Generally, keep calm. Even if you do nothing and just rest and keep warm, your body will remove the stone safely and effectively. And it usually doesn't take long: about 15–30 minutes (maximum 3 hours). Once the pain and nausea subside, have a good sleep for as long as your body needs. When you wake up, drink some warm water or warm meat stock. For a few days after passing a stone, eat only foods included in the first or second stages of the GAPS Introduction Diet, to allow full healing in your gall bladder and your gut. Following the GAPS Diet long term will prevent this situation from ever happening to you again.

Many people ask about *chronic hepatitis B infection*, which is readily diagnosed by our mainstream medicine, leading to lots of testing and pressure to take pharmaceutical medications (which do not cure the condition, but are suggested to 'control' it). Hepatitis B virus is quite common; a large percentage of humanity is infected with it. We do not yet know everything about this virus by any means! Many perfectly healthy people have this chronic infection, which is often found by chance. So, I recommend not worrying about this virus. The human body is a home for many viruses, most of which we haven't yet researched. Some 8-10% of our genome is of viral origin.[13] The fact that we are able to diagnose the presence of one of these viruses in the body doesn't necessarily mean that it is dangerous and needs to be attacked. Keep your body clean of man-made pollution and feed it properly, and your liver will function nicely, no matter how many different viruses may be present.

It is beyond the scope of this book to look at all liver diseases. If you ensure that your bile flows freely, then you are allowing your liver to cleanse itself on a regular basis. This will prevent many liver problems. The first sign of a congested liver is a headache, particularly migraine. A tendency for nausea is another sign. If the liver congestion lasts too long, the person can develop slight jaundice: yellow discoloration of the skin and the whites of the eyes. Drinking plenty of homemade fermented beverages can be very helpful, such as beetroot kvass, vegetable medley, other varieties of kvass and homemade kombucha. Be careful with drinking too much plain water, as natural electrolytes are important for the liver to function. Too much water dilutes electrolytes and can increase their removal from the body through the kidneys.[14] Always add raw lemon, cider vinegar, or some natural salt to the water. Coffee enemas for adults, daily consumption of GAPS 'shakes' and gradual increase of fat in the food will, over time, help your bile to flow normally. There are some herbs that can be used to assist the liver: dandelion leaves and root, chicory root, turmeric, peppermint, greater celandine, milk thistle seed and other.[15] And, of course, it is important to do your best in reducing the toxic load on your liver by avoiding alcohol and tobacco, personal care products, other man-made chemicals, radiation and electromagnetic pollution.

The lungs

Our lungs are the second most important detoxifying organ in the body (after the liver) for the water-soluble toxins. The blood, having been filtered by the liver, goes directly to your heart, which then pumps it straight to the lungs. For the fat-soluble toxins our lungs are the *first* detoxifying organ, because fat-soluble toxins generally bypass the liver and come directly to the lungs via the lymph.

The lungs are very well equipped for this function. Many toxic substances, particularly those that can be converted into gases, are eliminated through the lungs. Other toxins and pathogens are 'swallowed up' by immune cells in the lungs (macrophages and microphages) and are eliminated through the so-called *mucociliary escalator*, made up of epithelial cells lining our breathing passages.[16] These cells have tiny hairs on their surface which all point up; they push all the debris up the breathing passages to be coughed out. These are some of the normal ways for your lungs to remove toxins out of your body.

Unfortunately, in a person with abnormal gut flora these natural functions may not cope with the volume and character of toxins coming to the lungs. The damaged gut wall lets through a river of toxins and pathogens into the bloodstream and the lymph. The liver may not be able to cope with the sheer volume of toxicity, so many toxins escape back into the blood and are carried to the lungs.[17]

Lymph is the carrier of fats and fat-soluble substances, and the lungs are the first organ in the body to receive this flow of fats. Why did Mother Nature design it this way? Because the lungs require large amounts of fats, fat-soluble vitamins, cholesterol and other fat-soluble substances to function, and saturated fats are particularly important for lung health. This is what the late Mary Enig, the world expert on fats, had to say on this subject: "When it comes to our lungs, the very important phospholipid class, called lung surfactant, is a special phospholipid with 100 percent saturated fatty acids. It is called *dipalmitoyl phosphatidylcholine* (*DPPC*) and there are two saturated palmitic acid molecules attached to it. When people consume a lot of partially hydrogenated fats and oils, the trans fatty acids are put into the phospholipids, where the body normally wants to have saturated fatty acids, and the lungs may not work effectively."[18] Hydrogenated fats and oils with trans fatty acids come from cooking vegetable oils, used extensively today for cooking food. Lung surfactants (DPPC and other) are essential structural components of lung tissue. They are made out of 80-90% saturated fat, cholesterol and about 10% protein.[19] A key element of DPPC is an amino acid choline, which we get in good amounts from eating eggs and liver. Without surfactants the lungs are not able to fill with air; they can collapse. Premature babies have deficiency in pulmonary surfactants, and it used to be one of the main causes of their death until a *natural surfactant therapy* was developed. These babies are given purified surfactant from the lungs of animals, which saves their lives.[20] Not only premature babies can have deficiency in surfactants, but all people with lung disease (pneumonia, bronchitis, COPD, asthma, cystic fibrosis, cancer and other). So, in any pulmonary disease, acute or chronic, it is natural animal fats, protein and cholesterol that will provide real help. Foods rich in these nutrients are essential!

Being so dependent on fats makes the lungs vulnerable to fat-soluble toxins. Mercury, lead, aluminium and some other toxic metals, many industrial chemicals and toxins manufactured by abnormal gut flora are fat-soluble and get carried by the lymph. When the lungs have to handle too much toxicity coming from the gut, particularly toxins they have not been designed to handle, they can get damaged.[21] This can lead to any lung disease: asthma, emphysema, chronic obstructive pulmonary disease (COPD), chronic bronchitis, infections and cancer. With any chronic lung problem, first and foremost I recommend looking at the state of the person's digestive system. The gut is a powerful source of health and disease in the lungs! By treating the digestive system we can lay the ground for perfect health in the lungs, just as with elsewhere in the body.

Just like other organs in the human body, lungs have their own microbiome.[22] Research in this area is young, but some bacterial groups have been identified (largely *Proteobacteria, Firmicutes, and Bacteroides*). Apart from bacteria there are many other members of the microbial community in the lungs of a healthy person, such as fungi (particularly *Pneumocystis* genus), archaea and other creatures.[23] This normal lung flora plays an important role in the health of this organ, and its composition changes when a disease develops. There is no doubt that the activity of the lung microbiome plays a vital role in every lung disease.

Let us have a look at one of the most common lung diseases – asthma.

Asthma

Asthma is a GAPS condition. It develops because of abnormal gut flora and a damaged gut wall, which lets toxins through for the lungs to deal with.[24] At the same time, the immune system is out of balance, creating atopy (which we have discussed in the chapter *Immune System*). The first asthma attack usually happens in childhood, though it can happen at any time in our lives after we damage our gut flora. The majority of people develop their first asthma attack after eating ice cream or a similar high-fat processed substance.[25] The fats in ice cream will carry fat-soluble toxins (chemicals added to the ice cream) directly into the lymph and to the lungs. On top of that, sugar in the ice cream will feed the pathogenic flora in the gut and get converted into toxins, many of which will also be carried to the lungs. The immune system is likely to attach its own cells and complexes to the toxins, ready to start inflammation or an allergic response.[26]

As these toxins and immune complexes get into the lungs, they inflict damage to the lung tissue and bronchi. Mother Nature has created a good method for dealing with such a situation, called *bronchospasm*. During bronchospasm the smooth muscles in the bronchial walls contract and close up the damaged part of the breathing passages, so it can be repaired.[27] The repair process usually takes from a few minutes to quarter of an hour, and once the damage is repaired, the bronchus opens up again. This experience can feel alarming as you get short of breath and start wheezing. However, it does not last long, and at the end of it your lungs are as good as new. Natural bronchospasm is not dangerous, particularly in childhood, because the body keeps enough lung tissue open to compensate for the closed part. So, it is important to keep calm and still, and allow the body to do its work.

Bronchospasm is essential. Imagine that a big accident on a motorway has damaged the road surface. In order to repair the motorway it has to be closed, so the builders can do the work. The same thing happens in the lungs: the damaged part of the lung gets closed up by bronchospasm, so the body can repair it. This process has worked perfectly well for us for millions of years until anti-asthma medications were invented. These drugs stop the bronchospasm: they do not allow the bronchial motorway to close up. Imagine builders trying to repair a motorway while lorries and cars are going past them at 70 miles per hour? They cannot do it! The same thing happens in the lungs when anti-asthma medication is used: the body cannot heal and repair the damaged airway.[28]

Asthma is the most common long-term medical condition amongst children in the world.[29] How do children develop asthma? Here is the typical scenario: a child gets its first bronchospasm, usually in the second year of life and very often after eating an ice cream (or something similar, full of sugar, fats and chemicals), which is rapidly converted into a toxic flood coming from the gut to the lungs. The child gets short of breath and starts wheezing. The parents call an ambulance and rush to the hospital. A diagnosis of asthma is made and the child is prescribed an inhaler with an anti-asthmatic medication designed to stop the bronchospasm. As a result of using this medication, the child's damaged airway is left unrepaired after an asthma attack. In a few days the child eats another ice cream and another part of his bronchial tree gets damaged the same way. The body knows that the previous part of the lung is damaged, so it uses bronchospasm to try and repair both parts of the lung at the same time. Anti-asthma medication is used again, and the child finishes up with two parts of the lungs damaged and unrepaired. With the next asthma episode three parts of the lungs will be closed up by bronchospasm, making that episode more severe than the previous one and, if medication is used again, they do not get repaired. From episode to episode the child finishes up with more and more of his lungs damaged, and not repaired. This process continues until enough of the lung closes up with the next asthma attack to make it life-threatening. In old medical books asthma was always described as a benign and self-limiting condition; it did not require any treatment and doctors never saw deaths from asthma. Today asthma has become a deadly disease and we have to thank the wide use of anti-asthmatic medications for that.[28]

What should the parents do when their small child gets the first wheeze?

When your child gets his first asthma attack, don't rush him to the hospital! Instead wrap him up in a blanket and sit him on your lap. Keep him warm, keep him calm, make him feel safe and give him some hot water or mild camomile tea using a teaspoon. The crisis will pass in minutes; and you will watch your child happily playing again as if nothing has ever happened. But most importantly, your child's lungs will feel as if nothing has happened, because they were allowed to heal the damage and bring themselves back to normal.

Make a note of what has triggered this asthma attack and avoid it. Often it is something sugary, fatty and processed (such as an ice cream), that pathogens in the gut can quickly convert into a toxic flood to absorb through the child's damaged gut wall. In the long run you need to concentrate on healing the child's digestive system: healing and sealing the gut lining and normalising the gut flora. As the toxicity in the body drops, the liver and lungs will do their jobs properly, without the lungs having to initiate bronchospasm anymore.

What about a child who has had asthma for a while and is taking medication for it?

Don't stop the medication. Start working on healing the child's digestive system using the GAPS Nutritional Protocol. As the gut starts healing, you will observe that your child's asthma attacks become less frequent and milder. At this stage start reducing the dose of the medication gradually, and with mild attacks try not to use it at all. As the gut heals, the asthma attacks will stop and there will be no need for the medication anymore.

What about adults with chronic asthma who have been taking medication for many years?

It may take them longer to recover than it would a child. It is important not to stop medication abruptly, because asthma in adults can be a deadly disease. Start working on healing your gut and changing your gut flora first, without changing your medication. As the flow of toxins from the gut to the lungs reduces, you will find that you need to use less and less medication with your asthma attacks, and with milder attacks you can skip it altogether. Gradually and slowly you will be able to remove medication completely, but it is important not to force this process and listen to your body.

In my clinical experience asthma is quite easy to treat with the GAPS Nutritional Protocol. Apart from asthma, people with this condition often have many other health problems: digestive symptoms, allergies, learning disabilities, mental illness, autoimmune disease and hormonal problems. While we are working on those other conditions, asthma very often quietly disappears.

Conclusion: our bodies are beautifully designed! The liver and the lungs guard the body from anything harmful that can come through the gut. At the same time, these organs take first pick of the nutrients coming from the digestive system. Why? Because the liver and lungs work very hard and require high-quality nutrition. A GAPS person does not digest or absorb food well and develops multiple nutritional deficiencies. This situation puts the liver and the lungs in peril, making them weak and unable to fulfil their functions optimally. These organs are part of a very important system in the human body, called the detoxification system. This system cleans our bodies all the time, dealing with by-products of our own metabolism and toxicity coming from outside. When the liver and the lungs are overwhelmed by toxins coming from the unhealthy gut, our detoxification system doesn't work very well, it can even break down. When this happens, the body starts accumulating toxins. As a result of accumulating toxicity we have another problem developing in the Western world – parasite infestations. Let's have a look at it.

Toxins and parasites

In Nature there are neither rewards nor punishments; there are consequences.

Robert Green Ingersoll

Toxicity and parasites always come together, hand in hand. The more industrialised we humans become, the more toxins we accumulate in our bodies. To date, more than 100,000 new chemicals have been invented by humanity, chemicals which do not exist in Nature.[1] Our food is laced with agricultural poisons and chemicals added by the food industry. The air we breathe, the water we drink, the medications we take, the clothes we wear, the buildings we live in, the technologies we use all pollute our bodies and create a toxic load, which we have to live with.

The mother's body unloads toxins into the child during pregnancy.[2] Our children then live and grow up in a world full of man-made toxicity, the level of which is increasing every year. Children born with a high toxic load have a compromised constitution; they are not fit to survive an ever-increasing list of commercial vaccinations, processed and GMO foods, bottle feeding, medications, pollution and other toxic influences without further damage. In the industrialised modern world generations of people have been born with an ever-increasing toxic load. They have grown up with more toxicity, coming from the environment. Every year the level of toxicity accumulating in human bodies grows, providing one explanation for the constant increase in health problems worldwide.[3]

So, what are we to do with this situation? How do we clean a contaminated body, let alone heal it? Well, it is Mother Nature who does the cleaning and the healing because our bodies are part of Nature. We need to watch how she does it and actively assist this process.

Next time you come across a piece of soil contaminated with industrial chemicals, pay attention. When industry moves away and the soil is left alone, how does Mother Nature clean it and heal it? First and foremost, moulds and lichens will develop on that soil – members of the fungi family. Why? Because fungi are well equipped to absorb and neutralise toxins; cleaning up dirty places is their mission in Nature.[4] It may take a few years for this family to do its job, and once the place is clean enough plants will join the fungi: stinging nettles, dandelions, thistles, docks and other so-called weeds. These are plants which can grow on a very malnourished poor-quality soil, with a fair amount of toxins remaining in it. The plants and fungi will attract animals, insects and microbes, which will enrich the soil and put some life into it. After a few years of the weeds, the insects, the microbes and the animals enriching the soil and cleaning it up, other plants may be able to grow there – plants which require better-quality soil. And so it continues for quite a few years until that patch of industrially damaged soil heals and recovers fully. It becomes what a healthy soil is supposed to be – a rich community of microbes, worms, insects and other creatures living in a medium of organic matter and minerals, a soil which is able to sustain life. Only when this process is complete can trees, bushes, vegetables and fruit start growing on this soil.

Something very similar happens in the human body contaminated with man-made chemicals. It is inevitable that this person will have systemic fungal overgrowth: moulds, lichens and candida will grow in order to clean this body up! Every baby born with a heavy toxic load has fungal overgrowth. Every child or adult, whose body is contaminated with toxins, has fungal overgrowth: in their digestive system, on mucous membranes, in the inner organs, on the skin and everywhere else in the body. Unfortunately, while doing the cleaning job, fungi produce by-products of their own metabolism, causing symptoms. The child or the adult affected will have a 'foggy' brain, lack of energy and stamina, lethargy and hundreds of different unpleasant symptoms in every organ and system: eczema, asthma, allergies, autoimmune disease, pains and aches in muscles, bones and joints, digestive symptoms, restless legs, etc. – a so-called 'candida' syndrome.

Attacking fungi with antifungal medication or natural antifungal substances often proves to be counterproductive, because the toxins which these fungi are holding are released back into the body. This can make the person even more unwell.[5] As we discussed in previous chapters, the relationship between fungi and toxins is documented with mercury: candida inside your body absorbs mercury and holds it. As a result, your body is protected from mercury to a degree. So, your organism has to make a choice between toxic effects from fungi and mercury poisoning. Mercury is much more toxic than fungi, so the body decides that it is less damaging to have a fungal overgrowth. If you attack candida, without making sure that mercury is removed at the same time, this very toxic metal gets released back into your system and can make you even more ill. Apart from mercury, many other toxins are handled by fungi in our bodies: other toxic metals, petrochemicals, agricultural chemicals, solvents, plasticisers, etc.

When you stop attacking candida it will promptly grow back! Why? Because your own body will invite it back! When the body doesn't have good tools for dealing with a particular chemical, it will delegate this job to another living creature. Make no mistake: your body knows which fungus, worm, fluke, protozoa, virus, bacterium or other life form can eat and neutralise a particular chemical. Depending on the mixture of toxicity you have accumulated, your body will 'invite' a particular mixture of living creatures to handle those chemicals.[6] Some of them may come from outside, but some may arise from inside – from your own microbiome. These living creatures will neutralise the chemicals and absorb them into their own bodies. And once that job is done, your body will escort those guests out (with thanks!). They will leave and take away the toxins that were making you ill, so your body can get on with healing the damage. This can only happen if your exposure to those chemicals has stopped. But, if the chemicals are constantly coming into your body, then the 'job' can never be done, and those living creatures can never leave your body. You get a chronic infestation, and that is when we start calling these creatures 'parasites'. 'Parasite' is probably not the right name for this community of life forms. 'The cleaning company' is probably a more appropriate name.

Fungi, such as candida, received the name 'parasite' a long time ago, despite the fact that a healthy body is full of them. All worms ever found in the human body have been called 'parasites'. Yet we now know that they are essential for keeping our immune system healthy and well balanced. We even have a new form of therapy today, called *the helminth therapy*, where specific worms are deliberately introduced into the body.[7] This therapy can produce surprisingly good results.

Instead of attacking fungi and other 'parasites', it is best to try and add more microbes to the system in order to assist and speed up the cleaning of your body. This is what we do in the GAPS Nutritional Protocol. We eat fermented foods, which are teaming with beneficial fungi, bacteria and other microbes. One of the best remedies for fungal overgrowth anywhere in the body is kefir. Kefir grains are a natural balanced community of various microbes: fungi, bacteria, viruses and more, living in their own biofilm. Kombucha scoby is another natural community of microbes. Homemade kefir and kombucha are wonderful sources of a large group of beneficial fungi. Regular consumption of kefir and fermented vegetables and beverages will speed up the fungal stage of cleaning, which your body *has* to go through. On top of that, various microbes which live in fermented foods will eat pathogenic microbes in your body and reduce their load. Remember that the human body is full of microbes (and other living creatures). We cannot get rid of them! The sensible thing to do is to replace the pathogenic creatures with beneficial ones and increase their diversity. And the rule is: the more the merrier!

But let us come back to how the human body cleanses itself by using living creatures. As the fungal stage of cleansing goes on, other creatures populate the human body as well: creatures which feed on fungi and toxins. Various bacteria, protozoa, viruses, worms and other smaller and larger life forms, which we call 'parasites', proliferate in the digestive system and everywhere else in the body. They are an essential part of the 'cleaning' process, just like the fungi. The more chemically contaminated the human body is, the more 'parasites' it will have. One of these situations is Lyme disease, which is reaching epidemic proportions in the world.

Lyme disease

The vast majority of people affected have a so-called *chronic* Lyme disease, where the person does not remember being bitten by a tick and is suffering from a long list of chronic symptoms. Testing for this disorder is unreliable and there is no mainstream treatment worth considering. Chronic Lyme disease is a classic example of a chemically contaminated body which is going through the natural process of 'cleaning up', involving many microbes and other life forms. Scientists are looking at glyphosate (the chemical in the common herbicide *Roundup*) as one of the major causative chemicals in Lyme disease.[8] This toxic chemical is very widely used by our industrial agriculture. It is in all our food (including many organically produced foods) and its increasing use is perfectly correlated with epidemics of Lyme disease and other chronic illnesses in the world. The most contaminated population in the world is likely to be in North America, where glyphosate is particularly widely used, and where the numbers of people suffering from chronic Lyme disease are the highest.[9] This is just one chemical; there are thousands of others, plus electromagnetic pollution, GMO 'food' and other abominations that we humans are creating on our planet at an increasing rate.

People who have been bitten by a tick and have developed a classic *acute* Lyme disease are treated with antibiotics. This treatment works for a proportion of these people, but in many the disease becomes chronic despite the aggressive antibiotic treatment. The more we research Lyme disease, the more we realise that it is not just *Borrelia burgdorferi* that is the cause of the disease, but a plethora of various microbes living as a community in the body of the person.[10] This community can include candida and other fungi, bartonella, babesia, ehrlichia, anaplasma, micoplasma, tularaemia, rickettsia, viruses, protozoa, worms and other creatures. The symptoms of chronic Lyme disease are caused by all of these creatures, and now a new name is being given to this situation – *MSIDS (Multiple Systemic Infectious Diseases Syndrome)*.[11] That is why, in many cases, attacking borrelia with long-term antibiotics does very little to heal the person. In fact, it adds another pollutant to the body, which encourages more 'parasites'. The person's body has to be 'decontaminated' in order to start removing the parasitic load. Only natural methods of treatment work in this situation: nourishing your body properly (so it is able to clean itself), restoring your gut flora and your immune system, herbs, supplements and other natural approaches. Please, look in the chapter A–Z for more information on Lyme disease.

Mother Nature does not do anything fast, because it does things *properly*! The process of cleansing and removing parasites can take many years and requires full co-operation and active assistance from the person, which in turn requires proper information. The person has to stop polluting his or her body, eat a correct diet and take active steps in cleansing. If we don't do that, then the body will invite all sorts of living creatures to do these jobs for it.

Cancer

When a clump of toxicity has accumulated in a particular area of the body, the 'parasites' attracted to that toxin can settle in that area for a long time, particularly if the toxin keeps coming in. When we, humans, move to a new place, what do we do? We build a home to live in, and we look for various resources we may need. The parasite does the same thing: it makes a home for itself by building a nest. The body builds a thick protein capsule around this nest to protect it from the immune system. The protein it uses is native to your body, so the immune system cannot 'see' the nest. Then the parasite builds an extensive network of blood vessels around the nest to provide itself with food and other resources, and your body cooperates with this process fully. Your cells in that area are already weakened by the accumulation of toxicity, they cannot protect themselves from the parasite. So, this creature uses these cells as building material for the nest, mutates them, adds its own genetics to them, changes their structure and makes them work for itself. What are we talking about? We are talking about tumours, which can be benign or malignant. It has been observed many times by researchers and medics that cancers are inhabited by parasites: viruses, fungi, bacteria, protozoa, flukes and worms.[12] A tumour can be seen as a parasitic nest.[13] We don't know if these creatures cause the cancer, but they take part in the whole process, which begins from accumulation of carcinogenic chemicals, radiation, pollution and other toxic products of human activity. Remember, microbes exchange genetics between one another and they can do it with our human cells too. Cancer cells are hybrids, partly human and partly belonging to the parasites.[14] That is why they don't work and are rejected by the body. These mutant microbial/human cells proliferate and multiply as microbes do – very fast – and that is how a typical cancer grows.

With every generation these cells mutate more, becoming less and less human and more microbial.[15]

I believe that a parasite does not invade a human body without the body's permission. We are not helpless victims of parasites; our bodies are well equipped to deal with them! The human body has evolved on this planet together with all the creatures we call parasites. They are everywhere, contact with them is absolutely unavoidable! We all have them, and we have co-existed with them perfectly happily for millions of years. So what happened? We created an environment which pollutes our bodies on an unprecedented scale. Do we really believe that we can pollute and damage our environment and remain 'clean' ourselves? To deal with this pollution our bodies need the help of other creatures. It appears that, whatever the main 'parasite' may be in the tumour, there is always at least one other parasite present – yeast, candida or another fungal species. This is logical: fungi are universal cleaners in Nature, they are always present in 'dirty' places. The inevitable presence of fungi in any toxic place in the body can change the energy production in the cells. Instead of the normal process of using glucose, fat or protein for producing energy, your cells start fermenting glucose, producing alcohol, lactic acid and other unhealthy by-products. In oncology this is called the *Warburg's effect*: cancer cells use anaerobic fermentation, which is abnormal for healthy human cells, but is the normal way for fungi to produce energy.[16]

Future research may discover that every tumour is populated not by one or two, but by a large variety of living life forms – parasites. It is a fact that surgery is a major cause of metastasising (spreading) cancer to other parts of the body. If cancer is a parasitic nest, then it is obvious that cutting it open will allow eggs and larvae into the bloodstream to be spread around. That is why the majority of surgical procedures in oncology are followed by radiation or chemotherapy in the hope of stopping this process. Unfortunately, these methods destroy the person's immune system and detoxification system, so the body is no longer able to deal with the situation in a natural way. It is beyond the scope of this book to continue talking about cancer. All we need to understand is that none of it can happen if the person has a strong detoxification system and a powerful immune system. They will not allow the body to get polluted in the first place, so the body will not need to invite other living creatures to deal with the pollution. And whatever creatures already live in our bodies will be kept in a healthy balance, so they bring us only benefits. Please read more on the subject of cancer in the chapter *GAPS Ketogenic Diet*.

The official definition of a parasite states: a parasite is an organism which lives in or on another organism (its host) and benefits by deriving nutrients at the other's expense. Based on this definition, can our gut flora and the rest of the human microbiome be viewed as a parasite living inside us? The official definition of a parasite is based on the long-held proposition that this world is ruled by the 'survival of the fittest'; that everything in this world is eating and destroying each other and 'only the strongest survive'. But there is another position, which considers the world to exist on *co-operation*, where every living thing is creating an environment, a habitat and a source of food for everything else around. If you observe healthy natural environments, which still exist on our beautiful planet, you will see that they are healthy and thriving due to the co-operation of all the forms of life in that habitat: microbes, soil community, plants, insects, animals and other. For example, herds of zebra in Africa graze peacefully next to a family of lions. Both the zebra and the lions live in one habitat – the vast African grassland. Recent research has established that lions and other predators are a necessary part of the grasslands' ecosystem; they keep herbivorous animals in tight herds and keep them moving across the savannah.[17] This ensures proper maintenance of grasslands and the health and survival of the whole ecosystem. Without the lions, zebra will quickly destroy the grassland. Predators are 'shepherds' of herbivorous animals in Nature! Without them the grasslands deteriorate rapidly, leaving both zebra and the lions without a habitat. This co-existence of zebra, lions and grasslands in the wild is not survival of the fittest but intelligent co-operation! The theory of 'survival of the fittest' is based on a lack of understanding of the *full picture*. But, unfortunately, it prevails in our natural sciences and modern medicine: as soon as we find a microbe or another creature around us or inside us, we want to kill it, without a second thought. This attitude has created many problems for our planet and humanity, one of which is an epidemic of abnormal gut flora.

Western medicine is woefully inadequate in its ability to identify or deal with parasites. Parasitology – the science of studying parasites – is a 'Cinderella science' receiving very little funding or attention. The typical mainstream testing of stool for parasites is mostly a waste of time. Generally speaking, it is not a good idea to rely on a mainstream doctor to deal with parasites. Alternative medicine may offer some better ways of testing for parasites and dealing with them, but there is hardly any research in this area and the results can also be disappointing.

When we try to handle parasites, it is essential to deal with both the pollution and the creatures themselves! But, most importantly, we must equip the body with full resources to deal with the situation on its own. Remember, it is your own body that has to cleanse and heal itself! Anything we do from outside can only provide assistance. Following the GAPS Nutritional Protocol will provide your body with the necessary resources to deal with the pollutants and the parasites effectively. To this foundation you can add other treatments (herbs, sauna, homeopathy, essential oils and many other), which will help your body to clear the toxicity and the parasites associated with it.

Conclusion: We have a growing incidence of parasitic infestations in the industrialised world. The reason for this epidemic is industrial contamination of the planet and our bodies; contamination which we, humans, have created and continue creating at an increasing rate. I believe that microbes, worms and other 'parasites' play the role of cleansers in Nature; they are well equipped to absorb and neutralise various toxins. If your body is unable to handle the toxicity on its own, it will 'invite' those creatures to deal with the contamination. The only way for us to be free from parasites is to decontaminate our bodies and reduce our exposure to industrial toxicity as much as possible. To do that effectively we must change our environment! In order for the human body to handle toxicity on its own, without the help of other creatures, it is essential for us to look after its immune system and detoxification system.

Our bodies are part of Nature; we are just one form of life in this amazing ecosystem of trillions of life forms living on one beautiful planet. All life forms on the planet depend on each other and affect each other, and we humans are no exception. One comes to the conclusion that humanity has to learn a hard lesson! And, until that lesson is learned, increasing numbers of people all over the world will suffer from a large toxic load and large numbers of 'parasites', which always come with those toxins.

GAPS Nutritional Protocol will allow your body to maintain a powerful detoxification system to keep itself clean. It will feed and maintain a strong immune system to ward off microbes and parasites, and to keep them in balance. This protocol can be used as a very effective prophylactic measure to protect yourself and your family from the contamination and parasites which are becoming more prevalent in our modern world. People with parasitic infestations should use this protocol as a baseline treatment to give their body the best chance to decontaminate itself and remove parasites. In many people just following the GAPS Protocol is enough to deal with the problem. Some people need to add other modalities to this baseline, such as homeopathy, herbs, chelation of toxic metals, natural detox treatments and other. Please, read more about parasites and how to deal with them in the chapter A–Z.

Bones and teeth

The part can never be well unless the whole is well.

Plato

Nutrition is the most important basis for the health of our teeth and bones! The majority of GAPS people have dental problems and osteoporosis. Let us see why.

The teeth have a similar structure to the bones in our bodies. Under the microscope all bones can be described as 'bookshelves': the 'shelving' is made out of protein, mainly collagen, while the minerals (calcium, magnesium, boron and other) are the 'books', filling the 'shelves'. Bone loss and dental decay are usually not due to the lack of books, but to the lack of shelving! Modern diet, full of processed foods, does not provide nutrients for building strong 'shelving' in the bones and teeth. When the shelves are broken and weak, the books have nowhere to stand, so calcium and other minerals just get washed out from the bones and teeth. There is no point providing more minerals for a person with osteoporosis or tooth decay! We must build the shelving first by providing the body with building materials to produce lots of collagen.[1]

Collagen is a protein; it is made from amino acids, which come into the body when we eat meat, fish, eggs and dairy. Plant foods are unable to provide us with enough amino acids suitable for building collagen (read more about this in the chapter *Vegetarianism*). It is particularly nourishing for our bones and teeth to eat foods rich in animal collagen: ligaments, skin and joints of animals, chicken feet and skin, skin of fish, well-cooked offcuts and fascia and other collagen-rich tissues. When we boil these tissues in water we create a stock which is very rich in collagen-forming amino acids (meat stock). Drinking this stock and making soups and stews with it will provide your body with a very good amount of nourishment for your bones and teeth. Another important nutrient for forming collagen in the body is vitamin C. Scurvy – vitamin C deficiency – presents with symptoms of severe collagen deficiency: bleeding gums and easy bruising (blood vessels are made from collagen to a large degree) and teeth falling out (ligaments, which hold your teeth in place, are made from collagen). Liver is a good source of vitamin C, as well as many other nutrients which will provide your bones and teeth with excellent nourishment. Fermented and fresh vegetables and fruit also provide vitamin C for us.

Nothing is static in the human body; every tissue is constantly renewed. It is known that the human skeleton completely renews itself every 10 years: the old bone tissue is broken down and removed, and new tissue is created in its place. Not only do they get renewed all the time, but the bones and teeth also change their shape and form, depending on our age and lifestyle. As we grow, produce children, work and grow older, the shape of our skeleton changes substantially to adjust to new stages in our lives; this process is called bone remodelling.[2]

What builds and maintains the structure of our bones and teeth? What is responsible for the bone turnover and remodelling? There are two groups of cells in bone tissue, called osteoblasts and osteoclasts. They fulfil these complex functions for us. *Osteoblasts* are the builders of the bone (in the teeth their equivalent is called *odontoblasts*). They are the creators: they build those 'bookshelves' and fill them with 'books', they maintain the structure and function of the whole 'library'. They are central to the bone tissue, and every cell has long 'arms', which 'hold hands' with the adjacent cells, forming an amazing lattice structure of bone. Every cell is communicating information and passing nutrients to all the other cells and surrounding tissues. *Osteoclasts* are the destroyers of the bone; they produce substances which dissolve the bone structure and dismantle it, allowing the new bone to take its place. The balance between the activity of osteoclasts and osteoblasts is maintained very carefully by the body. Availability of the right nutrients, brain activity, our immune system, hormones, neurotransmitters and a multitude of other factors are involved in bone metabolism and structure.[3]

Both groups of cells are born, do their work and then die: osteoclasts live about two weeks, while osteoblasts live about three months. Newly born osteoclasts and osteoblasts replace the dead ones. This is a wonderful process of cell regeneration that all the cells in our bodies go through. Here we come to an interesting point: these cells are born in the bone marrow. Our bone marrow is the maternity unit for many cells in the body: practically all our blood cells, immune cells, endothelial cells, fibroblasts, stem cells and many other are born in the bone marrow. It has two parts to it: red bone marrow and yellow bone marrow or stroma; and it is in the stroma that osteoclasts and osteoblasts are produced. The stroma of the bone marrow is a very high-fat organ, which requires ample supplies of animal fats and fat-soluble vitamins to function well. Research has accumulated a lot of evidence that without fat-soluble vitamins (D, A, E and K2), as well as animal fats, we cannot build the bone mass in our bodies.[3,4] The three fat-soluble vitamins (A, D and K2) work as a team in depositing calcium, phosphorus and other minerals in the bone and tooth structure: vitamins A and D make sure that the right proteins are produced by the body, while vitamin K2 activates them.[4] The cells, which build and maintain our bones, come from the bone marrow which requires these nutrients. These nutrients are essential for all cell regeneration in the body! Your body cannot give birth to any cell without animal protein, animal fat and fat-soluble vitamins.[5] So, in order to treat osteoporosis and tooth decay, as well as other forms of bone loss in the body, it is essential to consume good quality high-fat meat, fish, eggs and dairy. These foods will provide all the necessary building materials for making collagen, producing osteoclasts and osteoblasts and building strong bones and teeth.

Your teeth constantly heal and rebuild themselves. When we chew acidic foods and brush our teeth, the enamel of the teeth loses minerals. But between meals and during sleep the enamel gets remineralised by saliva and the microbial community of the mouth. If the person is not eating well, remineralisation may not be able to keep up with the loss of minerals, and patches of weak enamel form. These patches of low mineral content in the enamel of the tooth are called *caries incipiens*.[6,7] Our mainstream dentists are trained to drill these patches out and fill the resulting cavity with synthetic materials, which leads to a lifetime of drilling and filling. Holistic (biological) dentistry recommends not doing that, because the body can heal these patches of demineralised enamel. All we have to do is change our diet, making sure to consume enough good quality protein, fat and fat-soluble vitamins.[7]

The fact that teeth can be healed is not new. Weston A. Price in the early twentieth century demonstrated that tooth cavities can be healed through supplementation of vitamins A, D and a K2 in the form of cod liver oil and high-vitamin butter oil.[8] He described the case of a 14-year-old girl who healed 42 open cavities in 24 teeth after seven months of supplementation. His research has been repeated in the following decades with the same positive results. Unfortunately, our mainstream dentistry is not informed about this research. So, when decay begins in your tooth, don't rush to damage it irreversibly by drilling-and-filling, but instead try to heal this damage by changing your diet and taking appropriate supplements.

Processed 'foods' do not provide building materials for the bones and teeth. On the contrary, many processed foods are known to destroy the bone and tooth structure. Soft drinks (pops), which contain phosphoric acid and other acids are particularly known for that. A lot of tooth decay and bone loss in our young people is due to consumption of these drinks.[9] Processed carbohydrates (things made from flour, sugar, soya and vegetable oils) drain nutrients from the body and create an environment for accelerated bone loss and tooth decay. All processed foods damage our bone health, as well as the health of the rest of the body.

Osteoporosis, or thinning of the bone structure, is very common in the Western world among people of all ages, from small children and teenagers to young adults and older people.[10] This is not normal! Only a short time ago (30 years or so) this condition used to occur only in elderly women (because oestrogens are necessary for maintaining the bone mass in women and oestrogen levels decline after menopause). Breaking a wrist by slipping and falling on an outstretched hand used to be called 'the trauma of menopausal women', because it is a symptom of osteoporosis. The vast majority of patients who suffered this trauma were, indeed, women of older age. Today this trauma is common amongst young men and women, as well as children, which shows that a large proportion of our young population has osteoporosis! A healthy bone has elasticity, it has an ability to bend slightly and absorb the shock of any trauma. In a healthy person it would take a very strong force to break a bone. Slipping on a wet floor and falling on your outstretched hand should not provide a force strong enough to break the bones in your wrist, unless you have osteoporosis. In people with osteoporosis bones become brittle and prone to breaking by fairly minor forces. Osteoporosis is due to lack of protein (collagen) in the bones. In order to prevent osteoporosis and to treat it we need to eat collagen-rich foods on a daily basis (animal foods), fat-soluble vitamins and foods rich in vitamin C (liver and fermented, as well as fresh, vegetables and fruit).[11]

When collagen is in poor supply, the person is prone to developing another common problem: *periodontal disease*. Our teeth are not fixed solidly to our jaws, instead they are loosely fitted into the surrounding tissues (called *periodontium*). Every tooth has ligaments (called *Sharpey's fibres*) which anchor the tooth firmly in the surrounding tissues, while giving it the ability to slide and spring slightly when we chew food.[12] It is important for teeth to have this flexibility, because it allows us to chew hard foods without breaking our teeth. These ligaments are made from collagen and get loose or destroyed when a person is not getting proper nutrition to produce collagen. On top of that many GAPS people develop a collagen disorder, when their collagen gets damaged by inflammation and autoimmunity. As a result, the tooth is not fixed well to the surrounding tissue anymore, it becomes loose and can even fall out. In the Western world some 70–80 percent of adults suffer from periodontal disease and, apparently, the numbers are growing. *Receding gums* are part of the same problem.[12]

An opposite condition to osteoporosis is *osteomalacia* (*rickets* in children), where the 'shelving' in the bone structure may be there, but the 'books' are missing: not enough calcium settles in the bones to give them the necessary rigidity. As a result, the bones become soft and can bend. In order for calcium and other minerals to settle in the bones we need vitamin D – the sunshine vitamin.[13] The first sign of rickets in a small child is reluctance to start walking. Normally babies start walking around the age of one year. If your baby is older than that and is reluctant to start walking, make sure to expose your baby to sunlight as much as possible in order to provide vitamin D. A few days of sunbathing will fix the problem and your baby will walk. There should be no clothes on the baby when sunbathing. If it is not possible to sunbathe, start supplementing cod liver oil and ask your doctor for a vitamin D supplement. Vitamin K2 is also essential for bone mineralisation.[14] It comes from high-fat animal foods and fermented foods; high-fat cheese is a good source of this vitamin in the Western world, while fermented soy products are a good source in the East (natto in particular). Breastfed babies receive this vitamin from the mother's milk, if the mother is not deficient in fat-soluble vitamins. Bottle-fed babies may be deficient in this vitamin, so steps need to be taken to provide it. Supplementing good quality cod liver oil (vitamins A and D) and butter oil (vitamin K2) is the best policy.[15]

A growing percentage of children in the Western world have *crowded teeth*, because of nutritional deficiencies they suffered during pregnancy.[15] If a pregnant woman does not get enough fat-soluble vitamins (A, D, K1, K2 and E), animal fats and animal protein (from meats, liver, fish, eggs and dairy), while eating lots of bread and other processed carbohydrates, her child will be born with small jaws, which do not have enough room to accommodate growing teeth.[16] Not only does dental health suffer, but some children finish up with narrow (sometimes even closed up) nasal passages, causing mouth breathing and chronic sinus infections. These children end up having operations, dental treatments and wearing braces on their teeth. Braces have become a common feature in modern children, which is very sad. These children have abnormally small jaws and their teeth don't have enough room to grow. Unfortunately, the standard treatment is to remove some teeth and put a brace on the jaw to squash it and make it even smaller. Due to this practice, used by mainstream dentistry for a few decades now, we see many people today (young and middle aged) with very narrow faces and small jaws. Holistic dentists are working on a new approach to this problem in children: they try to widen the jaw surgically to give the growing teeth room.[16] These children finish up with more attractive faces and a nicer smile – the way they were supposed to be born. Unfortunately, this operation is not possible in all children.

Weston A. Price was the first dentist to demonstrate that maternal diet during pregnancy is the reason for narrow faces and small jaws (with overcrowded teeth).[15] Many women nowadays follow a very deficient diet during pregnancy, which does not provide enough building materials for the child's body to form bones properly. Recently the situation has become even worse because of erroneous mainstream advice given to pregnant women to avoid foods rich in vitamin A. The reason for this is that processed foods are widely fortified with synthetic vitamin A, which has caused an excess of this chemical in the Western population. Synthetic vitamin A, particularly in excess, can cause damage to the foetus (as well as many other health problems in people). As usual, instead of advising pregnant women to stop eating processed foods, our mainstream medicine tells them not to eat natural foods rich in vitamin A, liver in particular.[17]

Liver provides *natural* vitamin A (which cannot be compared to the synthetic one) in combination with other fat-soluble vitamins, the full spectrum of B vitamins, vitamin C, protein and many other nutrients, all of which are absolutely essential for a growing foetus.[18] Eating liver on a daily basis used to be the duty of all pregnant women in most traditional cultures around the world! People knew, through experience, that eating liver would make sure that her baby was born beautiful and healthy. Today doctors tell pregnant women to avoid eating liver, while allowing them to consume plenty of synthetic vitamin A in processed foods. This misguided advice will result in new generations of children in the Western world with even more narrow faces and jaws, crowded teeth and dental braces, narrow nasal passages, mouth breathing and plenty of suffering as a result. Apart from the facial bones, other bones in the body may not form properly in the baby: the pelvis, the spine and the rib cage. For example, narrow pelvis in girls has become very common, presenting problems with childbirth later on. A narrow rib cage (leading to frequent chest problems) and chronic spinal problems are also, very often, the result of poor maternal diet during pregnancy.[19] The new epigenetic research adds another dimension to this problem: the damage is passed through generations. The poor diet of a mother during her pregnancy can damage not only her child, but also her grandchildren and even great grandchildren. The damage can last for three generations! The industrialised world has been eating a very poor diet indeed for at least three generations now, which is why we have such an epidemic of narrow faces, crowded teeth, narrow nasal passages (with mouth breathing) and other problems with proper bone formation.[20]

Our digestive system begins from the teeth. When we chew our food it is broken down into smaller pieces and mixed with saliva. Enzymes in the saliva start digesting carbohydrates in the mix. It is important for us to chew our food well to digest it properly. However, this depends on the state of the teeth! Unfortunately, tooth decay is a big problem in the world. When you chew your food with teeth that are chronically infected or contain toxic chemicals (put there by the dentist), these toxins are mixed with your food and swallowed.[21] The first place to suffer will be the gut itself. But, when these toxins absorb into your bloodstream, they can cause problems anywhere else in the body.

A very important element for keeping our mouths healthy is saliva. It is an amazing liquid equipped with antimicrobial elements, minerals, proteins, vitamins, lipids and other substances to keep the pH in the mouth normal, remineralising and healing our tooth enamel and maintaining the right microbial community in the mouth.[22] Unfortunately, some 400 commonly prescribed pharmaceutical medications reduce the production of saliva, making the mouth dry.[23] This makes the whole mouth environment abnormal and causes tooth decay, gum disease and other mouth problems. Amalgam fillings and other dental materials can do the same. Chronic stress and food additives can also reduce your saliva production. In a healthy body some 1.5 l (2½ pt) of saliva is produced every day.[24] People with an excessive histamine production in the body (so-called histadelics) produce much more saliva than normal and, as a result, rarely suffer from tooth decay.[25] Despite the fact that histadelics often live on a high-sugar diet, their excessive saliva production protects them from tooth decay.

Our teeth are covered with a very special film called the *pellicle*. It is a microscopic mesh made out of proteins, lipids, vitamins, minerals and other nutrients coming from our saliva and food.[24] Pellicle makes our teeth slippery, lubricating them and protecting them from mechanical damage. Research shows that the more natural fats a person consumes with food the stronger the pellicle becomes.[26] Eating good amounts of natural fats allows us to build a robust structure for our teeth. We can also brush our teeth with olive oil, coconut oil or other natural fats, instead of commercial toothpaste, making our pellicle stronger and better at protecting and healing our teeth.[27] A whole community of microbes make their home on the pellicle, adding their own substances and building a biofilm on the teeth. As long as this community is properly balanced and healthy, they take care of the health of our teeth, gums and other parts of the mouth.[24]

Unfortunately, our mainstream dentistry is trained to fear and attack microbes in the mouth: it tells us that tooth decay is due to the activity of these microbes. Based on this belief all sorts of mouth rinses, toothpaste and other chemical concoctions are recommended. The only reference to nutrition in mainstream dentistry is to sugar, because the microbes feed on sugar, producing acids which can damage the enamel of the teeth. The fact that the teeth are unhealthy because they are made from poor building materials, due to the person's poor nutrition, is not considered in dentistry today. Yet almost one hundred years ago, Weston A. Price and other prominent dentists established that it is our nutritional status which predetermines our dental health![28] His original research has shown that, when people had enough vitamins A, D and K2, the bacterial count in their saliva dropped dramatically and the minerals moved from the saliva into the tissues of the teeth. During a deficiency of these nutrients the bacterial count in the saliva became high, and minerals leached from the teeth into the saliva.[28,29] Further research in the following decades confirmed these findings. Vitamin K2 is particularly important in this process as our salivary glands concentrate this vital substance in large amounts. It is an interesting fact that, after the pancreas, our salivary glands have the highest concentration of K2 in the body.[29] Any dental decay is a sign of deficiency of this vitamin! If your teeth are made from quality materials, microbes in the mouth will have no chance of damaging them! Microbes have been in human mouths for all of our existence on this planet. Yet anthropology shows that, until we started replacing natural nutrient-dense foods with flour, sugar and other processed foods, tooth decay in humans was almost non-existent. Today, due to lack of proper nutrients in the diet for building healthy teeth, the majority of our population has damaged teeth.[30] Tooth decay is rampant and people have all sorts of dental treatments, fillings, crowns, implants, etc.

The problem is, the microbial theory produces very lucrative businesses selling all sorts of products to try and eradicate microbes in the mouth. Any thinking person would realise that one cannot eradicate microbes from the mouth! They are a normal part of our mouth ecology, an essential part. Our mouth flora plays a very important role in maintaining the health of all the organs in the mouth, but just like everywhere else in the body, this flora has to be balanced. Using antimicrobial mouth rinses, mainstream toothpaste and other chemical concoctions will only damage the balance of microbes in the mouth and add toxic chemicals to the mix.[31] One well-researched poison, which is present in most commercial dental products, is fluoride. It causes multiple damage in the human body. But the most obvious place where it is visible in a large proportion of the Western population is in their teeth. Fluorosis or mottling of the teeth has become very common.[32] Next time you talk to people pay attention: you will see white spots on their teeth, often accumulating around the edge of the tooth. This is fluorosis – accumulation of toxic fluoride in the tooth enamel. This is the damage we can see, but many people also accumulate fluoride in their bones, which we cannot see, but which undoubtedly contributes to bone diseases, bone cancer in particular.[33] There is plenty of information available on the toxic effects of fluoride; please research it and avoid toothpaste and other products which contain this poison.

God bless our modern dentistry! Without it the majority of the modern population would have very few teeth in their mouths. However, most materials used by modern dentistry are toxic. We swallow them for weeks after visiting a dentist. Mercury from amalgam fillings, for instance, leaches into saliva all the time they are in the mouth. Mercury is one of the deadliest toxins in the world, and the modern high-copper amalgam fillings leach more mercury than the previous formulas did.[34] The introduction of this new high-copper amalgam formula correlates very well with an epidemic of multiple sclerosis in the Western world, and other chronic illnesses.[35]

The more we chew our food with damaged teeth, full of toxic substances, the more these substances are released into the food and swallowed. People with amalgam fillings in their teeth usually have stomach problems: indigestion, reflux, gastritis, belching, etc.[36] Mercury, accumulating in the stomach walls, forces the body to grow a population of fungi and other microbes to neutralise this poison.[37] Fungal overgrowth in the stomach ferments carbohydrates in food, producing a lot of gas. Both mercury and microbial overgrowth cause inflammation in the stomach. On top of that, many microbes produce substances which can paralyse the muscles in the stomach wall, causing stomach paresis and poor emptying. People with an overgrowth of microbes in the stomach usually have low stomach acidity, because these microbes impair stomach acid production. Stomach acid is essential for us to digest food properly. People with low stomach acidity often have food allergies and intolerances, and nutritional deficiencies, because they cannot digest their food well enough.

It is essential to look at the teeth of any person with stomach problems! Not only mercury, but many other toxins can be leaching from your root canals, fillings, bridges, crowns, dental implants and other artificial dental materials. Not only will your stomach suffer, but the rest of your digestive system too. Many people develop diarrhoea, constipation, abdominal pain and flatulence because of toxicity coming from their teeth.[38]

Root canals are a source of chronic infections in the body.[39] There is no such thing as a 'clean' root canal, no matter how well your dentist did the job. The structure of any tooth is porous: it has millions of tiny canals in its dentin (called *dentinal tubules*), which are impossible to access and to keep microbe-free. The tooth itself is dead because the blood vessels and the nerve, which were giving it life, have been destroyed. All dead things in Nature are quickly populated by microbes to break them up and convert them into a source of building materials for other life forms. That is Nature's law! A root-canalled tooth is a dead body left to decay inside you. Most root-canalled teeth are populated by anaerobic infections, which are capable of producing very powerful poisons: a few parts per million can be enough to make the person ill.[40] These poisons not only leach into the saliva and get swallowed, but many absorb into the bloodstream directly from the tooth. It is a known fact that a chronically infected tooth can cause chronic fatigue, chronic arthritis, fibromyalgia, heart disease, kidney damage, mental problems and neurological illness (multiple sclerosis and neuropathy in particular).[41] Of course, many people have root canals and are not ill, because the immune system is coping with the situation and protecting the body from the infection in the tooth. In this case, it may not be necessary to remove the infected tooth. However, for people with stomach problems, other digestive problems, chronic fatigue, multiple sclerosis and any other chronic degenerative disease it is imperative to remove all infected teeth, which means all root canals have to be removed! Weston A. Price (1870-1948), arguably the most prominent and enlightened dentist in the history of humanity, had a personal tragedy connected to an infected root canal. His only son Donald died from an infected root canal filled by his father. This led Weston A. Price to undertake intensive research into dental causes of chronic and acute diseases in the human body. Unfortunately, mainstream dentistry is largely unaware of this research.

Dental implants often harbour an infection, leaching toxins into the saliva and the bloodstream. The standard dental implants are made from two pieces: an implant and a screw with the artificial tooth attached to it. The implant is fitted into the bone first and, in a few weeks, the tooth is screwed into it. No matter how tightly the tooth is screwed into the implant, there is always a large enough space for microbes to set up home there. By-products of their activity can be very toxic.[41] As the by-products are swallowed, they can cause chronic digestive problems and other chronic diseases. The implant in the majority of cases is made out of titanium – a metal which can cause many health problems in itself.

Having metals in the mouth is dangerous, and any biological or holistic dentist will tell you that. They will do their best to remove all metals and replace titanium implants with porcelain (zirconium). Metals in your teeth can create problems in the whole body, not only in the mouth. Allergies to metals are common, and a phenomenon called *oral galvanism* can do a lot of damage. In this situation an electric current runs between metals in the mouth. This electricity can damage your nervous system and immune system and contribute to any chronic disease in the body.[42]

Another problem, which can cause a lot of chronic illness in the body, is a *cavitation*. Cavitations are hollow spaces which form in the jawbone after a tooth has been extracted incorrectly.[40] These spaces are usually filled with crumbly necrotic tissue and almost always populated by anaerobic infections. There is a ligament at the tip of the root which must be removed when a tooth is being extracted. If this ligament has not been scraped out, a cavitation may form.[40] Holistic dentists are familiar with this problem and know how to find cavitations and how to deal with them. Unfortunately, conventional dentists may not even be aware of this problem.

Another fact, which our mainstream dentists may not be aware of, is that our immune system works on seven-day cycles.[40] The reason for this is that many groups of immune cells live seven days, die and then are replaced by newly born cells. If your body gets exposed to something toxic (a large amount of mercury released into your system during an amalgam removal, for example), a large group of immune cells will memorise that toxin and deal with it. But in seven days this group of cells will die. The replacement cells will take some time to learn the new information and start dealing with the toxin. While they are getting up to the task your body is unprotected. That is why people usually feel worse on the 7th, 14th, 21st, 28th and 35th days after exposure to a particular toxin. Holistic dentists are aware of this phenomenon thanks to the teachings of the late Dr Hal Huggins, a modern pioneer in holistic dentistry, who described the cyclical nature of the immune system and explained how to use it in dentistry.[40] Some cancer-treating doctors are also aware of this phenomenon; they use chemotherapy or radiation, taking into account when the immune system is the strongest in the patient.[43] A battery of tests needs to be performed in order to assess the person's immune cycles. The usual tests measure C-reactive protein and white blood cells. Every seven days there will be a peak and then a drop in the numbers. It is best to remove amalgam fillings or do any other toxin-producing treatments on the days when the immune system is at its peak or coming to the peak. Unfortunately, the majority of our medical profession and dentists are unaware of this phenomenon. So, it is up to the patient to inform them and to ask for the tests to be done. If your dentist removes your second amalgam 7, 14, 21 or any other multiple of seven days after removing the first amalgam, your chances of developing a chronic disease are much higher, because your immune system may be at its lowest and will not be able to protect you from the mercury onslaught.[40]

Modern dentistry is a major cause of chronic degenerative illnesses in the world! So, generally speaking, it is a good idea to work with a holistic or biological dentist, particularly for a GAPS person. There are many details and nuances to removing amalgam fillings correctly, dealing with infected teeth, cavitations and other dental problems. Holistic dentists are trained to deal with those situations in a way that will not cause chronic health problems in the body. Holistic dentistry is more expensive than a conventional dental treatment. However, by working with a holistic dentist you prevent many health problems developing later on, which will save you a lot of suffering and expense in the future.[41] Unfortunately, there is a shortage of holistic dentists in most countries. But it is demand for them that will remedy this problem!

In conclusion: the health of our bones and teeth is the direct result of the food we eat. These are living organs with their own blood supply, nerve supply and immune systems. They renew themselves all the time, and proper building materials must come from your diet for this process. It is not normal for any person, young or old to have osteoporosis! It is not normal to have narrow faces and crowded teeth! And it is not your dentist's job to keep your teeth healthy! It is our modern diet and lifestyles that have created these problems. The real way to have healthy teeth and bones is to nourish your body properly, to provide plenty of high-quality building materials for your bones and teeth.

Here are a couple of clinical examples to demonstrate what we have been talking about.

"In the five months after starting the GAPS Diet I have noticed that my teeth changed colour. They were marble with denser lines, shaped like tree branches from the root area up and more transparent areas in between. At first it scared me, but I soon realised that my teeth were not getting worse, because they used to be very sensitive and now they have lost this sensitivity, which is something I could not even dream about! And my gums started to grow, which is an unbelievable story for a periodontist! Then I searched in FAQs on your website gaps.me and found an explanation for what was happening to my teeth. My teeth were filling with calcium! Currently I have just a few transparent spots on my teeth and my gums are still growing. I hope that my bones are filling up with calcium as well." **O.O., Australia**

Maria (the name has been changed), 64 years old, has been suffering from chronic fatigue, multiple sclerosis, severe digestive problems, psoriasis, many allergies and severe sensitivity to electromagnetic devices for years. She tried many treatments – mainstream and alternative – without much improvement. GAPS Nutritional Protocol brought a lot of healing for her and she felt strong enough to address the state of her teeth. She started working with a holistic dentist, who removed eight amalgam fillings and four root canals from her mouth. Three cavitations were found in her jaw bones, which had to be surgically cleaned out, and all of them were found to have chronic anaerobic infections in them and remnants of amalgam fillings. The dental work took three years to complete, as Maria needed time to recover from every treatment. But, with every treatment her overall health improved: her energy levels increased, her symptoms of multiple sclerosis started reducing, allergies subsided and she was less sensitive to chemicals and electronic devices. When the dental treatments had been completed, she truly started to recover from all of her illnesses with the use of the GAPS Nutritional Protocol.

Problems down below

Chronic cystitis

People with abnormal gut flora have a river of toxicity flowing through their damaged gut wall into the blood and the lymph. Toxic chemicals produced by pathogenic microbes, undigested foods, immune complexes and alive microbes circulate around the body of a GAPS person, doing a lot of damage. At some point the body eliminates them, and one of the major routes for removing them is urine. The GAPS person's urine is full of toxicity, which changes every day depending on what the person has been eating and the activity of their abnormal gut flora.[1] When this toxic urine accumulates in the bladder it causes inflammation in its walls – cystitis. The typical symptoms of cystitis are discomfort or pain in the bladder area, uncomfortable or painful urination, frequent urination (often with small amounts of urine) and urgency. Many people develop bed-wetting at night, and some people may wet themselves a little when laughing, lifting something heavy or straining. Typically, testing finds no infection in the urine because chronic interstitial cystitis is not caused by infections. It is caused by toxic chemicals which come from the activity of abnormal gut flora in the person.[2] Our mainstream medicine doesn't seem to be aware of this cause of cystitis yet. Chronic interstitial cystitis is a common condition, particularly in women. Many men also suffer from it, as well as a growing number of children.

Bed-wetting is very common amongst children with abnormal gut flora, and quite a few adults have this problem too. When your body is in a deep sleep and a small amount of toxic urine accumulates in the bladder, it may empty to protect itself without waking you up. GAPS is the major cause of bed-wetting! In order to deal with bed-wetting permanently, we need to change the gut flora of the person and heal the gut, which will take time. Short term it is a good idea to wake the child up a few times during the night to go to the toilet.

Many plant foods contain substances which are very irritating for the urinary tract.[3] These are oxalates and salicylates. In a person with healthy gut flora these substances get digested and absorbed in the right shape and form and do no harm. But in GAPS people they do not get digested properly before they absorb through the damaged gut wall. Circulating around the body they cause a lot of damage in many organs and systems. After that they leave the body in urine, making it very irritating and damaging for the bladder and urethra. Foods rich in oxalates and salicylates are greens, nuts, berries, fruit, tea, coffee, chocolate, spices, many vegetables (particularly raw), many other plant foods, wine and beer. These foods have to be removed from the diet of a person with chronic cystitis, bed-wetting and other problems in that area. Working on healing the gut and changing the gut flora with the GAPS Nutritional Protocol will eliminate all these problems eventually. So, at some point you will be able to start reintroducing foods with oxalates and salicylates back into the diet. If you try to introduce any of these foods and your urinary problems come back, this is the signal your body gives that it is not ready for these foods yet. Stay away from them for a few weeks longer and then try again. Doing the GAPS Introduction Diet for a few months will speed up the healing in your gut wall and allow you to introduce these foods sooner. Always introduce one food at a time, starting from small amounts. It is possible that you may never be able to reintroduce some of these foods, such as spinach, for example.

Your bladder, urethra and the prostate gland in men are populated by a mixture of microbes – their own flora.[4,5,6] This flora comes from the groin, which in turn largely originates from your bowel. In a person with abnormal gut flora, the flora in those areas is likely to be abnormal too, creating inflammation and producing many toxic substances. Urine full of toxins will damage your bladder flora even further. GAPS Nutritional Protocol will work on the gut flora and heal your digestive system, which will clean up your urine. But, in order to heal the urinary system completely, it is important to work on restoring local microbial flora in the bladder and the urethra. In order to do that I recommend an old traditional practice.

How to restore local microbiome in the groin, bladder, urethra and genital organs. Keep a jar with fresh kefir in your bathroom. Every day, after your usual bath or shower, apply a small handful of kefir all over your groin. Let it dry a little before dressing. This simple procedure will populate that area with beneficial microbes, which will eliminate pathogens and heal the damage. The culture will travel up the urethra into the bladder over time. Women with vaginal problems can introduce some of this kefir into their vagina at the same time (use your fingers or a cotton wool ball soaked in kefir).

Clearing the bowel with the use of an enema can be very helpful in bringing down acute cystitis, because after an enema the amount of toxicity in the body drops dramatically.[7] Add a cup of homemade whey to the enema to populate the bowel with beneficial flora. It is helpful to drink plenty of fermented beverages and water with lemon. Mixed herbal teas, particularly herbs with diuretic properties, can be helpful. Supplements with cranberry, an herb *Uva Ursi* and D-mannose can also bring relief. But long term we need to normalise the gut flora and digestion. We need to heal and seal the gut wall, so toxins stop absorbing through it. Then urine will become clean and the bladder will have a chance to heal itself.

Chronic cystitis is the most common urinary tract problem in GAPS people. For information on less common problems, please look in the *Chapter A–Z, Kidney Problems.*

Female problems

The female reproductive system has a rich microbial flora.[8] At the moment of birth, a female baby acquires her mother's vaginal flora. Until puberty the pH in the vagina is close to 7.0, which encourages a very diverse microbial flora (*Staphylococci, Coryneforms, Peptostreptococci, Bacteroides, Clostridia, Eubacteria* and other). During puberty the vaginal wall starts secreting glycogen – a sugar that encourages the growth of *Lactobacilli.*[9] They dominate the rich microbial population of the vagina and reduce pH down to 3.5–4.5, making it hostile to pathogenic microbes. After menopause, vaginal pH returns back to pre-puberty levels.

For a long time it has been assumed that female reproductive organs above the vagina are sterile. However, recent research has demonstrated that the cervix, uterus, fallopian tubes and ovaries are populated by their own microbial flora.[8,9,10] More than 278 genera of microbes have been identified in the uterus alone. During pregnancy the placenta is richly populated by its own microbial flora, which the baby acquires and so it is born with already established species of microbes in its digestive system, on the skin and the rest of the body.[11,14] Ovaries and fallopian tubes have their own flora, dominated by *Lactobacilli* and, interestingly, the flora in one ovary can be different from the other in the same woman.[12]

This microbial flora in the reproductive organs protects the woman from infections and disease. However, in our modern world that flora can get damaged by regular antibiotic treatments, contraceptive pills, consumption of agricultural chemicals and other influences.[15] As a result, pathogenic flora may start dominating, and that always leads to health problems. Abnormal flora in fallopian tubes can lead to sterility (a woman cannot get pregnant). Abnormal flora on the ovaries and fallopian tubes can lead to endometriosis, infertility and other problems. Abnormal flora in the uterus can prevent pregnancy and cause stillbirths or miscarriages.[12,13] Abnormal placental flora is associated with poor pregnancy outcomes, such as excessive gestational weight gain and premature births.[13] Abnormal flora in the cervix and the vagina can cause many problems in that area.[14]

Abnormal flora in the vagina (which includes the cervix) makes it unprotected from infectious microbes, and the pH in the vagina changes. As a result, various bacteria, fungi, viruses and other microbes can get in and cause infections with abnormal discharge, itching, burning, swelling, pain, ulcers, unpleasant odour and other symptoms. Thrush – a yeast infection – is particularly common and can become chronic. It is very important for a woman to look after her vaginal flora! To do that, keep a jar with fresh raw kefir or sour cream in your bathroom and apply a small handful all over your groin on a daily basis. This can be done after your usual shower or bath. This simple measure will prevent many problems in that area. It is particularly important to do this during pregnancy, because pregnancy is a natural state of immune suppression. If a woman has a predisposition to thrush or any other vaginal problem, it is likely to become more active during pregnancy.[12] A regular vaginal douche with fresh whey from homemade kefir or yogurt will populate that area with beneficial flora, reduce pH and remove vaginal thrush and other common infections. Not only will the whey provide beneficial microbes, but many healing substances and vitamins for the vaginal lining and the cervix. Keeping your vagina well populated by beneficial microbes in pregnancy will also prepare your birth canal for the baby. During normal (vaginal) birth babies acquire a lot of their body flora, including gut flora, from the mother's vagina.[14] Preparing the birth canal for the baby's arrival was a standard practice in traditional societies. Women used their homemade kefir, yogurt, whey and sour cream to prevent any problems in their reproductive organs. And they used this simple practice to protect their men as well (often without the men's knowledge): they would apply kefir to their groin before intercourse, thus transferring beneficial microbes onto their husband's sexual organs. In menopause sour cream has been used to prevent vaginal dryness, which is the best remedy for this problem, because it provides healing fats, vitamin A, D and K and other beneficial substances for the vaginal lining. In our modern world women would do well to bring these practices back and teach their daughters and granddaughters to use them.

Male problems

In boys and young men with GAPS *inguinal hernia* is fairly common (part of the bowel descending into the scrotum). During foetal development testes travel down into the scrotum from quite a distance away – somewhere near the kidneys. As they descend, the testes pull a sack behind them, called the inguinal sack, which is supposed to close down during birth. In some boys it stays open, which can lead to an inguinal hernia. Surgery will close up the inguinal sack and remove the hernia. However, I believe that GAPS collagen disorder is an important factor in this problem (please read about it in detail in the chapter *Immune System*). It creates weakness in the abdominal wall predisposing the child to hernias.

The most common problems in older men are with the *prostate gland.* The prostate gland is a small male endocrine organ (about the size of a walnut) sitting underneath the bladder on the front wall of the rectum. The wall of the rectum and the capsule of the prostate gland form one structure, which is porous and allows substances to be transferred between the bowel and the prostate gland.[16] Recent research has discovered that certain microbes in the gut flora produce androgens (male sex hormones), which penetrate through the wall between the rectum and the prostate and affect the function of the prostate gland.[17] In a person with healthy gut flora this process is healthy and normal. But in a person with abnormal gut flora, which unfortunately includes a growing proportion of men in the Western world today, this process goes wrong. Androgens get converted into oestrogens and other substances by the pathogenic microbes, which absorb into the prostate gland and initiate inflammation (prostatitis), enlargement and prostate cancer.[18,19,20]

Prostate cancer is the most common cancer in men and the incidence is growing every year. It has been established that oestrogens drive prostate cancer and may even cause it in the first place.[19] Levels of these hormones in the prostate cancer tissues were found to be high, and some mechanisms of how they cause cancer have been already researched.[19,20] The researchers were not sure where these oestrogens come from in prostate cancer patients, because blood levels of oestrogens were never found to be high enough to explain the high levels of these hormones in the prostate gland itself. Now we may have an explanation: the hormones may be coming from the man's gut, across that little wall which the prostate gland shares with the rectum.[21,22]

Another obvious way for the excessive oestrogens and other toxins to get to the prostate gland is urine.[23] The prostate gland is positioned underneath the bladder and the urethra goes right through it. People with abnormal gut flora absorb a plethora of chemicals, which are produced by the microbes in the gut. Many of these metabolites leave the body in urine.[24] Many oestrogenic compounds produced by the abnormal gut flora will follow this route, getting directly into the prostate through the urine. Every time a man urinates, these toxic and damaging chemicals will affect the prostate gland, causing inflammation, enlargement and, eventually, cancer.

Prostate problems are most common in men aged 50 and older. In order to protect yourself, it is essential to look after your gut flora. By consuming a correct diet, fermented foods and probiotics you will make sure that your gut flora provides the right mix of hormones for your prostate gland, directly through the rectum/prostate wall and through the urine. Your urine, which passes through your prostate many times a day, will be clean and have only healthy metabolites in it. Your gut flora will provide the prostate gland with a healthy mix of hormones and other substances, nourishing it and protecting it from anything damaging.

Enlargement of the prostate gland (benign prostatic hyperplasia – BPH) is very common; it affects one in three men after the age of 50 in the Western world. It is not due to ageing, because healthy men age comfortably without prostate problems. It is due to inflammation in that area restricting the flow of urine.[21] In my opinion, this inflammation is caused by the same mechanisms that cause chronic interstitial cystitis. The urine of a person with abnormal gut flora is full of toxic chemicals. Metabolites produced by pathogenic microbes in the gut, undigested foods, immune complexes, salicylates and oxalates, and a plethora of other irritating and damaging molecules absorb through the damaged gut wall into the bloodstream, circulate around the body and then leave the body in urine. This toxic damaging urine causes chronic inflammation in the bladder, urethra and the prostate gland.[25] The longer this situation goes on, the more chronic the inflammation in that area becomes, and eventually it can lead to cancer. The urinary tract of a man is populated by microbial flora. This flora will get altered by the flow of toxic urine and become abnormal, which will contribute to the whole problem.

For every man who is suffering from enlargement of the prostate gland or prostatitis (inflammation of the prostate), I strongly recommend going on the GAPS Diet. The typical symptoms are: restricted urine flow, leading to slow and incomplete urination, having to strain to empty the bladder and painful or uncomfortable urination. You may want to start from the Full GAPS Diet and do the Introduction Diet at some point later. Initially it is important to stay away from foods rich in salicylates and oxalates, as they have a strong irritating ability for the urinary tract. Later on, as your gut flora improves and your gut wall heals itself, you may be able to reintroduce some of those foods. On the GAPS Nutritional Protocol your urination will become normal and all the symptoms will disappear. Many men with prostate problems choose to stay on the Full GAPS Diet for the rest of their lives, eating other foods only occasionally (when on holiday or visiting friends). The Full GAPS Diet is ideal for ageing people. Not only will it keep your prostate gland healthy, but all the other organs and systems in your body will stay healthy and allow you to age comfortably and gracefully. Ageing is not a disease! It is a normal stage in our lives, and it should be healthy.

In conclusion: in this chapter we have focused on the most common female and male problems in GAPS people. It is beyond the scope of this book to focus on all existing problems in this area. However, whatever your individual problem may be, consider the role of the microbial community, which lives in our urinary system and reproductive organs. And consider the fact that the bowel (with its very large microbiome) is very close by. Microbes are everywhere inside us; they are in the majority and always take part in every function or dysfunction in the body. It is impossible to be microbe free, so we must create the right environment in the body for the healthy balanced microbial community to thrive in every organ and tissue. A healthy microbial community will keep your urinary system and reproductive organs healthy and well, at any age.

GAPS behaviour

From caring comes courage.

Lao Tzu

Recent research has discovered that our gut flora can dictate our behaviour.[1] Behind every emotion there is a chemical storm in the body: production of hormones, neurotransmitters, enzymes and other active substances. Emotions are chemicals, and our gut flora produces plenty of chemicals! Many emotions, motivations, likes and dislikes, outbursts and other behaviours are not ours; they come from the microbial activity in our gut. GAPS patients have abnormal gut flora; it is taken over by pathogenic microbes. These microbes produce toxic chemicals which absorb and get into the brain.[2] The toxic brain can produce all sorts of symptoms, which may not be severe enough to diagnose a mental illness, but serious enough to affect the person's life. Many GAPS people are depressed to a degree, have emotional instability and may suffer from mild anxiety. All of this affects the person's behaviour and interaction with others. As a result, a GAPS person in a family is often a difficult person to live with.

When a collection of particularly toxic chemicals accumulates in the brain, the brain can develop a cleansing procedure: it initiates a cluster of activity that helps it to 'burn' these toxins out and eliminate them.[3,4] This activity manifests as tantrums, all sorts of fits and attacks, all the way to epileptic seizures. The subject of epilepsy has been covered in the first GAPS book (*Gut and Psychology Syndrome*). Here we are going to talk about less known and less understood reactions.

Let us start from temper tantrums. Both children and adults with GAPS are prone to emotional instability and tantrums, when they can become angry, tearful, aggressive and inconsolable, shouting, screaming, crying, lashing out, throwing objects, throwing themselves on the floor, running away, etc. These kinds of behavior usually appear without any particular reason, and they can be triggered by any trivial thing. For example, a little girl is screaming, scratching, lashing out and kicking all the way to school because a 'wrong-colour' ribbon has been attached to her hair. A little boy throws himself to the floor screaming, kicking, inconsolable because a 'wrong toy' has been given to him on his birthday. A woman is in a rage, crying and shouting obscenities for an hour at her husband and children, because they bought the 'wrong kind' of bread in a shop. A man running away in anger kicks a wall, breaking bones in his foot, because of a trivial domestic disagreement. The magnitude of the reaction does not match the trigger ('the reason') for this reaction, and nothing can console the person. As one parent of a GAPS boy, who had frequent temper tantrums, put it: 'this is some sort of a fit, he just has to go through it! Nothing we try to do can stop the tantrum. We just have to leave him to it, and let him go through the motions!' This behavior is due to toxic chemicals, produced in the gut of the GAPS person, which get into the brain and cause the fit. The person is not in control of this situation; that is why nothing can console or pacify him or her. Until the brain has 'burned' the chemicals, the person will continue with the tantrum.[4]

Some of these reactions can take the form of a panic attack, when the person feels a sudden rush of intense anxiety and fear. Physical symptoms of a panic attack can aggravate the fear: heart palpitations, nausea, trembling, dizziness, shortness of breath, profuse sweating, ringing in the ears and numbness in different parts of the body. The toxicity in the brain leads to the activation of the sympathetic nervous system and production of large amounts of stress hormones.[5,6] A panic attack, due to intense fear, can cause irrational and inappropriate behaviour: desire to run away and hide, various irrational fears, and a feeling that you are dying or having a heart attack. Once the brain has cleared toxicity the attack stops. Usually it takes 20–30 minutes, but can go on for longer.

Apart from panic attacks GAPS people can have other 'attacks', such as sudden episodes of impulsive, aggressive, violent behaviour or angry verbal outbursts triggered by trivial situations. The reaction is always grossly out of proportion to the 'reason' for it. The chemical load the brain is trying to clear can lead to domestic abuse, road rage, damage to possessions and property and other grievous behaviour. During the episode the person can be mean and unpleasant. But, when the chemicals have cleared, the person can become sweet and nice, feel ashamed of their behaviour and beg for forgiveness.

GAPS people are known to have pathological reactions to alcohol, cannabis, prescription drugs and other toxins.[7,8]

Here is a clinical example of a pathological reaction to alcohol:

John has always been a GAPS person, suffering from digestive problems and allergies. He is quite shy and finds it difficult to make friends. He has just started university, and in the first week of studies he was invited to a party by one of his fellow students. The party took place at this student's home. At the party John was given a glass of strong alcoholic drink, which he had never had before. Sometime after that John went outside, found an axe in the back garden and ran

inside the house waving it madly, shouting and trying to attack people. It is lucky that the guests managed to contain John and take the axe away from him. He had to be tied to a post in the garden for three hours before he calmed down and was safe to be released. John had very vague memories of this episode.

This was a seizure, a fit caused by the reaction of John's brain to alcohol. John was not in control of his behaviour, he could not even remember it well. Smoking cannabis (marihuana) can cause such reactions too. It has become widely available in the Western world and is now a major trigger of psychosis in young people.[7] I have no doubt that the majority (if not all) of the youngsters who react with psychotic symptoms to this plant are GAPS people. Their bodies are too toxic to be able to handle cannabis, alcohol or other drugs without the brain generating major symptoms.

During a fit or a tantrum many GAPS people are skilled at hurling accusations at those around them, which can make their parents or careers feel responsible for their suffering. It is important to understand that accusations, tantrums, fits, attacks, mean and aggressive behaviour are due to a chemical storm in the brain of the person. It is not anybody's fault, and the patient cannot help it! A calm and compassionate attitude is all that is required to weather these storms. Anything the person says during the fit should not be taken seriously. Very often they don't even remember what they have said. As the person works on the GAPS Nutritional Protocol these episodes will happen less and less, and eventually disappear altogether.

Living with a GAPS person in a family is always a challenge. Other members of the family have to understand that *it is easier to keep the GAPS person on the GAPS Diet than not*! The diet will remove the fits, tantrums, attacks and other behavioural problems. Though the diet may seem like hard work at first, it is easier to live with a calm, pleasant person than with a mean, irrational, depressed and, at times, aggressive one.

Many of these behaviours are caused by addictions to foods. Let us talk about this in more detail.

Food Addictions

Man cannot discover new oceans unless
he has the courage to lose sight of the shore.

Andre Gide

Our gut flora dictates our food preferences.[1] Whatever group of microbes you have dominating your gut, they will 'demand' their perfect foods, giving you an irresistible desire for them. GAPS people have abnormal gut flora and, as a result, have an abnormal relationship with food. Cravings for sweet and starchy foods are typical for most people with abnormal body flora. Bread, pasta, sugary drinks, biscuits, cakes, sweets, pizza, breakfast cereals, chocolates, chips and crisps are the foods to which many GAPS people limit their diet, because the most common pathogens overgrowing in their gut love these foods. This situation is particularly pronounced in GAPS children. If your child is fussy with food, refusing proper meals and instead demanding sugary and starchy alternatives, this is a clear sign that your child has GAPS. Fussy eating is a major symptom of this condition.

What is driving the desire for processed foods that harm us? There are solid physiological reasons for being addicted to those foods, and gut flora plays a crucial role in this addiction. The microbes in your gut are clever: they feast on the processed carbohydrates and convert them into many toxic substances.[2] Some of those substances are in the form of opiates and endorphins – chemicals which give the brain a pleasure signal.[3] So, the brain wants more, and it becomes addicted to those chemicals. As a result, the foods that harm you become your 'favourite' foods. You become an addict. 'But I don't take drugs or abuse alcohol'. You don't have to! Your own gut flora is producing those addictive substances for you every time you enjoy your 'favourite' foods. For example, yeast overgrowth in the digestive system converts everything made from flour and sugar into alcohol.[4] It is a very common situation in people after taking antibiotics. If you have yeast overgrowth you don't need to consume alcohol to have all its damaging effects on your body; the alcohol is produced in your gut every time you eat bread, sugar, potatoes, breakfast cereals or any other carbohydrates.

It is a fact that grains and sugar are addictive. Sugar is, arguably, the most addictive substance on this planet![5] Many people in our world are addicted to bread, pasta, pizza, cakes, chocolates, soft drinks, snacks and other foods made from flour, sugar and everything containing it, potatoes and everything made from them, and other processed carbohydrates. But, because 'everybody is eating them', people don't realise that these foods are addictive. On top of that, many processed foods, snacks and treats contain addictive chemicals, which are deliberately added to make these foods 'irresistible'.[6]

Apart from producing opiates and endorphins to make your brain addicted to carbohydrates, pathogenic gut flora produces a plethora of other chemicals that affect your whole body.[7] These chemicals make your brain 'foggy', so you cannot concentrate well enough to realise what is happening to you. They affect your mood and emotions, making them unstable. They can cause anxiety, depression, obsessions, oppositional-defiant behaviour and any other form of unstable or abnormal mental function, clouding your judgement and ability to perceive the state your body is in.

For many people, addiction to sugar, flour and other processed carbohydrates begins in early childhood. Sugar addiction is the basis for developing other addictions later on: addictions to alcohol, drugs, tobacco, work, sex and dangerous reckless behaviour.[8] Sugar addiction is also the most common basis for developing mental illness in children and adults. I would recommend reading an autobiography by Stephen Fry, a popular British actor, where he describes with precision and great sense of humour his sugar addiction from early childhood and what it led to.

How do GAPS children become addicts? In the first GAPS book (*Gut and Psychology Syndrome*) I described the fussy eating in GAPS children. It is a typical symptom of GAPS: these children are trapped in a vicious cycle of cravings and dependency on the very foods that hurt them. In effect, these children are drug addicts; the 'drug' is produced by abnormal flora in their gut when it is feasting on processed carbohydrates. As these children grow up, the food addictions do not disappear, instead they can develop into a more serious situation. In my experience, every adult who is suffering from an addiction to drugs, alcohol or anything else has started as a child addicted to sugar and other processed carbohydrates. Let us discuss how that happens.

Many GAPS children have mild symptoms and do not get diagnosed with any particular condition. They go through childhood with some mild problems in learning and social skills: they are not good at academic subjects or sport at school and they find it difficult to make friends. They often have physical problems, such as allergies, asthma, poor immunity, poor digestive function, poor eyesight, clumsiness and hyper-mobile joints. And they are fussy with food, preferring processed carbohydrates to anything else. Because their symptoms are mild, teachers and parents are keen to make excuses for them, and the medical profession avoids giving them any diagnostic labels, though dyslexia, dyspraxia and ADD/ADHD are common. When they reach adolescence, this group of children is prone to developing addictions to drugs, alcohol, tobacco or anything else. Why does that happen? There are two reasons for it: one psychological and another physical.

The psychological reason: these children grow up with poor social skills, other children don't want to play with them, and they often get bullied. As a result, their self-worth and self-esteem suffer. When they become teenagers, these children will do anything to fit in with their peer group, to have girlfriends and boyfriends, and to be invited to parties. Trying drugs and reckless dangerous behaviours attract attention; and this is the route these children often take to be popular.

The physical reason is based on how our major neurotransmitters are produced – serotonin, dopamine and GABA (Gamma Amino-Butyric Acid).[9] They are largely produced in the digestive system. After that they get transported to the brain to be used by different brain structures. GAPS is a digestive disorder; in these children their gut is unable to produce normal amounts of those neurotransmitters. When we don't have enough serotonin and dopamine, we become depressed, negative and apathetic. When we lack GABA, we can develop anxiety, poor sleep and inability to relax. These children have grown up with these symptoms, but they might have been mild enough to be dismissed as personality traits or individual character.

I believe that we are born to be happy! How do we achieve the state of complete happiness, joy of life, exhilaration? In part, by our brain receiving a fountain of neurotransmitters to hit a certain level. Because of a lack of neurotransmitter production in the gut, GAPS children may have never had this feeling; they went through childhood having some form of depression or anxiety. Illicit drugs (heroin, morphine, cannabis, etc), abuse of alcohol and tobacco, dangerous reckless behaviour and other addictive activities can raise the levels of neurotransmitters in the brain for a few minutes, producing that 'fountain'. That is the first time our youngster may experience the joy of life, the exhilaration of being lifted out of depression and apathy. It is the moment when they might realise that this is what life is about! And they want that feeling again; and who can blame them. That is when the physical addiction to the drug, alcohol or anything else they tried starts developing.

Addictions have reached epidemic proportions in the Western world. In order for any addict to recover, he or she needs to focus on their gut: they need to drive out pathogens and rebuild a healthy microbial community, restore the integrity of the gut wall and nourish and rebuild their bodies. But, when they begin the GAPS Diet, every addict realises that the addiction they have (drug, alcohol, tobacco, etc) is only the outer layer of the problem; underneath it there are food addictions to sugar, flour, potato and other processed carbohydrates. Those food addictions must be faced and removed in order to recover from the drug addiction, alcoholism or any other addictive activity. Here is a quote by a person who recovered from drug and alcohol abuse: *All alcoholics have GAPS! ...and the drug addicts, the sex addicts, and the gambling addicts have GAPS! ...and the food addicts, the bulimics, the anorexics – fat people and skinny people alike. They all have GAPS! This is what we have! This is it!* (Gerald, from the book GAPS Stories, p.189).

In my first GAPS book I described a behavioural approach to dealing with fussy eating in a child (chapter *It's feeding time. Oh no!*). It is much harder to deal with an adult in your charge, and even harder to deal with yourself! Every time you have a desire for a particular food, which you know is not allowed on the GAPS Nutritional Protocol, stop and think: *is it my body asking for this food or those pathogenic microbes in my gut demanding it?* More often than not, you will realise that it is your abnormal gut flora commanding you. Don't underestimate your gut microbes; they outnumber you by ten in the number of living cells, and by hundreds in the volume of their genetics! And your addicted brain will be ever so inventive in trying to persuade you to give in, giving you all sorts of excuses and reasons for why you should eat your addictive foods.

This letter from a GAPS person is a good example of what we are discussing.

In the food store I would just wander around aimlessly trying to remember what I was supposed to be purchasing.... with the smell of bread being pumped through the air con, stimulating the pleasure centres of my brain, convincing me that a bit of bread couldn't hurt. After all I am sure I must be a carb person!!!.... said with the certainty of an addict!!! Just this once won't hurt!

It is important to know, when following the GAPS protocol, that we are addicted to certain foods. This makes us feel the urge to move quickly through the process to bring in those foods. We will fall off the protocol and eat the things that are not on the recommended list, and we will always have an excuse....it was my birthday....I didn't want to offend the host....I felt miserable after a hard day....etc!!! There is always going to be a good excuse not to stick to the protocol. However, after about the 500th time (in my case!) of cheating we might just begin to notice how painful that momentary slip was. When finally we dare to review it properly by really thinking it through, we begin to see that the cake that lasted for two minutes in the mouth, wasn't worth the five days of discomfort. It takes a long time to see this for what it is.

Like any addict in recovery we also do substitution. When sugar in the form of sucrose, or starchy food is out, we switch to fruit (and honey)! We eat lots of fruit, as 'it must be good for us, because we are supposed to have between 5 and 15 portions per day'! Many of us will find, as I did, that this substitution takes us off course. We need to understand and address the addictive mind and notice its behaviours.

Not understanding the depths of this 'addiction' caused me to take a very circuitous route through my own healing. It wouldn't have taken me so long had I realised the source of these behaviours, and had I known the importance of sticking completely to the protocol and addressing the addictions head on. I can easily say this now with my beautifully crystal-clear brain, and my focus, and my high energy, and my stable mood, and my freedom from addiction.... I know, I did it! it's possible! But it is hard, very hard! You also have the nagging of microorganisms inside you that are fully in support of you eating that cake, chocolate, ice cream.... they just love the undigested residues. They will give you such an appetite for their favourite foods. We think we are in control at least of our own appetite.... we are not!

Most of the population is addicted to something, but they think that they are not. The drug addict and the alcoholic, when going through recovery, have to realise and acknowledge to themselves and others that they are addicts, and once they get that realisation they can begin to heal. Being aware of what is driving the desire and the resulting behaviours puts us back in control. (Katrina's story of recovery from rheumatoid arthritis and Crohn's disease on www.DoctorNatasha.com).

Conclusion: GAPS people have to understand that their abnormal gut flora turns them into addicts. It is a difficult fact to accept! It is not easy to admit to yourself that you are not in control of your food desires and preferences, and that in your belly there is somebody who is actually in charge. Only by facing this fact is it possible to overcome addictions to sugar, chocolate and items made from flour, potatoes and other processed carbohydrates. Only when you stop eating these 'foods' can you begin to recover from any chronic illness! So, overcoming an addiction to processed carbohydrates and other foods is essential and must be done at the beginning of your healing journey. It is vital to explain this to people who are close to you, so they do not undermine your efforts inadvertently. Having supportive family and friends around you, who fully understand what you are going through, is invaluable!

FOOD

What GAPS people should eat and what should be avoided

I eat and therefore I know food! That is what many people think. We grow up accepting the opinions of our family members and society about what food is 'good for us'. When we get ill, it doesn't occur to many of us that the food we have been eating may have something to do with the illness. Many people think: *How can food possibly have anything to do with my illness? I have been eating it all my life!* Only when I formally studied nutrition did I realise just how much there is to know about food. And when I started using food as medicine for my patients, I realised that there is nothing more powerful in the world in its effect on human health than food! People eat three times a day, sometimes more often. Every morsel of food you put into your mouth changes everything in your body: your metabolism, your hormonal balance, your electrolyte balance, your sympathetic/parasympathetic nervous system balance and much more. GAPS Diet over the years has earned a strong reputation for helping people to recover from debilitating health problems – physical and mental. The basis of the GAPS Diet has been described in my previous GAPS book, *Gut and Psychology Syndrome,* which focused on the functioning of the brain. In this book we are focussing on the rest of the body, but the diet remains the same. For those people who are not familiar with my previous GAPS book, it is necessary to repeat some of the essential information presented in it.[1]

Foods to avoid

To understand what foods to avoid we need to look at how foods are absorbed in our digestive tract. The absorption of digested food happens in the small intestine, mainly in its first two parts: the duodenum and jejunum. The walls of these parts of the digestive system form tiny finger-like protrusions, called villi, to increase the absorptive surface. These villi are lined by cells, called **enterocytes**.[2] These are the cells which absorb our food and pass it into the bloodstream to nourish our bodies. The importance of these cells to our health simply cannot be overestimated.

These cells are born at the base of the villi and through the course of their short life travel to the top of the villi, slowly getting more mature on the way. When they reach the top of the villi they are shed, because by then they have performed so much work that they have become old and worn out. This process of constant renewal of enterocytes is ruled by the beneficial microbes which live on them.[3] As already mentioned in the chapter on gut flora, the beneficial microbes ensure that enterocytes are healthy and capable of performing their jobs. When the beneficial microbes are not there and the absorptive surface of the intestine is populated by pathogenic microbes instead, the enterocytes cannot be healthy and cannot perform their duties. Animal research shows that, in the absence of healthy microbes, enterocytes change their shape, and their travel time to the top of the villi becomes too long, which can turn them cancerous. But most importantly, they become unable to perform their jobs of digestion and absorption of food.[2,3] Let us have a look at how enterocytes handle different groups of nutrients: carbohydrates, proteins and fats.

Carbohydrates

All carbohydrates are made of tiny molecules, called *monosaccharides*. There are many of them, but the most common ones are *glucose, fructose* and *galactose*. These *monosaccharides* or *monosugars* can easily penetrate the gut lining; they do not need digestion. Glucose and fructose are found in abundance in fruit and vegetables. Honey is largely made of fructose and glucose and does not require much digestion. Galactose is found in soured milk products, such as yogurt, kefir, sour cream and cheese.[4] *Monosugars* are the easiest carbohydrates for us to digest and should be the main form of carbohydrate in the diet of any person with a chronic health problem. In any chronic illness the gut is under stress and we have to be kind to it.

The next size carbohydrates are *disaccharides* or *double sugars*, made out of two molecules of monosaccharides. The most common ones are *sucrose* (the common table sugar), *lactose* (the milk sugar) and *maltose* from digestion of starch. These *double sugars* cannot be absorbed without quite a bit of work on the part of enterocytes. The tiny hairs (microvilli) on the surface of enterocytes, called the brush border, produce enzymes called *disaccharidases,* which break down the double sugars into monosaccharides to be absorbed.[4] This is where the biggest problem lies for people with abnormal gut flora. The sick enterocytes lose their ability to produce brush border enzymes. As a result, double sugars, like sucrose, milk sugar lactose and products of starch digestion cannot be split into monosugars, and hence cannot be absorbed. They stay in the gut becoming major food for pathogenic bacteria, *Candida* and other microbes, getting converted into a river of toxic substances which damage the gut wall even further and poison the whole body. Deficiencies in disaccharidases almost always accompany digestive disorders and many chronic illnesses, where the person may not have any digestive symptoms (for example, rheumatoid arthritis, multiple sclerosis and other autoimmune disease).[5,6] So, double sugars or disaccharides have to be out of the diet for GAPS children and adults in order not to feed abnormal flora. It is essential to allow your gut wall time to recover by shedding off sick enterocytes and building a layer of healthy ones.

We have mentioned maltose – the result of *starch* digestion. Apart from sugar (sucrose), starch is the main form of carbohydrates we consume. All grains, most legumes and some root vegetables (potato, yams, sweet potato, Jerusalem artichoke, cassava and parsnips) are rich in starch. Starch is made of huge molecules with hundreds of monosugars connected into long strands with many branches. Digestion of starch requires a lot of work on the part of the digestive system and, even in healthy people, due to its complex structure a lot of starch goes undigested.[4] Undigested starch provides a perfect food for pathogenic flora in the gut, allowing it to thrive and produce its toxins.

Whatever starch does get digested results in molecules of *maltose.* Maltose is a double sugar which cannot be absorbed without being split up into monosugars by the enterocytes. In a person with abnormal gut flora, enterocytes are not able to split double sugars, so maltose falls prey to the microbes. To allow the enterocytes to recover and to stop feeding abnormal gut flora, starch has to be out of the diet for GAPS children and adults. It means no grains or anything made out of them, no starchy legumes and no starchy vegetables. Clinical practice shows that, when the gut has been given a long enough period without double sugars and starch, it has a good chance of recovery. Once this recovery takes place, many people can start having grains and starchy vegetables again without any ill effects.

Of course, nothing in Nature is black and white. Most fruit, particularly when unripe, contain some sucrose, which is a double sugar. That is why it is very important to eat *ripe* fruit. Most vegetables and some fruit contain a little bit of starch. However, the amounts of sucrose and starch in fruit and non-starch vegetables are tiny compared to grains, legumes, starchy vegetables and table sugar. In the majority of people with digestive disorders and chronic degenerative conditions their gut lining can cope with these tiny amounts of sugar and starch from ripe fruit and non-starch vegetables.

Proteins

As a result of digestion in the stomach and duodenum by protein-digesting enzymes, proteins reach enterocytes in the form of peptides. Peptides are small chains of amino acids, and normally should not be absorbed until they are broken down into single amino acids.[4] This process is accomplished by enterocytes. On their hairy surface (the brush border) healthy enterocytes have peptide-digesting enzymes, called *peptidases*. Each peptidase is specific to a certain peptide chain and even to a certain chemical bond in this chain. These enzymes break the peptides down into single amino acids, which then get absorbed. In a child or adult with abnormal gut flora enterocytes are sick. They are unable to produce many peptidases or to accomplish this last step in protein break down and absorption of amino acids. At the same time the pathogenic bacteria, fungi and viruses damage the gut wall, allowing undigested peptides to leak through. The two most researched proteins which do not get broken down properly and get absorbed as peptides are *gluten* from grains and *casein* from milk. Some of these peptides have a structure similar to opiates and are called *gluteomorphins* and *casomorphins*.[7] They absorb and get into the brain in a similar fashion to opiates. The research into gluteomorphins and casomorphins was originally focused on autism and schizophrenia, where these substances have been shown to cause many mental symptoms characteristic for these disorders. In a person without such severe conditions undigested gluten and casein can cause depression, memory problems, inability to focus, sleep problems and other mental symptoms common amongst people with any chronic illness.[1]

Apart from gluten and casein, there are many other proteins in food which are not digested properly, absorb as peptides and cause problems in the body. We haven't researched all of them yet, but what we do know is that the most difficult for humans to digest are proteins from plants. Grains, beans, pulses, nuts and other plant matter contain many proteins which are indigestible for us and their amino acid composition is inappropriate for the human physiology. The most researched plant protein is gluten, and we are rapidly coming to the conclusion that the majority of humanity cannot digest it well.[8] On top of that, gluten has an ability to damage the gut wall's integrity, making it leaky and porous. When gluten absorbs undigested it is able to cause a plethora of health problems, from mental symptoms to arthritis, nephropathy and autoimmune disease. Depending on the person's general state of health and constitution, tolerance of gluten can vary dramatically, from full-blown celiac disease to a few mild symptoms. Bread (a major source of gluten in the diet) is a well-established staple in the world, and it may never occur to many people that their chronic headaches, arthritis, psoriasis, depression, allergies and other health problems are caused by consuming bread day after day.[9]

In the meantime, proteins are essential for us to have. The best sources of easy-to-digest and very nourishing proteins are eggs, meats, fish and well-fermented milk products. Proteins from these animal foods have the right amino acid composition for the human body to thrive on.[10] For GAPS children and adults it is important to eat easily digestible proteins to make work as easy as possible for their digestive systems. The way we cook meats and fish has an effect on their digestibility: boiled, stewed and poached meats and fish are much easier to digest than when fried, roasted or grilled. Eggs are one of nature's treasure chests of excellent quality protein, vitamins, minerals and many other useful nutrients.[11] Unless the patient shows a clear allergy, eggs should be an important part of the diet. We will talk about dairy products shortly.

Fats

To be digested and absorbed, fats require bile. The enterocytes do not have to do much work in absorbing fats. That is why clinical practice shows that natural fats in the diet, animal fats in particular, are well tolerated by people with digestive disorders. However, many people with chronic illnesses find it difficult to digest fats. In previous chapters we discussed the very common reason for poor fat digestion – gall stones accumulating in the liver and obstructing the bile flow. Apart from gall stones, there may be another problem in a person with abnormal gut flora. The gut lining is a mucous membrane. Any mucous membrane, when under attack from pathogens, produces a lot of mucus to protect itself. In people with digestive disorders mucus production can be excessive. These large amounts of mucus interfere with digestion of food, including fats. Mucus coats food particles and does not allow bile and digestive enzymes to get to them. As a result, a lot of fat goes undigested and often comes out as pale greasy stools. This impaired absorption of fats causes deficiencies in fat and fat-soluble vitamins: A, D, E and K. Clinical experience shows that, when starch and double sugars are out of the diet for a long-enough period, the production of mucus normalises and gall stones are naturally removed. As a result, the absorption of fats and fat-soluble vitamins normalises.

To summarise:

A GAPS patient has to avoid:

- All grains and anything made out of them: wheat, rye, rice, oats, corn, maize, sorghum, barley, buckwheat, millet, spelt, triticale, bulgur, tapioca, quinoa, couscous (some of them are not strictly grains, but are commonly perceived as such). Grains contain starch and other complex carbohydrates, proteins (gluten, hordein, secalin and other) and substances, called antinutrients, which are very difficult to digest and which can damage the gut lining and other tissues and organs in the human body.[12-15] These substances have been found to cause harm in healthy individuals, let alone in people with damaged gut flora and a sensitive digestive system. There is no doubt that removing grains is a must for a person with any chronic degenerative illness, physical or mental. This will remove a lot of starch and all gluten from the diet. In fact, removal of all grains makes the diet truly gluten free.[16]

- All starchy vegetables and anything made out of them: potato, yams, sweet potato, parsnip, Jerusalem artichoke, cassava, arrowroot and taro. Apart from starch, potatoes (and other starchy vegetables) contain antinutrients which can have a damaging effect on many organs in the human body.
- Sugar and anything that contains it. Sugar is a perfect food for pathogenic microbes in the gut. There can be no healing in the digestive system or anywhere else in the body without complete avoidance of table sugar. We will talk about sugar in more detail shortly.
- Starchy beans, legumes and pulses: soya beans, mung beans, garbanzo beans, bean sprouts, chickpeas, faba beans and many other varieties. There is no clear division between beans, legumes and pulses; these three names are often used interchangeably. Apart from starch, beans, legumes and pulses contain many antinutrients and are generally difficult to digest.[17] Some of them are allowed on the GAPS Diet, providing that they are properly prepared before consuming them. However, they can only be introduced when enough healing has happened in the digestive system of the person, which for many people means avoiding them for a year or longer.
- Lactose and anything that contains it: fluid or dried milk of any type, commercially produced yogurt, commercially produced buttermilk and sour cream, processed foods with added lactose. Lactose is a perfect food for pathogenic microbes in the gut and must be avoided by any person with a chronic illness.[18] When we ferment milk for 24 hours, we make it lactose free, because the fermenting bacteria love eating lactose. Homemade yogurt, kefir, sour cream and cheese are lactose free and are an important part of the GAPS Diet.

Antinutrients are substances in natural foods that have the ability to damage the human body, to impair digestion of food and cause nutritional deficiencies. They are almost exclusively found in plant foods, particularly in their seeds (grains, beans, pulses, legumes, seeds and nuts).[12–17] When plants produce seed, these are their babies. They don't want them to be eaten by other creatures; they want them to survive and grow. In order to protect them and make them unattractive for eating, plants put special substances into their seed – antinutrients. Some are designed to block vital enzymes in our bodies and are called enzymes inhibitors (protease inhibitors, lipase inhibitors, amylase inhibitors and other). They can impair digestion, protein synthesis, functioning of hormones and neurotransmitters and other important functions. Lectins are a group of antinutrients which can damage the immune system, the gut wall, the joints and many other organs. Another antinutrient in seeds, called phytic acid, binds to vital minerals and makes them unavailable for the body to use, particularly calcium, magnesium, iron, copper and zinc. Oxalates and oxalic acid are another group of antinutrients which bind minerals in the body. On top of that they can cause many unpleasant symptoms and reactions (such as behavioural abnormalities, painful urination and chronic cystitis). Green leafy vegetables are particularly rich in oxalates. Glucosinolates found in brassica vegetables (broccoli, cauliflower, cabbage and Brussels sprouts) bind iodine and can contribute to thyroid problems. Polyphenolic compounds, alkaloids, salicylates, saponins, tannins and flavonoids in plants can all cause problems, particularly when the person is unable to digest them[12-17]. GAPS people have a damaged digestive system and cannot handle many antinutrients. That is why plant foods present the biggest challenge for this group of patients. We have to remove the worst offenders out of the diet, such as grains, and we have to prepare vegetables and seeds (beans, nuts and other) carefully to make them more digestible.

Apart from these foods there is another category of products to avoid – processed 'foods'. Let us talk about this subject in some detail.

No processed foods, please!

We live in an era of convenience foods, which are also very processed foods. When Mother Nature made us, humans, she provided us with every food we need to stay healthy, active and full of energy. However, we have to eat these foods in the form Nature made them. It is when we start tampering with natural foods that we start getting into trouble. Any processing changes the food's chemical and biological structure. Our bodies were not designed for these changed foods! The more food is processed, the more nutrient depleted and chemically altered it becomes. Apart from losing its nutritional value, processed food loses most of its other properties: taste, flavour and colour. To compensate, various chemicals are added: flavour enhancers, colours, various E-numbers, additives and preservatives.[19–29] Many of these chemicals have been conclusively shown to contribute to many chronic health problems, physical and mental. Natural foods do not keep very well, so the industry has to change them to prolong their shelf life. So, natural foods get subjected to extreme heat, pressure, enzymes, solvents and countless number of other chemicals, fats get hydrogenated and proteins get denatured. Natural foods get changed into various chemical concoctions, which are then packaged nicely and presented to us as 'food'. This 'food' is made to suit commercial purposes where health considerations never enter the calculation. The manufacturers are obliged to list all the ingredients on the label. However, if the manufacturer uses an ingredient, which has already been processed or is made from processed substances, the manufacturer is not obliged to list what that ingredient was made from. So, if you are trying to avoid something in particular, like sugar or gluten for example, reading an ingredient list may not always help you.

If we look at supermarket shelves, we will see that the bulk of processed foods are carbohydrates. All those breakfast cereals, crisps, biscuits, crackers, breads, pastries, pastas, chocolates, sweets, jams, jellies, condiments, sugar, preserved fruit and vegetables, frozen precooked meals with starches and batter are highly processed carbohydrates. We will examine some of them in detail. But first, let's look at them as a group.

All carbohydrates in foods get digested and absorbed as monosugars, largely as glucose. Nature provides us with plenty of carbohydrates in the form of fruit, vegetables and grains. When we eat them in a natural untampered form, the carbohydrate in them gets absorbed slowly, producing a gradual increase in blood glucose, which our bodies are designed to handle. Processed carbohydrates get absorbed very quickly, producing an unnaturally rapid increase in blood glucose.[30] Blood glucose is one of those factors which our bodies go to great lengths to keep within certain limits, because both high and low values are harmful. A rapid increase in blood glucose, called **hyperglycaemia**, puts the body into a state of shock, prompting it to pump out lots of insulin very quickly to deal with the excessive glucose. As a result of this overproduction of insulin, about an hour later you will have a very low level of blood glucose, called **hypoglycaemia**. Have you ever noticed that after eating a sugary breakfast cereal in the morning you feel hungry again in an hour? That is hypoglycaemia. What do people usually have at that time in the morning to satisfy their hunger? A biscuit, a chocolate bar, a coffee or something like that, and the whole cycle of hyper-hypoglycaemia begins again. This up and down blood glucose roller coaster is extremely harmful for adults and children. It has been proved that a lot of hyperactivity, irritability, inability to concentrate and learn, aggression and other behavioural abnormalities in school children and adults at work are a direct result of this glucose roller coaster.[31,32] The hyperglycaemic phase produces the feeling of a 'high' with hyperactive and manic tendencies, whilst the hypoglycaemic phase makes the person feel unwell, often with a headache, bad mood, tantrums, aggression and general fatigue with excessive sweating. Fear of the hypoglycaemic symptoms can make the person dependant on sweet things and chocolate, making it very difficult to remove processed carbohydrates from the diet.

Another important point about processed carbohydrates is their detrimental effect on the gut flora. Processed carbohydrates feed pathogenic bacteria and fungi in the gut, promoting their growth and proliferation. Apart from that they make a wonderful gluelike environment in the gut for various worms and parasites to take hold and develop. These creatures convert carbohydrates into toxic substances, which go into the bloodstream and literally 'poison' the person. The more processed carbohydrates the person has, the more 'toxic' he or she becomes, and the more physical and mental symptoms we see.[33–35]

In the previous chapters we have looked in detail at the state of the immune system in GAPS patients. Compromised immunity plays an important role in development of GAPS. By negatively altering the gut flora, processed carbohydrates play an important role in damaging the person's immune system. However, on top of that, there is ample evidence showing that processed foods, particularly processed carbohydrates and sugar, directly weaken the functioning of macrophages, natural killer cells and other white blood cells and undermine systemic resistance to all infections.[36-38] Immune-compromised people who have sugary drinks and crisps daily will worsen their immune system's condition by these food choices.

As if all that is not enough, processed carbohydrates are the cause of our biggest health crisis in the modern world: the epidemics of heart disease, obesity, diabetes, dementia (Alzheimer's disease) and cancer. By constantly increasing the blood glucose levels, processed carbohydrates cause a chronic condition in the body called *Metabolic Syndrome*, which is the basis for all these health problems.[39] To learn about it, please, look in the *chapter A–Z, Metabolic Syndrome* and read my book *Put your heart in your mouth. What really causes heart disease and what we can do to prevent and even reverse it.*[40]

Let us have a look at some of the most common forms of processed carbohydrates.

Breakfast cereals

They are supposed to be healthy, aren't they? That is what numerous TV advertisements tell us. Unfortunately, the truth is just the opposite.[41,42]

- Breakfast cereals are highly processed carbohydrates, full of sugar, salt and other unhealthy substances. A bowl of breakfast cereal will start your day (or your child's day) with the first round of the blood sugar roller coaster bringing a plethora of unpleasant symptoms.
- Being a great source of processed carbohydrates, breakfast cereals feed pathogenic bacteria and fungi in the gut, allowing them to produce a new portion of their toxins perpetuating the vicious cycle of GAPS.
- What about fibre? The manufacturers claim that with a bowl of their product you will get all the fibre you need. Unfortunately, it is the wrong kind of fibre for GAPS and non-GAPS people alike. The fibre in breakfast cereals is harsh on the gut and full of health-damaging antinutrients. On top of that, fibre feeds pathogenic microbes in the GAPS gut causing inflammation and digestive symptoms.[43]
- An interesting experiment has been performed in one of the food laboratories. They analysed the nutritional value of some brands of breakfast cereals and the boxes in which these cereals were packaged. The analysis showed that the box, made of wood pulp, had more useful nutrients in it than the cereal inside.[44] Indeed, breakfast cereals have very low nutritional value. To compensate, the manufacturers fortify them with synthetic forms of vitamins, claiming that by eating your morning bowl of this cereal you will get all your daily requirements of those vitamins. Well, the human body has been designed to recognise and use natural vitamins, so synthetic vitamins have a very low absorption rate – most of them go through and out of your digestive tract without doing you any good. Whatever amount of vitamin does get absorbed is often not recognised by the body as food but gets taken straight to the kidneys and excreted in urine. We have a new syndrome in our modern pill-popping society – a 'syndrome of expensive urine'.

So, no matter what the advertisements say, there is nothing healthy in breakfast cereals for anybody, let alone a GAPS person.

Crisps (potato chips) and chips (French fries) and other starchy snacks

Crisps, chips, popcorn and other snacks are highly processed carbohydrates with a detrimental effect on the gut flora.[41] But that is not all: they are saturated with vegetable oil which has been heated to a very high temperature. Any plant oil that has been heated has substances called trans-fatty acids, which are unsaturated fatty acids with an altered chemical structure.[45] What they do in the body is to replace normal fatty acids in cellular structure, making the cells dysfunctional. Consuming trans-fatty acids has a direct damaging effect on the immune system. Cancer, heart disease, eczema, asthma and many neurological and psychiatric conditions have been linked to trans-fatty acids in the diet. For the full story about fat processing please look in the chapter: *Fats: the good and the bad.*

Some years ago, another strong argument appeared against consuming crisps and chips: the acrylamides story.[46–48] In the spring of 2002, the Swedish National Food Administration and Stockholm University reported that they found highly neurotoxic and carcinogenic substances in potato crisps, French fries, bread and other baked and fried starchy foods. These substances are acrylamides. Scientists in Norway, UK and Switzerland have confirmed this finding. They have also found acrylamides in starchy foods, fried or baked at high temperatures. Recently, instant coffee has been added to the list of foods containing these highly dangerous substances. The World Health Organisation, United Nations Food and Agriculture Organisation and the US Food and Drug Administration have developed a plan to identify how acrylamides are formed in foods and what can be done to eliminate them, since they can cause cancer, neurological damage and infertility. Acrylamides are so harmful to health that there are certain maximum limits set for these substances in food packaging materials. For years government agencies paid a lot of attention to controlling the amounts of acrylamides in plastic food packaging, but nobody looked at the food inside that packaging. Now it has been discovered that some foods inside these plastic packets have incredibly high amounts of acrylamides, way above all allowed limits. The acrylamides story provides another reason to avoid crisps, chips and other starchy snack foods and all other processed 'foods'.

Flour made from wheat, rye, maize and other grains

Cutting out gluten is widely recommended for coeliac disease, mental illness and other chronic diseases; gluten-free products made from gluten-free flour have become a staple for people with an increasing list of health problems. But, let us have a look at grain flour as a whole, with gluten or without it. Grains contain many fragile substances which get damaged by grinding them into flour, and which get further damaged by oxidation while the flour is being stored.[49] Flour is a highly processed substance. In the West, it arrives at bakeries in pre-packaged mixes for different kinds of breads, biscuits and pastries. These mixtures are already processed, with the best nutrients lost. Then they are 'enriched' with preservatives, pesticides to keep insects away, chemical substances to prevent it absorbing moisture, colour and flavour improvers and softeners, just to mention a few. The producers take the gluten out of these mixtures to make gluten-free products. You still get all the processed carbohydrate with all the chemical additives in it, but this time without gluten. Once swallowed, a piece of bread turns into a gluelike mass, which feeds parasites and pathogenic bacteria and fungi in the gut, contributing to the general toxic overload. Flour is the main ingredient in most processed foods in the world, wheat flour being the most common. Being staples around the world, grains are also the number one cause of food allergies and intolerances: maize in South America, rice in Asia and wheat in the rest of the world.[44]

Sugar and anything made with it

Sugar was once called 'the white death'. It deserves 100% of this title.[50–54] The consumption of sugar in the world has grown to enormous proportions and it is a highly processed substance. Sugar is everywhere and it is hard to find any processed food without it. Apart from causing the blood glucose roller coaster and having a detrimental effect on the gut flora, it has been shown to have a direct damaging effect on the immune system, which is already compromised in GAPS patients. On top of that, to deal with the sugar onslaught, the body has to use available minerals, vitamins and enzymes at an alarming rate, finishing up being depleted of these vital substances. For example, to metabolise only one molecule of sugar the body requires around 56 molecules of magnesium. Consumption of sugar is a major reason for widespread magnesium deficiency in our modern society, leading to high blood pressure, neurological, immune and many other problems.[55,56] A person with a chronic illness is already deficient in magnesium and many other vital nutrients and should not have sugar in any form. Cakes, sweets (candy), and other confectioneries are made with sugar and flour, as the main ingredients, plus lots of chemicals like colours, preservatives, flavourings, etc. It goes without saying that they should be out of the diet of any person with health problems

Soft drinks are a major source of sugar in our modern diets, not to mention all the chemical additives.[57-59] A can of soda can contain from 5 to 10 teaspoons of sugar. Fruit juices are full of processed fruit sugars and moulds. Unless freshly pressed, they should not be in your diet either. As the population started to learn about the harmful effects of sugar on the human body, industry started coming up with other sweeteners to replace sugar. All of them are synthetic chemicals or highly processed substances and are incompatible with good health. For example, aspartame, a sugar replacement in so-called 'diet' drinks, has been found to be carcinogenic and neurotoxic and should be avoided by all children and adults.[60-63] Its consumption has been connected with the development of multiple sclerosis in particular.

No Soya, please!

Soya is very big business, particularly in the USA. A large percentage of the industry uses genetically modified soya (some 95% of all soya produced in the world is genetically modified).[64] Soya is cheap to produce and is very profitable. It can be found in many processed foods, margarines, salad dressings and sauces, breads, biscuits (cookies), pizza, baby food, children's snacks, sweets, cakes, vegetarian products, dairy replacements, infant milk formulas, etc. Is there a problem with that? Let us have a look at some facts.

1. Traditionally soya has been used in Japan and other Eastern cultures as a whole bean fermented as soy sauce, tofu, miso, tempeh, natto and other recipes.[65] Soya beans are very hard to digest and contain a lot of antinutrients harmful to health, so traditional cultures have taken time and care to process soya beans to make them digestible and to remove antinutrients. Unfortunately, none of that wisdom made its way to the West. The form in which soya is used in the West is called *soya protein isolate*.[66] How is it made? After their fibre has been removed with an alkaline solution, the soya beans are put into large aluminium tanks with an acid wash. Acid makes the soya beans absorb aluminium, which will remain in the end product.[64] Aluminium has been linked to dementia and Alzheimer's disease and, indeed, there has been a lot of publicity recently linking soya consumption with these mental disorders.[67,68] After the aluminium-acid wash the beans are treated with many other chemicals including nitrates, which have been implicated in cancer development.[65] The end product is an almost tasteless powder, easy to use and add to any food. All Western soya products are made from this highly processed powder, which is included in most processed foods, bread, soya milk products and soya infant formulas.
2. Soya is a natural goitrogen; it has an ability to impair thyroid function.[65,71] Due to various toxins found in GAPS patients they are, almost without exception, hypothyroid, which means that their thyroid function is already impaired. Low thyroid function has very serious implications for adults and children. Having soya products in the diet would damage thyroid function even further.
3. Soya beans have a very high concentration of phytates.[73,74] These are antinutrients, found in all grains as well, particularly in their bran. Phytates have a strong ability to bind to minerals, preventing them from being absorbed, particularly calcium, magnesium, iron and zinc. Children and adults with chronic disease are already deficient in these vital minerals. Adding soya to their diet would make these deficiencies

worse. Other antinutrients have been found in soya, such as enzyme inhibitors and lectins.[64,66,69]

4. Soya is a powerful allergen. Ample research has demonstrated that Western soya products cause many forms of allergies and other immune abnormalities in children and adults.[64] For sensitive people, particularly people with eczema, asthma, hay fever and allergies *it is important to look for soya-free eggs, meat and milk*. This means that animals must not be fed soya in any form. Truly soya-free foods may be difficult to find, as the majority of soya produced goes into animal feed, including nutritional supplements for animals. A farmer may not be able to avoid soya completely unless he makes his own animal feed. Sensitive people may need to find such farmers and buy eggs, meat and milk directly from them. Unfortunately, in my experience, eggs, meat or milk may be labelled soya-free in a shop, but are not truly so.
5. Initially soya gained popularity in the West as a treatment for menopause because it contains natural oestrogens or phytoestogens.[70,71,72] We now know that these substances are not useful for menopausal women and are downright dangerous for the rest of the population, particularly for small children. There is growing concern among health professionals about the amount of phytoestogens infants and small children might be getting from soya milk and infant formulas. [75,76] Any person with a degenerative illness, whether child or adult, already has abnormal hormonal balance in the body. Adding another interference in the form of phytoestogens is not a good idea.
6. More research is coming out showing that Western soya products are implicated in cancer, heart disease, diabetes, mental illness and learning disabilities, autoimmune disease and many other chronic illnesses.[64-76]

What about soya in the natural traditional form as a soy sauce, tofu, tempeh, natto, etc.? For the first few years of following the GAPS Diet soya should be avoided in all forms. When full recovery has been achieved, traditional soya products can be slowly added into the diet.

Soya, sugar and wheat flour are so insidious that it can be very hard to find any processed food on the supermarket shelves without them. Any patient with a chronic illness, mental or physical, should have no processed foods at all in his/her diet. All foods should be bought fresh, as close to the way Nature made them as possible, and prepared at home. A digestive tract is a long tube. What you fill that tube with has a direct effect on its well-being. A GAPS digestive system is damaged and very sensitive. You cannot trust any food manufacturer to fill it for you. Instead fill your digestive system (or the gut of a child or an adult in your care) yourself with freshly cooked nourishing food, where you are in control and in charge of what the exact ingredients are and how they are prepared. Eating out a lot is a very unhealthy practice and has to be severely limited (that includes takeaway meals). You have no idea how your food was prepared and what ingredients were used.

Here is an alphabetic list of foods that have to be avoided on the GAPS Diet.

Foods to avoid

Acesulfame
Acidophilus milk
Agar-agar
Agave syrup
Algae
Aloe vera (once digestive symptoms have gone, you can introduce it)
Amaranth
Apple juice
Arrowroot
Aspartame
Astragalus
Baked beans
Baker's yeast
Baking powder and raising agents of all kind, apart from pure bicarbonate of soda
Balsamic vinegar
Barley
Bean flour and sprouts
Bee pollen
Beer
Bhindi or okra
Bitter gourd
Black-eye beans
Bologna
Bouillon cubes or granules
Brandy
Buckwheat
Bulgur
Burdock root
Butter beans
Buttermilk
Canellini beans
Canned vegetables and fruit

Carob
Carrageenan
Cellulose gum
Cereals, including all breakfast cereals
Cheeses, processed and cheese spreads
Chestnuts and chestnut flour
Chevre cheese
Chewing gum
Chickpeas
Chickory root
Chocolate
Cocoa powder
Coffee, instant and coffee substitutes
Cooking oils
Cordials
Corn
Cornstarch
Corn syrup
Cottage cheese
Cottonseed
Couscous
Cream
Cream of tartar
Cream cheese
Dextrose
Drinks, soft
Faba beans
Feta cheese
Fish, preserved, smoked, salted, breaded and canned with sauces
Flour, made out of grains
FOS (fructooligosaccharides)
Fructose
Fruit, canned or preserved
Garbanzo beans
Gjetost cheese
Grains, all
Gruyère cheese
Ham
Hot dogs
Ice cream, commercial
Jams
Jellies
Jerusalem artichoke

Ketchup, commercially available
Lactose
Liqueurs
Margarines and butter replacements
Meats, processed, preserved, smoked and salted
Millet
Milk from any animal, soya, rice, canned coconut milk
Milk, dried
Molasses
Mozzarella cheese
Mung beans
Neufchatel cheese
NutraSweet (aspartame)
Nuts, salted, roasted and coated
Oats
Okra
Parsnips
Pasta, of any kind
Pectin
Postum
Potato
Potato, sweet
Primost cheese
Quinoa
Rice
Ricotta cheese
Rye
Saccharin
Sago
Sausages, commercially available
Semolina
Sherry
Soda soft drinks
Sour cream, commercial
Soya
Spelt
Starch
Sugar or sucrose of any kind
Tapioca
Tea, instant
Triticale
Turkey loaf
Vegetables, canned or preserved

Wheat
Wheat germ
Whey, powder or liquid
Yams
Yogurt, commercial

Recommended foods

The GAPS Diet is designed to heal and seal the gut wall and normalise the digestion of food. This is a nutrient-dense diet and will remove nutritional deficiencies in your body quite quickly. As the digestive wall seals itself, the river of toxicity that used to flow from your gut into your body will stop. This will allow your body to clean out remaining toxins and start repairing itself. No matter how far away from the gut your particular set of symptoms may be, healing and sealing the gut wall must be the first step in your recovery. The roots of our health are in our gut! In order to lay a solid foundation for healing from any chronic illness it is essential to attend to those roots first. That is why I recommend the GAPS Diet as the basis for healing from any chronic disease, both physical and mental. We have had a look at what we must avoid. Now let us look at what we are going to eat on a daily basis.

Meat and fish

All fresh or frozen meats, game, organ meats, poultry, fish and shellfish are recommended.

Meats and fish are an excellent source of nutrition. Contrary to popular belief it is meats, fish and other animal products that have the highest content of vitamins, amino acids, nourishing fats, minerals and other nutrients which we humans need on a daily basis.[77] All this nutrition in meats and fish also comes in the most digestible form for us humans. I find it misleading to see vitamin tables in some books on nutrition showing that plants provide all our vitamins. First of all, the form in which plants contain these vitamins is difficult for us to digest. Secondly, if you compare the amounts of vitamins in meat, fish or other animal products with plants, it is the animal products which are at the top of the list.[78-80] Let us have a look at some of them.

Vitamin B1 (thiamin): the richest sources are pork, liver, heart and kidneys.

Vitamin B2 (riboflavin): the richest sources are eggs, meat, milk, poultry and fish.

Vitamin B3 (niacin): the richest sources are meat and poultry.
Vitamin B5 (pantothenic acid): the richest sources are meats and liver.
Vitamin B6 (pyridoxine): the richest sources are meat, poultry, fish and eggs.
Vitamin B12 (cyanocobalamin): the richest sources are meat, poultry, fish, eggs and milk.
Biotin: the richest sources are liver and egg yolks.
Vitamin A: the richest sources are liver, fish, egg yolks and butter. We are talking about the real vitamin A, which is ready for the body to use. You will see in many publications that you can get vitamin A from fruit and vegetables in the form of carotenoids. The problem is that carotenoids have to be converted into real vitamin A in the body, and a lot of us are unable to do this, because we are too toxic, or because we have an ongoing inflammation in the body.[79] So, if you do not consume animal products with the real vitamin A, then you may develop a deficiency in this vital vitamin despite eating lots of carrots. Vitamin A deficiency will lead to impaired immunity, eye problems and impaired learning and development.[77] GAPS people cannot convert carotenoids into the real vitamin A and must consume it in a ready-made form from animal foods. Many processed foods are fortified with synthetic vitamin A, which does not work in the body and is generally toxic.[81]
Vitamin D: the richest sources are fish liver oils, eggs and fish (particularly livers and fish eggs). The Western world is in the midst of a vitamin D deficiency epidemic and the food industry is starting to fortify processed foods with this vitamin. Just as with any other synthetic vitamin it does not work. Only natural foods and exposure to sunlight can provide humans with real vitamin D.[82]
Folic acid derivatives: the richest source by far is liver. Green leafy vegetables are considered a good source, though they contain much less folates and are more difficult to digest. It is easier for the human digestive system to extract nutrients from animal foods. Folic acid derivatives are particularly essential to have in pregnancy in order to prevent neural tube defects in the baby. That is why every traditional culture made sure that pregnant women ate liver regularly in order to provide plenty of folates, as well as many other nutrients, in the biochemical form which is easy to digest and assimilate.[83]
Vitamin K_2 (menaquinone): the richest sources are organ meats, full fat cheese, good quality butter and cream (yellow and orange from pastured animals), animal fats and egg yolks. Amongst its many functions in the body this vitamin is essential for normal calcium metabolism, its deficiency leads to deposition of calcium in soft tissues and initiation of inflammation, while the bones and teeth do not get

enough calcium. Apart from the high-fat foods an important source of this vitamin is our own gut flora: the probiotic microbes in the gut produce and release vitamin K_2. Fermented foods are full of vitamin K_2 as the bacteria produce it in the process of fermentation; natto (fermented soya beans) is one of the richest plant sources.[84]

Two well-researched vitamins which meats and fish do not appear to provide, as far as we know, are vitamin C and vitamin K_1 (phylloquinone); they have to come from vegetables and fruit. However, recent research indicates that animal liver is a good source of vitamin C.[85] Fruit, apart from avocado and lemon, generally interferes with the digestion of meats and should be eaten between meals. Vegetables, however, combine well with meats and fish and would provide any missing nutrients.

The majority of GAPS patients are anaemic. It is essential for people with anaemia to have red meats on a regular basis (lamb, beef, game and organ meats in particular) because these foods are the best remedy for anaemia. They not only provide iron in the haem-form: the form which the human body absorbs best, they also provide the B vitamins and other nutrients essential for treating anaemia. Meats also promote better absorption of non-haem iron from vegetables and fruit, while vitamin C from vegetables and greens promotes absorption of iron from meat. Large epidemiological studies show that eating red meat is associated with a much lower incidence of iron deficiency and anaemia in different countries of the world.[86]

An absolute resuscitation for an anaemic person (and any other nutritional deficiency) is eating liver. Liver is a true powerhouse of nutrition.[87] No matter what the nutrient, you will find it in abundance in liver, including all the nutrients which GAPS people are deficient in. Making sure that the GAPS patient eats some liver on a regular basis will do immeasurably more for his or her nutritional status than the best and the most expensive supplements in the world. An anaemic person should eat some liver and other organ meats every day until anaemia is gone. After that a piece of liver should be eaten once a week at least.

Make sure that you buy meats and fish fresh or frozen, but not preserved, as preserved meats and fish have a lot of additives (E numbers, preservatives, starches, sugar, the wrong kind of salt, lactose and other ingredients) which will not allow the digestive system to heal. Ham, bacon, delicatessen meats and all commercially available sausages are preserved meats and should be avoided. Sausages are a popular food. I recommend finding a local butcher who will produce pure meat sausages for you. The only ingredients in these sausages should be full fat minced meat, salt and pepper. If you wish to add some fresh garlic, onion or fresh herbs to the mince, that is fine. It is important to emphasise that no commercial seasoning or sausage mix should be added. Many commercial seasonings for sausages contain a flavour enhancer MSG (monosodium glutamate), which GAPS people must not consume.

Meat, bone or fish stocks are wonderful nutritional and digestive remedies.[87] When you cook meats, bones and fish in water a lot of nutrients get extracted into the water. Use these stocks for making soups, stews and simply as a warming therapeutic drink with and between meals. In the recipe section you will find detailed instructions on how to make meat, bone and fish stocks. It goes without saying that all commercially available stock granules and cubes are to be avoided. They do not possess any of the healing properties of a homemade meat stock and are full of detrimental ingredients. Meats cooked in water are easier to digest for a person with a sensitive digestive system. Avoid lean meats; our physiology can only use meat fibres when they come with the fat, collagen and other substances that a proper piece of meat will provide. GAPS people need plenty of animal fats, so choose pieces of meat with a good fat covering. When we eat poultry it is important to eat the skin and the fats, as well as the meat. When we eat fish it is essential to eat the skin as well as the meat; that is why fish must always be descaled before cooking.

The best meat comes from animals which were allowed to live the way Mother Nature designed them to live – grazing freely on organic pasture in the sunlight. However, buying organic meat can be expensive. I have had many patients with very limited funds who bought any meat they could find, and they healed! Animals have powerful detoxification systems, which work constantly on neutralising agricultural toxins. That is why eating a piece of non-organic, conventionally raised meat is infinitely safer than eating vegetables which have been sprayed with chemicals. Animal liver does not accumulate toxins, it neutralises them. So, in my clinical experience, eating liver is safe and very beneficial whether it came from organic or non-organic animals. Buying meats does not have to be expensive. I recommend my patients to find a good local butcher and buy meat from him regularly. When a friendly relationship is established, many butchers are happy to provide large bags of bones and offcuts for free, to make meat stock, bone broth and soup. These offcuts and bones are the most nourishing parts of the animal and, typically, they are discarded because the majority of people want to buy pure muscle (steaks, chops, etc). Organ meats are not a popular food in the Western world, so your butcher may be happy to sell liver, tongue, heart and other organs to you very cheaply, or even give them to you for free (as long as you have already paid for some other meat, of course!). I also recommend buying meat in bulk directly from farmers or smallholders. When you buy a whole lamb, half a pig, a dozen chickens, or a quarter of a cow you will pay a lower price overall, and you can make sure that the animals have been raised naturally. You will get all the bones, muscle, organs and other tissues of the animal; nothing will be discarded. To ensure a good dinner on a daily basis, just purchase a second-hand chest freezer and fill it up with meat. Instead of rushing to shops looking for meat, all you have to do is to get a piece out of your freezer in the morning to defrost for dinner, or cook a frozen piece in water to make soup, or put a frozen piece of meat into your slow cooker in the morning (with some water, salt and spices), so by dinner time it will be ready to eat. Buying meat in bulk directly from the farmer saves a lot of time and effort, and means that you can buy home-raised healthy animals at a lower price.

Eggs

Eggs are one the most nourishing and easy-to-digest foods on this planet. Raw egg yolk has been compared with human breast milk, because it can be almost 100% absorbed without needing digestion. Egg yolks will provide you with most essential amino acids, many vitamins (B1, B2, B6, B12, A, D, biotin), essential fatty acids, zinc, magnesium and many other nutrients, so necessary for healing.[86] Eggs are particularly rich in vitamin B12, which is vital for normal development of the nervous system and immunity. The large majority of GAPS patients are deficient in B12, and hence anaemic.

Egg yolks are very rich in cholin – an amino acid essential for the nervous system and the liver to function. Cholin is a building block of a neurotransmitter called acethylcholin, which the brain uses for cognitive or learning processes and memory amongst its many functions.[88] Cholin supplementation is recommended for people with neurological damage, memory loss and poor learning ability. Cholin is also prescribed to people with liver problems. GAPS patients almost invariably benefit from extra cholin in their diet. Egg yolks, particularly uncooked, provide the best food source of cholin.

Sadly, based on some faulty 'science' and commercial publicity, eggs have been made unpopular despite their wonderful nutritional value. This happened because eggs contain cholesterol. In the last few decades there have been a number of clinical studies confirming that consuming eggs has nothing to do with heart disease or atherosclerosis.[89] In fact, people who consume eggs show a lower risk of these health problems. We will talk in some detail about cholesterol and its role in the body in the chapter on fats. But, to learn what causes heart disease and how to prevent and even reverse it, please read my book *Put your heart in your mouth*.

I suggest getting your eggs from a source you trust. Free-range organic eggs are the best because the hens have much better nutrition, are not fed antibiotics and agricultural chemicals and are exposed to sun, green pasture and fresh air. Free-range organic eggs are also better from another important point of view – the concern about *Salmonella*. According to the National Egg Marketing Board around one in 7000 eggs may harbour *Salmonella*. These are the numbers for battery eggs laid by hens in cages. Salmonella-infected eggs come from an infected hen. Free-range organically reared hens are much less likely to have *Salmonella,* as they possess much healthier immune systems. Raw egg yolks are more nourishing than cooked. However, if you feel unsure about the source of the eggs you bought, then cook them any way you prefer. *Salmonella* is destroyed when eggs are cooked thoroughly. Try to find a good supply of natural organic eggs from pastured birds, so it is safe for you to consume egg yolks raw.

Egg whites are usually cooked, simply because most of us don't like the taste of raw whites. Though one case of biotin deficiency has been described where a person lived on a self-fashioned diet of raw egg whites,[86] there is no conclusive evidence as to why we should not eat them raw as well. However, when it comes to egg allergy, whites are usually the part of the egg which the majority of sufferers react to, because the whites contain very complex proteins and antigens. Egg yolks contain single amino acids, which virtually do not need digestion. That is why a lot of people with egg allergy can tolerate egg yolks if carefully separated from the whites.

If you suspect a real allergy to egg, which can be dangerous, before introducing it do the **Sensitivity Test**. You need to test egg yolks and egg whites separately. Take a drop of raw egg yolk (carefully separated from the white, so there is no contamination) and place it on the inside of the patient's wrist. Do it at bedtime. Let the drop dry on the skin before letting your patient go to sleep. In the morning check the spot: if there is an angry, itchy red reaction, avoid egg yolks for a few weeks, and then do the test again. If there is no reaction, then go ahead and introduce egg yolks gradually, starting with a small amount. Do the Sensitivity Test with the raw egg white in the same way on a separate night.

If a GAPS child or adult has a true allergy to eggs and must avoid them, you will find delicious egg-free recipes in the recipe section of this book. If there is no allergy, eggs should be a regular part of your diet. I generally recommend that a GAPS child consumes 2-6 uncooked or lightly cooked egg yolks per day (with or without the whites) and an adult 4-8 egg yolks per day with or without the whites.

Milk and dairy products

The GAPS Diet permits lactose-free dairy products. Lactose is a milk sugar with a double molecule. It is present in fresh milk and many commercially available dairy products. According to various sources, from 25% to 90% of the planet's population cannot digest lactose due to a lack of the lactose-digesting enzyme, called lactase.[90] Children and adults with GAPS and people with gut problems most certainly cannot digest it and have to avoid it. Well-fermented milk products, such as kefir, yogurt, soured cream and natural cheese, are largely free of lactose, because in the process of fermentation the fermenting bacteria consume lactose as their food.

Apart from lactose, milk contains other substances which GAPS people may have a problem with. The most researched substance is the milk protein casein. When a person cannot digest it well, it can absorb in the form of casomorphins – peptides with an opiate structure, which are found in the urine of autistic, schizophrenic, depressed and other patients.[91] Casomorphins come from inappropriate digestion of casein. They absorb through the damaged gut lining into the bloodstream of the GAPS person, cross the blood-brain barrier and affect the functions of the brain. And, indeed, when dairy products are completely removed from the diet of some (not all) autistic children or schizophrenic patients, we observe an improvement in the clinical picture, sometimes quite dramatic. There is a debate about what particular form of casein is the problem. The group of proteins called beta-caseins have received most attention. For example, Cade and other researchers have shown that in an unhealthy digestive system they convert into beta-casomorphin-7, which gets taken up by 32 areas of the brain, many of which are responsible for vision, hearing and communication.[92]

Another problem with dairy is its great ability to create allergies and intolerances. Real allergy to milk is one of the most common allergies in existence, because dairy products have a wide range of antigens (various immunoglobulins). According to various research papers it is the main reason for infantile colic. Even in breastfed babies, if the mother consumes dairy products, the child may develop colic due to sensitivity to dairy antigens being passed through the mother's milk. In many cases when the breastfeeding mother stops consuming dairy foods the colic in her baby goes away.

All this information is correct if you do not take into account a wonderful natural process, called fermentation. When milk is properly fermented at home, a large percentage of the proteins get pre-digested, immunoglobulins get broken down and lactose is consumed by the fermenting microbes. Fermentation makes milk much easier for the human gut to handle. On top of that, fermenting bacteria produce lactic acid, which has a healing and soothing influence on the gut lining. Many important vitamins are produced during fermentation (B vitamins, biotin, vitamin K2 and others) and active enzymes.[93] Unfortunately, commercially available fermented dairy products are not fermented long enough to make the milk suitable for GAPS patients. On top of that they are often pasteurised after fermentation, which kills the probiotic microbes, destroys enzymes and vitamins and changes the structure of proteins, fats and other nutrients in the product. That is why *only home-fermented dairy products* are recommended for GAPS people. In my experience, the majority of GAPS children and adults tolerate homemade yogurt, sour cream and kefir perfectly well as part of their GAPS Introduction Diet. Whether or not you are sure you belong to this group, I recommend doing the Sensitivity Test to see if there is a real allergy to dairy. Take a drop of your homemade yogurt, sour cream or kefir and place it on the inside of the patient's wrist. Do it at bedtime. Let the drop dry on the skin, before letting your patient go to sleep. In the morning check the spot: if there is no reaction, then go ahead and introduce dairy as part of the GAPS Introduction Diet. If there is an angry red reaction, then there is an allergy. In that case you will have to do the Introduction Diet without dairy, and later in the diet you can try to follow the *Dairy Introduction Structure* using the Sensitivity Test at every step. The Dairy Introduction Structure has been described in detail in the chapter *The Full GAPS Diet*.

The good news for many sensitive patients is that dairy products do not have to be out of the diet forever. As the gut lining heals many GAPS patients, who used to react to dairy, stop reacting and are able to introduce yogurt, sour cream, kefir, cheese and butter. Dairy products are delicious and give the diet a nice variety; it is worth working on introducing them! But before we start, it is important to find the right supply of milk.

What is the right supply of milk? We have to find milk from native breeds which have not been extensively crossbred by agricultural science. Did you know that the vast majority of milk products in Western supermarkets come from the Holstein-Friesian breed, which has been selectively bred to produce very large animals, yielding at least three times more milk than any native breed? [94,95] These animals are prone to illness and infection and so are given antibiotics, hormones and other drugs regularly. A large percentage of them have mastitis at any time, suffer from arthritis and die from cancer. [95] An unhealthy animal produces unhealthy milk! Modern science has accumulated a mountain of research to show that dairy products can cause disease in humans: from allergies, autoimmunity and heart disease to mental illness and cancer. Almost all of that research has been done on milk products from these modern breeds of cow! In the GAPS Diet we do not use their milk, which excludes most dairy products available in the supermarkets. We buy milk directly from organic farms with more robust breeds, such as Jersey, Guernsey, Ayrshire, Shorthorn and British Friesian, or from native breeds in different parts of the world.

Milk from other animals is often better tolerated by sensitive patients than cow's milk. The most readily available is goat's milk and, again, we want milk from natural breeds on organic pasture. Ewe's milk, donkey milk, deer milk, horse milk and camel milk are available in some countries and can also be used. There is some research showing many health benefits from consuming milk from these animals. In traditional cultures milk from all animals has largely been consumed in a fermented form: yogurt, sour cream and cheese – exactly what we do in the GAPS Diet.

Once you have found a farm where you can get organic milk from natural breeds of animals, make sure to buy this milk raw! This is milk straight from the animal which has not been pasteurised, homogenised or tampered with in any other way. This milk can be called 'alive' because it is full of enzymes which will digest this milk for you, leaving very little work for your digestive system. Many people who cannot digest lactose can handle raw milk without any problems. Raw milk is full of 'alive' vitamins, amino acids, proteins, essential fats and many other nutrients in the biochemical shape and form which our bodies need.[94,95]

When we pasteurise milk, we destroy these nutrients; we alter their biochemical structure, which makes them difficult for us to digest and assimilate and, as a result, they cause allergies and other problems.[96] Homogenisation is when the milk is forced through a fine mesh to break down the fat globules. This is done purely for cosmetic purposes and takes the milk one more step away from its natural state, making it more processed.

For thousands of years people used to give their babies raw milk straight from the animal, with great benefits and no problems. We started getting problems only when we started giving our babies processed dead milk. In many countries of the world people still give their babies raw milk. They know that the baby must not have milk which has been pasteurised, boiled, homogenised or processed in any other way because the baby would get sick. Vets in Western countries know very well the harmful effects of processed milk and do not recommend giving it to cats, dogs or any other animals. Incidentally, all these animals thrive beautifully on raw milk. For some reason human health has not received such detailed attention – we are not told about the harm processed milk can do to our health.

Why do we pasteurise our milk? Because years ago there was a risk of getting some serious infections from raw milk. However, these infections only come from infected cows and goats. If the animal is healthy and is regularly examined by a veterinarian there is no risk of getting any infection from the milk. In fact, salmonella, E. coli and many other harmful microbes cannot survive in raw milk, they get destroyed by beneficial bacteria, enzymes and immune complexes naturally present in the milk.[94-96] If these pathogenic microbes get into pasteurised milk however, they thrive because the enzymes and beneficial bacteria have been destroyed by pasteurisation. That is why we still get serious outbreaks of infection through drinking pasteurised milk. Because most milk in the West gets pasteurised, farmers are not obliged to look after their cows' health rigorously enough: if the cow is ill and passes any infection into her milk pasteurisation will destroy that infection.

Fortunately there are dairy farmers who take a more conscientious approach: they look after the health of their animals and, as a result, are able to provide their consumers with organic raw milk without any risk of infections. For an updated list of these farmers please look at *www.westonprice.org* and *www.realmilk.com*. When you have found a local supply of organic raw milk from healthy cows or goats, make all your yogurt, kefir and sour cream from raw milk and cream and buy raw butter. If it is impossible for you to find raw organic milk, try to find pasteurised organic milk from natural breeds of cow or goat. When we ferment pasteurised milk the fermenting microbes will put some life back into it.

GAPS patients cannot drink milk without fermenting it first. However, once the digestive system of the person has healed, all homemade fermented raw milk products are well tolerated and cheese has been introduced, many GAPS people find that they can start drinking raw organic milk. As with all dairy products, start gradually with a tiny amount. It goes without saying that all milk available in our shops is 'dead' and should never be consumed by GAPS people as milk. In order to make it useful for us we have to make it 'alive' again by fermenting it with beneficial microbes.

One more important point about dairy: adding whey, yogurt and kefir does miracles for those who are prone to diarrhoea. Different substances in sour milk products, lactic acid in particular, soothe and strengthen the gut lining, slow down food transit through the intestines and the bowel and firm up the stool. So, if your patient is prone to diarrhoea, follow the GAPS Introduction Diet and introduce fermented milk products right from the beginning. Constipation, however, is a different matter. If you or your patient are prone to chronic constipation, introduce sauerkraut juice and juice from fermented vegetables from the start but be cautious with dairy. In my experience, people with chronic constipation do well with high-fat dairy products, such as ghee, butter and sour cream, but not with high-protein dairy, such as yogurt, whey, kefir and cheese: high-protein dairy can aggravate constipation. This may not be the case in every constipated person, as all of us have a unique gut flora, but in my experience it happens in more than half of the cases.

Non-starch fresh vegetables

French artichoke, beets, asparagus, broccoli, Brussels sprouts, cabbage, cauliflower, carrots, cucumber, celery, green beans, marrow, courgette (zucchini), aubergine (eggplant), garlic, onions, kale, lettuce, mushrooms, parsley, green peas, peppers of all colours, pumpkin, runner beans, squash, spinach, tomatoes, turnips, watercress.

Frozen vegetables can be used, as long as they are not coated with starch, sugar or anything else. All vegetables should be peeled, deseeded and cooked until diarrhoea, abdominal pain and other digestive symptoms have completely cleared. After that raw vegetables can be slowly introduced with meals or as snacks.

There is a plethora of publications on the virtues of eating vegetables, so we will not concentrate on this subject here. However, one point is important: organic vegetables are better than non-organic. I had patients who were getting persistent diarrhoea from eating particular vegetables until they switched to organic ones. A GAPS patient's sensitive digestive system would undoubtedly react to pesticides and other chemicals in non-organic vegetables.

If you are sensitive to nightshade foods (tomatoes, aubergine/eggplant and peppers), then initially avoid them. As you complete the Introduction Diet, you may find that you do not react to them anymore. Introduce them gradually and one at a time.

All ripe fruit, including berries

Fruit can be fresh, cooked or raw, dried (no sorbates, no sulphites, sugar, starch or anything else added), and frozen (providing there is nothing added to the fruit). If the patient has diarrhoea or abdominal pain, avoid fruit initially. As the diarrhoea settles, start introducing cooked fruit (peeled and deseeded prior to cooking). When the stool becomes consistently normal, then you can slowly introduce raw fruit as a snack between meals. It is not a good idea to have raw fruit with the meals as the fruit may interfere with the digestion of meats. The fruits that do combine with meats fairly well are lemons, fresh lemon juice, avocado and sour-tasting varieties of apple.

Fruit should be ripe, as unripe fruit has too much starch. For example, bananas should have brown spots on their skins. As the fruit ripens, the starch gets converted into monosugars, which are easy to digest.

Avocado is a wonderfully nutritious fruit and combines well with meats. It is easy to digest and is particularly rich in nourishing oils. Make sure it is ripe and serve it with meats, fish, shellfish and salads. Delicious drinking smoothies can be made with avocado (please look in the recipe section).

Berries are wonderful powerhouses of nutrition. They are rich in vitamins, minerals and a whole host of anti-cancer and detoxifying substances. All sorts of edible berries are allowed on the diet: strawberries, blueberries, raspberries, blackcurrants, redcurrants, white currants, blackberries, elderberries, sea buckthorn, etc. However, do not give them to a person with diarrhoea or abdominal pain. When the diarrhoea has cleared completely, introduce cooked berries gradually. If cooked berries are well tolerated then go ahead with raw berries. In some cases, when the digestive tract is too sensitive, you have to remove the seeds by putting your cooked berries through a sieve.

Many people with chronic disease have an overgrowth of yeast in their bodies, which always includes the digestive tract. Yeast feeds on sugars in the fruit, producing gas and giving the person unpleasant symptoms: belching, bloating, flatulence, cramps and stool abnormalities. That is why for many people it is sensible to avoid fruit, particularly in the initial stages of the diet. Many GAPS people find that they have to avoid fruit for most of their lives. However, what has to be taken into account is that yeast in the gut holds toxins. When we eat fruit, yeasts grow into the fruit very fast and transfer some toxins into its fibrous mass. The fibre is indigestible for humans and takes these toxins out of your body in the stool. That is why fruit has a cleansing effect on the human body. If you would like to have a cleansing episode, do it only when you have access to organic, ripe and very fresh fruit. This means picking berries from the bushes yourself and eating them immediately, or picking an apple which has ripened fully on an organic apple tree. Fruit from supermarkets is unsuitable, because it has been produced commercially, picked unripe and has had to travel long distances to get to you. Even when labelled 'organic' commercial fruit is not health-giving for GAPS people.

Nuts and seeds

Walnuts, almonds, brazil nuts, pecans, hazelnuts, cashew nuts, peanuts, sunflower seeds, pumpkin seeds and sesame seeds. Nuts and seeds should be bought in their shells or freshly shelled. They should not be bought roasted, salted, coated or processed in any other way. Peanut butter with just peanuts and salt is allowed, providing the person is not allergic to peanuts and his or her digestive system is ready to tolerate them. A lot of peanut allergy is due to contamination with moulds and their toxins, so make sure to get good quality peanuts. Blanched ground almonds (nut flour) can be purchased for baking in health food shops. As soon as almonds are ground into flour, they start oxidising and losing their nutritional value, which is why it is recommended that you keep almond flour in the freezer. It is best to buy whole almonds and process them into flour at home. Coconut flour is also available on the market, but there is no industry standard on how it is produced. Some recovering GAPS people can tolerate commercially available coconut flour, but more sensitive people should make their own at home.

Nuts and seeds can be highly nourishing when we are able to digest them. They are rich sources of minerals, amino acids and fats: magnesium, selenium, zinc, omega-6 and omega-3 oils. Epidemiological studies show that people who regularly consume nuts and seeds have lower rates of heart disease, cancer and many other degenerative diseases.[97] The GAPS Diet uses nuts and seeds extensively. But all nuts and seeds must be prepared properly to make them digestible for humans and to neutralise antinutrients. Please, look in the Recipe section for how to prepare nuts and seeds. They have a high fibre content and should not be introduced until the diarrhoea and abdominal pain have settled. After the diarrhoea has cleared, baking with properly prepared nuts, ground into flour or paste consistency, can be introduced. When baked products with nuts and seeds are well tolerated, then raw nuts can be gradually and slowly introduced as snacks between meals.

Sunflower seeds, pumpkin seeds and sesame seeds also should not be used until diarrhoea has settled. They are best soaked in water for 12–24 hours and sprouted or fermented. This way they are much easier to digest and are more nourishing. Sprinkle your soaked and sprouted seeds on salads and ready-made dishes. You can add them to your baking mixtures and grind to use as flour. You can use tahini (creamed sesame seeds), almond butter, hazelnut butter, peanut butter and pumpkin seed butter in your baking, providing they are pure, without any additives, and you buy them as fresh as possible.

Beans, legumes and pulses

Dried white (navy) or haricot beans, lima beans (dried and fresh), string beans as well as lentils and split peas. Apart from the ones mentioned, all other legumes are too starchy to give to GAPS patients and should be avoided. With all dried beans, lentils and peas it is very important to prepare them properly. They must be soaked in water for at least 12 hours (preferably longer), then drained and rinsed well under running water to remove any harmful substances. After soaking, many traditional cultures have fermented or sprouted them before cooking. Do not use commercially available bean flours, as the beans are not properly prepared before grinding them into flour. In cases of nut allergy, properly prepared, cooked and mashed white (navy) beans can be used instead of nuts in baking. Beans, lentils and peas should be avoided until diarrhoea and other digestive symptoms have cleared completely.

Beans, lentils and other legumes are generally hard to digest, as they contain many antinutrients and starches. That is why it is important not to rush with introducing this group of foods into your patient's menu, and it is essential to soak them long enough, wash them thoroughly, ferment or sprout them, and cook them well. Please, see the Recipes section for how to prepare beans, legumes and pulses properly.

Honey

Natural honey is allowed. Cold-pressed honey is preferable, as it is unprocessed. Many producers heat honey in order to speed up the process of extraction from the honeycomb, which damages it. Honey is sweeter than table sugar and contains monosaccharides which the GAPS digestive system can handle. Use honey as a sweetener. In the initial stages of the diet try to limit all sweet things, including honey, because they may encourage growth of yeast in the gut and unbalance your blood sugar level.

Honey has been created by the forces of Nature; it carries within itself Nature's infinite wisdom. Before the introduction of sugar in the 17th century honey was the only sweetener which humans used in their diet. Starting from the end of the 17th century sugar, being cheaper and more available, gradually replaced honey in people's diet, starting an era of sugar-related health problems. Honey is far more natural for our bodies and, far from damaging health, has a lot of health-giving properties. It has been used as food and medicine for thousands of years.[98–105]

In Greek mythology honey was considered a 'food fit for gods'. There are dozens of books written about the health-giving properties of natural honey. It works as an antiseptic and a healing agent, providing vitamins, minerals, amino acids and many other bio-active substances. Depending on the variety of flowers providing the pollen, different flavours and compositions of nutrients and bio-active substances can be found in the honey. Apart from its chemical composition, honey has a complex biophysical structure, which carries the unique energy pattern of the bee colony which produced it. This energy pattern is important for the honey's healing ability and must not be altered by heating, application of chemicals or radiation. Traditionally honey has been used to treat digestive disorders, chest and throat infections, arthritis, anaemia, insomnia, headaches, debility and cancer. It can be applied therapeutically to open wounds, eczema patches, skin rashes, skin and mouth ulcers and erosions. [98–105]

Beverages

A GAPS child or adult should drink water, freshly pressed juices and meat/fish stock.

For an adult weak tea and coffee without milk is allowed. Tea and coffee must be freshly made, not instant. A slice of lemon in tea is beneficial. Herbal teas are allowed as long as they are made from fresh or dried single herbs and not from commercially available herbal tea bags. Freshly made ginger tea is a good digestive.

Some milk replacements are allowed: homemade almond milk and homemade coconut milk. Please look in the recipe section for how to make them.

Drinking water is a very healthy habit, but it is not advisable to drink tap water unless it is filtered. Tap water is chlorinated and damages the gut flora balance. It is best to drink bottled mineral water or filtered water. A GAPS person's day should always start with a glass of still mineral or filtered water, cool or warm to personal preference. A slice of lemon or a teaspoon of apple cider vinegar in the water is beneficial. The same should be drunk between meals. Drinking a lot of water with meals is not advisable, as it may interfere with digestion. It is better to drink warm homemade meat stock with meals, which stimulates production of digestive juices in the stomach. Drinking anything cold arrests digestion, so during meals it is important to drink warm beverages.

Freshly pressed fruit and vegetable juices are highly recommended. They will speed up the detoxification processes in the body and support the liver. You will need to have a good juicer at home. A juicer often comes with a recipe book, but you can experiment with your own mixtures and combinations (look in the recipe section). For more on juicing look in the chapter *Detoxification for People with GAPS*.

I do not recommend any commercially available juices, unless they have been freshly pressed. Commercial juices are pasteurised, which destroys a lot of nutrition in the juice and turns it into a source of processed sugar. Some commercial juice labels do not mention added preservatives, sweeteners and other substances. Most commercially available juices are prone to having moulds and fungi in them, which GAPS people very often react to. It goes without saying that all cordials and other soft drinks have to be out of the diet.

Alcoholic beverages are best avoided by people with GAP Syndrome as they add more toxicity for the liver to deal with. However, on rare occasions a small amount of dry wine, gin, Scotch whisky, bourbon and vodka are permissible. Beer has to be completely avoided as it has a high carbohydrate content.

Fats and oils

Animal fats and dairy fat (butter and ghee) are the best fats for GAPS people. They provide all the right nutrients for restoring immunity, gut and nervous system.[106] GAPS people need to consume them in ample amounts. In fact, the more animal fats your patient consumes, the quicker you will see recovery.

Animal fats are the best fats to cook with because they do not change their chemical structure when heated. All cooking oils or vegetable oils are full of harmful damaged fatty acids and should be avoided.[106] Cooking should be done with butter, ghee, pork dripping, beef fat (lard), lamb fat, goose fat, duck fat or chicken fat. If you roast a duck, collect the fat from the baking tray, put it through a sieve or cheesecloth and you will have a large jar of excellent cooking fat. If you roast a goose you will have even more. You can bake with these fats too if you have any concerns about using butter and ghee in your baking. If you can find natural non-hydrogenated coconut oil, you can use it for cooking and baking. Unfortunately, many brands of coconut oil available in the West are hydrogenated and best avoided.

Avoid all commercially available oils apart from virgin cold-pressed olive oil. It is not a good idea to cook with it, as heating will destroy a lot of nutrients and damage some unsaturated fatty acids in it. Use it as a dressing on your ready-to-serve meals, salads and vegetables in ample amounts. Other cold-pressed oils, such as flaxseed oil, evening primrose oil, avocado oil, etc., are very beneficial but, again, should never be heated and should be bought fresh (as they oxidise quite quickly).

Avoid all artificial fats like margarine and butter replacements. Avoid all foods cooked with these fats.

For a detailed explanation about fats and oils please look at the chapter: *Fats, the Good and the Bad*.

Salt

Only a small percentage of all salt production goes for human consumption. More than 90% of all salt produced is used for industrial applications: making of soaps, detergents, plastics, agricultural chemicals, PVC, etc.[107] These industrial applications require pure sodium chloride. However, salt in Nature contains many other elements: in fact, natural crystal salt and whole sea salt contain all the minerals and trace elements which the human body is made of. In this natural state salt is not only good for us, but essential.[108,109] However, because industry requires pure sodium chloride, all the other elements and minerals are removed. We consume this under the name of 'table salt' and, of course, all our processed foods contain plenty of it.

This kind of salt comes into the body like a villain, upsetting our homeostasis on the most basic level. Our bodies have been designed to receive sodium chloride in combination with all the other minerals and trace elements which a natural salt would provide. Pure sodium chloride draws water to itself and causes water retention, with many consequences, such as high blood pressure, tissue oedema and poor circulation.[107-111] As the body tries to deal with the excess of sodium chloride, various harmful acids and gall bladder and kidney stones are formed. As sodium in the body works in a team with many other minerals and trace elements (potassium, calcium, magnesium, copper, zinc, manganese, etc.), the levels of those substances get out of normal balance. The harmful results of table salt consumption can be numerous and serious. That is why most medical practitioners, including mainstream doctors, tell us not to consume table salt.[112]

Our planet has plenty of good quality salt for us to consume. Throughout human history, salt has been highly valued: it used to be called 'the white gold' and the Roman Empire paid its soldiers with salt (hence the word 'salary'). Natural salt is just as fundamental to our physiology as water is.[107-112] We need to consume salt in its natural state: as a crystal salt (such as Himalayan crystal salt) or as a whole unprocessed sea salt (such as Celtic salt). There are a number of companies around the world which can provide you with good quality salt.

Can we trust organic labels on the supermarket shelves?

It is a very sad fact, but we cannot! Organic production is being rapidly taken over by the agrochemical industry all over the Western world. We now have a new term: 'fauxganic' produce or fake organic.[113]

Some 80% of all 'organic' poultry and eggs in American stores now come from CAFOs (Concentrated Animal Feeding Operations) – large factories, where chickens are kept in cages, fed artificial feed and never see the light of day. Over half of all 'organic' milk sold in American supermarkets comes from huge certified 'organic' CAFOs, where cows live on concrete and never see pasture. At the same time, real organic milk producers are going out of business because they cannot compete with the large producers of the fake organic.[113] Hydroponic vegetables and fruit now dominate the 'organic' market: tomatoes, peppers, lettuce and berries grown without plants ever touching the soil, using artificial chemicals and under artificial light. Cheating and downright lies are dominating the whole industry, while the public is largely unaware of what is going on and still trusts the organic label. According to NOFA (Northeast Organic Farming Association) the real organic farmers are becoming an endangered species. They list $250 million worth of fake organic grain imports into the USA and estimate that $6 billion in annual 'organic' sales are fake organic.[113] This situation is happening not only in America, but in other Western countries too.

This development is not surprising. The demand for organic food has grown enormously and is still growing. In the USA alone in 1990 the organic food market was worth $1 billion; by 2017 it has grown to $43.7 billion and is estimated to grow to $70.4 billion by 2025. Of course, industrial chemical agriculture wants a 'piece of that pie'! This industry has an unsurpassed ability to manipulate the agricultural policies of Western governments and, in the last decade, it has successfully changed organic laws and regulations to suit its commercial agenda.[113–117]

Where does this leave us, the consumers? What can we do to make sure that we get real organic food? Certainly not by going to the supermarkets! If you want to find fake 'organic' produce, the supermarket is the place to go. We have to buy food directly from the farmer: we need to visit the farm, meet the farmer, see the gardens and the animals and ask questions about how they are looked after. By buying food directly from honest organic farmers we support the real organic sector while supplying our families with real food. Many people are already doing this; they are forming co-operatives, where families take turns in driving outside the cities to organic farms and bringing food for the whole group. Many people are starting to grow their own produce and keep chickens, goats and other animals. The results are always worth the effort! Better health and a happier lifestyle come from eating good honest food, meeting good honest people, making good honest friends and being closer to the land and Nature.

Recommended foods

Almonds, including almond butter and oil
Apples
Apricots, fresh or dried
Artichoke, French
Asiago cheese
Asparagus
Aubergine (eggplant)
Avocados, including avocado oil
Bananas (ripe only, with brown spots on the skin)
Beans, dried white (navy) or haricot, string beans and lima beans, properly prepared
Beef, fresh or frozen

Beetroot (beets)
Berries, all kinds
Black, white and red pepper: ground and peppercorns
Black radish
Blue cheese
Bok choy
Brazil nuts
Brick cheese
Brie cheese
Broccoli
Brussels sprouts
Butter
Cabbage
Camembert cheese
Canned fish in oil or water only, preserved in glass jars
Capers
Carrots
Cashew nuts, fresh only
Cauliflower
Cayenne pepper
Celeriac
Celery
Cellulose in supplements
Cheddar cheese
Cherimoya (custard apple or sharifa)
Cherries
Chicken, fresh or frozen
Cinnamon
Citric acid
Coconut, fresh or dried (shredded) without any additives
Coconut milk
Coconut oil
Coffee, weak and freshly made, not instant
Collard greens
Colby cheese
Courgette (zucchini)
Coriander, fresh or dried
Cucumber
Dates, fresh or dried without any additives (not soaked in syrup)
Dill, fresh or dried
Duck, fresh or frozen
Edam cheese
Eggplant (aubergine)

Eggs, fresh
Filberts
Fish, fresh or frozen, canned in its juice or oil in glass jars
Game, fresh or frozen
Garlic
Ghee, homemade
Gin, occasionally
Ginger root, fresh
Goose, fresh or frozen
Gorgonzola cheese
Gouda cheese
Grapefruit
Grapes
Haricot beans, properly prepared
Havarti cheese
Hazelnuts
Herbal teas
Herbs, fresh or dried without additives
Honey, natural
Juices, freshly pressed from permitted fruit and vegetables
Kale
Kiwi fruit
Kumquats
Lamb, fresh or frozen
Lemons
Lentils
Lettuce, all kinds
Lima beans (dried and fresh)
Limburger cheese
Limes
Mangoes
Meats, fresh or frozen
Melons
Monterey (Jack) cheese
Muenster cheese
Mushrooms
Mustard seeds, pure powder and gourmet types without any non-allowed ingredients
Nectarines
Nut flour or ground nuts (usually ground blanched almonds)
Nutmeg
Nuts, all kinds freshly shelled, not roasted, salted or coated
Olive oil, virgin cold-pressed

Olives preserved without sugar or any other non-allowed ingredients
Onions
Oranges
Papaya
Parmesan cheese
Parsley
Peaches
Peanut butter, without additives
Peanuts, fresh or roasted in their shells
Pears
Peas, dried split and fresh green
Pecans
Peppers (green, yellow, red and orange)
Pheasant, fresh or frozen
Pickles, without sugar or any other non-allowed ingredients
Pigeon, fresh or frozen
Pineapples, fresh
Pork, fresh or frozen
Port du Salut cheese
Poultry, fresh or frozen
Prunes, dried without any additives or in their own juice
Pumpkin
Quail, fresh or frozen
Raisins
Rhubarb
Roquefort cheese
Romano cheese
Satsumas
Scotch, occasionally
Seaweed fresh and dried, once the Introduction Diet has been completed
Shellfish, fresh or frozen
Spices, single and pure without any additives
Spinach
Squash (summer and winter)
Stilton cheese
String beans
Swedes
Swiss cheese
Tangerines
Tea, organic and weak, freshly made, not instant
Tomato purée, pure without any additives apart from salt
Tomato juice, without any additives apart from salt

Tomatoes
Turkey, fresh or frozen
Turnips
Ugli fruit
Uncreamed cottage cheese (dry curd)
Vinegar (cider or white); make sure there is no allergy
Vodka, very occasionally
Walnuts
Watercress
White navy beans, properly prepared
Wine dry: red, rosé or white
Yogurt, home-made
Zucchini (courgette)

TREATMENT

A journey of a thousand miles begins with a single step.

Lao-Tzu

For all the conditions which we have talked about in this book, you will find many treatments proposed – natural and conventional. Every GAPS person is an individual with his or her own unique constitution and individual set of circumstances. That is why there is no treatment that fits all. Imagine that you are planning to make a cake. Before thinking about the cherries you are going to use to decorate it, you first have to bake the cake. Healing your gut with the GAPS Nutritional Protocol is baking the cake. Other treatments, such as chelating of toxic metals, anti-parasitic treatments, infrared sauna, hyperbaric oxygenation, acupuncture, naturopathic and chiropractic treatments, homeopathy, physiotherapy, hypnotherapy, herbs, bio-identical hormones, etc. are the 'cherries on the top'. They can all be very helpful, and every GAPS patient decorates his or her 'cake' with their own individual 'cherries'. However, clinical experience shows that for many people there is no need for the 'cherries', just implementing the GAPS Nutritional Protocol can be enough for their recovery. So, bake your cake before thinking about the cherries, as they can be expensive and non-productive if you use them too early. First, lay a good foundation for your recovery with the GAPS Nutritional Protocol.

The human body has an incredible ability to heal itself, given the right help. If a tree gets ill, we must attend to its roots before attending to its leaves and branches. As we discussed in previous chapters, the roots of our health are in our digestive system, so that is where we have to start in order to allow the body to heal all its 'branches and leaves'. Once your digestive system starts working properly, you will be amazed by how quickly many of your symptoms, far removed from the gut, start melting away: your joints and muscles stop hurting, the PMS goes away, your skin clears, your energy comes back, you start sleeping well, your memory and ability to concentrate improve, you find long-lost stamina to accomplish your daily tasks, your constant colds become a thing of the past, your asthma disappears, you realise by the middle of summer that you have had no hay fever this year, your headaches go away, your chronic cystitis vanishes, etc. As they disappear, the symptoms which you or your doctor have never connected with the state of your digestive system, will tell you that you have done the right thing in healing your gut.

Mother Nature does not work fast. It can be very fast getting ill, but to recover always takes longer. Everybody is different, but for the majority of GAPS people it takes at least two years to heal their gut. No matter what chronic illness you have to deal with (physical or mental), to lay a good foundation for recovery I recommend following the GAPS Nutritional Protocol.

GAPS Nutritional Protocol

After years of trying I began to learn why the GAPS Protocol was so clever, and that there was no way around it! There was no way to argue with it, unless I chose to be right and forever unwell!

Katrina, recovered from Crohn's disease and rheumatoid arthritis

GAPS Nutritional Protocol has evolved through personal experience with my own family and clinical experience with many thousands of children and adults around the world. During the last twenty years it has become an international movement with patients helping themselves and their families to recover from all kinds of chronic illnesses.

What does this protocol involve?

1. Diet. GAPS conditions are essentially digestive disorders. The digestive system is a long tube; what you fill that tube with has a direct effect on its well-being. That is why diet is the most important and the number one treatment. Everything else takes second place.
2. Supplementation.
3. Detoxification and lifestyle changes.

Let us look at each of these three elements in detail.

GAPS DIET

The GAPS diet was originally based on the SCD (the Specific Carbohydrate Diet). SCD was invented by a renowned American paediatrician Dr Sidney Valentine Haas in the first half of the 20th century. Dr Haas and his colleagues spent many years researching the effects of diet on celiac disease and other digestive disorders. The results of this research were published in a comprehensive medical textbook *The Management of Celiac Disease*, written by Dr Sidney V. Haas and Merrill P. Haas in 1951.[1] At that time the diet, described in the book, was accepted by the medical community all over the world as a cure for celiac disease, and Dr Sidney V. Haas was honoured for his pioneer work in the field of paediatrics. Unfortunately, in the following years celiac disease was redefined as a gluten intolerance or gluten enteropathy and the SCD was considered outdated. It was revived by the late Elaine Gottschall, who discovered the work of Dr Haas in 1958, when her little daughter was suffering from severe ulcerative colitis and learning problems. Following the success of the SCD with her daughter, Elaine Gottschall has, over the years, helped thousands of people, suffering from Crohn's disease, ulcerative colitis, celiac disease, diverticulitis and various types of chronic diarrhoea. She devoted years of research into the biochemical and biological basis of the diet and published a book in 1994, called *Breaking the Vicious Cycle. Intestinal Health Through Diet.*[2] SCD has a large following around the world and I have been using it in my clinic for many years. Having accumulated valuable clinical experience, I had to make several adjustments in the diet appropriate for my patients. Through the years my patients named their dietary regime – the GAPS Diet.

Implementing the diet

Over the years the GAPS Diet has become known all over the world, helping children and adults to recover from very serious health problems, and the diet has continued to evolve to suit more and more complex patients. Some people do well with following the *Full GAPS Diet*, which is the easiest to implement and is very suitable for following as a permanent lifestyle. Many people have to go through the *GAPS Introduction Diet*, which is more difficult to follow, but it achieves deeper healing of the gut and the rest of the body. People with particularly severe digestive problems, severe mental illness and some severe physical diseases have found great help following the *No-Plant GAPS Diet* for a while. At the most severe end, patients with cancer, multiple sclerosis, Lyme disease and other very serious health problems have found *GAPS Ketogenic Diet* to be the most appropriate approach for them. Then there are people who need to eat more plant matter to feel well; these people enjoy the *More-Plant GAPS Diet*. In some situations, having a rest from solid food is what is needed; in these cases we can follow the *GAPS Liquid Fast*.

The full spectrum of the GAPS Diet:

- GAPS Introduction Diet
- The Full GAPS Diet
- The No-Plant GAPS Diet
- GAPS Ketogenic Diet
- More-Plant GAPS Diet
- GAPS Liquid Fast

Let us have a detailed look at each approach.

GAPS introduction diet

The Introduction Diet is designed to heal and seal the gut lining quickly. It achieves this aim by providing three factors:

1. Large amounts of nourishing substances for the gut lining: amino acids, gelatine, glucosamine, collagen, fats, vitamins, minerals, etc. – all the substances, which your gut lining is made from. As we have discussed in previous chapters, your gut lining renews itself all the time by shedding off old and worn out cells and giving birth to new ones. In order to produce healthy new cells, your gut lining needs very special nourishment, which this diet will provide in abundance.
2. The majority of GAPS people have inflammation and ulcerations in their gut lining, which they may not be aware of, as they do not always produce particular symptoms. Your gut lining may be sore and very sensitive. GAPS Introduction Diet is very gentle; it removes fibre and any other substances which may irritate or damage your gut and interfere with the healing process.
3. The cell regeneration process in the gut lining is ruled and orchestrated by the beneficial microbes which normally live on its surface.[3,4] Without their presence there can be no healing! GAPS Introduction diet provides probiotic microbes in the food right from the start.

The very name Introduction Diet implies that we begin with this diet. However, ***not everybody has to start from the Introduction Diet!***

I recommend that most GAPS patients follow the Introduction Diet at some stage in their healing, because it will give you the best chance to optimise the healing process in the gut and the rest of the body. However, this diet is very demanding and can be difficult to follow. Depending on your lifestyle and circumstances you may want to start from the Full GAPS Diet and do the Introduction Diet later. If you are a good cook, your kitchen is set up well and you have found a supply of all the necessary ingredients, you may be ready to do the Introduction Diet from the beginning. Unfortunately, many people are not in this group: they need to organise their lives and their kitchen to start doing a lot of cooking, find suppliers of the right foods, take a break from a busy job, take the child out of school (or wait for a long school holiday), etc.

Here are the usual situations when it is sensible to start from the Full GAPS Diet and plan to do the Introduction Diet later.

- If you are travelling and working away and are not set up to cook, it is easier to start from the Full GAPS Diet. You can eat out on the Full GAPS Diet and the choice of allowed foods is much wider. Later on, in about six months or a year, you may be able to get organised to follow the Introduction Diet.
- When we are trying to heal a person where compliance may be an issue, it is sensible to start from the Full GAPS Diet. About a year down the road a lot of healing will be achieved and the person may be ready to go through the rigours of the Introduction Diet and comply with it. Many teenagers and young people are in this group. They have pocket money and are under peer pressure. Trying to implement the Introduction Diet with this group is often impossible, so I recommend starting from the Full GAPS Diet. Make sure that your teenager is involved in cooking his or her meals to establish a proper sensory relationship with food. Children generally are more likely to eat what they have cooked themselves, rather than what somebody else has cooked for them. As your teenager starts healing and seeing results, he or she is more likely to become ready to comply with the Introduction Diet.
- People with chronic constipation do better starting from the Full GAPS Diet. This group of people usually rely on fibre supplementation to pass any stool at all. On the Introduction Diet we remove fibre, which is likely to make this person even more constipated. When constipation is resolved on the Full GAPS Diet, you can then attempt the Introduction Diet to achieve deeper healing.
- People without serious digestive symptoms can start from the Full GAPS Diet. In some cases they recover from their illnesses without having to go through the Introduction Diet at all. I have had such patients with depression, ADHD and autoimmune disease. However, this group is fairly small. The majority of people have to go through the Introduction Diet at some stage in their healing, and often not just once.

Following the Introduction Diet fully is absolutely essential for people with serious digestive symptoms: chronic diarrhoea, abdominal pain, bloating, reflux, blood or mucous in the stool, ulcerative colitis, Crohn's disease, acute or chronic gastritis, acute or chronic enterocolitis, oesophagitis and other serious digestive disorders. This diet will reduce the symptoms quickly and initiate the healing process in the digestive system. Even for healthy people, if you or your child gets a 'tummy bug' or any other form of diarrhoea, following the Introduction Diet for a few days will clear the symptoms quickly and permanently, usually without needing any medication.

People with food allergies and intolerances should go through the Introduction Diet in order to heal and seal their gut lining. The reason for allergies and food intolerances is so-called 'leaky gut' when the gut lining is damaged by unhealthy microbial flora. Foods are not digested properly before they get absorbed through this damaged gut wall and cause the immune system to react to them. Many people try to identify which foods they react to. However, with damaged gut wall they are likely to absorb most of their foods partially digested, which may cause an immediate reaction or a delayed reaction (a day, a few days or even a couple of weeks later). As these reactions overlap with each other, you can never be sure what exactly you are reacting to on any given day. Testing for food allergies is notoriously unreliable: if you were tested twice a day for two weeks, you would find that you are 'allergic' to everything you eat. As long as the gut wall is damaged, and stays damaged, you can be juggling your diet, forever removing different foods, and never get anywhere. From my clinical experience it is best to concentrate on healing the gut wall with the GAPS Introduction Diet. Once the gut wall is healed, the foods will be digested properly before being absorbed, which will remove most food intolerances and allergies. If there is a particular food you react strongly to, it makes sense to remove it while you are working on healing your gut wall with the GAPS Introduction Diet. Once the gut heals, you may be able to reintroduce that food into your diet.

If you suspect an anaphylactic-type allergy (which can be dangerous) to any particular food, before introducing it do **the Sensitivity Test**. Take a drop of the food in question (if the food is solid, mash and mix with a bit of water) and place it on the inside of your wrist at bedtime. Let the drop dry on the skin before going to sleep. In the morning check the spot: if there is an angry red reaction, avoid that food for a few weeks, and then try again. If there is no reaction, go ahead and introduce it gradually starting from a tiny amount. Always test the food in the state you are planning to eat it: for example, if you are planning to introduce raw egg yolks, test the raw egg yolk and not the whole egg or cooked egg.

Depending on the severity of your condition, you can move through the Introduction Diet as quickly or as slowly as your symptoms will permit. On the first two stages most of your digestive symptoms will start subsiding (diarrhoea, abdominal pain, bloating, etc). When you move to the next stage, if any of those symptoms return, this is the signal that your gut is not ready for the new foods to be introduced. Go back to the previous stage and stay on it longer, before trying to move to the next stage. Once enough healing has happened in your gut, you will be able to move to the next stage without any of the old symptoms returning. For example, you may move through the First Stage in one or two days and then spend two weeks (or longer) on the Second Stage. *The Second Stage will provide all the necessary nourishment for your body to thrive on, so there is no rush to move from it.* Some people stay on the Second Stage of the Introduction Diet for a year or even longer feeling well and improving all the time. For some patients I recommend staying on this stage of the Introduction Diet more or less permanently, such as with severe cases of cerebral palsy, Down syndrome, severe autism, Rett syndrome and similar conditions.

Implementing the GAPS Introduction Diet

Start the day with a cup of still mineral or filtered water. Take your probiotic. Make sure that the water is warm or at least at room temperature, not cold, as cold will send a wave of contractions along your digestive tract and aggravate your condition. Only foods listed are allowed: you must not have anything else. On the First Stage the most drastic symptoms of abdominal pain, diarrhoea and bloating will quickly subside. If, when you introduce a new food, you get diarrhoea, abdominal pain or any other symptoms, then you are not ready for that food to be introduced. Wait for a week and try again.

First stage:

Homemade meat or fish stock. Meat and fish stocks provide building blocks for the rapidly growing cells of the gut lining and they have a soothing effect on any areas of inflammation in the gut. That is why they aid digestion and have been known for centuries as healing folk remedies for the digestive tract. Do not use commercially available soup stock granules or bouillon cubes. They do not heal the gut, as they are highly processed and full of detrimental ingredients. There is a confusion about meat stock and bone broth; you will find detailed information on this subject in the chapter *What We Shall Eat And Why, With Some Recipes*. We focus on the *meat stock* in the GAPS Nutritional Protocol. Chicken stock is particularly gentle on the stomach and is a very good starting point. To make good meat stock you need joints, bones, a piece of meat on the bone, a whole chicken, feet and giblets from chicken, goose or duck, whole pigeons, pheasants or other inexpensive meats. It is essential to use bones and joints, as they provide the healing substances, not so much the muscle meats. Ask the butcher to cut large tubular bones in half, so you can get the bone marrow out of them after cooking.

- Put the bones, joints and meats into a large pan and fill it up with water, add natural unprocessed salt to your taste at the beginning of cooking and about a teaspoon of black peppercorns, roughly crushed. Bring to boil, cover and simmer on a low heat for 2.5–4 hours (if using a slow cooker, cook overnight). You can make fish stock the same way using a whole fish or fish fins, bones, skins and heads; fish stock takes about 1–1.5 hours. After cooking take the bones and meats out and sieve the stock to remove small bones and peppercorns. Strip off all the soft tissues from the bones to add to soups later. It is important to eat all the soft tissues on the bones. Extract the bone marrow out of large tubular bones, while they are still warm, by banging the bone on a thick wooden chopping board. The gelatinous soft tissues around the bones and the bone marrow provide some of the best healing remedies for the gut lining and the immune system; you need to consume them with every meal. If you are making fish stock, take off all the soft tissues from fish bones and heads and reserve for adding to soups later. The meat or fish stock will keep well in the fridge for at least 7 days, or it can be frozen. Keep drinking warm meat stock all day with your meals and between meals. Do not use microwaves for warming up the stock or anything else, use a conventional stove (microwaves destroy food and make it carcinogenic).[5,6,7] It is very important for you to consume all the fat in the stock and off the bones as these fats are essential for the healing process. Add some probiotic food into every cup of stock you drink (the details about introducing probiotic foods follow).
- Homemade soup with your homemade meat or fish stock. Please look for some recipe ideas in the chapter *What We Shall Eat And Why, With Some Recipes*. Here we will go through some details, specific for the Introduction Diet. Bring some of the meat stock to boil, add chopped or sliced vegetables, choosing from onions, carrots, broccoli, cauliflower, courgettes, marrow (zucchini), squash, pumpkin and leek, and simmer for 25–35 minutes. You can choose any combination of available vegetables, avoiding very fibrous ones, such as all varieties of cabbage and celery. All particularly fibrous parts of vegetables need to be removed, such as skin and seeds of pumpkins, marrows and squashes, stalk of broccoli and cauliflower and any other parts that look too fibrous. You can add a handful of homemade fermented vegetables and cook them in the stock to make soup (together with the fresh vegetables). Fermented vegetables have been pre-digested by microbes during fermentation and cooking will make them even easier to digest. Cook the vegetables well, so they are really soft. When vegetables are well cooked, add 1–2 tablespoons of chopped garlic, bring to boil and turn the heat off. Eat this

soup with the bone marrow, meats and other soft tissues which you took off the bones. You can blend the soup using a soup blender or have it as it is. Add some probiotic food into every bowl of soup (the details about introducing probiotic foods follow). You should eat these soups with boiled meat and other soft tissues off the bones as often as you want to all day. Once you have made a large pot of soup, it will keep in the fridge for 5-6 days, so you can warm up some of it when you need. This can be very helpful for those of you who suffer from fatigue and find frequent cooking strenuous.

- **Probiotic foods** are essential to introduce right from the beginning. These can be dairy based or vegetable based. To avoid any reactions, introduce probiotic foods gradually, starting from 1–2 teaspoons a day for 2–5 days, then 3–4 teaspoons a day for 2–5 days and so on, until you can add a few teaspoons of the probiotic food into every cup of meat stock and every bowl of soup. Start by adding juice from your homemade sauerkraut, fermented vegetables or vegetable medley into your cups of meat stock and bowls of soup. Do not add the vegetables themselves yet, as they are too fibrous. Look in the chapter *What We Shall Eat And Why, With Some Recipes* for how to ferment vegetables. Apart from providing probiotic bacteria, these juices from fermented vegetables will help you to restore normal stomach acid production. Make sure that the food is not too hot when adding the probiotic foods, as the heat would destroy the beneficial probiotic bacteria.

  Apart from some rare exceptions, juice from fermented vegetables is well tolerated by GAPS people. Dairy-based fermented foods are a different matter. In my experience a large percentage of GAPS people can tolerate well-fermented homemade whey, yogurt or sour cream right from the beginning. However, some cannot. So, before introducing dairy, do **the sensitivity test**. Test whey first from dripping your homemade yogurt (dripping will remove many dairy proteins). If there is no reaction on the sensitivity test, then try to introduce whey. Start from 1 teaspoon of whey per day, added to the soup or meat stock. After 2–5 days on 1 teaspoon of whey per day, increase to 2 teaspoons a day and so on, until you are having ½ cup of whey per day with meals. At this stage try to add 1 teaspoon per day of homemade yogurt (without dripping), gradually increasing the daily amount. In parallel with the yogurt you can try to introduce homemade sour cream (fermented with yogurt culture), it has a beautiful fatty acid profile for your immune system and gut lining. After yogurt introduce homemade kefir. Kefir is far more aggressive than yogurt and usually creates a more pronounced die-off reaction. That is why I recommend introducing yogurt before starting on kefir. If you had no reaction to yogurt, then you may be able to introduce kefir almost from the beginning. For those who clearly react to dairy, please look at Dairy Introduction Structure (p. 179). If you have been consuming yogurt, kefir and other fermented dairy products prior to doing the GAPS Introduction Diet and have no negative reactions to them, then continue having them in your usual amounts; you do not have to start from one teaspoon per day.

Adding whey, yogurt and kefir does miracles for those who are prone to diarrhoea. Different substances in sour milk products, lactic acid in particular, sooth and strengthen the gut lining, slow down food transit through the intestines and the bowel and firm up the stool fairly quickly. So, if you are prone to diarrhoea introduce fermented milk products right from the beginning. Constipation, however, is a different matter. If you are prone to chronic constipation introduce sauerkraut juice and juice from fermented vegetables from the start but be cautious with dairy. In my experience people with constipation do well with high-fat dairy products, such as ghee, butter and sour cream, but not with high-protein dairy, such as yogurt, whey, kefir and cheese: high-protein dairy can aggravate constipation. This may not be the case in every constipated person, as all of us have a unique gut flora, but, in my experience, it happens in more than half of the cases.

- Ginger, mint or camomile tea with a little honey between meals. To make ginger tea, grate some fresh or frozen ginger root (about a teaspoonful) into a small teapot and add boiling water, cover and leave for 3–5 minutes. Pour through a sieve.

In extreme cases of profuse watery diarrhoea *exclude vegetables. Drink warm meat stock with probiotic foods every hour (preferably whey, sour cream or yogurt; if dairy is not tolerated, then juice from fermented vegetables), eat well-cooked gelatinous meats and fish (which you made the stock with) and consider adding raw egg yolks gradually. Do not introduce vegetables until the diarrhoea starts settling down. When the gut wall is severely inflamed, no amount of fibre can be tolerated. That is why do not rush to introduce vegetables (even very well cooked). If diarrhoea persists, please look at the No-Plant GAPS Diet* or *GAPS Liquid Fast.*

Second stage:

- Keep eating the soups with bone marrow, boiled meats or fish and other soft tissues off the bones (particularly gelatinous and fatty parts). Keep drinking the meat stock and ginger tea. Keep adding some probiotic food into every cup of meat stock and every bowl of soup: juices from sauerkraut, juices from fermented vegetables or vegetable medley, and/or homemade whey, sour cream and yogurt.

- Add raw organic egg yolks. If there is any concern about egg allergy, do the sensitivity test first with raw egg yolk. It is best to have raw egg yolks added to every bowl of soup and every cup of meat stock. Start from 1 egg yolk a day and gradually increase until you consume an egg yolk with every bowl of soup. When egg yolks are well tolerated add soft-boiled eggs to the soups (the whites cooked and the yolks still runny). Before introducing egg white, if you have any concerns about egg allergy, do the sensitivity test first with raw egg white. There is no need to limit the number of egg yolks per day, as they absorb quickly almost without needing any digestion, and will provide you with wonderful and most needed nutrition. Get your eggs from a source you trust: fresh, free range and organic.
- Add stews and casseroles made with meats and vegetables. Avoid spices at this stage, just make the stew with salt and fresh herbs. The stew needs to be cooked slowly and for a long time (2.5 hours minimum) so the meats and vegetables are well cooked (look for the *Italian Casserole* recipe in the chapter *What we shall eat and why, with some recipes,* for example). The fat content of these meals must be quite high: the more animal fats you consume, the quicker you will recover. Add some probiotic food into every serving.
- Keep increasing daily amounts of homemade sour cream, yogurt and kefir, if introduced. Increase the amount of juice from sauerkraut, fermented vegetables or vegetable medley.
- Try to introduce fermented fish, starting from one piece a day and gradually increasing. Look for the recipe in the chapter *What we shall eat and why, with some recipes.*
- Introduce homemade ghee. If dairy has been introduced, you can start from a few tablespoons per day and gradually increase. If dairy products have not been introduced yet, then start from 1 teaspoon a day and gradually increase.

Third stage:

- Carry on with the previous foods.
- Add ripe avocado mashed into soups, starting from 1–3 teaspoons and gradually increasing the amount.
- Add pancakes, starting from one pancake a day and gradually increasing the amount. Make these pancakes with three ingredients: 1) organic nut butter (almond, walnut, peanut, etc); 2) eggs; 3) a piece of fresh winter squash, marrow or courgette (peeled, deseeded and well blended in a food processor). Make a mixture the

consistency of pancake batter. Gently fry small pancakes, using ghee or any animal fat which you have rendered yourself: fat from goose, duck, pork, lamb or beef. Make sure not to burn the pancakes, use low heat.

- Egg gently fried or scrambled with a generous amount of ghee, goose fat, pork fat or duck fat. Serve it with avocado (if well tolerated) and cooked vegetables. Cooked onion is particularly good for the digestive system and the immune system: melt 5 tablespoons of duck fat or ghee in the pan, add sliced large white onion, cover and cook for 20–30 minutes on low heat until soft, sweet and translucent.
- Introduce the sauerkraut and your fermented vegetables. You have been drinking the juices from these vegetables for a while now, so your gut should be ready for the fibrous cabbage itself. Start from a small amount, gradually increasing to 1–2 tablespoons of sauerkraut or fermented vegetables per meal.

Fourth stage:

- Carry on with the previous foods.
- Gradually add meats cooked by roasting and grilling (but not barbecued or fried yet). Avoid bits which are burned or too brown. Eat the meat with cooked vegetables and sauerkraut (or other fermented vegetables). Drink a cup of warm meat stock with this meal (add some probiotic food to the meat stock).
- Start adding cold-pressed olive oil to the meals, starting from a few drops per meal and gradually increasing the amount to 1–2 tablespoons per meal.
- Introduce freshly pressed juices, starting from a few spoonfuls of carrot juice. Make sure that the juice is clear, filter it well. Drink it slowly diluted with warm water or mixed with some homemade yogurt. If well tolerated gradually increase to a full cup a day. When a full cup of carrot juice is well tolerated try adding juice from celery, lettuce and fresh mint leaves. You should always drink the juice on an empty stomach, so first thing in the morning and the middle of afternoon are good times.
- Try to bake bread with flour made from almonds or any other nuts and seeds (sunflower and pumpkin); this flour needs to be fermented prior to baking. The recipe (please look in the chapter *What we shall eat and why, with some recipes*) requires only three or four ingredients: 1) fermented nut/seed flour; 2) eggs; 3) some natural fat (ghee, butter, goose, pork or duck fat); 4) optional – a piece of fresh winter squash, marrow (zucchini) or courgette (peeled, deseeded and finely sliced) and some salt to taste. Start from a small

piece of bread per day and gradually increase the amount. Watch your stool while introducing this bread: if you get loose stools, then you are not ready for this step.

Fifth stage:

- If all the previous foods are well tolerated, try to add cooked apple as an apple purée: peel and core ripe cooking apples and stew them with a bit of water until soft. When cooked add a generous amount of ghee and mash with a potato masher. If ghee has not been introduced yet add duck, pork or goose fat. Start from a few spoonfuls a day. Watch for any reaction. If there is none, gradually increase the amount.
- Add raw vegetables, starting from softer parts of lettuce and peeled cucumber. Make sure to chew raw vegetables very well. Watch your stool: if you get diarrhoea or constipation, then consider yourself not ready for this step yet. Again, start from a small amount and gradually increase if well tolerated. After those two vegetables are well tolerated, gradually add other raw vegetables: carrot, tomato (if nightshades are tolerated), onion, cabbage, etc.
- If the juice made from carrot, celery, lettuce and mint is well tolerated, start adding fruit to it: apple, pineapple and mango. Avoid citrus fruit at this stage.

Sixth stage:

- If all the introduced foods are well tolerated, try some peeled raw apple. Gradually introduce raw fruit and more honey. Chew your fruit very well, as digestion of all carbohydrates begins in the mouth with the action of the saliva.
- Gradually introduce baking cakes and other sweet things allowed on the diet. Use dried fruit as a sweetener in the baking.

As I mentioned before, you may be able to move through the Introduction Diet faster or slower depending on your individual symptoms. Most indicative are abdominal pain and the stool changes: let the diarrhoea start clearing before moving to the next stage. You may have to introduce some foods later than in this programme depending on your personal sensitivities. Make sure that you carry on consuming soups and meat stock at least once a day after you complete the Introduction Diet.

As we remove fibre from the diet some people go through a stage of being constipated. As an immediate remedy for constipation I recommend using enemas. Regular enemas will not only manage constipation for you, but allow your body to detoxify sooner though removing old stale matter from the bowel. To learn about enemas, please look at the chapter *Bowel Management*.

When the Introduction Diet has been completed and when most pronounced digestive problems have gone, move into the Full GAPS Diet.

The Full GAPS Diet

If you have gone through the GAPS Introduction Diet before moving into the Full GAPS Diet, then you will be quite experienced already on how to use this healing protocol. Just expand your diet according to the lists of allowed and not-allowed foods, which you will find at the end of this chapter.

If you have decided to start from the Full GAPS Diet, then please carefully study the Introduction Diet first, because it will give you essential information about the most important elements of this nutritional protocol – meat stock, soups and fermented foods. These foods need to be introduced on the Full GAPS Diet from the very beginning.

Many delicious recipes can be used on the Full GAPS Diet, including baking breads, cakes and desserts. However, keep in mind that, as pleasant as they are, you do not start from them. About 85% of everything you eat daily should be made out of meats (including organ meats), fish, meat and fish stock, eggs, fermented dairy and vegetables (some well cooked, some fermented and some raw). Baking and fruit should be limited to snacks between meals; they should not replace the main meals. If you are starting from the Full GAPS Diet, baking and fruit should be kept out of the diet for a few weeks, and then introduced slowly and gradually watching your symptoms: your body will let you know if you are ready for them. If you are not ready, symptoms, which started disappearing when you avoided fruit, nuts and baking, will return when you introduce them. Homemade meat stock, soups, stews and natural fats are not optional – they should be your staples.

Everything you eat must be cooked at home from fresh ingredients. You need to completely avoid all non-allowed foods for two years at least. This means avoiding all grains, sugar, potatoes, parsnips, yams, sweet potato and anything made out of them. The flour in your cooking and baking can be replaced with ground almonds, coconut flour (or any other nuts, sunflower and pumpkin seeds ground into flour consistency); these flours need to be fermented prior to baking. The chapter *What we shall eat and why, with some recipes* will provide you with all the necessary information on how to bake with these flours.

Introduce fermented foods. If they have already been introduced, then slowly increase their amounts. You can ferment vegetables, fruit, milk and fish (please look in the chapter *What we shall eat and why, with some recipes*). You can make fermented beverages using kombucha or natural microbes, which live on fresh organic fruit and vegetables (beet kvass, for example). Eating fermented foods with every meal will help you to digest the meal without using supplements of digestive enzymes. Make sure to introduce all new fermented foods into the diet gradually starting from 1–2 teaspoons a day, because they can produce a die-off reaction.

The best foods for the GAPS person to buy are eggs, meats and fish, shellfish, fresh vegetables and fruit, nuts and seeds, garlic and olive oil. Meat and fish need to be bought fresh or frozen, not smoked, canned or processed in any other way, and cooked at home. As well as eating the vegetables cooked it is important to have them raw in the form of salads and sticks. In this form they will provide you with valuable enzymes and detoxifying substances, which will help in digesting meats. Raw fruit should be eaten on their own, not with meals, as they have a very different digestion pattern and can make work harder for the stomach. For most GAPS people it is a good idea to avoid fruit at the beginning. When your digestive symptoms have gone or reduced substantially you may be ready to eat some fruit as a snack between meals.

It is very important for a GAPS person to have plenty of natural fats in every meal from meats (animal fats), butter, ghee, coconut and cold-pressed olive oil. The fat content of the meal will regulate the blood sugar level and control cravings for carbohydrates. Cooking should be done with animal fats, which you have rendered yourself from meats (see the chapter *What we shall eat and why, with some recipes*). They will provide you with a plethora of nutrients to heal your immunity, nervous system and gut; the bulk of all fats you consume should be animal fats. Use generous amounts when cooking with them; the more animal fats you consume, the quicker you will recover. Plant oils must be cold pressed and of good quality. The most stable and reliable plant oil is cold-pressed olive oil. It is easily available and is a good source of vitamin E and other antioxidants. If you wish you can use other cold-pressed oils, such as hemp oil, walnut oil, avocado oil, pumpkin oil, etc. Never heat these oils, use them as a dressing on ready served meals. Plant oils are quite fragile: they are easily damaged by light, heat and oxygen. If you taste or smell any rancidity then do not use the oil (no matter how much you paid for it). Coconut oil is very stable and good for cooking and adding to ready meals. Organic ghee is another stable fat and very good for cooking and adding to dishes.

If you get any form of diarrhoea, go back to the first or second stage of the GAPS Introduction Diet for a few days: meat stock, soups, meat and vegetable stews, fish, eggs, fermented dairy and well-cooked vegetables, until the diarrhoea completely clears. After the stools have been normal for a few days introduce raw vegetables slowly, one at a time and starting from small amounts. When vegetables are introduced, try to introduce nuts, oily seeds and fruit gradually.

It is important for you to balance meals according to your body's needs. Please read the chapter *One man's meat is another man's poison* to understand this issue fully. Every one of us is a unique individual with a unique metabolism. Nobody in the world can dictate to you what proportions of protein-rich foods (meats, fish, eggs and dairy) to vegetables you need to eat at every meal. Only your body knows that, and it will let you know through your senses how to choose your foods on a daily basis.

Do not use a microwave oven, as it destroys food and makes it carcinogenic.[5,6,7] Cook and warm up food using a conventional oven and stove.

As you progress through the GAPS Diet you will become an expert on how your body responds to food in its own individual way. This is a unique and very valuable knowledge, which can serve you well for the rest of your life. That is why it is a very good idea to keep a diary through the Introduction Diet and beyond, where you record the whole process of food introduction and your individual symptoms and reactions.

The Full GAPS Diet needs to be followed for about two years. Some people with milder conditions can start introducing non-allowed foods in about a year; others have to adhere to the diet strictly for many years, and some for the rest of their lives. When your health problems are gone and you have been well for six months at least, you may be able to consider coming off the GAPS Diet. At that stage please look at the relevant chapter in this book. However, for many people the Full GAPS Diet has to become a permanent lifestyle.

If you are starting from the Full GAPS Diet, it is very important to introduce dairy products correctly. Here I would like to give you a structured approach on how to introduce dairy for a person who started from the Full GAPS Diet.

Dairy Introduction Structure

This structure is for:

1. those who have shown an allergy to dairy products on the Sensitivity Test, and as a result could not introduce dairy products during the GAPS Introduction Diet.
2. those who have chosen not to follow the GAPS Introduction Diet but start with the Full GAPS Diet. The Introduction Diet allows the gut to heal and recover more quickly. That is why we are able to introduce fermented dairy products from the beginning as part of the Introduction Diet. Some people, particularly those without severe digestive problems, decide to implement the Full GAPS Diet straight away. In this case it is advisable to follow this Dairy Introduction Structure.

Milk fat, which contains virtually no milk proteins or lactose, is generally well tolerated by most people, even those who show an allergy to other dairy products. Pure milk fat is called ghee or clarified butter. It is easy to make at home from organic butter (please look in the chapter *What we shall eat and why, with some recipes*). If you buy ghee make sure it does not contain preservatives and other additives. To make sure that your ghee is pure it is best to make it at home. Ghee contains a lot of valuable nutrients and is excellent for cooking and baking. Some people with severe dairy allergy cannot tolerate even ghee and have to avoid it. However, in my experience, the majority of GAPS children and adults have no reaction to ghee and can use it in their diet right from the beginning. If your patient has shown a reaction to yogurt, kefir and sour cream on the Sensitivity Test, you may be able to introduce ghee in the second stage of the Introduction Diet. Do the Sensitivity Test to your ghee first before introducing it.

After ghee the first dairy product to add to the diet is butter. Butter is virtually pure milk fat and contains only very small amounts of whey, which at a certain stage in the diet the patients can usually handle. Butter should be bought organic, because non-organic butter contains a lot of pesticides, hormones and antibiotics, which non-organic cows consume. For sensitive individuals I generally recommend trying to introduce butter after 6 weeks on the diet. Doing the Sensitivity Test will let you know if your patient is ready for this step. It is preferable to have unsalted butter, because it is processed salt that is usually used to preserve butter, and often other chemicals are added to the salt (flow agents and other additives). I would like to emphasise here that butter and ghee contain a lot of valuable nutrition for children and adults and should not be avoided, unless there is an anaphylactic-type allergy. Butter and ghee provide various fatty acids with important health-giving benefits, vitamins A, D, E, K2, beta-carotene and other nutritious substances in an easy-to-digest form.

Once ghee and butter are introduced well, in 6–12 weeks' time a gradual introduction of protein-containing lactose-free milk products is possible: yogurt, sour cream, kefir and cheeses. As the gut flora gets established and the digestive system heals, many GAPS patients are able to digest milk protein without absorbing it in the opiate-like form of casomorphin. However, all patients are different. Some are ready for this step in a few months, some require much longer. It is critical to proceed very carefully and slowly, introducing milk protein-containing foods one at a time and starting with tiny amounts, watching for any reaction. Any signs of regression in a child or an adult with GAPS would indicate that he/she may not be ready. It may be an increase in joint pain, sleep disturbances, anxiety, mood alterations and hyperactivity, bed-wetting in a potty-trained child, eczema flare-up or worsening allergies. Every patient will have symptoms typical for him or her. In some cases, dairy proteins have to be avoided indefinitely, particularly in long-standing cases of mental illness, cases complicated by epilepsy, autoimmune disease, severe asthma and severe eczema. The first protein-containing milk products that can be introduced are homemade yogurt and sour cream.

In a clinical setting some patients report that milk from other animals is much better tolerated than cow's milk. So, initially you may want to try making your kefir or yogurt from goat's milk, ewe's milk or camel milk. If it is not possible to find alternative milk in your area, try making yogurt from cow's milk. The majority of my patients use it with good results. A very important point here is to use only organic milk, as there is a noticeable difference in the clinical observations of the effects of non-organic and organic yogurt. People who react to non-organic yogurt often tolerate an organic one perfectly well, because non-organically reared animals have to consume a whole array of chemicals from antibiotics to pesticides, most of which finish up in the milk. It is best to find *raw* organic milk from native breeds of cow, goat or another animal reared on organic pasture.

It is important to introduce homemade yogurt gradually, starting with one teaspoon a day and slowly increasing the daily amount to one or two cups a day. The reason for this is that yogurt provides alive probiotic bacteria, which can cause a die-off reaction. *What is a die-off?* As these probiotic bacteria attack and kill pathogens in the gut, those pathogens release toxins. These are the toxins which make the person ill. In every person the die-off symptoms are very individual. Introducing probiotic foods gradually allows us to control the die-off symptoms (you can learn more on this subject in the chapter on probiotics). As you introduce yogurt, it can be added to homemade soups and stews, served as a dessert with fruit and honey or mixed with fruit smoothies and drinks. You can drain yogurt through a cheesecloth to produce thicker yogurt or cottage cheese. At the same time as yogurt you can introduce sour cream (fresh cream fermented with yogurt culture); it will provide excellent nutrition for the immunity and nervous system. Just as with yogurt, introduce sour cream gradually, starting with one teaspoon per day. Yogurt and sour cream will give a nice variety to the diet. However, I would repeat that the patient's digestive system has to be ready for them! So, do not rush with this step!

Once the GAPS patient can tolerate homemade yogurt and sour cream without any problem, kefir can be introduced. Kefir is similar to yogurt but uses a much more powerful combination of fermenting bacteria and fungi. You can get kefir starter from commercial companies or use kefir grains, which are available online. Kefir usually produces a more pronounced die-off reaction than yogurt. This is why I recommend introducing yogurt first before trying kefir. GAPS patients are affected by pathogenic yeasts, candida in particular. Introducing beneficial yeasts in kefir will help to take pathogenic yeasts under control. You can ferment cream with kefir culture and introduce it at the same time as the kefir made from milk. Just as with yogurt, start with one teaspoon per day and gradually increase the daily amount of kefir. Continue consuming good amounts of yogurt and sour cream (fermented with yogurt) while introducing kefir.

Once yogurt, sour cream and kefir have been introduced well, natural organic cheese can be tried. It has to be said that cheese is one of the more difficult dairy products to introduce as it provides a very concentrated milk protein. Cheese is also a great breeding ground for yeasts and moulds, which a lot of GAPS people cannot tolerate. Some GAPS patients find that they can have homemade yogurt without any problem but can never have cheese. However, in the majority of cases, providing that their digestive system has had a good chance to heal, GAPS children and adults can enjoy a good variety of natural cheeses, like cheddar and parmesan. As with kefir and yogurt, introduce cheeses one at a time, starting with a very small amount (no more than one mouthful) and watching the patient's reaction.

In a few months after safely introducing cheese many patients find that their digestive system is in a good enough state to handle commercially produced live natural yogurt (with no additives), sour cream and crème fraiche. At the end of the second year on the diet, fresh cream can be added to the list and some people can start drinking raw organic milk from native breeds of animals on organic pasture.

Dairy Introduction Structure – the summary

Step 1: avoid all dairy for 4–6 weeks. This will allow your body to clean out all debris from commercial dairy products. It takes that amount of time because commercially processed dairy foods accumulate in the body! This cleansing may bring many improvements in your health, which will demonstrate that you used to react to commercial dairy products.

Step 2: introduce homemade ghee made from organic raw butter. It is preferable to use cultured butter. Cultured butter has been churned from fermented cream; it has no lactose in it and any protein remaining will be pre-digested by fermenting microbes. Please look in the chapter *What we shall eat and why, with some recipes* for how to make ghee. Have one teaspoon of ghee with a meal. Then wait for 2–3 days observing your symptoms. If nothing has happened (none of your usual symptoms have got worse and no old symptoms have returned), then gradually make ghee a regular part of your diet. In my experience the majority of people can tolerate ghee. If you reacted to it, then wait for a few months and try again. When enough healing has taken place in your body, many things will change and you may be able to start tolerating dairy, as well as other foods you cannot tolerate now.

Step 3: introduce raw organic cultured butter (butter, churned from fermented cream). Try a teaspoon with a meal and then observe your symptoms for 2–3 days. Butter has a little protein in it and may have tiny amounts of remaining lactose. Hopefully, by this point, enough healing has happened in your body to tolerate that amount. If there is no reaction, then gradually make butter a normal part of your diet. Once cultured butter is well tolerated, try ordinary butter (made from cream which has not been fermented). Butter and ghee are wonderful foods which will bring many benefits for your health. It is worth introducing them!

Step 4: Introduce homemade yogurt and sour cream made from raw organic milk and cream using yogurt culture. Please look in the chapter *What we shall eat and why, with some recipes*. Introduce gradually, starting from one teaspoon per day. Gradually get up to fairly large amounts per day (a cup at least), being guided by your taste buds and your desire for these foods. Add them to your soups and stews, vegetables and salads, or eat them with a little honey or dried fruit.

Step 5: Introduce homemade kefir and sour cream made from raw organic milk and cream using kefir culture. Please look in the chapter *What we shall eat and why, with some recipes*. Kefir is more powerful than yogurt and produces a more pronounced die-off reaction, but will bring much more healing when fully introduced. Start from one teaspoon per day and gradually increase.

Step 6: Make cottage cheese by dripping homemade yogurt or kefir through a cheesecloth overnight. Again, introduce gradually.

Step 7: Now you can try commercially available, natural, traditionally made cheese. Usually at this stage there are no problems, and fairly quickly you will be able to have all sorts of cheeses from different traditions of the world, including beautiful creamy Italian and French cheeses.

After two years on the diet a lot of GAPS people find that, on an occasional basis, they can have any natural dairy product without any apparent problems, including cream and cheeses off the allowed list. However, I recommend limiting these products to occasional use and staying safe with those milk products which are allowed on the diet. At this stage some people can gradually introduce raw milk and raw cream into their diet without any problems.

A typical menu on the Full GAPS Diet

Start the day with a glass of still mineral or filtered water with a slice of lemon or a teaspoon of apple cider vinegar. It can be warm or room temperature to personal preference. If you have a juicer you can start the day with a glass of freshly pressed fruit/vegetable juice.

A good juice to start the day is 40% apple + 55% carrot + 5% beetroot (all raw of course). You can make all sorts of juice mixes, but generally try to have 50% therapeutic ingredients: carrot, small amount of beetroot (no more than 5% of the juice mixture), celery, cabbage, lettuce, greens (spinach, parsley, dill, basil, fresh nettle leaves, beet tops, carrot tops, dandelion leaves, etc), white and red cabbage, and 50% of some tasty ingredients to soften the taste of therapeutic ingredients: pineapple, apple, orange, grapefruit, grapes, mango, etc. You can have these juices straight or diluted with water.

When the juice is ready you can add to it 1–2 raw eggs (both the yolk and the white) and 2 tablespoons of homemade raw sour cream or coconut oil (or any homemade animal fat, melted and cooled to room temperature). Whisk the whole mixture and it will turn into the consistency of a milkshake. My patients call it ***'The GAPS shake'***. This mixture can replace a meal for you if you are in a hurry. But most importantly it will help your liver to remove gall stones. Many GAPS people have an accumulation of gall stones in the biliary ducts in the liver, which slows down the bile flow and impairs digestion of fats. Many people have had their gall bladder removed, which also makes fat digestion problematic. If you find it difficult to digest fats, then having GAPS shakes twice a day will resolve this situation by improving your bile flow and removing gall stones from your liver. First thing in the morning and the middle of the afternoon are good times, because juices and GAPS shakes need to be consumed on a fairy empty stomach. They will remove gall stones gently and slowly, and over time improve your digestion of fats.

Every day our bodies go through a 24-hour cycle of activity and rest, feeding and cleaning up (detoxifying). From about 4 a.m. till about 10 a.m. the body is in the cleansing or detoxification mode. Having fresh fruit and vegetables, water with lemon or cider vinegar, freshly pressed juices or GAPS shakes and probiotic foods will assist in this process. Loading the body with other food at that time interferes with the detoxification. That is why many of us do not feel hungry first thing in the morning. It is better to have breakfast around 10 a.m. when your body has completed the detox stage and is ready for feeding. At that stage we usually start feeling hungry. Children may be ready for their breakfast earlier than adults, and sometimes adults are ready for a hearty breakfast early in the morning. Follow your hunger and it will tell you what to eat and when.

Breakfast choices

- Eggs cooked to personal liking. They can be served with meat and vegetables, some cooked, some fresh as a salad (tomato, cucumber, onions, celery, any fresh salad greens, etc.) and some fermented. It is nice to have an avocado with your eggs. The yolks are best uncooked and the whites cooked lightly. Use plenty of cold-pressed olive oil as a dressing on the salad and eggs. You can mix a tablespoon of pre-soaked or sprouted sunflower and/or sesame and/or pumpkin seeds with the salad. You can add some cooked meat, fish, bacon (made with salt only) or sausages. Sausages must be made of pure minced meat and fat with only salt and pepper added (you can also add chopped onion, garlic or fresh herbs). Make sure that there is no commercial seasoning, chemical additives or MSG (Monosodium Glutamate) in the sausages. I recommend finding a local butcher who will make pure meat sausages for you to order. If diarrhoea is present, then the vegetables should be well cooked and the person should not have seeds at this stage. Serve a cup of warm homemade meat stock as a drink.

- Avocado with meat, fish or shellfish, vegetables raw, fermented and cooked, lemon and cold-pressed olive oil. Serve a cup of warm meat stock as a drink with food.
- Homemade soup, served with sour cream and gelatinous meat.
- Pancakes made with nut flour (nuts ground into flour) or coconut flour. The flour needs to be fermented prior to making pancakes. These pancakes are delicious with some butter, sour cream and honey, or as a savoury snack. If you blend some fresh or defrosted berries with honey, it will make a delicious jam to have with pancakes. You can have them with an herbal tea with lemon, ginger tea or fresh mint tea.
- Any of the home-baked GAPS goods: muffins, fruit cake or bread.

Lunch

- Homemade soup or stew with sour cream and meat or fish.
- Meat, fish, shellfish and raw or cooked vegetables. You can add avocado. Use olive oil with some lemon squeezed over it as a dressing. Serve a cup of warm homemade meat stock as a drink.
- Any meat/fish dish made with vegetables and probiotic foods.

Dinner

One of the dishes from the lunch or breakfast choice.

For snacks between meals you or your patient can have fruit, nuts and home-baked products. If you want something before bed, serve a cup of hot meat stock, homemade yogurt, kefir or sour cream with a bit of honey. You can also try Russian custard (please see the chapter *What we shall eat and why, with some recipes.*).

No-Plant GAPS Diet

Many medics would agree that in recent years our patients' symptoms are getting more complicated and more severe. Numbers of babies and children with FPIES (Food Protein Induced Enterocolitis Syndrome), babies and children with type one diabetes, children and adults with Crohn's disease and ulcerative colitis, people with severe mental illness and autoimmune diseases are growing rapidly. When trying to help some of these patients, I have discovered that their digestive systems were so damaged that even the first stage of the *GAPS Introduction Diet* was not gentle enough. Despite only having very small amounts of well-cooked vegetables they continued suffering from diarrhoea, abdominal pain and vomiting. So, the logical step was to remove all plant matter from the diet. Not a leaf, not a speck of anything from the plant kingdom was allowed. It was a difficult path to follow, but the patients tried it, and we started getting results! Diarrhoea started disappearing, vomiting stopped, sleep improved, the malnourished patients started putting on weight and the children started growing. Behaviour started improving and many individual symptoms started disappearing.

The first group of patients that followed the No-Plant GAPS Diet were babies with FPIES. The next group were children with ulcerative colitis and adults with mental illness. One patient with severe rheumatoid arthritis tried it with very good results. Having accumulated some experience, I now recommend this approach to any person who has tried the GAPS Introduction Diet and the Full GAPS Diet and is still struggling with digestive symptoms or any other chronic symptoms. I now have patients who have been on the No-Plant GAPS Diet for four years and longer and they are thriving. This experience has demonstrated, that it is perfectly safe and healthy for human beings to live without eating any plants at all! In other words, humans can live entirely on animal foods with excellent health; plants appear not to be essential for us. Please, read more about this in the chapter on vegetarianism.

Animal foods provide excellent quality proteins and fats for our bodies. However, some people may be concerned about carbohydrate intake on the No-Plant GAPS Diet. It may sound surprising, but animal foods do contain carbohydrates. To start with, I would like to introduce you to a very special molecule called glycogen. This molecule is an animal equivalent of starch and is stored in muscles, liver, blood cells (both white and red), kidney and brain tissue of animals. Both starch and glycogen are concentrated stores of glucose, and glycogen is packed with glucose molecules even more compactly than starch. Animal liver contains 5–6% of glycogen, while muscle (meat) can contain 1–2% of the muscle mass.[8] This carbohydrate content is what makes meats fermentable. The traditional ancient practice of dry curing meats (salumi – pancetta, salami, dry cured hams and other) is based on the fermentable carbohydrate (glycogen) content of the meats. Indeed, glycogen was first discovered through the fermentation of liver tissue by Claude Bernard (1813–1878), a famous French physiologist.[9] Glycogen is much easier for humans to digest than starch and other carbohydrates from plants; the net result of sugars absorbed from glycogen is probably higher than we absorb from a starchy meal.

Apart from glycogen, the gelatinous parts of meats and joints – the connective tissue (ligaments, joint capsules and fascias) – contain molecules where proteins and sugars are combined together (glycoproteins, proteoglycans and glucosaminoglycans).[8] These connective tissues also provide a considerable amount of carbohydrate. Cooking gelatinous meats in water for a few hours makes these molecules easy to digest and absorb, and in the GAPS Diet we place a strong emphasis on consuming these gelatinous meats daily. So, a person on the No-Plant GAPS Diet will not be without carbohydrates! Of course, compared to plants the amount of carbohydrate in animal foods is much smaller. However, from a clinical perspective and observation this small amount is quite enough. These patients not only thrive on purely animal foods, looking and feeling well, but recover from severe debilitating illnesses.

Where do patients on the No-Plant GAPS Diet get their vitamin C? For a long time, it has been assumed that we can get vitamin C only from plants. However, recent research has showed that we can get a good amount of this vitamin from eating animal liver.[10] Also, the juice of fermented vegetables provides bio-available vitamin C.[11] The fact that patients thrive on the No-Plant GAPS Diet and show no signs of any nutritional deficiency whatsoever demonstrates the fact that we, clearly, don't know everything about vitamin C yet!

For a long time, it has been assumed that carbohydrates are the most important foods for our gut flora. However, recent research has discovered that the decisive factor in the health of our gut flora is dietary protein.[12] It provides nitrogen for the gut microbes, which is something carbohydrates cannot provide. Carbon and nitrogen are considered to be two essential elements for the microbes in the gut. It is the balance between carbohydrates and protein in food that is important for our gut flora and this balance is likely to be very individual for every person. The clinical success of the No-Plant GAPS Diet shows that animal foods alone *can* provide the right balance of carbohydrates and proteins for the gut flora of people with severe digestive problems, mental illness and some severe physical problems. Animal foods are much easier for us humans to digest than plant matter. Plants can be quite harsh on a damaged digestive system. The foods that are consumed on the *No-Plant GAPS Diet* are healing and rebuilding for the gut lining and, obviously, provide the right mixture of nutrients for the gut flora to thrive. Without well-functioning gut flora there can be no healing in the gut! The fact that my patients recover so well on the *No-Plant GAPS Diet* shows that the gut flora was able to thrive and do its work in their digestive systems without any plant matter at all.

It is a good idea to work with a Certified GAPS Practitioner if you would like to try the No-Plant GAPS Diet. You will find a full list of these practitioners on www.gaps.me. I recommend trying this extreme end of the GAPS Nutritional Protocol in the following conditions: babies with FPIES and failure to thrive, children and adults with recently diagnosed type one diabetes, severe forms of ulcerative colitis, Crohn's disease and other inflammatory bowel disease, severe cases of mental illness and any other disorder where the Full GAPS Diet and the GAPS Introduction Diet did not achieve full results. Transfer to the No-Plant GAPS Diet gradually from the previous regime the patient was following. For example, a breastfed baby should continue breastfeeding while starting to follow this diet (while the mother needs to follow the Full GAPS Diet to provide breast milk of the right quality). If the person is already on the GAPS Diet, then transferring to the No-Plant Diet can happen quite quickly.

How to implement the No-Plant GAPS Diet

1. Start from meat stock made with a whole bird and giblets (chicken, duck, goose, pheasant, pigeons, turkey, etc.), a joint of lamb, joint of pork, fresh fish (with heads and skin), rabbit, horse, donkey, goat or game. Use whatever meats are easily available in your area. Beef is poorly tolerated by the majority of patients (because it has similar antigens to cow's milk), so I recommend introducing it later, when the digestive system has healed to a degree. For many patients (not for all) we have to find corn-free and soy-free chicken (not fed any grains or soy), because grain and soy antigens seem to finish up in the meat and affect very sensitive patients. Put the whole bird or a joint of meat into a pan, add 4–5 l (7–8¾ pt) of filtered water and a tablespoon of natural salt, bring to boil, reduce heat, cover and simmer for 2–4 hours. When ready, strain the stock by pouring it through a sieve into a clean dry pan. Start from a few teaspoons of this stock per day and gradually increase the amount to a few cups per day. After a few days of having meat stock, start blending into it the gelatinous parts of meats (which

you used to make the stock): the skin, fat, ligaments with a bit of brown meat off the body, legs and wings of poultry, fatty gelatinous parts of the lamb or other joints of meat, bone marrow, the skin and soft fatty parts of fish (the skin must be descaled before cooking the fish). Gradually make the stock thicker; this is your patient's 'soup', which he or she will need to eat daily for a long time (several times a day). Gradually start giving the meats with fat and gelatinous parts to your patient (from the joints you used for making the stock) as a separate meal, so they can chew it themselves. They should drink a cup of clear meat stock with these meats. Fat content of all meals must be high, so use fats naturally present on the meats and in the stock. Always extract bone marrow from large bones and add it to the soups.

2. While working on the meat stock, find a regular supply of raw organic milk from a goat, ewe, donkey, camel or reindeer. Cow's milk is too allergenic for this sensitive group of people and should be avoided at this stage. Get kefir grains (you can buy them online) and start fermenting the milk following the recipe in this book. After at least two weeks of meat stock and gelatinous meats, start adding 1–2 drops of kefir into the soup (make sure the soup has cooled down a little so as not to destroy the beneficial microbes in the kefir). Observe your patient for a few days on this amount of kefir. In many patients it produces a die-off reaction, which can manifest as a skin rash, eczema, behavioural problems, depression, headaches, poor sleep, nausea and vomiting, heart racing and palpitations or any other individual symptoms. Some amount of die-off has to be tolerated, but it needs to be kept within tolerable limits. If the die-off is too harsh, stop the kefir, wait a few days for the die-off symptoms to disappear and start from one drop of kefir per 3–4 days. As soon as this small amount of kefir is tolerated, gradually and slowly start increasing it to at least one cup per day. Add it to all soups and give it to your patient to drink as it is. If kefir produces a very strong reaction you may want to start from homemade yogurt. Yogurt generally produces a milder die-off reaction than kefir.
3. While working on kefir or yogurt make vegetable medley following a recipe in this book. If you find kefir too difficult to introduce, replace it with the liquid from this recipe. Start from 1–2 drops of the vegetable medley liquid per day. Many patients call it their 'vegetable tonic'. It is a probiotic drink and will also produce a die-off reaction. Depending on the severity of the die-off, increase the amount of this liquid gradually to several tablespoons per day. If kefir is well tolerated, you can introduce this tonic fairly shortly after introducing kefir. Both will provide a good mixture of probiotic microbes for healing your patient's digestive system.

4. Once kefir or yogurt is well tolerated, start fermenting raw cream from the same animals (a goat, ewe, donkey, camel or reindeer; not cow). Use some of your kefir as a starter for making sour cream. Introduce it gradually starting from a tiny amount per day. Sour cream provides wonderful fats and fat-soluble vitamins for the immune system and the brain of your patient. You cannot overdose on it, so add it to soups and other meals.
5. Introduce raw egg yolk starting from 1–2 drops per day. Make sure that the eggs come from healthy organic chickens which are kept on green pasture under the sun and are not fed any soy. Separate the yolk from the white very carefully. For people who may have egg allergy I recommend doing a *Sensitivity Test* beforehand: take a drop of raw egg yolk and apply it to the wrist of your patient at bedtime. Let it dry on the skin. In the morning check if there is any reaction on the spot. Red, swollen and itchy reaction means that we cannot introduce this food yet. If there is no reaction on the skin, put a drop on the lip and ask your patient not to lick it off. If there is a true allergy to egg, the lip will become swollen and red in a few minutes. People with egg allergy usually react to the egg white, while the yolk can be safely introduced. Eggs are a wonder food, full of nourishment, particularly when we consume them raw. If it is tolerated, gradually increase to 6-8 raw egg yolks per day. Later on, in the majority of patients, we can introduce raw egg whites too, starting from a tiny amount and gradually increasing.
6. Introduce organ meats: liver, kidney, tongue, brain, heart, tripe and intestines. Initially cook them in water with natural salt and introduce gradually. Once introduced you can cook them following your favourite recipe.
7. Introduce fresh fish and shellfish available in your area. Make sure that they are cooked with water and salt only, nothing else. Make sure to descale the fish before cooking it, because some of the best nutrients in fish are in the skin and just under it. Make sure to consume all the soft tissues from the head of the fish (they are rich in oils and fat-soluble vitamins).
8. I do not recommend bone broth on the No-Plant GAPS Diet, only fresh meat stock. Please read carefully in the chapter *What we shall eat and why, with some recipes* about the difference between the two and how to prepare them. Bone broth is irritating for this group of very sensitive patients. However, this doesn't seem to apply to all of them. Some patients could tolerate bone broth. If you would like to try it, introduce it quite a bit later in the diet, after the meat stock and all other foods are well tolerated.
9. I would like to emphasise that it is essential to use plenty of natural salt in the food! When we reduce carbohydrates in the diet the body

excretes a lot of sodium, which in itself is not bad because a lot of excess water and toxins are removed together with sodium. However, sodium is an essential mineral for us. Your body will not allow you to develop severe deficiency in sodium, but mild deficiency can cause aching muscles, low energy, constipation, feeling a little dizzy and other problems. Meat stock (made with natural salt) is an excellent way to replenish sodium and other minerals in the body. The more homemade meat stock you drink every day, the better you will feel. Also, liquid from the vegetable medley (cabbage tonic) is very rich in minerals. Let me emphasise that only *natural* salt must be used! Natural, unprocessed salt contains some 92 minerals and trace elements, all of which are essential for us. Salt in the shops has been processed with most of these vital substances removed, it causes disease and should not be consumed by anybody. You can find natural rock salt or sea salt online or in health shops.

These are the only foods that are allowed on the No-Plant GAPS Diet. I have had some parents in my clinic who worried about the lack of variety in their child's diet. If you think about it, humanity has evolved eating quite a limited list of foods that could be found in their local area. And every season imposed its own limitations on the variety of foods: what was available in the summer was not available in the winter. A human baby consumes mother's milk only for many months and thrives on it, without demanding any variety. From my experience, children and adults can heal and grow very well on a very limited list of foods, as long as these foods are wholesome and homemade. The No-Plant Diet is not for life, it is only temporary. When the person heals from the illness, we can introduce plants and widen the choice of foods.

This is a case study of a little boy with ulcerative colitis and learning problems who stayed on the No-Plant GAPS Diet for three years.

James was a typical GAPS child. He had acquired abnormal gut flora from his parents at the start of his life. As a result, he suffered from diarrhoea, abdominal pain, feed refusal, nausea and vomiting. In the first 18 months of his life he had many courses of antibiotics for recurrent ear infections, which damaged his gut flora even further. This affected his development: James was hyperactive and aggressive with poor social skills and poor ability to learn. At the age of three years he was diagnosed with ulcerative colitis. Mainstream medications and alternative treatments were not bringing any real progress. At the age of six years he was suffering from severe diarrhoea with blood and mucous in his stools, abdominal pain, asthma, hay fever, anaemia

and a learning disability. James was small for his age and looked very pale and malnourished. He was taking medications for ulcerative colitis and hay fever.

The parents agreed to try the No-Plant GAPS Diet for James. Having suffered for most of his life James was very compliant with his new diet. He started consuming meat stock, boiled meats, fresh fish, raw eggs and homemade meat jelly. Raw goat's kefir was gradually introduced, starting from a few drops per day. In a few weeks James had improved dramatically: his stools became normal, abdominal pain became rare and the parents started reducing his medications (sulfasalazine and antihistamins). James' academic ability improved and he started making some friends at school. Every increase of the daily amount of kefir produced a die-off reaction, when James would become aggressive, very tired and have heart racing and palpitations. The fat content of the diet was gradually increased, using ghee, goose fat and other animal fats. Fish oil was gradually introduced.

After six months on the diet all medication had been stopped. James had normal stool and no abdominal pain, he had put on weight and started growing.

After eight months on the diet sour cream (made from raw goat's cream) and organ meats (liver, kidney, heart and tongue) were gradually introduced. The introduction of every new food produced a reaction with abnormal behaviour, fatigue, heart racing or a skin rash.

After one and a half years on the No-Plant GAPS Diet asthma, environmental allergies and hay fever were gone and James looked very healthy. He was growing well and started playing sports. Threadworms were found in the stool and James started getting constipated. The parents started doing enemas at bedtime and James was given diatomaceous earth (DE) to address parasites, starting from a tiny amount and gradually increasing. James passed about 60 gallstones (green in colour and floating) and many worms after starting DE and enemas. After passing the gall stones James was able to tolerate much more fat in his diet. He passed many different parasites in his stools with the help of the enemas, some large (up to 10 cm/4 in long) and filled with blood, some looking like large black slugs, some looking like mushrooms (brown and white, rubbery, 3–4 cm/1¼–1½ in diameter) and some white worms and larva.

After two years and four months on the No-Plant GAPS Diet mainstream tests for ulcerative colitis came back negative. James had no inflammation in his digestive system, no symptoms and had been off all medication for two years. The only plant-based food he was having was 1.5 teaspoons of liquid from a homemade vegetable medley (cabbage, garlic and beetroot fermented in brine). This liquid was

introduced very gradually starting from a few drops per day. All the other food James was eating was of animal origin.

After three years of strict avoidance of all plant foods one clove of roasted garlic per day was successfully introduced, followed by one drop of olive oil per day. These foods provoked a die-off reaction and many more parasites came out in stools (liver flukes and long white worms). The garlic and olive oil resolved constipation and enemas have been stopped. James started producing normal daily stool. Seven months later other vegetables were gradually introduced: cooked courgette (zucchini), broccoli, spinach, cauliflower, raw avocado and raw garlic. James continued eating a high-fat diet with cooked meats, fish, eggs and fermented raw goat's milk and cream.

Four years from the beginning of the No-Plant Diet James is doing very well. He is eating all the vegetables allowed on the GAPS Diet, apart from the nightshade family (tomato, aubergine/eggplant and peppers). He is eating baked apples with sour cream, fermented vegetables and commercially produced cheese (cheddar, camembert, brie and parmesan). But the bulk of his diet is still animal foods: meat stock, meats, fish, eggs and fermented dairy. Generally, James is very well, looks healthy, is doing well at school, playing sports and has a few good friends. He is enjoying his life and has no signs of ulcerative colitis or a learning disability. Overall, he has spent three years eating only animal foods.

How to come off the No-Plant GAPS Diet

While your patient is on this diet prepare fermented vegetables: sauerkraut, vegetable medley, kimchi and other recipes. The longer these vegetables ferment the easier they will be to digest. In fact, the best sauerkraut is last year's one: the cabbage is well pre-digested, histamine is largely gone and it has the best chance of being tolerated by sensitive patients. Initially ferment at room temperature. Once the mixture stops producing gas, move it to a cool, dark place where it will continue maturing.

1. Make a soup by cooking a teaspoon of well-fermented vegetables in the meat stock. If you are dealing with a particularly sensitive person, start from a tiny amount of fermented vegetables per litre of meat stock. Cook this soup well, for 30 minutes at least. Let your patient eat a bowl of this soup, making a note in your diary. Watch for any reactions to this first bowl of soup for 3–4 days. If there are no reactions, gradually make this soup part of daily diet. Gradually increase the amount of fermented vegetables in the soup.

2. Roast some garlic, peel it and try to blend a tiny amount with the meat stock. Again, make a note in the food diary and watch for any reactions for 3–4 days. If there are no reactions, gradually introduce roasted garlic.
3. If garlic and soups with fermented vegetables are tolerated and have been introduced, try to cook some courgette (zucchini) without the skin or seeds, broccoli or cauliflower in the meat stock, starting from a tiny amount. Again, make a note in the food diary and watch for any reactions for 3–4 days. If there are no reactions, gradually introduce. Make sure to introduce one vegetable at a time, slowly and patiently. All vegetables must be organic and, even better, grown yourself in your own garden.
4. Congratulations! Your patient is now on the first stage of the *GAPS Introduction Diet*. From now on, follow the stages.

Case study of a baby with FPIES.

FPIES (Food Protein-Induced Enterocolitis Syndrome) is a new variation of food allergy/food intolerance. Typically it happens in breastfed babies in the first year of life, when the child develops diarrhoea, vomiting and dehydration. Testing finds that the child is allergic to most protein in foods (cow's dairy, soya, egg, meat, grains, many vegetables and often breast milk). Typically the child is put onto an elemental formula (where protein has been broken down into single amino acids) and the parents are told not to give the child any food with protein in it, only some vegetables. Often immune-suppressing medication is used, but there is no effective mainstream treatment available. Children with FPIES may finish up with failure to thrive and mental and physical disability.

Laura was exclusively breastfed from birth. At 12 weeks of age she developed diarrhoea with blood in her stool. The doctor advised stopping breastfeeding and put Laura on an elemental formula, but diarrhoea did not stop. When tried with solids Laura developed projectile vomiting, lethargy and acid stools. Tests revealed that Laura was allergic to most proteins in foods and diagnosed with FPIES. At the age of 18 months she was still on elemental formula and suffering from diarrhoea, vomiting and anaemia. She was not growing or developing.

We put Laura on the No-Plant GAPS Diet with some fermented cabbage juice. After four months on this diet Laura was thriving; she started putting on weight and developing. Her diarrhoea and vomiting stopped. Then she developed eczema. We suspected that she reacted to cornfed chickens. The mother found corn-free chicken for making Laura's soups and her eczema cleared up.

Laura has been on her diet for three years now and is doing very well. By now she has got to the third stage of the GAPS Introduction Diet, so her food choices are still quite limited. However, she is healthy overall, has normal mental and physical development and is a beautiful thriving child.

The No-Plant GAPS Diet is at the extreme end of the GAPS Nutritional Protocol. It is difficult to follow and should be attempted only in situations when nothing else has worked. Great determination and full compliance are required to follow this diet. Many people ask if this diet is ketogenic. Let us address this issue.

GAPS Ketogenic Diet

Ketones (acetoacetate, beta-hydroxybutyrate and acetone) are water-soluble substances produced in the body when it uses fats for making energy. In a normal healthy state our bodies can use both glucose and fats, depending on the composition of our meals, activity level and other factors. Having ketones in the blood is normal, because fat is the preferred source of energy for most organs and tissues in the human body. Every time your body burns its own fat for energy, ketones are produced and they can also be used for energy production.[8]

The mainstream medical profession is trained to fear ketones because of a very dangerous situation which can happen in diabetic people, called ketoacidosis. During ketoacidosis the person has very high levels of both glucose and ketones in the blood. High levels of glucose in the blood are always dangerous! During ketoacidosis the body cannot use glucose for producing energy and uses fats instead (hence ketones are high), leaving glucose to do a lot of damage. This situation happens largely in type one diabetes and in people with very advanced type two diabetes, because their normal mechanisms of energy production are broken. In people who don't have diabetes, ketones are produced routinely by the liver to maintain a low level of these substances in the blood. When the body starts using fat exclusively for producing energy it goes into a state of *physiological ketosis,* which is perfectly normal and healthy and has nothing to do with diabetic ketoacidosis.[8]

By changing our diet, we can deliberately switch the body to using fats as a source of energy instead of using glucose. Ketones are produced as a result of this type of energy production, so the diet is called a ketogenic diet. Ketogenic diets have been gaining popularity over several decades now. They are being used successfully for treating cancer, epilepsy, Lyme disease, chronic fatigue syndrome, obesity, mental illness and other severe health problems.[13,14] When following a ketogenic diet it is essential to measure your ketone levels regularly to achieve the target of 0.5–3 mmol/L in the blood. Ketone levels can be measured in blood, breath and urine, and various measuring devices are available online or in pharmacies. Using urine is the least expensive way of measuring ketones, but it is considered to be less reliable than measuring ketones in blood and breath. Measuring ketones in the breath is becoming the most popular method; it is reliable and non-invasive.

Surprisingly, the No-Plant GAPS Diet may not necessarily be ketogenic. It depends on the person's constitution and metabolism. Some people move into ketogenic state easily and quickly, other people do not. One of the major reasons for that is the individual composition of our gut flora. Many microbes in the gut are able to produce glucose from proteins and fats.[15] They manufacture glucose for themselves and can release enough of it into the general bloodstream of the person to sabotage all efforts to get into ketosis. GAPS people have abnormal gut flora, which can be the reason why some of them find it difficult to get into physiological ketosis.

The rules of a ketogenic diet are limiting carbohydrates and protein, while eating large amounts of fat. On the No-Plant GAPS Diet carbohydrate consumption is very small. However, protein consumption can be high. Our bodies are able to convert protein into glucose through a process called gluconeogenesis. So, in order to get into ketosis, we need to gradually reduce protein while replacing it with fats. Coconut oil and ghee are the two most helpful fats for getting the body into physiological ketosis, because they contain medium-chain fatty acids which do not need much digestion and absorb quickly. I do not recommend MCT oil as it is highly processed and not natural for the human body to consume. GAPS Nutritional Protocol is based on natural foods first and foremost; we avoid all artificial inventions.

In my experience, for the vast majority of GAPS people there is no need to get into ketosis; just following the standard GAPS Diet will provide all the necessary tools for healing. When would we need to move into ketogenic state on the GAPS Diet? One situation where this has been found useful is cancer.[14,16] Many cancer cells cannot use fats for producing energy. They must have glucose to live and grow. When we move into ketosis cancer is starved of energy. This approach has been found to be successful in many cancer sufferers, though not all. Epilepsy has been treated with a ketogenic diet for a long time now; it works in many cases but not for everybody.[15] People with other health problems around the world are trying ketogenic diets for treatment of Lyme disease, severe autoimmune conditions, obesity and diabetes, and some find it useful. But, apart from cancer, I don't feel that it is really necessary for the majority of GAPS people to be in ketosis to recover from their health problems.

It is beyond the scope of this book to focus on the ketogenic diet in detail. There are very good sources of this information available; please study them well before moving into physiological ketosis. It is important to measure ketones in your blood or breath daily, so you will need to invest in an appropriate device and record all your measurements meticulously. If a person, who has been on the GAPS Diet for a while, feels that they may achieve more improvements in their health by getting into physiological ketosis, then it is possible to do that.

How to move into physiological ketosis on the GAPS Nutritional Protocol

1. Move into the No-Plant GAPS Diet first and settle into it for a few weeks. It will help you to get into ketosis slowly and gradually.
2. Then start reducing protein (meat, fish and eggs) gradually and increasing fat consumption, focussing on organic raw coconut oil and organic ghee. Add increasing amounts of these two fats to every cup of meat stock you consume and try to drink 5–6 cups a day.
3. Make sure that all the meals you eat have a high fat content. Focus on animal fats, but you can also add plenty of good quality olive oil to your meals. Snack on high-fat cheese adding a good slab of butter to it. You can also snack on fresh nuts and oily seeds (sunflower, pumpkin and sesame) if your digestive system is ready for them; it is always a good idea to soak, sprout or ferment nuts and seeds to make them more digestible.
4. Replace kefir and yogurt with homemade sour cream.
5. Don't forget to use plenty of natural salt in all your meals to keep your sodium stores replenished. Ketogenic diets remove large amounts of water and sodium out of the body.[16]
6. Drink plenty of water and add 1 tablespoon of cider vinegar or squeeze half a lemon into every cup of water you drink. They will help your body to balance its pH, as ketosis can make your body quite acidic.
7. Keep in mind that the health of your gut is the most important target for you! As you are trying to get into ketosis don't lose sight of that. It is important to adhere to the lists of allowed foods on the GAPS Nutritional Protocol and not forget to have plenty of meat stocks, gelatinous and organ meats and fermented foods.

There are many good recipe books for following a ketogenic diet, which will help you to make your diet enjoyable. You will need to find your own individual proportions of fats to protein to stay in ketosis. Depending on the composition of your gut flora these proportions can be very different from what works for other people and from what the books may say. Because of the activity of the gut flora it may take time for a GAPS person to get into physiological ketosis and make it stable.

The More-Plant GAPS Diet

Every human being is unique with a unique constitution and metabolism. There are people who need to eat more carbohydrates to feel well. And even people who thrive on mostly animal foods have periods when their bodies ask for more plant matter. The chapter *One Man's Meat is Another Man's Poison* goes more deeply into this subject. We must learn to listen to our bodies and give them what they need, and these needs change all the time. The GAPS Diet is flexible, and it is possible to eat plenty of plants when your gut is ready for it. This particularly applies to the so-called 'carbo type people' according to the concept of *metabolic typing* (see chapter *One Man's Meat is Another Man's Poison*). This type requires larger amounts of carbohydrates in their diet. People with this kind of metabolism may feel well on the GAPS Diet for a while, but then start feeling that they do not get enough carbohydrates and are not tolerating large amounts of animal fats. You may also feel that you do better on low-purine meats (white meats and fish) and low-fat dairy or no dairy at all. The true 'carbo type' people are rare, but if you feel that you may belong to this group, please research *metabolic typing* and identify your unique nutritional needs.

In order to follow this form of the GAPS Diet make sure that you do not suffer from diarrhoea (particularly with blood and mucous in the stool) or abdominal pain. If any of these symptoms are present, then follow the GAPS Introduction Diet first before considering the More-Plant GAPS Diet.

Cooked plants are much easier to digest and are gentler on the digestive system than raw. If you feel that you need to consume more plant matter, focus on cooked plants. Vegetables can be cooked in meat stock to make soup, baked, stir-fried or steamed. If you find it difficult to digest animal fats, use olive oil or coconut oil in the amounts that appeal to you.

If you really miss starch, eat plenty of cooked winter squashes as well as cooked turnips, swedes, carrots and celeriac. These vegetables contain a small amount of starch but are allowed on the GAPS Diet. Listen to the messages from your digestive system when eating these vegetables; if you get bloating, diarrhoea, constipation or other symptoms, then you are not ready for starch, no matter how much you crave it. Stop eating them until your digestive system recovers and then try to introduce them again, slowly. Make sure to drink meat stock with your cooked vegetables and eat some fermented foods. If this group of vegetables is tolerated well by your digestive system and you have taken plenty of time to introduce them into your diet, then you can look in the chapter *Coming off the GAPS Diet* and start introducing potatoes and grains.

The same goes for fruit: cooked fruit is much easier to digest than raw. Apple purée, stewed berries, plums, pears and other fruit are much easier to digest than their raw counterparts. Make sure always to add some fat to your fruit in the amount that appeals to you (animal fat or a plant fat, such as olive oil or coconut oil). Some honey or dried fruit can be added for sweetness. The fat content of your cooked fruit will make sure that your body uses the sugars in the fruit appropriately and your blood sugar level stays within the normal limits. It is not a good idea for GAPS people to consume cooked fruit without added fat, and the more fat you can comfortably add, the better you will feel after eating the fruit. Adding spices, such as cinnamon, cardamom and nutmeg will make cooked fruit taste even nicer and assist in its digestion. Please, look at some recipes for fruit pies in the chapter *What we shall eat and why, with some recipes*. Adding properly prepared nuts to your fruit will balance carbohydrates in the fruit with some plant proteins and fats.

Beans, lentils and dried peas can become a regular part of the diet, as long as they are properly prepared and you can digest them. All these foods are seeds. Plants do not want their seeds eaten, which is why they equip them with substances, called antinutrients, which can damage the digestive system of an animal that eats them. Soaking, sprouting and/or fermenting beans, lentils and dry peas before cooking reduces the amount of antinutrients in them and makes these foods much more digestible. Please look in the chapter *What we shall eat and why, with some recipes* for how to prepare them properly.

Nuts and oily seeds, such as sunflower, sesame and pumpkin seeds, can be used to make breads, pies and desserts. They are also seeds and need to be prepared properly before cooking.

If you feel like eating raw vegetables, nuts and fruit, make sure that you can digest them. If your gut is not ready for raw plant matter, you will get bloating, crampy pain or abnormal stool for a few days after eating it. These symptoms are a signal for you to wait with the raw vegetables, nuts and fruit and focus on cooked plants instead.

Fermentation is a powerful way to make plant matter more digestible. Make sure to ferment all kinds of vegetables and consume some of them with every meal.

The More-Plant GAPS Diet is not vegetarian. We need to continue eating meats, fish, eggs and fermented dairy products. Depending on your unique metabolism you may favour low-purine meats and fish or enjoy high-purine foods. You need to find your own proportions of proteins to fats to carbohydrates by adjusting the amounts of animal foods to the amounts of plants in every meal. Some meals can even be vegetarian if that is what you desire. Adjust the proportions of plant to animal foods in every meal according to your body's needs, dictated to you by desire for food, smell, taste and satisfaction from eating food. Please, read the chapter *One Man's Meat Is Another Man's Poison* before commencing the More-Plant GAPS Diet.

GAPS Liquid Fasting

Rest is not idleness,
and to lie sometimes on the grass under trees on a summer's day,
listening to the murmur of the water,
or watching the clouds float across the sky,
is by no means a waste of time.

John Lubbock

Do you feel that your digestive system is tired and could do with a rest? Do you feel that your body has accumulated too many toxins? Is your appetite low and you don't feel like eating? Do you suffer from acute ulcerative colitis or Crohn's disease, when symptoms are not improving on the GAPS Introduction Diet or No-Plant GAPS Diet? Then perhaps it is a good idea for you to consider GAPS Liquid Fasting.

Fasting is one of the oldest and most effective ways of cleaning your body on the inside. Our bodies spend large amounts of energy on digesting and metabolising food. When we stop eating, the body re-directs its energy to other jobs, such as removing toxins and parasites, and healing itself. Fasting has an excellent record of curing all sorts of 'incurable' conditions – from rheumatoid arthritis to cancer. In people without serious illness, regular fasting will clean and rejuvenate the body and prevent disease. The aim of GAPS Liquid Fasting is to give our digestive system a rest by avoiding solid food and only drinking clear liquids.

I do not recommend water fasting for GAPS people as it is quite harsh on a body that is malnourished and filled with toxins. The purpose of the GAPS Nutritional Protocol is to heal the body, starting from healing the gut. We avoid solid foods, which gives the gut a good rest and allows it to direct its resources to healing itself. On a GAPS Liquid Fast we drink all kinds of clear liquids, not only water. Liquids rich in minerals, vitamins, enzymes, probiotics, fats and proteins will assist your body in going through the fast with maximum benefit and no side effects.

Who should be careful with fasting? Underweight and slim people should not fast longer than one day at a time (with a break of at least one month between fasting episodes). Your body simply does not have enough resources to accomplish a prolonged fast. The same goes for pregnant and nursing women. In the first few days of pregnancy, when a woman experiences nausea and has no appetite, the GAPS Liquid Fast can be quite helpful. But as soon as the nausea subsides, and the appetite returns, she should move to the Full GAPS Diet. People with acute ulcerative colitis and Crohn's disease may be underweight, but their gut simply cannot handle solid food, so they have to follow the GAPS Liquid Fast regardless of what their body mass is.

Who should consider fasting? When your body would like a rest from food, it will let you know by supressing your appetite. Listen to your body! If you don't feel like eating, then don't (this does not apply to people with anorexia nervosa, please read about this disorder in the first GAPS book *Gut And Psychology Syndrome*). Drink only liquids until your appetite for solid foods returns. For one person this can be one day, for another person a month. People with a high toxic load, people with stubborn symptoms, overweight people, patients with severe allergies and people who feel 'stuck' in their healing progress can find the GAPS Liquid Fast very helpful. People with severe digestive problems, such as acute ulcerative colitis and Crohn's disease, may benefit from a period of avoiding solid foods and consuming only liquids. It is safe for children older than three years of age to go on the GAPS Liquid Fast. Children are generally better connected to their bodies than adults and will refuse food when they have no appetite. Your child will let you know when to end the fast by showing interest in solid food. Be calm about it and just let your child be present at dinner table with the rest of the family, and he/she will start eating when ready.

What liquids do we consume on the GAPS Fast? You simply cannot drink too much when fasting; as soon as you finished one beverage, move to the next. Here is a list of liquids you should consume on a GAPS Fast.

- Meat stock. Drink it hot or warm and make sure to remove any solids, as the stock needs to be clear. Meat stock is a staple on the GAPS Diet; it has a powerful ability to help your digestive system rebuild itself and heal any damage. It provides collagen and other proteins, minerals, amino acids and a plethora of other building materials for your gut lining and the rest of the body. Make gelatinous stock by boiling joints and bones with ligaments and some meat, skin, feet and heads, adding some natural salt, black pepper and bay leaves to the water. You can also add your favourite spices, making sure that you can tolerate them. Vegetables can be added as well – onion, carrot, celery, cabbage, greens, etc. Meat stock should be cooked for a few hours: fish 1 hour, chicken and other poultry 1.5–2 hours, beef, pork and lamb 3–4 hours. When ready, add some freshly chopped garlic and parsley, strain and enjoy. There is no need to remove fat from the stock unless you feel that you cannot digest fat at the moment. I do not recommend bone broth on the GAPS Fast, as it is too rich in amino acids and can cause reactions in some people, particularly those who are new to the GAPS Nutritional Protocol. If you have been consuming bone broth before and are adapted to it, then you can add it to your list of liquids. Meat stock and bone broth are prepared quite differently and have a different nutrient composition and a different effect on the body; they should not be confused. On the GAPS Fast we consume homemade fresh meat stock. Make sure to have a cup of meat stock every hour or every few hours; the more meat stock you consume per day, the quicker you will heal.

- Vegetable medley is a wonderful remedy for fasting. It is rich in minerals, enzymes, vitamins, antioxidants, probiotics and many other substances to support your digestive system and other systems and organs in the body. During fasting we lose a lot of salt (sodium chloride). Vegetable medley is salty and will replenish your stores of this very important substance. If, for whatever reason, you are not able to have vegetable medley, then add some natural salt to every glass of water you drink (about ½ teaspoon per glass).
- Brine from home-fermented vegetables is another wonderful beverage, rich in minerals, enzymes, salt, lactic acid and other supportive nutrients. Use brine from fermented garlic, cucumbers, peppers, cabbage or any other mixture of vegetables you have fermented at home. Dilute it with water to your taste and enjoy. It is important to drink it slowly 'chewing' every mouthful. Vegetable medley and brine have powerful laxative properties, drinking them quickly can cause diarrhoea (often the same colour as the vegetable medley or the brine). Diarrhoea is welcomed during fasting. All major fasting clinics worldwide give their patients laxative salts to induce diarrhoea, which cleanses the bowel and removes large amounts of toxic matter from the body. Drinking brine or vegetable medley slowly will reduce the intensity of diarrhoea and make it more comfortable.
- Vegetable broth is another warm and comforting liquid, which is quite nice to consume on the GAPS Fast. It is made by slowly cooking all sorts of available vegetables in water for several hours or even overnight. Here is how to make it: fill a non-metal cooking pot (ceramic, glazed or glass) almost to the top with chopped vegetables (you can use parts of vegetables that are usually discarded – stalks of broccoli, cabbage and cauliflower, offcuts and skins of squashes, pumpkins, garlic and onions, etc), add some salt, black pepper, bay leaves and a source of acidity: a handful of any fermented vegetables

you have, brine from fermented vegetables or ½ cup apple cider vinegar. This is a good opportunity to use any of your less-successful fermented vegetables, which, perhaps, don't taste very good. Leave to simmer overnight on the stove or in the oven. In the morning strain the liquid (the vegetable broth) and discard the vegetables, add some freshly chopped garlic and parsley, strain and enjoy. Try to add some whey or vegetable medley to it.

- Herbal teas made from any mixture of herbs you like. Loose herbal teas are the best (not in tea bags!). To make them, pour boiling water onto dried or fresh herbs and leave in a warm place to steep for 5 minutes. Fresh ginger tea is very soothing and healing for the digestive system and other systems of your body. To make it, grate fresh or frozen ginger root, add boiling water and let it steep for 5 minutes. Pour through a strainer.
- Fresh whey from homemade kefir or yogurt. To make it, pour homemade fresh kefir or yogurt into a cheesecloth, tie the four corners of the cloth together and hang it overnight to drip into a bowl. The yellow liquid you will find in the bowl in the morning is whey. It keeps well in the fridge in glass bottles and is an excellent drink during the GAPS Fast. It is rich in probiotics and lactic acid and has a profound healing effect on the gut lining. It will balance the laxative effect of the vegetable medley and the brine from fermented vegetables as it has a firming effect on the bowel. Many people like it salty, so try to add some salt to whey according to your taste. You can dilute your whey with some water or have it as it is, and you can add it into every cup of your meat stock.
- Green juices made from vegetables: cucumber, celery, greens (lettuce, kale, swiss chard, parsley and any other greens available), garlic, ginger and lemon. I would not use fruit juices for fasting as they are too sweet. If you desire a little sweetness, add a little carrot to the green juice or some orange. Generally, sweet taste is not a good friend for GAPS people; sour taste is the good friend, particularly on the GAPS Liquid Fast.
- Natural mineral and spring water, still and carbonated (the bubbles of gas in the water improve its energetic properties). It is important to drink your water at room temperature or warm; drinking chilled water is stressful for the digestive system and will interfere in its ability to heal. Every cup of water should have a piece of lemon squeezed into it (drop the lemon itself into the glass after squeezing; it will contribute antioxidants, minerals and other beneficial substances to the water). Alternatively, you can add organic apple cider vinegar to the water (a tablespoon per glass). Fasting makes the body quite acidic and drinking plain water does not alleviate this

problem. Lemon and cider vinegar have the right mineral profile to help your body maintain a normal acid-alkaline balance. Make sure to buy your mineral water in glass bottles, not plastic! Plastic bottles leach toxic chemicals into the water. Do not use tap water! In most places around the world it carries a heavy load of man-made chemicals.

As you can see, you have a good choice of liquids to drink during your GAPS Liquid Fast. Have them all available to you every day and choose what you want to drink. Listen to your body, it will tell you what it wants by giving you a desire for a particular beverage. All these choices will also allow you not to feel hungry during fasting. Don't drink anything cold; all beverages should be consumed warm, hot or at room temperature.

How do we know if we drink enough liquids during fasting?
We watch our urine: it needs to be clear and pale in colour, and there should be a normal to larger than normal volume coming out of you. If your urine is dark and concentrated, then you are not drinking enough water and your kidneys are struggling to remove toxins. If it is difficult to drink more liquids than you are already consuming, then do an enema. It will allow your body to replenish missing water and remove a large amount of toxicity, reducing pressure on your kidneys.

How long should one fast for?
It is very much up to you how long you should fast. Some people fast one day, others can fast three weeks or even longer (no more than 42 days, please!). The length of the fast very much depends on what your lifestyle will allow and what your body tells you. If you can rest undisturbed, sleeping as much as you need and not having too many responsibilities, then you can accomplish a long fast at home. If you are looking after a family, working or have other responsibilities, be kind to yourself and fast only for the period of time that feels comfortable to you under the circumstances. When we fast, the body directs its resources to cleansing, removing toxins and repairing accumulated damage. All of this can make you feel quite tired and sleepy; fasting is a parasympathetic activity. You may need to do enemas every two days or possibly even daily to keep your bowel empty, which will take time. Planning the length of your fast very much depends on how much time you have available to focus on yourself and allow your body to relax. Some people manage to fast at home, but for other people it is optimal to go to a fasting clinic or a retreat; this allows you to leave all your responsibilities behind and focus on rest and healing.

If you go to a clinic, make sure to take with you a few bottles of vegetable medley and brine from your fermented vegetables, a few bottles of whey, a small bottle of cider vinegar, a bag of organic lemons and, depending on the length of your stay at the clinic, ingredients for making another batch of vegetable medley (a large glass jar, fresh beetroot, garlic, cabbage, dill seed, natural salt and a knife for slicing the vegetables). Most fasting clinics provide good quality water, juices and vegetable broth. A clinic may not provide a facility for you to make meat stock; if it does, then make sure to bring all the ingredients with you. Alternatively, you may want to make the meat stock at home and bring it with you frozen (in 1 cup bags). You will need to ask the clinic to provide you with some freezer space, where you can keep your meat stock. You will also need a facility to defrost and warm up 2–4 cups for yourself daily.

Enemas during fasting

It may sound surprising, but during fasting your bowel will keep removing solids despite the fact that you are not eating any. Many toxins leave the body this way and your bowel may need assistance in removing them as soon as they accumulate. So, enemas are an important part of any fasting protocol. It is recommended to have an enema every other day, but some people find it helpful to have them daily.

It is best to clean the bowel with the basic enema solution. Here is how to make it: put 1 teaspoon of bicarbonate of soda (aluminium free) into a glass jug and add about a cup of boiling water. Once the bicarbonate of soda stops releasing gas add 1 teaspoon of natural salt and mix to dissolve it. Then add enough cool water to bring it up to one litre (about a quart) making sure that the solution is close to body temperature. Use this basic solution for cleansing your bowel. If you have a headache or feel particularly sluggish, then after using all the basic enema solution, do a coffee enema. Make sure that there are no more solids coming out of you before putting the coffee in. Please, read about enemas in the chapter *Bowel Management*.

Consuming vegetable medley and brine from fermented vegetables can cause diarrhoea, which is beneficial during a fast. If, on any particular day, you have diarrhoea and there aren't many solids coming out of you, then you don't have to do an enema on that day. During fasting we often feel tired and sleepy; doing an enema in that state can be a laborious task. At some point your bowel will start producing solid or semisolid stool despite having the vegetable medley or brine. If you feel well after passing such stool, then you don't need to do an enema. This is a signal that your bowel has cleaned itself from the old debris and started restoring its normal function; an enema may be an unwelcome interference at that time. Drinking whey, vegetable medley and brine will provide probiotics, enzymes and healing substances to allow the bowel to start restoring its normal microbial community; we should allow it to do this work.

What should we do during the fast? We should rest, sleep, read, meditate and watch pleasant happy films. We must stay in a parasympathetic mode; that is when healing and repair happen in the body. That is why fasting is usually a solitary activity! Human company often introduces topics of conversation and emotions which move us out of the parasympathetic state. The company of a loved one who is fasting with you can be comforting, but other people are better avoided. Working may not be a good idea during fasting, as it can introduce stress which will move you into the sympathetic state. Perhaps, this is the time to attend to calm and pensive work, which you didn't have time for before.

It is not a good idea to do any strenuous exercise during fasting. Your body will use all its available resources on cleansing, healing and repair, so you are likely to feel quite tired and low on energy. Shiatsu, foot and head massage, Indian and Thai massage and other gentle forms of massage can be very pleasant and helpful. Gentle kinesiology, Bowen technique, Reiki, osteopathy and other relaxing and adjusting therapies are also good. Going to the sauna, resting in a jacuzzi, water massage, mud packs and gentle swimming in warm water are compatible with fasting. Sunbathing and relaxed swimming in the sea, river or a lake will assist your body in healing. Comfortable walking in Nature and breathing exercises can be quite healing too. Do only what feels good to you and comfortable for your body! Remember, your body is already doing a lot of work (cleansing and repairing itself), so don't force it to do any strenuous activity on top of that.

Coming out of the GAPS Liquid Fast: we follow the GAPS Introduction Diet starting from the first stage. Continue drinking whey and vegetable medley in your usual amounts while following the stages of the Introduction diet. It is also possible to move into the No-Plant GAPS Diet straight after the fast. This should be done by people who feel that their digestive system is not able to manage plants yet, such as people with Crohn's disease and ulcerative colitis.

Overall, you should not feel hungry or deprived on the GAPS Fast. It is a time for rest and contemplation. Your body and soul will thank you for it!

* * * *

This is the full spectrum of the GAPS Diet, which offers flexible choices for every situation. Having accomplished the GAPS Introduction Diet, we can go into the Full GAPS Diet, the More-Plant GAPS Diet and even into the No-Plant GAPS Diet. To go into the Ketogenic Diet we will need to go through the No-Plant GAPS Diet. When there is a need to repeat the Introduction Diet, we can dive into it from every variety of the diet. And when we feel like having a rest from solid food, we can accomplish the GAPS Liquid Fast.

You will gain good health on the GAPS Nutritional Protocol but may find that it is impossible for your body to ever leave it. Any amount of modern industrially produced food (or any other element of typical modern lifestyles) will be received by your body as an unacceptable abuse. One transgression may undo months of effort and make your life miserable again. For this group of people, it can be very hard to accept that they can never go back to their previous lifestyle. The Full GAPS Diet has to become your permanent diet, and there may be periods when you will have to go back to the GAPS Introduction Diet, the GAPS Liquid Fast or even to the GAPS No-plant Diet for a few weeks to deal with temporary problems. Adhering to the GAPS Nutritional Protocol for the rest of your life will keep you or your patient healthy and well.

For people with milder health problems there may come a time when they can move on from the GAPS Diet. Their bodies will heal well enough for these people to be able to introduce new foods.

Coming off the GAPS Diet

For the majority of people the strict GAPS Diet should be adhered to for at least two years. Depending on the severity of the condition, some people recover more quickly while others take much longer. You, or your patient, needs to have at least six months of normal digestion before you start introducing foods not allowed on the GAPS Diet. Do not rush with this step!

The first foods you will be able to introduce are new potatoes and fermented gluten-free grains (buckwheat, millet and quinoa). The chapter *What we shall eat and why, with some recipes* will explain how to ferment grains. Don't forget that potato is a nightshade plant. For people, who are sensitive to this family of plants, they need to try introducing tomato, aubergine (eggplant) and peppers first before trying potatoes.

Introduce one food at a time and always start with a small amount: give your patient a small portion of the new food and watch for any reaction for 2–3 days. If there are no digestive problems returning, or any other typical-for-your-patient symptoms, then in a few days try another portion. If there are no reactions, gradually increase the amount of the food. These are starchy foods, so do not forget to serve them with good amounts of fat (butter, ghee, olive oil, any animal fat, coconut oil, etc.) to slow down the digestion of starch. Do not rush with the introduction of these new foods, it may take several months to do it properly.

Once new potatoes and fermented grains are introduced, try to make sourdough at home with good quality wheat or rye flour. You can make pancakes or bread with homemade sourdough (please, look in the chapter *What we shall eat and why, with some recipes*). Once homemade sourdough is tolerated well, you may be able to buy commercially available good quality sourdough breads.

At that stage you may find that you or your patient can digest buckwheat, millet and quinoa without fermenting them prior to cooking. Gradually you will find that you can introduce various starchy vegetables and properly prepared grains and legumes.

YOUR PATIENT WILL NEVER BE ABLE TO GO BACK TO THE TYPICAL MODERN DIET FULL OF SUGAR, ARTIFICIAL AND PROCESSED INGREDIENTS AND OTHER HARMFUL 'FOODS'. USE THE YEARS OF FOLLOWING GAPS NUTRITIONAL PROTOCOL TO DEVELOP HEALTHY EATING HABITS FOR LIFE!

In conclusion: at first glance the GAPS Diet appears to be hard work. However, it is a very wholesome and healthy diet and will allow you to rebalance your gut flora, heal and seal the gut lining and lay a strong foundation for good health for life. It means that many GAPS people do not have to adhere to a special diet for the rest of their lives: once the digestive system starts functioning normally, they can gradually introduce most wholesome foods commonly eaten around the world. Some people achieve this target in two years, some take longer – it depends on the severity of the condition and the age of the person.

Once introduced, the GAPS Diet is no more difficult than any normal cooking and feeding the family. And shopping is very simple: just buy everything fresh and unprocessed.

To complete this chapter on the GAPS Diet I would like to add one more point, last but not least: the emotion and the mood during our mealtimes.

GAPS mealtime ritual

"Food is a subtle thing.' 'One must not only know what to eat, but when and how.' 'And what to say while you're eating. Yes, my dear sir. If you care about your digestion, my advice is – don't talk about news or medicine at table. And, God forbid – never read newspapers before dinner!"

Mikhail Bulgakov, The Dog's Heart

We have talked a lot about *what* we should eat. Now let us address a very important issue: in what state should we eat our food.

It has been said many times that 'we are what we eat'. But, no matter how good your food is, if you are not able to digest or assimilate it properly, it will not do you much good. The part of the human nervous system that is responsible for proper food digestion and assimilation is called the autonomic nervous system. It has two branches which generally work in opposition to each other: sympathetic and parasympathetic. We must be in a parasympathetic state in order to digest our food well and really benefit from it. In our modern world we need to make a special effort to get into the parasympathetic state before consuming food. It is particularly important for people with any digestive problems and any chronic degenerative disease.

Imagine a modern family gathering for dinner: the father is still thinking about work, the daughter is texting her friends on a social network, the son's head is in his latest computer game and he is slightly annoyed at being taken away from this activity, the baby has just woken up from a nap and is cranky. The mother worked hard to prepare the meal and put it on the table, but the family is not even thinking about it. So, she is anxious that they may not like it and will not eat it. Everyone is in a sympathetic state somewhere on the second floor of their stress houses (please, read about this in the chapter *Healing*)! Are they going to digest this food well? No! The sympathetic state shuts down the digestive system, reduces appetite and directs the body's resources and energy to dealing with stressful daily tasks.

So, what do we do? We need to make sure that the whole family switches into the parasympathetic state before starting to eat. We need to put their minds on food. How can we do that?

In many cultures around the world people used to say a prayer before every meal. Today that tradition has largely been lost. It is not clear if the prayer put people into a parasympathetic state, but it certainly put their minds on food. Here is a little rhyme I suggest for you, dear reader! It can help you and your family to put your whole attention on the food and jump-start your digestive process. May I suggest that the whole family sits around the table (laden with GAPS food, of course!) and says this with as much enthusiasm as they can muster (maybe even holding hands):

I am hungry! I want food!
Food that's beautiful and good!
I'll enjoy it, every bite!
My digestion is just right!
So, I say: Good Appetite!

Finish the rhyme with a deep intake of breath (a group breath-in) smelling the food and then noisily breathing out as a group. The deep breath-in and a deep breath-out has a magical ability to put our bodies into a parasympathetic state. Finishing this little rhyme with laughter will help even more. Try to make it your mealtime routine, a mealtime ritual.

If this rhyme is not to your liking, then I invite you, dear reader, to make up your own rhymes and songs that will resonate with you and your family. Just keep in mind that every phrase needs to be an affirmation, as in this little rhyme, no hesitation or 'maybe' or 'we wish' or 'we hope' or 'we believe'. Your subconscious mind must have a firm command in the present tense in order for it to switch on your parasympathetic nervous system. This rhyme needs to take your mind away from everything else you have been doing before dinner and put your mind firmly on food, on enjoying it and digesting it well.

Once the meal has begun, make sure not to discuss any stressful topics at the table. All conversation should be directed to creating and maintaining a parasympathetic state. Use silly jokes, discuss light subjects and happy plans and employ any other joyful topics of conversation, which will encourage laughter, imagination and a cosy feeling of a happy family. Let your children remember their family meal times as happy occasions for the rest of their lives! Occasions which have never been spoiled by tense discussions of problems and things to do. There are plenty of other times to discuss those, but not at mealtimes, please!

Good appetite and enjoy your food!

What we shall eat and why, with some recipes

Have you ever wondered what a 'balanced meal' means? The mainstream will tell you that it is proportions of carbs to protein and fat. No, that is not what it means! It means that all your taste buds are singing praises to the meal you eat. Our taste buds are specialised: some perceive sweet, some sour, some salty, some astringent, some pungent and some bitter. All these tastes should be present in the meal. So, when you make a meal, add some sweet vegetables (carrots and beets for example), some bitter (celery leaves, dark-green leaves, aubergine/eggplant, courgette/zucchini, spices and herbs), some chillies, garlic, onion or herbs for a pungent taste, some natural salt and seaweed, broccoli, cauliflower, asparagus and turnip for an astringent taste, and some fermented vegetables, vinegar or lemon for the sour taste. These guidelines will produce balanced, delicious and satisfying meals for you. But, of course, the most important parts of any meal are the meat and the fat, which are perceived on a very deep level!

Use non-toxic kitchenware. No aluminium or non-stick (Teflon) pans or pots, please! Avoid plastic. There are questions about stainless steel, but it is infinitely better than non-stick kitchen ware or aluminium, and it is affordable for the majority of people. So, pans and pots should be made from glass or stainless steel. Enamelled pans, clay and earthenware pots and oven trays can be used. Cast iron, particularly enamelled can be used. Use spatulas and ladles made from wood or stainless steel. Use glass storage jars and bowls. No microwave ovens or induction hobs, please! Use a conventional stove heated by gas, electricity, wood or oil. Cutlery can be made from stainless steel, silver, wood or china. Unfortunately, nothing manmade is perfect in this world, but we have to find practical solutions which work. So, make sure that everything that touches your food is made from materials which do not transfer anything toxic into the food. As new materials are invented all the time, keep researching this subject and asking questions before bringing anything new into your kitchen.

This chapter will provide the reader with some basic GAPS-compliant recipes. However, the GAPS Nutritional Protocol has been used by people all over the world since 2004. Many wonderful GAPS recipe books have been published in different languages over the years and new books are coming out. Typically, these books are written by people who have recovered from severe health problems with the use of the GAPS Diet and by parents of GAPS children. You will find an up-to-date list of such books on *www.gaps.me* in the *Resources* section.

We will go through different food groups in order of importance.

Contents

1. MEAT STOCK AND SOUPS

Homemade meat stock is the staple of the GAPS Diet. The more meat stock a patient consumes, the quicker they recover. Meat stock contains all the necessary nutrients for your gut lining to rebuild itself from quality materials and to heal and seal all the holes in the gut wall (the so-called 'leaky gut'). The human body renews itself all the time: all cells and structures in our bodies live a short life. As they wear out, they get removed and replaced with newly born cells and structures; this is how our bodies renew themselves and heal any damage. The gut lining has a very rapid cell and tissue turnover, which gives us a real opportunity to rebuild it. In order for the gut wall to rebuild itself, building materials are required. The meat stock and soups, which we make on the GAPS Diet, provide all the necessary building materials for your gut to produce healthy robust cells and other structures to rebuild itself anew.

I would like to bring to the reader's attention that we are talking about *MEAT STOCK, not bone broth*! I do not recommend bone broth on the GAPS Diet for one year at least, for some people much longer (several years). Bone broth is made from bare bones (often cooked bones, left from previous meals) cooked for a long time in water with some acid. It is rich in minerals and amino acids, but in the GAPS Nutritional Protocol we need much more than that!

Meat stock is very different: it is always made from *raw* pieces of animal carcass with bones, joints, fascia, cartilage, fat and a good amount of muscle on it. To make meat stock we use a whole bird (chicken, duck, pheasant or any other bird) with the skin on and preferably with feet, neck, giblets and head too, or a joint of pork, lamb, beef or game (neck, ribs, tail, spine, feet, head, leg, shoulder, shank, etc). To make fish stock we use the whole fish with the skin, head, tail, skeleton and fins. Use all the parts with tough, chewy tissues to make meat stock – the parts that require long cooking in water to make them soft enough to be eaten and digested. So, pure lean muscle (such as a steak meat) is not suitable. The meat stock takes a few hours to make and it provides a meal for a family with well-cooked meat and a delicious stock or broth, which is good to drink and for making soup.

Why meat stock?

Properly made meat stock aids digestion and has been known for centuries as a healing folk remedy for the digestive tract and the rest of the body. What is it in the meat stock that makes it so healing and nourishing? It is full of minerals, vitamins, amino acids and various other nutrients in a very bio-available form, but most importantly it is rich in collagen, elastin, proteoglycans, glycoproteins, hyaluronic acid and other molecules which form *THE CONNECTIVE TISSUE* of all animals (including humans).[1] Most of our bodies are made from connective tissue: the structure of our bones and muscles, joints and skin, fascia and fat tissues, cartilage and ligaments, all capsules and supportive structures of our internal organs (the stroma of an organ), all our blood vessels and the supportive structures of our nervous system, large parts of our heart and lungs, and many other organs and tissues. Our gut is a long tube made largely out of connective tissue: in order to heal it we need large amounts of all the elements of connective tissue as building materials.

In GAPS people their connective tissue is in a poor shape: it holds many toxins, it is made from poor quality materials and is damaged by the immune system (please, read more about it in *Collagen Disorders* in the chapter *Immune System*). In order for the person to recover from any chronic illness, we must rebuild their connective tissue from quality materials, which can only come from the connective tissues of healthy mammals, birds and fish. For millennia, in every culture around the world, people used every morsel of an animal for making homemade meat stock, transferring vital elements of the connective tissue of the animal into the liquid during cooking. By consuming this liquid people maintained the very structure of their own bodies – their connective tissue – keeping their bodies strong and supple, their skin smooth and beautiful, their bones dense and non-brittle, and their blood vessels clear and elastic at any age.

When homemade meat stock cools down in the fridge it turns into a jelly due to high amounts of collagen and other elements of the connective tissue in it. Collagen is the most ubiquitous protein in the human body: about a third of all protein in your body is collagen.[2] In order to heal from any disease, we need large amounts of collagen. The pieces of the animal carcass, which were used for making the meat stock, are rich in collagen and should be consumed as part of the soup. After cooking, the connective tissue is soft and falls off the bones easily. We use every bit of these soft tissues by cutting them into bite-size pieces and putting them into our soups: the ligaments and muscles, arteries and nerves, cartilage and skin, fat and bone marrow, glands and organs, fascia and joint capsules. So, the GAPS soup contains gelatinous meat stock and pieces of gelatinous meats – a powerhouse for rebuilding the patient's connective tissue – the very structure of the patient's gut wall and the whole body. At least one cup of homemade meat stock or a bowl of soup, made with this meat stock, should be consumed every day by a GAPS person! Every person with a chronic illness has unhealthy connective tissue made from poor-quality materials. Rebuild your connective tissue out of high-quality materials and watch how your body and your health will transform!

Once you have made your meat stock, it will keep well in a refrigerator for at least a week or it can be frozen for longer storage. You can make soups, gravies and stews with this meat stock or warm up a cup of it to drink with meals or between meals. If you make sure that you always have some meat stock in your fridge, you will find that it is very easy and quick to make a nourishing meal for the whole family. Just cook some vegetables in it for 15–20 minutes. When the vegetables are soft, add those bite-size pieces of connective tissue to the pot and you have a warming and nourishing soup. This soup will also keep in the fridge for a week at least. Do not take fat out of the stock; it is important to consume the fat together with the stock, unless you have a problem with digesting fats. We work on proper digestion of fats in the GAPS Nutritional Protocol, so at some point you will be able to have any amount of fat and digest it well.

You need meats, joints, skin, bones and organs to make a good meat stock. Beef, lamb, pork, game, poultry and fish are all highly suitable and will make stocks with different flavours and different nutritional compositions. So, make sure that you alternate between different meat stocks to provide a whole spectrum of nourishment. It can be very inexpensive to make a good quality meat stock as you use the parts of the animal which butchers usually sell cheaply or give away for free. The meat and bones can be fresh or frozen and there is no need to defrost them prior to cooking. Apart from bones, joints, skin and meats all you need is a large pot, clean water and a bit of salt and pepper.

How to make meat stock

Lamb, pork, beef or game

Any joint with bones and cartilage in it, tough connective tissues (ligaments and joint capsules), blood vessels and nerves, fascia and skin (on pork), fat and a good amount of muscle meat. You can use one large piece or several smaller pieces, fresh or frozen. Wash the meats with cool water in order to remove any oxidised substances on the surface, which naturally form when meat is stored for a while (particularly in plastic). Place the meats in a large pot, add 1–2 teaspoons of black peppercorns (crush them slightly using pestle and mortar), add salt to taste and fill the pot with water. The proportion of water to meats should be approximately 3:1 to cover the meats. Heat to boiling point, then cover the pan, reduce the heat to a minimum and simmer until the meats are soft and come off the bones easily (typically for 3–4 hours). When ready, pour the stock through a sieve into a separate pan to remove any small bones and peppercorns, leaving the meats in the pot. Make sure that the separate pan is dry and clean; pour the meat stock while hot to kill any microbes in it. This will make sure that your stock will keep in that pan for a long time without spoiling. You can make soup with this stock or keep it in the fridge for later.

When the meats have cooled enough to be handled, take all soft tissues off the bones and cut them into bite-size pieces. If you are planning to make soup straight away, these pieces should be added to the soup at the end, when the vegetables have cooked. If you are planning to make soup later, then keep these meats in the fridge. Alternatively, the meats can be served as the main part of dinner or lunch.

Remove the bone marrow from large bones. In order to do that, make sure large tubular bones are cut in half prior to cooking. After cooking, bang the bone on a thick wooden chopping board. Make sure that the bone has not cooled down completely, it should be quite warm for the bone marrow to come out easily. It is delicious to eat while hot with some salt and pepper, or it can be mashed with a fork and returned to the meat stock. Bone marrow is a natural folk remedy for the immune system and should be consumed by GAPS people as often as possible.

Chicken stock (and other poultry)

Chicken stock is a favourite for many people: it is delicious and easy to make. Use a whole chicken, fresh or frozen. Very valuable parts of the bird for making good stock are the skin, the feet, the neck, the head and the giblets (rich in the connective tissues, so healing for the gut lining and the whole body). If you can get these parts, then add them to the pot with the whole chicken. Always wash all the meats with cool water prior to cooking in order to remove any oxidised substances on the surface, which naturally form when meat is stored for a while (particularly in plastic).

Put all the chicken parts into a large pot, fill it up with 2–4 l (4.2–7 pt) of water, add salt and heat it to boiling point. Cover the pan and reduce the heat to a simmer. Simmer for 2 hours until the meats are soft and come off the bones easily. For a commercial chicken 1.5–2 hours of cooking is usually enough. For a home-reared free-range chicken you may need 3 hours. Take the pot off the heat and pour the stock through a sieve into another pan. Make sure that the pan is dry and clean; pour the stock while hot to kill any microbes in it. This will make sure that your stock will keep in that pan for a long time without spoiling. You can make soup with this stock immediately or keep it in the fridge for later.

The chicken, cooked this way, is delicious and can be served for dinner with vegetables and a hot cup of your freshly made chicken stock. Let your family eat all the soft tissues on the feet, neck, head and carcass of the chicken and discover just how delicious they are. Alternatively, take all the soft tissues from the chicken and cut them into bite-size pieces. If you are planning to make soup straight away, these pieces should be added to the soup at the end, when the vegetables have cooked. If you are planning to make soup later, then keep these meats in the fridge. Nothing should be discarded from the cooked chicken! All soft tissues, including bone marrow, skin, fat, soft cartilage and every other morsel should be used.

Instead of chicken any other poultry can be used to make a delicious stock: duck, turkey or goose pieces, pheasants, pigeons, guineafowl, etc. Remember to use pieces with plenty of connective tissues: legs, wings, skin, neck, head, feet, giblets and carcasses. Commercial chickens, turkeys and other poultry are specifically bred to have large breasts, which become dry and tough when cooked too long. You may want to remove the breast meat from the raw bird before making meat stock, leaving the skin on the carcass. The skinless breasts can be used for other recipes later, when they are cooked differently to remain soft and juicy.

Fish stock

To make good fish stock you need the connective tissues of the fish: bones, fins, skins and heads with some meat left on the bones. So, buy your fish whole. It is essential to descale the skin of the fish prior to cooking! The skin is a very nutritious part of the connective tissue of the fish and should be consumed, never discarded. It is easier to descale the fish before gutting or cutting it, so make sure to do it yourself or ask your fishmonger to do it for you. When the fish is descaled it should be washed in cool water. If it is a large fish, you can cut the meat off the skeleton to cook as a separate meal, using the rest of the fish to make your fish stock. If you have small fish, descale them, wash and remove the guts prior to cooking.

To make a good stock we need at least 250 g (9 oz) of fish. Put the small fish or heads, bones, fins and skins of a large fish into a suitable size pan, add 1 teaspoon of black peppercorns (crush them slightly using pestle and mortar) and fill it up with enough water to cover the fish: the proportion of water to fish is about 3:1. Bring to the boil, reduce the heat to a minimum and simmer for 1–1.5 hours. Add salt to taste at the end of cooking. When ready, take the pot off the heat and pour the stock through a sieve into a dry, clean pan. Pour the stock while hot to kill any microbes in it. This will make sure that your stock will keep in that pan for a long time without spoiling. You can make soup with this stock immediately or keep it in the fridge for later.

When the fish has cooled enough to be handled, take all soft tissues off the skeleton (the skin, the meat and fat) and cut them into bite-size pieces to use for soup. If the bones are soft after cooking, you can use a food processor to grind all the fish solids into a soft paste, then add to the fish stock. Mix and strain through a sieve again. This will remove hard bones and make the fish stock much richer.

The basic soup recipe

The most important part of any soup is the meat stock! Homemade, delicious, rich meat stock, which turns the soup into a satisfying meal in itself. The decline in health of any nation can be timed to the moment when its people started using plain water instead of meat stock to make soup!

Never use commercially available soup stock granules or bouillon cubes. They are highly processed and full of detrimental ingredients. No healing will be gained from these commercial products.

To make soup bring some of your homemade meat stock to the boil, add chopped or sliced vegetables and simmer for 20–25 minutes, or until the vegetables are soft. You can choose any combination of available vegetables allowed on the GAPS Diet: onion, cabbage, carrot, broccoli, cauliflower, pumpkin, courgettes, marrow (zucchini), squash, leek, turnip, etc. If you are planning to blend your soup, then you can cut vegetables roughly into any size pieces. If you prefer not to blend, then make sure that you cut or dice your vegetables into small pieces before cooking. If your meat stock was made with lamb, pork or beef you can add a handful of dried French or Italian mushrooms for a wonderful flavour. It is customary to crush the dried mushrooms by hand before adding to the soup. For a chicken soup, cabbage and cauliflower generally don't seem to work very well, but onions, carrots, leaks, courgettes (zucchini), squashes, pumpkins and broccoli work beautifully.

Remember that all taste buds should be satisfied by your soup, so make sure to add some vegetables and herbs for bitter, pungent, sweet and astringent tastes. The meat stock is already salty. To satisfy the sour taste I strongly recommend adding a handful of homemade fermented vegetables: carrot, celery, cabbage, beetroot, greens, cucumbers, kimchi, etc. Nice-tasting successful ferments are good to add at the end of cooking. Less successful homemade fermented vegetables are particularly good to use for making soup and should be added at the beginning of cooking. These are vegetables which may not taste good to eat as they are, for example fermented celery, greens, beetroot, Brussel sprouts, etc. If you add them to your soup at the beginning of cooking, they will supply a wonderful sour taste and taste good when cooked in the whole mixture. Remember that probiotic microbes are beneficial to health even when dead. Cooked fermented vegetables will provide these microbes, as well as pre-digested vegetable matter and other beneficial substances.

When the vegetables are soft use a soup blender if desired. After that add bite-size pieces of the soft tissues taken off the bones after making the stock. Bring back to boil, add 1–2 heaped tablespoons of roughly chopped garlic and turn the heat off. Let the soup rest for a few minutes before serving.

You can serve your soup with any combination of the following:

- some chopped parsley, coriander (cilantro), dill and other greens
- some sauerkraut, fermented garlic or another fermented vegetable
- juice from fermented vegetables, such as the *Vegetable Medley* recipe
- hard-boiled egg or a soft-boiled egg, peeled and cut into pieces
- a generous spoonful of homemade sour cream, kefir, whey or yogurt
- red onion cut into very small pieces
- spring onion or chives cut into small pieces
- a spoon of cooked and ground liver

From this basic recipe you can improvise and develop your own recipes. Here are a few ideas.

Oxtail soup

1 kg (2½ lb) oxtail, fresh or frozen
200 g (7 oz) fresh cabbage, chopped into small pieces
1 large onion, finely chopped, or a large leek, sliced
1 large carrot, sliced
2 tablespoons dried French or Italian mushrooms
4 tablespoons homemade fermented vegetables (cabbage, carrot, greens or celery)
a handful of chopped garlic

Oxtail, cooked this way, is delicious and is good to eat as a main meal. It contains large amounts of connective tissue, which needs cooking in water for a long enough time to become soft. Many people, having tried oxtail for the first time, fall in love with this meat. It is considered to be a delicacy in traditional cultures.

Wash the pieces of oxtail with cool water. Place them in a stock pot and add 2–3 l (4.2–6.3 pt) of water, salt to taste and a teaspoon of black peppercorns (freshly crushed, using pestle and mortar or another device). The proportion of water to meat should be approximately 2:1 to cover the meat. Heat to boiling point, then cover the pan, reduce the heat to a minimum and simmer until the meats are soft and come off the bones easily (typically for 2–3 hours). When ready, pour the stock through a sieve into a separate dry clean pan to remove any small bones and peppercorns. Pour the meat stock while hot to kill any microbes in the pan. This will make sure that your stock will keep in that pan for a long time without spoiling. At this point taste the stock for salt and pepper and adjust if necessary.

To make soup, put all the vegetables into the stock, apart from the fermented vegetables and garlic. Cook for 20–25 minutes until the vegetables are soft and easy to chew, then add fermented vegetables. Bring back to the boil and take the pot off the heat. At this point add the garlic. If you are planning to put the meat into the soup, then take all the soft tissues off the bones and cut into bite-size pieces. Add them to the soup. Take the spinal cord out, chop and also add to the soup. Alternatively, the meat can be served in parallel with the soup and people can eat the meat on the bones using their hands.

Serve this soup with some sour cream, kefir or yogurt and some chopped parsley or dill.

A spring nettle soup

1½–2 l (3.1–4.2 pt) homemade meat stock (beef, pork, lamb or chicken)
large bunch spring nettles
2 tablespoons dried French or Italian mushrooms
1 medium onion
1 medium carrot
2 courgettes (zucchini) or ¼ peeled marrow or squash
2 tablespoons homemade fermented vegetables (carrot, greens or celery)
4 eggs, hard boiled

Young shoots of stinging nettles appearing in spring are full of wonderful nourishment. They are high in iron, magnesium, copper, zinc, vitamin C, carotenoids and other useful substances. For this recipe collect a large bunch of spring nettles. You will have to wear gloves and a long-sleeved shirt to do this. Rinse the nettles and shake the excess water off. Using scissors cut the leaves and tender shoots of the nettles into small pieces, discarding the hard stems. Reserve for the recipe.

It is good to use leftovers of homemade meat stock for this recipe, when the meats have already been consumed and so are not available.

Cut the marrow, squash or courgettes into small cubes, thinly slice the carrot and chop the onion. Bring the homemade meat stock to a boil. Add all the vegetables and the French or Italian dried mushrooms, crumbling them with your hands before adding. Simmer under a tight lid for 15–20 minutes. Add fermented vegetables at the end of cooking and bring to a boil again. Add your prepared nettles, mix and immediately take the pot off the heat. Serve with 1–2 tablespoons hard-boiled egg, cut into small pieces, and a spoonful of homemade sour cream, kefir or yogurt.

Russian borsch

2 l (4.2 pt) homemade meat stock (beef, pork or lamb)
1 medium onion, finely chopped
1 medium carrot, finely sliced
¼ medium-size white cabbage, finely sliced
2 medium-size beetroots, or 4 small beetroots, raw or cooked
2–3 tablespoons fermented beetroot, carrot, sauerkraut or another fermented vegetable
handful peeled cloves of garlic
1 finely chopped tomato
bite-size pieces of meats reserved from making the meat stock

If the beetroot is cooked (in water, not in vinegar):
Bring the meat stock to the boil and add the onion, carrot and cabbage. Cover and simmer for 20 minutes. In the meantime, slice the cooked beetroots into long thin strips and add to the soup. At the same time add fermented vegetables, chopped tomato and bite-size pieces of reserved meats. Mix well and simmer for another 5 minutes. Take the pot off the heat and add chopped garlic. Let it rest for 10 minutes. Serve with a large spoon of sour cream or homemade kefir or yogurt, adding some chopped parsley and/or a thick slice of hard-boiled egg.

If the beetroot is raw:
Wash the beetroot and remove any unsuitable bits. Slice into long thin strips by hand or using your food processor. Chop the onion, slice the carrot and the cabbage. Bring the meat stock to the boil and add the beetroot, onion, carrot and cabbage. Simmer for 20-25 minutes or until the vegetables are soft and can be cut through with a spoon. Add fermented vegetables, chopped tomato and reserved bite-size pieces of meats. Take off the heat and add chopped garlic. Let it rest for 10 minutes. Serve with a large spoon of sour cream, kefir or homemade yogurt, adding some chopped parsley and/or a thick slice of hard-boiled egg.

Fish soup

1 l (2.1 pt) homemade fish stock
1 large onion, finely chopped
1 carrot, thinly sliced
1 courgette (zucchini) or an equivalent amount of marrow or squash, peeled and cut into small cubes
1–2 tablespoons fermented vegetables (fermented carrot works well)
fish meat reserved from making the stock

Bring the fish stock to the boil and add all the vegetables. Simmer under a lid for 10–15 minutes until the vegetables are soft and take off the heat. Add the reserved fish meat. Serve with a spoonful of sour cream, kefir or yogurt and/or with a hard-boiled egg (sliced or chopped). It is traditional to add some freshly squeezed lemon juice (from half a lemon) to this soup and chopped dill, when serving.

If you would like to add more fish to the soup, you can use meat (skinless and boneless) of any available fresh raw fish. Cut the meat into bite-size pieces and add into the boiling soup in the last 5 minutes of cooking.

Meatball soup

400-500 g (14–18 oz) minced meat (a mix of pork and beef is best)
1–1½ l (2.1–3.6 pt) water or meat stock (beef, pork or lamb)
1 large onion, finely chopped
1 large carrot, thinly sliced
1 cup winter squash or courgette (zucchini), peeled and cut into small cubes
1 cup cabbage, finely chopped (optional)
2–3 tablespoons homemade fermented vegetables (carrot, celery, cucumber or other)
2 tablespoons chopped garlic
salt and black pepper to taste

It is best to ferment minced meat for a few hours before making this soup. Fermentation makes the meat easier to digest, particularly pork. Add 1-2 tablespoons of any homemade fermented vegetables to the meat and mix thoroughly using your hands, squeezing the meat between your fingers. Any less-successful ferments will do. Form the meat into a firm ball, cover and leave at room temperature for 2–4 hours.

Bring water up to the boil and add salt and black pepper to taste. You can use meat stock for this recipe to make it rich, but the minced meat will provide enough flavour, so this soup can be made with water. With your hands shape meatballs about 2 cm (¾ in) in diameter and add them, one at a time, to the boiling water. Make sure that the meat balls don't stick to each other. Cover and simmer on low heat for 30-40 minutes. Add all the vegetables, apart from fermented vegetables and garlic, cover and simmer for another 20 minutes until the vegetables become soft. At this point add the fermented vegetables and bring back to boil. Take off the heat and add the garlic. Serve with some sauerkraut, homemade sour cream, kefir or yogurt and finely chopped parsley or dill.

Winter squash soup

1½–2 l (3.6–4.2 pt) homemade meat stock (beef, pork, lamb, turkey or chicken)
1 leek, washed and sliced
a few rosettes of broccoli
½ medium-size buttercup squash or a 1/3 butternut squash or any winter squash with sweet orange flesh
3–4 tablespoons of fermented carrots
optional: some cayenne or chilli pepper to taste, ½ teaspoon dill seed or caraway seed
handful of garlic cloves, peeled and chopped

Peel and deseed the squash and cut it into chunks. Put the pieces of squash, leek and broccoli in your soup pan, add the meat stock, cayenne pepper, aromatic seeds and bring to the boil. Reduce the heat to a minimum, cover with the lid and simmer for about 30 minutes or until all the vegetables are soft. Add fermented carrots and bring to boil. Take off the heat, add chopped garlic and blend with a soup blender. You can add bite-size pieces of meats to the soup after blending it; bring the soup back to the boil if the meats were cold. Serve with a spoonful of sour cream, kefir or yogurt.

Meat jelly

2–4 pig trotters or a pig's head
1 large carrot
2 handfuls peeled and roughly sliced garlic
salt and black peppercorns

Put pig trotters or a head in a large pan, fill it with water to cover the meats, add salt and 2–3 teaspoons of black peppercorns, freshly crushed. Bring up to the boil, reduce heat to a minimum, cover with a lid and simmer for 3–6 hours, or until the meats are very soft and come off the bones easily. At the end of cooking, taste the salt in the stock and adjust.

In the meantime, cook a large carrot by steaming, cool it down and cut into thin slices.

When the meats are cooked, pour the stock through a sieve into a separate clean, dry pan. Let the trotters or head cool down. Take all the soft tissues off the bones (the skin, ligaments, muscles and other soft tissues) completely stripping the bones. Cut the meats into small pieces.

Lay the pieces of meat, the sliced carrot and the garlic in a large deep tray. You can add more or less garlic to your family's taste. Pour the meat stock in to fill the tray to ¾ to cover the meats. Sprinkle some chopped parsley or dill on top. Place the tray in the refrigerator for the jelly to set. You can also set this jelly in different dishes as individual servings.

This dish is wonderful to eat on a hot summer's day. It contains all the nourishing substances for your connective tissue and is considered to be a folk remedy for digestive problems.

2. FERMENTED FOODS

He, who does not eat fermented foods, should expect disease!

Sudanese proverb

Until the last hundred years or so food was seasonal, local and very perishable. People searched for a way to preserve food and found that fermentation – employing microbes to preserve the food for us – is the best way to make food keep for a long time, sometimes for years. All around the world people have developed different ways of fermenting food: vegetables, grains, nuts, beans, lentils, fruit, milk, meat, fish and even eggs.[3,4] In the Western world the best known traditional fermented foods are cheese and yogurt, sauerkraut, beer, vinegar, wine, soused herring, Mediterranean ham and salumi (salami, pancetta, fermented sausages, etc). Some Asian fermented foods are also known in the West, such as kimchi, miso soup and soy sauce. Apart from these commonly known foods, there are hundreds of less well-known fermentation recipes used by traditional cultures all over the world. Fermentation has become popular again in the last decade, and something beautiful is happening: traditional recipes from different countries are becoming available to the whole world through books and online publications. More than that: people now combine different traditional recipes, modifying them and creating new ways of fermenting food.

Apart from keeping food for longer, fermentation provided us with another major benefit: the food becomes much easier to digest and absorb. Microbes have an unsurpassed ability to digest plants and animal products, break down tough structures, release nutrients from these structures and create new nutrients (B vitamins and vitamin K2, for example). As a result, fermented foods have become far more nourishing for us than their raw counterparts. For example, a handful of sauerkraut (fermented cabbage) can provide almost twenty times more bio-available vitamin C than the same amount of raw cabbage![5] In raw cabbage vitamin C is locked in the cellular structure of the cabbage and our digestive system cannot extract it. In sauerkraut the microbes have extracted vitamin C and made it easy for us to absorb. It has been recorded that in the Middle Ages British sailing ships always had barrels of 'sour cabbage' on board to prevent 'bleeding gums' (scurvy). In those times people didn't know about vitamin C, but they knew how to prevent its deficiency during long sailing trips. Fermented vegetables and fruit can be some of the best vitamin C 'supplements' in the world.[3,4] Not only does this vitamin get released from the tough vegetable structure during fermentation, but so do many other nutrients. The whole plant structure is transformed into something that is much easier to digest and far more nourishing.

The third major benefit we get from eating fermented foods is the beneficial (probiotic) microbes which live in those foods. These microbes make little homes in the particles of food, where they are protected from the stomach acid. These particles of food carry probiotic microbes all through your digestive system, allowing them to do good work in all parts of your gut. Fermented foods are natural probiotics, bringing you alive and active beneficial microbes with all their healing abilities.[3–5] These microbes produce enzymes to help you digest food. They alter the pH and other parameters in your gut to encourage growth of other microbes and stimulate larger diversity in your gut flora. And they engage your immune system, making it more balanced, better educated and more capable of doing its complex jobs properly. Fermented foods are much less expensive than commercial probiotics, particularly when they are homemade, and can be quite effective as probiotic 'supplements', particularly in the maintenance stages of the programme.

The most common method of fermentation worldwide is *lactic-acid fermentation*. Lactic acid bacteria naturally live on all plants and animal foods and they love to eat carbohydrates. They are anaerobic and, if we create proper conditions for them, they do the work for us beautifully. Of course, the food needs to be natural and not covered with agricultural chemicals or anything else that can damage this community of microbes. As they grow and multiply in the food, they consume carbohydrates and produce lactic acid, which preserves the food and gives it acid taste. These microbes take some time to multiply and start producing lactic acid, so traditionally people added salt to their recipes to suppress any putrefactive microbes and give the lactic acid bacteria time to proliferate. That is why lactic-acid fermentation was often called 'salting' the food, as only salt was added. Using this method, we can ferment any mixture of vegetables, fruit, greens and spices, meats, milk, fish, grains, seeds, nuts and beverages. We use lactic-acid fermentation extensively in the GAPS Diet; every meal should have a small amount of fermented foods, raw and/or cooked.

Another way to ferment food comes from Asia and it is alkaline, using *moulds* and *Bacillus subtilis* for fermenting cooked beans and grains. The two moulds used traditionally are *rhizopus spp.* for making *tempeh* and *aspergillus spp.* for making *koji* and *miso*. Fermentation with moulds is not widely accepted in Western culture. If you are interested in exploring it, there are some good books to follow.[3,6]

Bacillus subtilis lives naturally in the soil and is a normal inhabitant of human gut flora. When we introduce it into food, it produces ammonia, which raises pH to an alkaline level of 8.0–9.0, preserving the food. It is used to make *natto* in Japan and *cheonggukjang* in Korea – two recipes for fermenting cooked beans and preserving them for a while.[6] We are going to use a modification of these recipes to ferment beans and other legumes in the GAPS Diet, which makes them easier for us to digest, breaks down antinutrients, preserves the beans and enriches their nutritional composition.

Sauerkraut-type fermentation

Sauerkraut is a fermented white and/or red cabbage, commonly consumed in Germany, Russia and Eastern Europe. It is a wonderful healing remedy for the digestive tract, full of digestive enzymes, probiotic bacteria, vitamins and minerals.[3–6] Eating it with meals improves digestion as it has a strong ability to stimulate stomach acid production. For people with low stomach acidity I recommend having a few teaspoons of sauerkraut (or juice from it) 10–15 minutes before meals or with meals. For children, initially add 1–3 tablespoons of the juice from the sauerkraut to their meals. You do not need to add any starter to the sauerkraut, as fresh cabbage has natural lactic acid bacteria living on it, which will do the fermentation for you. The best cabbage to use is from your own garden or someone's else's garden, where it has been grown without any chemicals. Cabbage from supermarkets, even labelled 'organic', is not the same.

Thinly slice a large white cabbage and add two shredded carrots. You can use red cabbage or a mixture of white and red. Add 2–3 heaped tablespoons of salt. Salt is essential as it will draw the juice from the cabbage during kneading. In addition, salt will stifle the putrefactive microbes in the initial stages of fermentation, until the fermenting bacteria produce enough lactic acid to kill the pathogens. You can add aromatic seeds or spices to the mixture: juniper berries, coriander seed, dill seed, caraway seed, fennel seed, black, red or green pepper corns, chilli peppers, paprika, greens and pealed cloves of garlic. Using your hands, mix and knead the mixture in a large bowl until a lot of juice comes out (it may take 5-10 minutes of kneading). If the cabbage is not juicy enough, add freshly made brine, old brine from other fermented vegetables or a little filtered water. Pack this mixture into a large wide-mouth glass jar, pressing it firmly so there is no air trapped and the cabbage is drowned in its own juice. Fermentation is an anaerobic process: if the cabbage is exposed to air, it will rot instead of fermenting. Leave 5 cm (2 in) or so empty space at the top, as the cabbage will expand during fermentation because of production of CO_2 gas. I recommend covering the top of the mixture with a fresh horseradish leaf, which will suppress the growth of mould. If horseradish leaves are not available, use a cabbage leaf to cover the top. Place some weight on top of the cabbage to make sure that the vegetables are always submerged in the juice. Some fermentation kits provide a glass ring to use as a weight. Alternatively, you can use a small glass jar of a suitable size, which will keep the cabbage submerged when the lid is closed (the lid will push the jar down). Make sure that this small jar has no label or lid and is clean and dry. Close the lid tightly and keep at room temperature in the dark. It is a good idea to stand the jar in a bowl or a tray in case any juice spills out during fermentation. Depending on the surrounding temperature it can take from one week to a month for the sauerkraut to be ready. When ready, sauerkraut has a sharp acid taste and there is no more gas coming from it. Some people find it difficult to eat sauerkraut on its own due to acidity, particularly people with sensitive teeth. Mixing sauerkraut with other foods helps to avoid this problem, so I recommend adding small amounts to all your salads, soups and stews. For children and people with sensitive teeth it is helpful to blend small batches of sauerkraut in a food processor and keep it in a separate glass jar in the fridge, to be added to meals.

Using this sauerkraut-type fermentation, you can ferment any vegetable or a mixture of vegetables. I invite you to experiment. Korean kimchi is becoming popular. It is just a variety of sauerkraut, where radishes, chillies, ginger, onion, garlic, greens and other available vegetables are added to the cabbage, kneaded well with salt to release juices and fermented. Koreans have many variations of kimchi depending on what vegetables are available, and in some places raw fish is added to the mixture before fermentation.

If you grow your own vegetables, always ferment the surplus (rather than wasting it): beetroot, carrots, celery, radishes, greens, etc. Always add spices and aromatic seeds to the vegetables: juniper berries, coriander seed, dill seed, caraway seed, fennel seed, black, red or green peppercorns, chilli peppers, paprika, greens and garlic. Juicy vegetables will release enough juice while kneading, so you will not need to add any water or brine. For drier vegetables and when you want to preserve their shape, you can add brine.

Fermenting with brine

To ferment whole Brussel sprouts, whole cucumbers, whole radishes, garlic cloves, whole cabbages, cauliflower and broccoli florets, whole apples and whole tomatoes you will need to make brine the day before.

How to make fresh brine for fermenting vegetables and fruit

Fill a large pot with filtered water, counting how many litres go in. Bring the water to boil and add natural salt: 70–90 g (2½–3½ oz) per 1 l (2.1 pt) of water. Mix until the salt has dissolved, then bring back to boil. Take the pot off the heat, cover and leave overnight to cool down completely. This brine will keep for a long time in glass bottles or glass jars at room temperature, so you can use it for several fermentation recipes.

Old brine left from last year's vegetables

It is good to use old brine from your fermented vegetables as a starter to ferment new vegetables. This old brine is rich in minerals, enzymes and probiotics and must never be discarded! It tastes beautiful and for centuries has been a folk remedy for food poisoning, any stomach upset, nausea and hangover. Pregnant women find it very helpful during those times when nausea is a problem. It can be consumed as it is or diluted with water. You can add it to your soups, stews and other dishes. Adding some of this old brine to new batches of vegetables will guarantee that your fermentation will go right.

Fermented cucumbers (dill cucumbers)

The cucumbers need to be small and very fresh. Wash the cucumbers and pack into a large wide-mouth glass jar (clean and dry), filling spaces between them with dill (stems, leaves and crowns), bay leaves, peeled cloves of garlic, black peppercorns, coriander seed and mustard seed. Leave 5 cm (2 in) of space at the top. Cover the cucumbers with a fresh horseradish leaf. If horseradish is not available, then cover with a few bay leaves. Fill the jar with fresh brine (cool or at room temperature). Close the lid tightly and leave to ferment in a cool place – around 12–18°C

(53–64°F). In a couple of days the cucumbers will already be delicious to eat but, if you leave them fermenting longer, they will keep for a few years. They are wonderful to add to salads, soups and stews. The brine is delicious and can be used for adding to soups and stews, as well as a folk remedy for stomach problems.

Using this recipe, you can ferment whole radishes, whole Brussel sprouts, whole garlic cloves, whole tomatoes, whole cabbages, whole apples, whole plums, broccoli, cauliflower, pieces of carrot, beetroot or a mixture of vegetables and fruit. Experiment, and you will find how easy and satisfying this recipe is. These preserves will keep several years, becoming even easier to digest year after year. Of course, the fruit and vegetables must be grown without any chemicals.

Vegetables fermented with added microbial culture

Using a commercial starter or homemade whey (from dripping yogurt or kefir) you can ferment vegetables and fruit. This method allows fermentation without adding any salt, which some people prefer. Companies which produce fermented vegetables choose to use a commercial starter, because they have to use vegetables from commercial growers (which can be contaminated with chemicals and not have a good population of lactic acid bacteria on them). By adding a microbial starter you can get guaranteed fermentation batch after batch, with the same look and taste.

Take any mixture of vegetables, for example some cabbage (white, red or any other variety), beetroot, garlic, cauliflower and carrot, slice them into bite-size pieces or shred them roughly, add some spices of your choice and pack into a 1 l (2.1 pt) glass jar. Take 500 ml (17 fl oz) of cold filtered water and dissolve in it the contents of the sachet of commercial microbial starter. Alternatively, add half a cup of your homemade whey to the water. Add this water to the jar until it completely covers the vegetables. It is important that the vegetables are completely covered by the water, because if they are left dry at the top, they will get mouldy. Don't forget to leave 5 cm (2 in) of space in the jar at the top, as the vegetables will expand during fermentation. Cover tightly with the lid and leave to ferment at room temperature for a week or longer.

Russian vinaigrette winter salad

1 large swede
4 fresh beetroots (large to medium-large)
2-3 large white or/and red onions
6 large carrots
4 large fermented cucumbers (dill cucumbers)

1 cup sauerkraut or kimchi
a handful of frozen peas
olive oil

Cook the swede and the carrots until a knife goes through them easily (they can be cooked together). You can steam them or simmer in a small amount of water. Cook beetroots separately by steaming until well cooked and a knife goes through them easily. Leave these vegetables to cool down.

You will need a large bowl made out of glass, glazed clay or china. I recommend cutting all the vegetables by hand, using a sharp knife, rather than using a food processor. Chop the onions into tiny pieces (about 5 mm/¼ in) and put in the bowl. Slice fermented cucumbers into tiny pieces and mix with the onions. Peel the swede and the carrots, cut into small pieces (about 10 mm/½ in cubes) and mix with the onions and fermented cucumbers in the bowl. Peel the beetroots, cut into small pieces and mix with the rest of the vegetables in the bowl. Add sauerkraut or kimchi and mix well. If the sauerkraut has large pieces of cabbage, it may be a good idea to blend it first in a food processor. Add peas to the mixture. Add plenty of olive oil and mix well. Leave at room temperature for an hour, after that keep in the fridge. This recipe will keep refrigerated for a week to ten days. It is delicious and a very good way to eat fermented vegetables every day. And remember, for a dish to be successful all tastes need to be present: the sweet, the sour, the salty, the bitter, the pungent and the astringent. This mixture of vegetables provides all of these tastes.

Fermented probiotic beverages

Using whey as a starter you can make delicious fermented beverages for the whole family. They will provide you with beneficial bacteria, enzymes and many nutrients, which the fermentation process releases from the fruit and vegetables.

Vegetable medley

This probiotic food will provide you with delicious fermented vegetables and a wonderful beverage to drink, full of great nutrition, enzymes and beneficial microbes. The liquid from this recipe is used in the No-Plant GAPS Diet and can be introduced quite early in the GAPS Introduction Diet.

In a 5-l (9-pt) enamelled pan or a large glass jar put a whole cabbage, roughly cut, a medium-size beetroot, sliced, a teaspoon of dill seeds or dill herb (fresh or dried) and a handful of peeled garlic cloves. The pan should be half filled with the vegetables. You can also add some coriander seed, caraway seed, black peppercorns, mustard seed or juniper berries. Add 2 tablespoons of good quality sea salt, a cup of kefir whey and top up with cool filtered water until the pan is full. If fermenting in a pan, float a glass plate on top of the brine to keep the vegetables completely submerged. If the vegetables are dry at the top, they can get mouldy. If you are fermenting in a glass jar, close the lid tightly (the CO_2 gas, released during fermentation, will expel oxygen from the jar and prevent moulds from growing). Leave to ferment for a few days to a week at room temperature. When ready, the vegetables will be soft and tangy and the liquid bright red and delicious. To stop the fermentation, move the pan (or the jar) into the refrigerator. You can add these vegetables to your soups and stews, drink the brine diluted with water with your meals or between meals and eat the vegetables with meat. When the brine and the vegetables start getting low, add fresh cabbage, beetroot and garlic, some salt to taste, top up with water and ferment at room temperature again. To this vegetable medley you can add a few rosettes of cauliflower, sliced carrot, Brussels sprouts and broccoli. You can have this vegetable medley going forever, as long as you keep feeding it with more fresh vegetables. The brine from this medley is an excellent remedy for any tummy upset, sore gums and sore throat.

Kefir or yogurt whey

The clear yellow liquid left after dripping your yogurt or kefir is called whey. It is a very nourishing beverage, an excellent source of enzymes and probiotic microbes and a traditional cure for gastritis, stomach ulcers and reflux. You can add it to freshly pressed juices, soups and stews. You can add some salt and spices to it and drink it as it is or diluted with some water. You can use it as a starter for fermenting vegetables, fruit, fish and grains (when you are ready to introduce grains). Detailed instructions for making whey are given later in this chapter.

Beetroot kvass

Beetroot kvass is an old digestive remedy, very easy to make. Using a knife, slice medium-size beetroot finely. Don't grate the beetroot in a food processor, as that will make it ferment too quickly, producing alcohol. Put the beetroot in a 2-l (4.2-pt) jar, add 1–2 level tablespoons of good quality sea salt, 1 cup of whey, 5 cloves of garlic, your favourite spices and aromatic seeds, 1 teaspoon of freshly grated ginger (optional) and fill up with water. Let it ferment for 2–5 days in a warm place. After that keep in the refrigerator. Drink diluted with water. Keep topping the water up in the jar so your kvass will keep going for a long time. When it starts getting pale then the beetroot is spent, so start again.

Kvass from other fruit and vegetables

You can make kvass from any combination of fruit, berries and vegetables, so try to experiment. Another good recipe is apple, ginger and raspberry kvass. Slice a whole apple including the core, grate ginger root (about 1 tablespoon) and get a handful of fresh raspberries. Put them all into a 1-l (2.1-pt) jar, add ½ cup whey and top up with water. Let it brew for a few days at room temperature, then keep in the refrigerator. Drink diluted with water. Keep topping up your brew with water until the fruit is spent, then start again.

Probiotic tomato juice

Blend 1 cup whey, 1–2 tablespoons thick tomato purée or tomato paste, 1 cup water and some salt and pepper to taste. Chill and enjoy!

Yogurt, kefir and sour cream

In the initial stages many (not all) GAPS patients tolerate goat's milk products better than cow's milk. I strongly recommend using only organic milk. If you cannot find organic goat's milk, then try cow's. The best milk to use is **raw** organic milk, which has not been pasteurised or processed in any other way. Milk sold in most shops in the world has been pasteurised, which changes the structure of the milk and destroys many useful nutrients in it. For a full discussion on raw milk, please, see *Milk and dairy products* in the chapter *Food. What GAPS People Should Eat and What Should Be Avoided*. A lot of milk on the supermarket shelves, apart from being pasteurised, has been subjected to a process called homogenisation in order to stop milk from separating in the bottle (a purely cosmetic purpose). This process breaks down the fat globules and changes the structure of milk even further, making it harmful for the body. Try to buy organic milk which has not been processed at all. If it is not possible to buy unpasteurised milk, try to buy milk which, apart from pasteurisation, has not been subjected to any other processing. If that is not possible then do your best to buy any organic milk labelled 'fresh'. Despite the fact that it has been pasteurised and homogenised, the fermentation process will do a lot to restore its nutritional value.

Goat's yogurt and kefir are more liquid than cow's yogurt or kefir. You can use it as a drink, or if you want to thicken it, you can drip it through cheesecloth. Sometimes cow's yogurt or kefir turns out to be quite liquid as well, so you can drip it through cheesecloth to make it thicker or to make cottage cheese and whey.

To make yogurt you need to introduce lactic acid bacteria into the milk and ferment it at a certain temperature (40–45°C/105–113°F). You can buy commercially available yogurt starters from many health food shops or small-holding suppliers. Alternatively, you can use commercially available *live* yogurt as a starter. After making their first yogurt, many people successfully perpetuate it by using it as a starter for the next batch. You can also keep the liquid left from dripping your yogurt, called whey, in a clean dry jar in your refrigerator to use as a starter for making the next batch of yogurt. If, at any point, your own yogurt or whey does not work, you need to begin again with a commercial starter or commercial live yogurt.

After yogurt has been introduced, I recommend introducing kefir. Kefir produces a more pronounced die-off reaction, which is why I recommend introducing it after the yogurt, which is quite a bit milder. Apart from good bacteria a healthy body is populated by many other microbes, including beneficial yeasts which normally protect the person from pathogenic yeasts, such as overgrowth of *candida albicans*. Kefir contains these beneficial yeasts (as well as beneficial bacteria and many other microbes), which help to take pathogenic yeasts under control.

Instructions for making yogurt

If you are using pasteurised milk bring 1 l (2.1 pt) of milk (goat's or cow's) close to the boil in a pan, stirring occasionally. You need to bring the milk close to the boiling point in order to destroy any bacteria which may linger in pasteurised milk and interfere with the fermentation. However, do not boil the milk, as this will change its structure and taste. Take the pan off the heat. Cover the pan with the lid and cool down by placing the pan in cold water until the temperature of the milk is around 40–45°C (105–113°F). If you do not have a suitable thermometer use your hand to determine the right temperature. Take a teaspoon of milk from the pan (using a clean dry spoon) and put the milk on the inside of your wrist. If it feels just slightly warm, then the temperature is right.

If you are using raw organic milk, *which has not been pasteurised* or processed in any other way, you don't need to heat it, so you can skip this step. Keep in mind though that raw milk has its own microbial population, so the fermentation process will be less predictable. Your yogurt may be more liquid or lumpy or sour than you expect. It is always best to consume dairy raw, but if you are dealing with a particularly fussy patient who would only accept a certain consistency of yogurt, then heat the raw milk close to the boiling point to make the fermentation more predictable. Gentle heating at home is not as destructive for the milk as commercial pasteurisation.

If you are using a commercial yogurt starter in powder form, you need to dissolve the powder in a little milk before adding it to the pan. If you are using your own yogurt or commercial live yogurt, add 1/3 cup to the milk. Stir well, cover with the lid and put in a warm place at 40–45°C (105–113°F). You can use a clean dry thermos for this purpose, a yoghurt maker, an electric plate, the top of your boiler or your airing cupboard (if it is warm enough). Ferment the yogurt for at least 24 hours.

After the fermentation is complete, move your yogurt to a clean dry glass jar, cover and refrigerate.

Instructions for making kefir

Kefir is similar to yogurt but much more powerful. Its origins, folklore and history make fascinating reading. Kafir is a complete balanced colony of some two hundred microbes living in their own biofilm, called kefir grains. Kefir grains look a little like cauliflower florets, but are soft to touch and slightly translucent. They live in milk and they need to be fed every 24 hours with fresh milk. If they are looked after well, they multiply quite quickly, producing more kefir grains, which can be shared with friends and neighbours. No laboratory in the world can make kefir: it is hundreds of years old and has been passed from person to person down to modern times. Some manufacturers dry kefir grains and turn them into powder, which is sold as a kefir starter. But the best kefir starter is the live grains, which you can get online or from somebody nearby, who makes kefir for their own family and can share a few kefir grains with you.

Kefir contains a balanced stable community of microbes (fungi, bacteria, viruses, etc), it is a powerful natural medicine for the digestive system, fungal overgrowth (thrush) anywhere in the body, skin problems and other maladies. It stimulates and rebalances the immune system, balances the gut flora and microbial flora elsewhere in the body, and makes milk more nourishing and much easier to digest. You don't need to pasteurise, boil or even warm up the milk for making kefir, it will work at any room temperature from warm to quite cold. Kefir grains will stay alive in the fridge for months, so they can be stored when you are away, as long as they are covered by plenty of fresh milk. Any microbes living in milk cannot stand up to kefir, so you do not need to sterilise the milk, no matter whether it is raw or pasteurised.

Kefir grains do not react well to metal or plastic, so use glass, wood, clay and cheesecloth (a polypropylene sieve is also acceptable). Fill a clean dry glass jar with fresh milk (cold or room temperature), add kefir grains, cover and leave in a dark place for 24 hours. In this time the kefir grains will turn the milk into 'kefir' – a sour, curdled yogurt-like product. To remove the kefir grains, pour the whole mixture through cheesecloth or a polypropylene sieve into a glass jug. Put kefir grains back into the same jar, fill the jar up with fresh milk, cover and put back into a dark place for 24 hours. It takes 3–5 minutes per day to make kefir, and the same glass jar will host this culture for you in perpetuity. You don't even need to wash the jar, unless it develops mould around the edges. This can be wiped off with a clean cloth.

Your jug now contains drinking kefir without the kefir grains. It is delicious to drink as it is, diluted with water, with some salt and spices or sweetened with honey and cinnamon. A cup of fresh kefir every day is one of the best preventative remedies for any illness.

Instructions for making whey and cottage cheese from yogurt or kefir

To drip yogurt or kefir, line a large bowl (glass or clay, not metal or plastic) with double layers of cheesecloth and pour your yogurt or kefir into it. Tie the four corners of the cheesecloth, turning it into a 'bag' with yogurt or kefir inside, and hang this 'bag' above the bowl for a few hours or overnight. Whey is a clear yellow liquid which drips out through the cloth. What is left in the cloth is cottage cheese, though depending on how long you leave your yogurt or kefir dripping, you can make a soft cottage cheese or thicker yogurt.

Cottage cheese can be used for baking, adding to salads and soups and as a dessert with honey, sour cream and fruit. Whey is an excellent remedy for gastritis or any other stomach problem. Diluted with water or any freshly pressed juice it makes an excellent probiotic beverage, and you can use it as a starter for fermenting other foods. Put it in a clean, dry glass jar and keep it refrigerated. If the whey was dripped from kefir, it will keep in the fridge for a couple of months at least.

Instructions for making sour cream

Homemade sour cream is delicious and nice to use in salads, soups, stews, in baking or as a dessert with some honey and berries. You can blend it with a little honey and frozen fruit or berries to make an instant ice cream. Sour cream has a wonderful profile of fatty acids, nourishing for the immune system and the brain, so use it liberally in your GAPS patient's diet. You cannot overdose on it!

It is best to make sour cream from raw organic fresh cream. If you cannot find this quality, then use pasteurised fresh cream. Use only glass, clay or wood to make sour cream (no metal or plastic).

For 1 l (2.1 pt) of cream use ½ cup of live kefir or yogurt or one sachet of commercial yogurt starter. Never put kefir grains into cream! When cream becomes sour it solidifies and you will not be able to remove the kefir grains! Use fresh drinking kefir, after straining it through a sieve to remove the grains.

If the cream is raw, pour it into a dry clean glass jar, add a little kefir, mix and leave for 24 hours to ferment at room temperature. If you would like to make it with a yogurt starter, you need to maintain a specific temperature necessary for yogurt: 40–45°C (105–113°F), using a yogurt maker, a hot plate or another device.

If the cream has been pasteurised and you are using fresh kefir as a starter, you may not need to heat the cream prior to fermentation. Just add some kefir, mix and ferment for 24 hours. If you are using yogurt starter, you may need to heat the cream prior to adding yogurt.

Making sour cream at home, particularly from raw cream, is an art and there may be variations in texture and taste in different batches. Raw cream contains its own microbial community, which will take part in fermentation, making the whole process less predictable. For the vast majority of people this is perfectly acceptable. If you need to produce sour cream of consistent taste and texture, you may have to heat the cream to remove any microbial presence. This makes the process predictable, particularly if you are making sour cream regularly for a fussy patient. Bring the cream to the boil constantly stirring, but do not let it boil. Cool down by placing the pan in cold water, keeping it covered at all times. If using a yogurt starter, you must keep the temperature at 40–45°C (105–113°F). Add the yogurt starter and ferment for 24 hours, maintaining the same temperature. If you are using kefir as a starter, you don't need to pay attention to temperature; it will ferment well at any room temperature.

Fermented legumes (beans, lentils and dried peas)

Legumes are seeds. Like all seeds they are difficult to digest, as they contain a plethora of indigestible and damaging substances, called antinutrients. Even people with a very healthy digestion struggle with legumes, unless they are properly prepared. Soaking, fermenting and sprouting them helps to improve their digestibility and make them more nutritious. GAPS people cannot digest this group of plants until enough healing has happened in their gut. That is why we avoid them for quite a while, sometimes for years, before trying to introduce them. When the person's digestive system is ready, we can try them after soaking and *double fermentation*, which pre-digests the beans well enough to be tolerated by a person with a sensitive digestive system.

Double-fermented beans

In this recipe you are going to employ lactic acid fermentation followed by alkaline fermentation. Lactic acid bacteria live naturally on legumes so you don't need to add them, though you can add some kefir to speed up the fermentation process. Alkaline fermentation is done by using *bacillus subtilis* from a Japanese fermented soya bean recipe, called *natto*. You need to get fresh natto or a natto starter, both of which are available online or in specialised shops; 2–3 tablespoons of fresh natto will be enough.

You can use dried haricot beans, which are allowed on the GAPS Diet. But, because you are using double fermentation in this recipe, you can use any mixture of beans, lentils or dried peas. Put 1 kg (2¼ lb) of legumes into a large bowl and add filtered water. Leave for 24 hours to soak; the beans will absorb water and become larger. Drain and rinse the beans under running water. Add fresh water again to cover the beans and leave for 3–4 days to ferment at room temperature. You may want to add a few tablespoons of kefir or whey from kefir to speed up fermentation. The water will start getting frothy and the smell will be slightly sour, as this is lactic acid fermentation. Discard the water and rinse the beans again. Put the beans into a large pan with boiling water, cover and simmer until the beans become soft. Drain the beans and cover to keep them hot.

Put fresh natto or natto starter into a large clean dry tray (glass or glazed) and pour a little boiling water into the tray. Mix the starter with the water and spread around the tray. Immediately add the hot beans into the tray and mix well with the starter. The heat shock is essential for bacillus subtilis to activate. The tray needs to be large enough to spread the beans in a thin layer (2–3 cm/¾–1¼ in thick). Cover the tray with cling film (Saran wrap) making sure that the plastic does not touch the beans, but keeps the moisture in. Place the tray in a warm, dark place at 37–45°C (99–113°F). Use an airing cabinet, a hot plate or another setup, which you will need to think about in advance. Leave the tray to ferment for 2–4 days, checking every day. The beans need to develop a slimy film and a strong smell of natto. At this point you can divide the beans into portions, put them into small bags and freeze. Add a bag of these frozen beans to your soups, minced meat or vegetable stew at the beginning of cooking. Don't worry about the smell and the texture of the beans; by the time the dish is cooked, the smell is not usually a problem anymore. Make sure to add a small amount of beans (no more than a cup) and cook them with vegetables, meat, salt, pepper and spices. The double fermentation of the beans will make sure that they are easy to digest, even for sensitive people.

It has to be admitted that processing legumes this way is laborious, and the resulting flavour may not be to everyone's taste. Also, some GAPS people find that they can never have legumes. Their digestive systems cannot cope with this group of plants, no matter how well they are prepared and processed. If you belong to this group of people and really want to consume legumes, you may have to look into ancient techniques for making miso, natto, koji and tempeh.[6]

Chilli with meat, vegetables and double-fermented beans

500 g (18 oz) full-fat minced meat (a mixture of pork and beef is best)
1 cup homemade fermented vegetables (cabbage, beetroot, celery, carrot, etc)
1 cup double-fermented legumes (can be frozen)
2–3 large onions
2–3 red/orange/green peppers
2–3 courgettes (zucchini) or an equal amount of fresh pumpkin
1–2 large aubergine (eggplant)
1 chilli pepper or chilli powder to taste
6 tablespoons of chopped fresh garlic
3 tablespoons tomato purée or a 200–300 ml (7-10 fl oz) tomato passata; can be replaced with 4–5 fresh tomatoes, roughly chopped
salt and black pepper to taste

Mix the minced meat with homemade fermented vegetables and leave at room temperature for 2–6 hours to ferment. Meat is digested best if it has been fermented prior to cooking, particularly pork.

Put the minced meat and fermented vegetable mixture in a large pan, cover with plenty of water (double the volume of the meat). Add fermented legumes, salt and pepper and bring to boil. Simmer for about an hour, mixing occasionally, until the meat is cooked well. Taste for salt and adjust. If the meat didn't have enough fat in it, add extra animal fat. It is the fat that will give it the best flavour. If all the water has absorbed into the meat and beans, add a little more; the mixture should be nicely moist with the consistency of a stew. Add all the vegetables, cut into large or small pieces (your choice), the chilli pepper and tomato purée. Mix well and simmer until the vegetables are soft and have absorbed a lot of fat and water. Mix well and take off the heat. Add chopped garlic and parsley. Let it rest for 15 minutes and serve. This is a complete meal, which doesn't need anything else served with it. It will keep in the fridge for a week at least.

Fermented fish

Fermentation of fish is traditional in many parts of the world. Soused herring in Holland, salted herring in Russia, gravlax in Scandinavia, bloaters in England and many different fermentation recipes in Asia (Korea, Japan, China and Vietnam) and Africa have served their populations very well for thousands of years. When we ferment fish instead of cooking it, we preserve valuable nutrients and the fish is pre-digested for us by microbes. If a person used to have reactions to fish but would like to try it again, start from fermented fish. This is the form we introduce fresh fish in the GAPS Introduction Diet.

Fermented herring or mackerel

3–4 very fresh large herrings or mackerel
1 small white onion
1–2 tablespoons salt per litre (1 quart) brine
1 tablespoon peppercorns
5–7 bay leaves
1 teaspoon coriander seeds
fresh dill or some dill seeds
1 cup kefir whey
a suitable glass jar

Skin the fish, remove large bones and cut into bite-size pieces. Peel and slice the onion. Put the pieces of the fish into the glass jar, mixing it with peppercorns, slices of white onion, coriander seeds, bay leaves and dill seeds or dill herb. In a separate jug dissolve 1 tablespoon of sea salt in some water and add half a cup of the kefir whey. Pour this brine into the jar until the fish is completely covered. If the fish is not covered just add more water. Close the jar tightly and leave to ferment for 3–5 days at room temperature, then store in the fridge. Serve with eggs, vegetables, fresh dill, spring onion and some homemade mayonnaise. Consume within 1–3 weeks.

Fermented sardines

5–7 very fresh sardines
1–2 tablespoons salt

1 tablespoon peppercorns
5–7 bay leaves
1 teaspoon coriander seeds
fresh dill or some dill seeds
1 cup kefir whey
a suitable glass jar

Descale the fish, cut off the heads and clean the belly out. Put into a glass jar or a glazed pan. Add all the other ingredients. Top up with water so the fish is completely covered. If you are using a pan, float a small plate on top of the fish to keep it submerged in the brine. Cover the pan or put the lid on the jar and let it ferment for 3–5 days at room temperature. When the fish is ready take the meat off the bones, cut into bite-size pieces and serve with eggs, fresh dill and some chopped red onion.

Fermented grains

Please, read the chapter *Coming Off the GAPS Diet* before using this recipe. After two years or longer on the diet, and when all digestive problems are gone, your patient may be ready to have some gluten-free grains: buckwheat, millet and quinoa. First try fermented grains, as the fermentation process will predigest them. To ferment buckwheat, millet or quinoa wash the grain, cover with water and add ½ cup of whey. Leave to ferment at room temperature for a few days: quinoa for 1–2 days, buckwheat for 2–3 days, millet for 5–7 days. When the fermentation is complete, drain the liquid out and cook the grain in homemade meat stock or water with some salt (for 1 cup of grain add 2 cups of meat stock or water). Bring the meat stock to the boil and add the grain, mix well, bring to the boil, cover and reduce heat to the minimum. Simmer for 20–30 minutes, stirring occasionally. When the grain is cooked all the liquid should be completely absorbed and the grain should be soft and fluffy. Serve it with meats and vegetables or bake with it, using it instead of flour. Introduce gradually, starting from 1–2 teaspoons a day and watching for any reaction. Do not forget to serve grains with plenty of natural fat: butter, ghee, olive oil, coconut oil or any animal fat. The fats will slow down the digestion of the grains and help to control the blood sugar at a normal level. This is particularly important for people who had poor blood sugar control before commencing the GAPS Nutritional Protocol. Always introduce one grain at a time, slowly and gradually, starting from buckwheat or quinoa. Millet is the hardest to digest for many people and should be tried last.

3. FATS FOR COOKING

Cooking (roasting, frying, baking, etc.) should be done with animal fats, because they are stable and do not alter their chemical structure when heated at usual cooking temperatures: pork fat, goose fat, duck fat, beef fat, lamb fat, butter and ghee. Coconut oil can also be used for cooking and baking. Particularly valuable is the fat from the inside of the animal's body: the fat surrounding the heart, kidneys, intestines and other inner organs. It can be sold under the name of suet (minced inner fat of beef or lamb) and, when melted in the oven, it produces a liquid fat called tallow. You can purchase many of these fats in shops. It is also easy to make many of these fats at home, which has an advantage: you know exactly what is in it. I would like to repeat here that animal fats are vital for a GAPS person to have in generous amounts daily. The more animal fats your patient consumes with breakfast, lunch and dinner, the quicker will be the recovery. For more information on this subject please look in the chapter: *Fats: The Good and the Bad*.

Ghee

Ghee is a clarified butter. It is traditionally used in many cultures around the world for cooking and baking. Butter can be used very effectively for cooking too. However, small amounts of whey in the butter often burn. Also, whey contains lactose and some milk proteins, which many GAPS patients have to avoid in the initial stages of the diet. Ghee on the other hand does not contain any whey, milk protein or lactose, just milk fat, and does not burn at normal cooking temperatures.

To make ghee, preheat your oven to around 100–110°C (212–230° F). Put a large block of organic, preferably unsalted, butter in an oven dish and leave it in the oven for 25–30 minutes. Carefully pour the golden fat from the top (ghee) through cheesecloth into glass jars, making sure that the white liquid at the bottom stays in the pan. Discard the white liquid. Keep the ghee in glass jars and refrigerate. Alternatively, you can melt the butter in a pan on the stove (making sure that it doesn't burn) and then filter it through cheesecloth.

With some varieties of butter the white liquid accumulates at the top. In that case put the dish in the fridge. As it cools down the ghee will become solid, and you will be able to pour the liquid off and wipe the rest of it with a paper towel.

Goose or duck fat

Roast a goose or a duck in the oven in the usual way. Take the bird out and pour the fat through cheesecloth or a fine metal sieve. Keep in glass jars and refrigerate. These fats can be used for all cooking, baking and frying; they give a nice flavour to roasted vegetables in particular. Use in liberal amounts.

Pork, lamb or beef fat

You can collect these fats in much the same way as the duck and goose fats. It is particularly good to use the internal fat layer from the animal, which the butcher often gives away almost free. You will be amazed by how much cooking fat you will collect from a fairly small piece. It is wise to use organic animals for this purpose, as fat is a natural body storage for various toxins. Investing in a large piece of organic fat once or twice a year will not cost you much and will last for many months.

Roast the fat on a fairly low heat (120–130°C/250–260°F) for 2–6 hours depending on the size of the piece. Pour the fat through cheesecloth or a fine metal sieve. Store in glass jars and refrigerate. Use for all cooking, baking and frying in liberal amounts.

Coconut oil is traditionally used for cooking in tropical countries. It contains largely saturated fats and hence is quite stable, not changing its chemical structure when heated. Make sure that you buy good quality natural organic coconut oil.

Tallow is one of the most healing fats in nature! It makes the best skin cream for dry or inflamed skin (in eczema, psoriasis or dermatitis of any kind) and it is very healing for our digestive system and all other organs and systems. You need inner fat from a grass-fed animal to make tallow, usually from beef or lamb (the fat from inside the body of the animal from around the heart, kidneys and digestive system). Melt pieces of inner fat in the oven for a few hours (or overnight) at fairly low temperatures: 100–110° C (212–230° F). Yellow fat will melt out – this is tallow. Pour it through a sieve into glass jars and refrigerate. Use for all your cooking. The crackling left in the oven tray is delicious and should also be used for cooking. You can blend it into a paste in your food processor or cut into smaller pieces and store in the fridge.

Tallow skin cream: fill a glass jar to 2/3 with tallow and let it cool down to a warm temperature. Add olive oil to fill the jar. Add 10–15 drops of your favourite essential oil (the majority of people prefer lavender oil). Mix well and put in the refrigerator. The cream will set and can then be kept at room temperature in your bathroom and used daily. It is wonderfully healing for any irritated or inflamed skin and works very well as a skin cream for your face, hands and other parts of the body.

Salo (Russian, Ukrainian and Eastern European) or Lardo (Italian). Salo is an under-skin pork fat, cured with salt, from home-reared pigs. The fat is often as thick as 10–15 cm (4–6 in) and the skin is left on. Once cured, salo keeps for about a year without spoiling and, traditionally, it is consumed raw. It can also be used for cooking, cut into bite-size pieces and melted in the pan. You can use it to fry eggs and cook vegetables or any dish with meat, fish, eggs and vegetables. When consumed raw, salo is very beneficial to health, as it provides raw uncooked fat for the body to use. Ukrainians traditionally attribute their good health and physical strength to eating salo daily.

This recipe will be helpful for people who rear their own pigs or who have access to large pieces of fresh under-skin pork fat. Trim all muscle off the fat. Lay a large cotton cloth on a counter and cover it with salt (about 1–2 cm/½–¾ in). Lay a slab of fresh raw pork fat, skin down, on that salt. Cover the slab with salt on all sides and spread 1–2 cm (½–¾ in) of salt on top of it. Lay another slab of fat, skin up, on top of the first piece. Cover it with salt on all sides. Wrap the slabs tightly in the cloth to keep the salt in and put in the fridge. Turn every day for 2 weeks, keeping it in a refrigerator. The salo will then be ready to eat. Brush the salt off (or rinse it off) and cut a thin layer off the edges to remove any discoloured or rancid parts. The salo inside will be slightly pink and taste delicious. Slice and enjoy! The skin, if soft, should be good to eat as it is, or it can be cut off and used for making soups or stews.

Salo will keep for weeks in a fridge. Make sure to keep it wrapped in cotton cloth; it should not have contact with plastic. If you would like to keep it for longer, put the whole thing (with the cloth on and salt inside) into a plastic bag and store it in a freezer. This way salo will keep for about a year without spoiling.

4. MEATS, ORGAN MEATS AND FISH

Meats, organ meats and fish are consumed daily on the GAPS Diet. They provide the easiest-to-digest and the best quality protein, fat, vitamins, minerals and even carbohydrates for the human body.

As we have already discussed in the chapter on meat stock, *we are not interested in the pure muscle mass of an animal (lean steak).* We are interested in pieces rich in connective tissue, containing plenty of collagen and fat in a mixture with some muscle fibres. Such pieces require long cooking (low and slow), usually with some water, to loosen the structure of tough connective tissue, to make it soft and easy to chew and digest. It has been common knowledge in traditional cultures for centuries that eating the lean muscle of any animal without fat and connective tissue is unhealthy.[4] Modern nutritional science keeps telling us that 'eating meat is unhealthy'. What they mean under the word 'meat' is the lean muscle of the animal, and that is what the majority of people in the West understand. In traditional cultures nobody eats lean muscle; the muscle fibres have always been consumed with fat and well-cooked connective tissue. So, when we say the word 'meat' in the GAPS Nutritional Protocol, that is what we mean – a proper piece of animal carcass containing the full spectrum of connective tissues, muscle, fat, bone, fascia, nerves, blood vessels, skin and all other tissues which belong to that piece of the animal. Nothing is trimmed off, as every tissue contributes something unique nutritionally.

Organ meats: brain, liver, kidney, spleen, heart, tongue, lungs, stomach, intestines and endocrine glands of the animal are many times more nourishing than the muscle of the animal.[2] For thousands of years people in traditional cultures valued organ meats above muscle, considered them to be a delicacy, and consumed them first when an animal was slaughtered.[4,5] The easiest way to cook organs is to mince them all together: heart, lungs, spleen, pancreas, oesophagus, diaphragm and large blood vessels should be minced with fat, which normally surrounds some of these organs (particularly the heart). Even stomach and intestines can be added to the mixture (they need to be cleaned well). The resulting mince is delicious and rich in valuable nutrients. It can be used for any recipe where minced meat is required, or it can be frozen to be used later.

Kidney can be added at the end of cooking to any meat dish (a stew, a soup, a chilli) or cooked vegetables, because kidney cooks very quickly. Using scissors, cut small pieces from the soft parts of kidneys, leaving the tough parts for mincing with the rest of the organs later. Add small kidney pieces into any hot dish, bring up to simmer and take off the heat. In this short time the pieces of kidney will cook and add a nice flavour to your dish.

In traditional societies liver was often consumed by the children, pregnant women and other people with high nutritional needs, because liver is the best source of most B vitamins, vitamin A and other fat-soluble vitamins, iron, many amino acids and proteins, enzymes, many other nutrients and even vitamin C.[5] Any person suffering from anaemia must eat liver daily, as it is the best cure for anaemia. Many people wonder if liver is 'toxic to eat, because it processes toxins'? Yes, the liver processes toxins, but it does not store them! If our liver was a storage site for toxins, we probably would not survive past the first few weeks of life! The liver does not store toxicity in its own structure, it neutralises toxins and sends them elsewhere in the body to be stored (often in the under-skin fat tissue). So, eating liver of animals is safe and essential, particularly for GAPS people!

Another concern people have about eating liver is parasites. Liver can be a natural home for some parasites, though a healthy animal should not have this problem. Freezing fresh liver for two weeks at least will kill any parasites that may possibly be present, so it is a good practice to cook only liver that has been frozen for two weeks.

In traditional societies there was a rule: whatever organ in your body is diseased, you need to eat the same organ from animals to heal yourself. If you have a kidney disease, eat kidneys from animals. If your pancreas is unhealthy, eat animal pancreases. If your heart is struggling, eat animal hearts. There is a lot of wisdom in this traditional practice: the animal organ will provide you with the full spectrum of specific building materials to heal and rebuild your diseased organ.

Birds: chicken, duck, goose, turkey, guineafowl, pigeon, pheasant and other are a very important part of the GAPS Diet. Again, *we do not eat the lean breast of the bird (pure muscle),* but focus on the whole carcass, particularly connective tissues and organs. The most valuable parts of any bird nutritionally are its skin, feet, neck, head, wings, legs, joints, cartilage and bones. These tissues need to be cooked in water for a few hours to make them soft and easy to digest. The lean muscle of the breast (particularly in commercial breeds of chicken) becomes dry and chewy if cooked too long. So, I recommend cutting it from the bird before cooking and reserving it for stir-frying or other dishes. The rest of the bird needs to be cooked for a few hours in water with some salt, pepper, herbs and vegetables to make delicious meat stock, very soothing and healing for a sensitive digestive system. After cooking, all the soft tissues need to be taken off the bones, cut into bite-size pieces and returned to the stock to make a rich healing soup. Organs (giblets) are very valuable nutritionally and should always be added to the pot when making the stock. After cooking, they too should be cut into bite-size pieces and returned to the stock.

Fish and shellfish are an important part of the GAPS Diet. The most valuable tissues of seafood are the skin, cartilage, heads and other parts rich in connective tissue. It is essential to descale the fish prior to cooking, so the skin can be eaten. The muscle of fish should be cooked very briefly, or even consumed uncooked, because long cooking makes fish muscle dry and chewy. Indeed, this is reflected in most traditional recipes where fish is cooked quite quickly or consumed raw (marinated, salted, dried or fermented). Fish stock is highly nutritious and healing and should be made from the skin, head, skeleton, fins and tail of large fish or from a few handfuls of small fish (descaled and gutted).

Like all other foods, meat digests best when it has been fermented prior to cooking and eating. This applies to pork in particular; there is something about fresh pork that can have a negative effect on our metabolism. We don't have enough research yet to say what exactly it is in pork that can damage our bodies, but when we ferment pork by salting it and leaving it to age, these negative effects disappear.[3,7] Traditional cultures around the world discovered this through experience; that is why many of them fermented pork before eating it. Good examples are traditionally made ham and sausages (jamon and chorizo in Spain, prosciutto in Italy, przut in Dalmatia, aged sausages in France, Poland, Russia and many other countries). In all these recipes pork is salted and then left to hang for some time to ferment. Once the meat is properly fermented it will keep for years without refrigeration, even in the summer heat of Mediterranean countries. Korean people ferment most of their meat before cooking. Traditionally made bacon, ham and sausages in the English-speaking world have also been salted and hung for a while to ferment.[3]

In the Western world the term that is often used instead of 'fermentation' is 'marinating'. When we marinade food, we leave it for a while mixed with some salt, herbs, spices and vinegar. During that time the natural microbes, which live on all fresh raw foods, become active and ferment the food a little, making it easier for us to digest. Many of my patients find it difficult to digest fresh meats, but when they start fermenting them prior to cooking this problem disappears. Fermentation predigests meats somewhat, adds flavour and makes the meat softer and juicier.

So, how do we ferment meat at home? Easy: just add some of your fermented vegetables to the meat and leave for a while before cooking it. This is particularly easy with minced and diced meat: just add a handful of fermented carrot, onion, garlic, pepper, squash or radish, cabbage or any other fermented vegetable you have at home, some salt (not too much, as fermented vegetables are salty already) and black pepper to taste, mix and leave in a glass, clay or wooden bowl. Do not use plastic or metal bowls, as fermentation will leach toxic substances out of them into the meat. Make sure to compact the meat, squeezing out as much air as possible, and then cover with a plate. You can also cover it with olive oil or any animal fat. Healthy fermentation is generally an anaerobic process (without oxygen), so the meat needs to be submerged in the mixture of fermented vegetables and juices. Besides, contact with air encourages yeasts to grow in the mixture, which in itself is not harmful but may alter unfavourably the texture and flavour of the meat. If you only have a few hours before cooking the meat, leave it at a room temperature. If you have a few days, leave it in the fridge covered with a plate. Cook the meat according to your recipe without removing fermented vegetables.

If you have a joint of meat, which you are planning to roast, you can ferment it too. Place the meat joint into a glass, clay or wooden bowl small enough to just about fit, cover with some of your fermented vegetables and fill up with salty water (brine) to cover the meat completely.

Float a small plate on top of the water to keep the meat submerged. Leave it in the fridge for a few days or at a room temperature for a few hours. When you are ready to cook it, remove from the brine and put in a preheated oven.

The beauty of using fermentation is that the meat will not spoil, even if you forget and leave it fermenting in the fridge for too long. The beneficial microbes in your fermented vegetables will not allow any pathogenic or putrefactive microbes to grow, so the meat is well preserved.

There are hundreds of wonderful recipes for cooking meats, fish and organs from all over the world. Here I would like to offer a small sample.

Italian meat casserole

This is an alternative way of making an excellent meat stock, as well as preparing a meal for the whole family. You can use any of the following: a leg or a shoulder of lamb, a joint of pork, beef or venison, 2 pheasants, 2–4 pigeons, 2 quails, a whole chicken or turkey legs. You need a large casserole with a lid for this dish. Put your meat joint or a whole bird(s) into the casserole, add water to fill 2/3 of the casserole, some salt, black pepper, chilli pepper, dried herbs to taste, bay leaves and a sprig of rosemary. I recommend adding a handful of homemade fermented vegetables (Brussels sprouts, carrot, cabbage, greens, celery, etc). Cover with a lid and put in the oven for 5–6 hours on low heat (140–160°C/285–320°F). If you have time, leave the casserole at room temperature for a few hours to ferment a little before putting it in the oven. Add various vegetables 40–50 minutes before dinner time: rosettes of broccoli and cauliflower, whole peeled small red or white onions, Brussels sprouts, pieces of swede or turnip and large pieces of carrot. When ready, take the meat and vegetables out and serve to your family. Pour the meat stock through a sieve and serve it in bouillon cups with the dinner. Meat stock, left from this dinner, will keep well in the refrigerator and can be used for making soups or warming up as a nourishing drink.

Stuffed peppers

6 large peppers (a combination of green, red, yellow and orange)
500 g (18 oz) full-fat minced meat (a mixture of ½ pork and ½ beef is best)
2 medium-size carrots
1 large onion
salt, black pepper, chilli pepper and spices to taste
a handful of homemade fermented vegetables (celery, cabbage, carrot, beetroot, kimchi, greens, etc)

Mix the minced meat with fermented vegetables and leave at room temperature for 2–6 hours. Grate or slice the carrots and chop the onion. Mix them with the meat adding salt, pepper and spices to taste.

Cut off the tops of the peppers and take out the seeds. Fill the peppers with the mixture of the meat and vegetables. Place the stuffed peppers upright in a pan. Your pan should allow all the peppers to stand upright and support each other. Add 3–4 cups of water to the bottom of the pan and cover it with the lid. Bring up to the boil, reduce the heat to a minimum and simmer for an hour. Serve a pepper per person with a ladle of the stock from the bottom (best to serve in a soup bowl). Add a tablespoon of homemade sour cream or yoghurt mixed with a clove of crushed garlic. Garnish with chopped parsley.

Meatballs

500 g (18 oz) full-fat minced meat (a mixture of pork and beef is best)
a handful of homemade fermented vegetables (celery, cabbage, carrot, beetroot, kimchi, greens, etc)
1 large onion
1 red pepper
1 courgette (zucchini)
2 tablespoons chopped fresh garlic
1 tablespoon tomato purée
salt, pepper
2–3 bay leaves

Mix the minced meat with fermented vegetables and leave at room temperature for 2–6 hours. To make the sauce, cover the bottom of the pan with 3–4 cm (1¼–1½ in) of water and mix in the tomato purée, salt and pepper. Bring to the boil. With your hands shape balls out of the mincemeat about 4-5 cm (1½–2 in) in diameter. Put the balls one at a time into the boiling sauce. Make sure that you use a large enough pan to fit all the balls in one layer. Cover with the lid and simmer on low heat for 30 minutes.

In the meantime, prepare the vegetables. Finely chop the onion and red pepper. Cut the courgette into cubes. Chop the garlic.

After cooking the meatballs for 30 minutes add the chopped onion, pepper and courgette, and mix with the sauce gently in order to preserve the shape of the meatballs. Cover and cook for another 25 minutes. Add the bay leaves and garlic. Cover and turn the heat off. Let it sit for 10 minutes before serving. Sprinkle with finely chopped coriander (cilantro) or parsley and serve with cooked vegetables.

Meat cutlets (burgers)

500 g (18 oz) full-fat minced pork
500 g (18 oz) full-fat minced beef or lamb
a handful of homemade fermented vegetables (celery, cabbage, carrot, beetroot, kimchi, greens, etc)
1 large onion, finely chopped
salt, pepper and spices

Mix the minced meat with fermented vegetables and leave at room temperature for 2–6 hours. Mix all the ingredients well with your hands and make oval shaped cutlets about 4–5 cm (1½–2 in) thick. Place the cutlets on a greased baking tray (use any animal fat for greasing) and bake in a preheated oven for about an hour at 180°C (355°F). Serve with cooked vegetables and a salad.

Fish cutlets

2–3 fairly large freshwater or sea fish (a mixture of different fish works very well)
a handful of homemade fermented vegetables (celery, cabbage, carrot, beetroot, kimchi, greens, etc)
1 egg
3–5 tablespoons butter (ghee, goose fat, duck fat, pork dripping or coconut oil)
1–2 cups shredded coconut
salt and pepper

Cut all the meat off the fish, remove skin and large bones. Use the bones, heads and skin for making a very nourishing fish stock (recipe in the *Meat Stock And Soups* section). Alternatively, you can buy fish fillets already without skin and large bones.

In the food processor put the meat of the fish, fermented vegetables, one egg, butter, salt and pepper to your taste and grind to make mince. If you have a meat mincer it will do the same job for you. Leave it at room temperature for 30–60 minutes. Mix well, using your hands, and make oval-shaped flat cutlets about 2 cm (¾ in) thick. Roll them in shredded coconut. Place the cutlets on a large oven tray, greased with fat. Add 1/3 cup of water and put into preheated oven. Bake for 20–30 minutes at 160°C (320°F).

Swedish gravlax

skinless and boneless salmon fillet
1 l (2.1 pt) water at room temperature
1½ tablespoons salt
1 tablespoon honey
juice from 2 fresh lemons
fresh dill and coarsely ground black pepper

The fish has to be very fresh. Cut it into 0.5-cm (¼-in) thick slices and place in a deep tray (any glazed or glass baking tray will do). Sprinkle with finely chopped dill and black pepper. Dissolve the salt and the honey in the water to make a brine; add the lemon juice. Cover the fish with the brine and leave at room temperature for 1–1½ hours. Take the fish out of the brine and serve with some lettuce, avocado and olive oil.

This dish works particularly well with wild salmon. Because the fish is not cooked, all the essential fatty acids and other nutrients are preserved. Refrigerate and consume within two days.

Marinated wild salmon – a variation of gravlax

6 boneless wild salmon fillets with the skin on (each fillet is the serving size for one person) or two sides of a large salmon with skin on
3–4 large lemons
1 heaped teaspoon natural sea salt
1 heaped teaspoon grainy mild mustard
½ teaspoon dill seeds or some fresh dill, chopped
coarsely ground black pepper to taste

The fish has to be very fresh. In a glass or glazed baking tray of suitable size lay three of the salmon fillets skin down. The fillets should fill the tray completely, fitted in tightly together. In a separate bowl make the marinade: cut the lemons in half, squeeze the juice and then scoop the flesh into the bowl. Add the rest of the ingredients and mix well. Don't worry if the lemon flesh is in chunks. Cover the layer of fish in the tray with all the marinade and lay the other three fish fillets on top skin up. Press the two layers of fish together with a heavy object so the marinade covers the fish completely. You can use another baking tray with something heavy in it or a slab of clean stone/granite. Leave in the fridge for 24 hours to marinade. Take the fish out and peel the skin off: it comes off fairly easily. Using scissors cut the fish into bite-size pieces and serve with avocado and some lettuce, using the marinade as a dressing. This dish is delicious and easy to digest. Because the fish is not cooked, all the essential fatty acids and other nutrients are preserved.

Baked beans or French cassoulet

500 g (18 oz) white navy (haricot) beans
1 whole duck
a handful of homemade fermented vegetables (celery, cabbage, carrot, beetroot, kimchi, greens, etc)
2 large onions, chopped
1 large carrot, sliced
1 tablespoon salt
2 tablespoons tomato purée or 500 ml (17 fl oz) pure tomato passata
cayenne pepper and black pepper
5–6 bay leaves, a sprig of rosemary, a teaspoon of thyme or oregano

Beans and other legumes are generally hard to digest, as they contain many anti-nutrients. Soaking and fermenting will make the beans easy to digest for the majority of people, even those with sensitive digestive systems.

Soak the beans in water for 12–24 hours, drain, rinse well in cold water and drain again. Cover the beans with boiling water to break their tough skins, cool down and then add 4–5 tablespoons of homemade whey, kefir or yogurt. Make sure that the beans are completely submerged in the water. Leave to ferment for 4–6 days at room temperature. Drain and rinse well. Now the beans are ready to be cooked.

Cut the duck into individual servings, separating the drumsticks, thighs, wings and pieces of carcass (leave the bones in). Cut the giblets into small pieces.

In a large clay or glass pot mix the beans and the duck pieces with all other ingredients. Add 1–2 l (2.1–4.2 pt) of water. If the duck is not fatty enough, add 300-500 g (11–18 oz) of butter or another animal fat (goose, duck, lamb, beef or pork). Cover the pan with a lid and put in the oven. Cook at 160–180°C (320–355°F) for 4–5 hours. Check occasionally. If the beans are getting dry, add more water. When ready, the beans and the duck should be soft and the water should have turned into a thick sauce.

Cool down a little and serve. The baked beans left from this meal will keep in the fridge for a long time and can be served with other dishes.

You can make this dish without the meat, in that case add plenty of animal fat (duck, pork, goose, beef, lamb, ghee, etc.). You can preserve this dish for about a year if you ladle it hot into sterilised glass jars and keep them refrigerated. To sterilise glass jars and their lids (metal or glass) place them in a cold oven and heat it to about 120°C (250°F) for 30–40 minutes. Do not put the lids on the jars for sterilising, but keep them separate.

Turkey casserole

turkey legs, wings, carcass and other pieces with the skin on (not skinless breast!)
1 l (2.1 pt) water
a handful of homemade fermented vegetables (celery, cabbage, carrot, beetroot, kimchi, greens, etc)
1–2 teaspoons salt
6–10 peppercorns, freshly crushed
cayenne pepper to taste
fresh or dried herbs: oregano, rosemary, bay leaves
a combination of available vegetables: choose from carrots, winter squash, pumpkin, courgette, marrow (zucchini), peeled small/ medium onions, cauliflower, broccoli, peppers, aubergine (eggplant) and Brussels sprouts

Put fermented vegetables, water, salt, tomato purée, peppercorns, cayenne pepper and herbs in a large casserole. Add the turkey pieces. Brush the parts of the turkey pieces not covered by the water with generous amounts of goose fat (or duck fat, ghee, pork fat, beef fat, lamb fat). Turkey is naturally quite lean, so add plenty of animal fat. Do not cover the casserole with the lid. Cook in the oven at 160–180°C (320–355°F) for 2–2½ hours. About 50 minutes before the end of cooking cut the vegetables into large chunks. Using your hands, rub generous amounts of fat over the vegetable pieces and add them to the casserole. Mix them well into the sauce and leave cooking. When the vegetables are cooked so a sharp knife goes through them easily, take the casserole out. Serve the meat and the vegetables with some freshly chopped parsley and garlic.

Basic liver pâté

100 g (4 oz) liver (calf, pork or lamb)
1 cup homemade sour cream (you can use commercially available sour cream or ghee)
salt and pepper to taste
a large handful of peeled garlic

Wash the liver, dry and cut into bite-size pieces. Constantly stirring, fry the liver in plenty of animal fat with salt and black pepper until medium rare (still pink inside, but no blood coming out). Take off the heat and cool down. Using a food processor, blend the liver with sour cream and garlic into a fine paste. Taste and adjust salt and pepper; this recipe needs quite a bit more salt and pepper than usual. When the pâté tastes perfect, fill glass jars or deep dishes and leave in the fridge to set. When set, pour some melted butter or ghee to cover the top (to prevent it from drying). Instead of butter or ghee, you can use gelatinous meat stock. This pâté will keep in the fridge for a week or it can be frozen. It is delicious with any meal and can be mixed into soups, stews, cooked vegetables and salads.

Liver in a clay pot

100 g (4 oz) liver (calf or lamb)
100 g (4 oz) lamb hearts
1 large onion
10 dried prunes with stones
1 large pot natural yogurt or sour cream (you can use your home made yogurt or replace with ½ cup of butter/ghee)
allspice, salt and pepper to taste

Wash the liver, dry and cut into bite-size pieces. Cut the hearts into bite-size pieces. Put the liver and hearts, finely chopped onion and prunes in a clay pot. Add salt, pepper and allspice to the sour cream or yogurt and mix well. Add to the clay pot and mix with the meats. Add a cup of water and mix. Cover the pot with the lid or foil. Bake in the oven for about 1 hour at 160–180°C (320–355°F).

Quick liver recipe

100 g (4 oz) liver
1 large onion
6–7 cloves of garlic
½ cup butter/ghee (or any animal fat)
fresh parsley or dill
salt and black pepper to taste

Wash and dry the liver and cut into bite-size pieces. In a frying pan melt the butter/ghee, add the sliced onion and fry slightly until the onions start turning golden. Add the liver, salt and pepper and stir-fry for about 4-5 minutes. Add chopped garlic, mix quickly and take off the heat. Sprinkle chopped parsley or dill on top and drizzle with olive oil. Serve immediately.

Liver pudding for babies and small children

100 g (4 oz) liver (calf, pork or lamb)
1 egg

4–5 tablespoons butter (or ghee, goose/duck fat)
1 medium-size onion
salt to taste
parsley

Wash the liver, dry with a paper towel and blend into a pulp in the food processor. Put through a sieve to remove any hard bits. Add salt, egg yolk, butter, finely chopped parsley and finely chopped onion. Whip the egg white stiff and fold into the mixture. Put the mixture into a suitable dish, cover with a sheet of baking paper and cook with steam. You can use a steamer or a large pan. To steam in a pan, put some water at the bottom of the pan and place the dish in it. Make sure that you don't have too much water in the pan, so it does not get into the dish with the liver. Cover the pan with a lid and put it on the stove. Steam for about one hour. Serve with baked winter squash and plenty of butter. Other cooked vegetables also complement this dish well.

Ox tongue

1 fresh ox tongue (not salted or treated in any other way)
salt and black pepper to taste
2 l (4.2 pt) water
a handful of fresh chopped garlic and chopped parsley

Wash the tongue, put into a pan and cover with water. Bring to a boil, cover and reduce heat to simmer for 1–2 hours, until the tongue is soft enough for a knife to go through it easily (like through soft butter). When ready, take the tongue out of the water and let it cool down just enough to be touched. As soon as the tongue is just cool enough, use your hands to peel off the skin (a tough whitish layer, which covers the tongue). If you allow the tongue to cool down too much, the skin will be very difficult to remove. Discard the skin (or give it to your dog or cat). Cut the tongue into pieces 3–4 cm (1¼–1½ in) thick and lay them in a deep glass dish (preferably with a lid). Add freshly crushed black pepper, garlic and parsley. Add salt to the stock left from cooking the tongue, tasting it (the stock needs to be a little more salty than normal). Pour this stock over the tongue pieces to cover them completely. The tongue has a tendency to dry up, so it is important to keep it submerged in the stock. Cool down and refrigerate. This dish is an absolute delicacy, and the majority of people fall in love with it from the first try! Serve with some mustard or horse radish.

Black pudding

1 kg (2¼ lb) fresh blood (or frozen)
Salt, black pepper, spices and herbs
300 g (11 oz) winter squash (without seeds), cooked in the oven and mashed
100 g (4 oz) sour-tasting berries, frozen or fresh (sea buckthorn, red currants, raspberries) – optional
a handful of fermented vegetables (celery, beetroot, carrot or cabbage)
2 large onions, finely chopped
500 g (18 oz) salo (lardo), tallow, beef fat, pork fat or goose fat

Fresh blood is collected on traditional farms when an animal is slaughtered. The blood is very valuable nutritionally and should not be wasted. Often, it is frozen for later use, so defrost it for this recipe.

Put the blood through a sieve to remove any impurities. If it is congealed, use your hands to break it into small pieces. Add salt, pepper, spices and herbs to your taste and mix well. This dish can take large amounts of herbs and spices, and it requires more salt than usual. Spices which work very well are: black pepper, chilli and paprika, coriander seed, dill seed, caraway seed, turmeric, fennel seed, juniper berries, dried oregano, rosemary fresh or dried, allspice, nutmeg, cinnamon and cumin.

Add chopped onion and cooked and mashed winter squash. Cut salo into bite-size pieces (p. 248) and mix in. If salo is not available, use other listed fats (melt them and mix in).

Grease a deep oven tray and pour in the mixture. Bake in the oven at 180°C (355°F) for 40 minutes. Use a dry knife to check if the pudding is ready; it should go through easily and come out dry. Cool down completely. Cut into square pieces about 10–15 cm (4–6 in) in size, put into individual bags and freeze for long storage.

Black pudding is part of a traditional English breakfast. It can also be added to any dish with meat or vegetables to increase its nutritional value and improve the taste.

5. CONDIMENTS

Most fresh salads can be dressed with olive oil and fresh lemon juice, yogurt, kefir or sour cream. Here is a small sample of a few more complicated condiments.

Ketchup

2 cups tomato juice
1–3 tablespoons white vinegar
honey to taste
bay leaf (optional)
salt and pepper to taste

Mix all the ingredients together, except the honey, and simmer on the stove until thick, stirring often to prevent sticking. When almost the desired thickness, add honey to taste and complete cooking. Ladle into sterilised jars and seal immediately, or place in small containers and freeze. (Recipe courtesy of Elaine Gottschall)

Guacamole

2 ripe avocados
juice 1 orange
1 clove garlic, crushed
small amount of water

In the food processor blend together all the ingredients. Use as a dip for vegetables and a side dish with any meal. There are many variations of this recipe. You can add chopped fresh tomato and onion, greens, herbs and olive oil.

Mayonnaise

1 whole egg
1 cup olive oil or slightly more
1 tablespoon white vinegar or fresh lemon juice
¼ teaspoon dry mustard powder
salt and pepper to taste
a little honey to taste

Blend in your food processor for a few seconds: egg, lemon juice (or vinegar), mustard, salt, pepper and honey. While the machine is running, add the oil in a fine stream. Do not add oil quickly; it should take at least 60 seconds. As mayonnaise thickens, the sound of the machine will deepen.

Suggestions:
Use to thicken gravy: add 2 tablespoons of mayonnaise to about 1 cup of meat stock and heat gently for 1–2 minutes, stirring constantly.

Use as a base for tartar sauce by adding ½ cup chopped dill pickles (unsweetened) and ¼ cup chopped onion.

Use as mock Hollandaise sauce by adding grated cheddar cheese (if well tolerated). Spread over vegetables such as cooked cauliflower or broccoli. Cover and heat in oven.

Mix with homemade yogurt (one part mayonnaise, one part yogurt) and use as salad dressing.
(Recipe courtesy of Elaine Gottschall)

Salsa

4 medium-size tomatoes
half a pepper (green, red, orange or yellow)
1 medium onion (white or red)
–3 cloves of garlic
dill and parsley
2–3 tablespoons of kimchi or any other fermented vegetables
olive oil
salt and pepper to taste

Put all ingredients in the food processor and chop coarsely. Can be served with meats and vegetables. You can also use it for cooking meats. To do that, bring salsa to simmer, add diced meat (beef, pork, lamb or chicken) and a generous amount of butter (or any animal fat), cover and simmer for 30 minutes.

Aubergine (eggplant) dip

2 aubergines
salt
3 medium-size tomatoes
3–4 cloves of garlic
1/3 cup olive oil
fresh dill or parsley

Cut the aubergines into 1-cm (½-in) thick slices, rub well with salt and any animal fat. Place on a baking tray and bake at 180°C (356°F) for 30–40 minutes, or until soft. Alternatively, you can bake whole aubergines until a knife goes through them easily. Cool down.

In the food processor blend together the baked aubergines, tomatoes, garlic, herbs and olive oil. Serve with meats and fish and as a dip with vegetables.

Fruit chutney

1 kg (2¼ lb) cooking apples
500 g (18 oz) plums
1 kg (2¼ lb) dried dates without stones (or/and dried figs)
3 peppers (green, red or yellow)
3–4 medium-size onions
2 cups apple cider vinegar
1 teaspoon black/green/red peppercorns, crushed
1–2 teaspoons aromatic seeds: cumin, coriander, dill, fennel, etc.
½ teaspoon cayenne pepper or chilli powder
1 teaspoon natural salt

In a large pan slowly bring the dates and ½ cup of water to the boil. When soft, mash the dates with a potato masher or use a soup blender. Then add apples, cored and cut into large pieces, plums without stones, peppers and onions finely chopped, vinegar and the rest of the ingredients. Mix well and put on a very low heat. Cook for 1–1½ hours stirring occasionally, or in a slow cooker for a few hours. As apples and plums get well cooked, they fall apart and mix into a rough paste with the rest of the ingredients. While the chutney is cooking, sterilise glass jars and their lids (metal or glass) by placing them in a cold oven and heating it to about 120°C (250°F) for 30–40 minutes. Do not put the lids on the jars while sterilising, but keep them separate.

Ladle hot chutney into the jars and close the lids. When cooled down, put in a refrigerator. Keep refrigerated and serve with meats and fish.

6. SALADS

Salads should be served when diarrhoea is no longer present.

To increase the nutritional value of your salads it is good to sprinkle coarsely chopped walnuts or oily seeds on top (sunflower seeds, pumpkin seeds or sesame seeds). Seeds should be soaked in water overnight and then sprouted for 2–3 days. Soaking and sprouting makes seeds more nourishing and easier to digest.

Beetroot salad

8 small beetroots or 4 large ones
1/3 cup shelled walnuts
4-6 cloves garlic
8 dried stoned prunes

homemade mayonnaise
1/3 teaspoon salt

Wash the beetroots and cook by steaming until a knife goes through easily. Alternatively, you can buy cooked beetroots (in water not in vinegar). Once cooled, grate the beetroot through a coarse grater. In the food processor chop together the walnuts, garlic and prunes. Mix well with the grated beetroot. Add salt, mayonnaise and mix. Enjoy with meats and vegetables.

Salad with cabbage and apple

100 g (4 oz) white cabbage
1 large apple
½ cup homemade yogurt or sour cream
1 teaspoon honey
a pinch salt
2 tablespoons raisins

Grate the cabbage. Peel, core and grate the apple. Slightly fry the raisins in butter to make them soft. Mix honey and salt with yogurt. Mix all ingredients together.

Salad with tomatoes and cucumber

2 tomatoes
1/3 long cucumber
1 stick celery
spring onion
dill or parsley
salt

Cut cucumber into ½-cm (¼-in) thick slices. Cut tomato into bite-size pieces and slice the celery into small pieces. Sprinkle with salt. Chop the spring onions, dill and parsley. Mix all ingredients and dress with cold-pressed olive oil.

Russian salad

½ long cucumber
1 large carrot, steamed
100 g (4 oz) cooked meat or sausages (leftovers are good)
1 onion

2 hard-boiled eggs
2 tablespoons sauerkraut or kimchi
fresh dill and/or parsley
1/3 teaspoon salt
mayonnaise
yogurt or sour cream

Cut cucumber and carrot into small cubes. Cut the meat and/or sausages into small cubes. Finely chop the onion. Peel and cut the eggs into small cubes. Finely chop dill and parsley. In a separate pot mix mayonnaise and yogurt in equal proportions and add salt. Mix all ingredients together.

Carrot salad

1 large carrot
1 tablespoon raisins
1 tablespoon coarsely chopped walnuts
yogurt

Slightly fry the raisins in butter to make them soft. Finely grate the carrot. Mix the carrot, raisins, walnuts and yogurt.

7. VEGETABLES

Cooked vegetables are nourishing, warming and easy to digest, they are gentle on the gut lining and should be a regular part of the diet. You can cook your vegetables by steaming, stir-frying, stewing, roasting, grilling or as a soup. Instead of boiling vegetables I recommend steaming them, as boiling removes a lot of nutrients into the water, which then gets thrown away. The best vegetables to steam are broccoli, cauliflower, Brussels sprouts, fresh green beans (runner beans, string beans, etc.) carrots, asparagus, French artichokes and beetroot. We can cook our vegetables without meat, but we must add good amounts of fat to them! It is the fat that will bring out all the tastes and extract beneficial nutrients from the vegetables, as many of them are fat-soluble. The best fat to use comes from animals: bacon fat, pork dripping, lard, tallow, lamb fat, goose fat, butter and ghee. Fat is essential for our bodies to be able to use minerals, vitamins, protein and many other nutrients. So, the more animal fat you can comfortably add to your meal, the more nourishment your body will get out of it.

If diarrhoea is not present, raw vegetables should also be a normal part of every meal. They provide a lot of active enzymes, which will help you to digest your food. Carrots, cucumber, tomato, greens, cabbage, onion, garlic, lettuce, baby spinach, celery, cauliflower can all be served as salads or cut into rosettes and sticks to eat with a dip (mayonnaise, guacamole, liver pâté, aubergine/eggplant dip, etc).

A nice way to cook cabbage

½ cabbage, finely sliced
1 large carrot, finely sliced
½ onion, finely chopped
1 tomato, finely chopped
1 tablespoon chopped garlic
salt and pepper to taste
a handful of fermented vegetables

Cover the bottom of the pan with homemade meat stock, add 3–5 tablespoons of any animal fat and bring to the boil. Add cabbage, carrot, onion, salt and pepper. Cover and cook on a low heat for 30 minutes. Add the chopped tomato and garlic, mix, cook for another 3 minutes and take off the heat. Mix in ½ cup of homemade kefir, yogurt or sour cream. Serve with meat.

Quick cooked vegetable mix

2 courgettes or ¼ medium-size marrow (zucchini)
1 large onion
10 cloves garlic
1 pepper (red, yellow or green or a combination of different coloured peppers)
1 tablespoon of tomato purée
salt and pepper
a handful of fermented vegetables

In a frying pan melt about 50–100 g (2–4 oz) of butter or any animal fat. Mix in sliced courgettes or marrow, onion, garlic, sliced peppers, tomato purée, season to taste with salt and pepper. Cover with a lid and leave for 10 minutes on minimum heat. Alternatively, you can stir-fry it on a low heat. Mix well and serve with plenty of cold-pressed virgin olive oil and freshly chopped dill or parsley. Enjoy with meat and fish.

Cauliflower 'potatoes'

1 large cauliflower cut into large pieces

¼ cup butter or ¼ cup homemade yogurt or sour cream
salt and pepper to taste
parsley and paprika garnish

Cook cauliflower until just tender. Drain.
Purée in blender or food processor. Add butter or yogurt, salt and pepper and blend thoroughly. Reheat and serve. Garnish with parsley and paprika.

The puréed cauliflower may be placed in a baking dish, sprinkled with grated cheddar cheese and heated in the oven until the cheese melts.
(Recipe courtesy of Elaine Gottschall)

Baked vegetables

You can bake any combination of the following vegetables:
onions, white or red, or shallots
peppers, red, yellow, orange or green
Brussels sprouts
courgettes or marrow (zucchini)
pumpkin
winter squashes
large mushrooms
turnips and/or swedes
aubergines (eggplant)

Peel the onion and cut into halves or quarters. Shallots do not need to be peeled, just bake them in their skins.

Cut the peppers into quarters, remove seeds.

Wash and clean the Brussels sprouts.

Peel and cut into large chunks courgettes, marrow and pumpkin.

Remove the seeds from the pumpkin and the marrow. Rub courgettes and marrow with salt.

Peel and slice winter squash, remove the seeds.

Peel the turnips and cut like potato chips/fries.

Cut the aubergine into chunks and rub with salt.

Rub very generous amounts of any animal fat on the vegetables, place them on a baking tray and bake at 180°C (355°F) for 20–40 minutes or until a sharp knife goes through easily. If there is a little gravy under the fat, adding it will give the vegetables extra good flavour. Serve with meat or fish.

8. BAKING AT HOME

In the GAPS Diet we can use nuts, oily seeds and cooked beans for making bread, cakes, muffins, pancakes, waffles and various deserts. The following nuts are allowed on the diet: almonds, walnuts, Brazil nuts, pecans, hazelnuts, pine nuts, cashews and coconuts. Strictly speaking peanuts are not nuts but legumes. However, they can also be used. Oily seeds: pumpkin, sunflower and sesame seed are allowed. We grind any of these nuts or seeds into flour consistency to replace flour made from grains. But, before we can use these new 'flours', we must prepare the nuts, seeds and legumes properly.

All nuts, legumes and grains are seeds. Plants equip their seeds with special chemicals, called antinutrients, to allow them to survive the journey through an animal's digestive system. If an animal consumes the seed whole without damaging it, the seed will travel through unchanged and land on the ground in its own perfect fertiliser (animal manure or bird droppings). This step is an important way for many trees, grasses and herbs to propagate and to spread to new territories. So, natural seeds are largely indigestible. If an animal chewed the seed before swallowing, the antinutrients would affect its digestive system negatively and, if absorbed, cause damage to the body. The human gut is particularly badly equipped to digest seeds and their many antinutrients: enzyme inhibitors, lectins, phytates, oxalates, salicylates and other. For thousands of years people in traditional cultures have realised this fact through experience, and developed ways of preparing seeds prior to eating them in order to destroy antinutrients and make seeds more digestible. These methods are soaking, sprouting and fermentation. Here I will give a summary of various techniques. These techniques are also described in detail in *The Complete Cooking Techniques for the GAPS Diet* by Monica Corrado, which I warmly recommend.

Mother Nature put nuts into shells to protect them from oxidation, light, moulds and other damaging influences. So, it is best to buy whole nuts in their shells. The second best is to buy them shelled, but whole, not broken into pieces or ground into flour. Walnuts and pecans cannot be shelled without breaking the nut into pieces, so it is best to buy these nuts in their shells and crack them at home. Nuts contain unsaturated fats which oxidise fairly quickly, making the nut smell and taste rancid. Walnuts, Brazil nuts and macadamia are particularly vulnerable to oxidation and should be bought in their shells. Cracking them at home just before using is the best way to consume these nuts. Pine nuts also go rancid quickly, however it is too laborious to shell them at home, so we can buy them shelled, but make sure to buy them as fresh as possible.

Almonds and hazelnuts are more resistant to oxidation and can be purchased shelled, as long as they are left whole and not broken into pieces. Cashew nuts are poisonous in their raw state and are processed using heat before being sold. So, all cashews available to buy are precooked and don't require a lot of processing at home. It is important to soak cashew nuts for 1–3 hours (maximum 6 hours), after which they can be used for baking or making deserts. If you buy almond flour or flour made from any other nut, make sure that it is fresh and was kept frozen. Unfortunately, many such flours are already oxidised to a degree, so it is best to avoid them. I do not recommend commercially available coconut flour: it is too harsh on the gut and there is no industry standard on how it is made. Coconut flour is easy to make at home and it is more digestible. Just buy natural desiccated coconut (shredded coconut) and grind it in a food processor.

The best flour to use for GAPS baking and deserts is made from fresh nuts, shelled at home. After shelling there are two ways of preparing them before using them in a recipe:

1. Grind nuts into flour (particularly if they are broken into pieces, such as walnuts and pecans). Add half cup of whey, kefir or yogurt, mix and add some water to make a porridge-like consistency. Make sure that the mixture is not dry on the top, because we are using lactic-acid fermentation, which is anaerobic. Cover with a cloth and ferment this mixture for 5–7 days. Mix it daily and add a little more water to keep the top covered, if necessary.
2. If the nuts are whole, such as almonds or hazelnuts, you can soak them and sprout. Soak for 12–24 hours, then rinse the nuts, drain and leave in a glass jar covered with a cloth. It is a good idea to remove the fibrous brown skins from the nuts after soaking, particularly for sensitive people. Keep rinsing the nuts every day. In a few days little shoots will appear at the growing point of the nut. After sprouting, grind the nuts into a paste consistency and use in your recipe. Sprouting may not be enough to make these nuts digestible, so after grinding them you may want to ferment them for a few days (as above).

If you would like to have some dry nuts for snacking, remove shells and then soak, sprout or ferment them. Drain and dry in a dehydrator or on the lowest setting in your oven. If you live in a sunny warm climate, you may be able to dry them in the sun outside.

Shelled sunflower seeds can be used with great effect for GAPS baking. It is important to soak them in water overnight, drain and then sprout for 1–3 days (until little shoots grow from them). At that point they can be ground into a paste and used for baking straight away (please, see some recipes in this chapter). Sprouted sunflower seeds can also be added to salads and other dishes, they are easy to digest, have a crunchy texture and taste beautiful. Shelled pumpkin seeds can be difficult to sprout, it is easier to ferment them. Grind them into flour and mix with some warm water, adding some whey, kefir or yogurt. Leave the mixture to ferment for a few days, then use for baking.

Nut or seed butter can be purchased in shops, often made out of hazelnuts, almonds, peanuts, other nuts and sesame seed (tahini). Just as with commercial nut flours, the seeds may not have been properly prepared before being ground into butter (though some companies do this nowadays). Rancidity can also be a problem with these products. Some people can tolerate them well, but for more sensitive people it is best to make nut or seed butter at home. The nuts or seeds need to be soaked in water, then sprouted or fermented and pulverised into butter, using a food processor.

Peanuts, white navy beans, lima beans and lentils are legumes and can be used for baking. They must be bought raw and unprocessed. To make them digestible, particularly for a GAPS person, they need to be properly prepared at home using soaking, sprouting and/or fermentation. After being fermented, beans and lentils should be cooked and then they can be used for baking instead of flour.

To prepare beans and other legumes, soak them in water for 12–24 hours, drain, rinse well in cold water and drain again. Cover the beans with boiling water to break their tough skins, cool down and then add a cup of your homemade whey, kefir or yogurt. Make sure that the beans are completely submerged in the water. Leave to ferment for 4–6 days at room temperature. Drain and rinse well. Bring a large pot of water to boil and add the beans, bring up to boil again, reduce heat and let them simmer for as long as it takes for the beans to become really soft. It may take a different time for different beans, from 30 minutes (in the case of some lentils) to a few hours. When the beans are really soft, drain the water and cool them down. Now they can be ground into a paste and used in recipes for baking. It is convenient to prepare a large batch of beans in advance this way, and then freeze them in small bags for future use.

With all legumes we must keep in mind that, even after proper preparation, many GAPS people still cannot digest them. If your digestive symptoms return after trying legumes, you may have to avoid them for another year or more before trying them again. For sensitive people, if you really want to try beans, please have a look at the recipe for *double-fermented beans* (p. 242).

Cocoa (chocolate, cacao bean and cacao powder) are not allowed on the GAPS Diet. Chocolate is much loved all over the world and some people introduce it successfully later on in the programme, when digestive symptoms have disappeared. Make sure that your patient's body is ready for this indulgence, as cocoa contains many substances which are irritating for the gut and which can upset the balance of blood sugar levels and neurotransmitters in the brain (causing migraine headaches, unstable mood and behaviour abnormalities). It may be necessary to ferment cocoa powder prior to using it in your recipes. In order to do that, mix cocoa powder with the nut flour (nuts which you have ground into flour consistency) and a cup of whey, kefir or yogurt. Add some water to make a porridge-like consistency and leave to ferment for a week before using in your recipe. Stir it once a day and make sure that it is covered with a little water (the surface of the mixture must not get dry), as this fermentation is anaerobic.

Humanity is addicted to bread! This addiction has two components: physical and psychological. By making your bread from nuts and oily seeds (instead of wheat flour or any other flour from grains), you remove the physical component of being addicted to processed carbohydrates and gluten. However, the psychological component remains: the comfortable feeling of cutting a loaf, smearing something on it, making toast or a sandwich and taking a bite. It is easy, quick and lazy. It is unconscious: done automatically without thinking about what you are eating and what your body needs to nourish itself properly. The majority of people acquire this habit in early childhood. Beware of this addiction! Observe people around you: bread constitutes a large part of everything they eat on a daily basis. Instead of making a bowl of soup, or cooking some eggs with bacon, or meat with vegetables, it is too easy just to cut a slice of bread. Substituting the GAPS-compliant bread for ordinary bread can maintain this addiction and bring your disease back in no time at all. To recover from a chronic illness and maintain good health afterwards involves overcoming addictions, particularly addiction to bread! It is important to focus on changing your eating habits completely, which involves eating GAPS bread only occasionally as a treat, and not relying on it as a daily substitute for proper meals.

Baked goods and deserts are a nice addition to the diet. However, the person's gut must be ready for these foods! Even properly prepared, seeds and nuts can be difficult to digest and can bring back symptoms which you have worked hard to remove. So, I recommend not rushing the introduction of these foods. We must also keep in mind that overindulging in nuts can unbalance the immune system, leading to activation of resident viruses (which are normal inhabitants of our bodies). Cocoa (chocolate, cacao beans) is also very powerful in this sense. The first indication of this imbalance is activation of papilloma virus, leading to the appearance of new itchy warts on your body (particularly in warm sweaty places, such as armpits and skin folds). The next step may be activation of herpes viruses, causing cold sores on the lips or elsewhere. If any of these symptoms appear, stop consuming nuts and seeds for a while and focus on rich soups and stews instead, to rebalance your immune system and allow it to take resident viruses under control.

The basic bread/cake/muffin recipe

2 cups properly prepared nuts, sunflower seeds or pumpkin seeds, ground into paste
¼ cup softened butter (or coconut oil, goose fat, duck fat or any other animal fat, homemade yogurt or sour cream)
3–6 eggs (depending on consistency of the nut paste)

How to prepare nuts for this recipe.
You can use your favourite type of nut or a mixture of nuts. You can add pumpkin seeds to the mixture of nuts. Cover the nuts with water and leave overnight to soak. Cashew nuts are an exception: they should not be soaked longer than 6 hours, preferably 1–3 hours.

In the morning drain the nuts and do one of the following: ferment the nuts as they are or grind into a paste and then ferment. Cover the nuts or the paste with warm water and add 1 teaspoon of whey, kefir or yogurt. Leave to ferment at room temperature for 1–6 days. Watch for mould developing on the top; if you see any signs of it, then the nuts have fermented long enough. Drain and use in the recipe.

If you are using whole almonds, you may want to sprout them a little before fermenting. Sprouting is easy: after soaking almonds overnight, drain them and leave in a glass jar in a light place to sprout. Make sure they stay moist, so rinse them once or twice a day. Two to three days are usually enough for tiny shoots to appear. To make almonds more digestible, it is a good idea to remove their brown skins after sprouting. At that point you can grind the almonds into a paste and use in your recipe. If you would like to make them even more digestible, cover the paste with warm water, a little kefir or yogurt and ferment for 2–3 days.

Blend all the ingredients in a food processor. You may want to add more or less nut paste and eggs to reach porridge-like consistency. Grease your baking pan with butter or ghee, line it with greased baking paper and put the mixture into it. Bake in the oven at 170°C (338°F) for 40–60 minutes. Check occasionally with a dry clean knife. If the knife comes out dry, then the bread is ready.

To make variations of this bread you can add some salt, pepper, dried herbs, tomato purée, grated cheddar cheese (if well tolerated), dried fruit, fresh or frozen berries, chunks of cooking apple, grated carrot or pumpkin, chunks of pumpkin (without the skin and seeds). If you want to sweeten the mixture, add a cup of dried fruit (dates, apricots, raisins, figs) and/or 2 ripe bananas. If the dried fruit is too hard for blending, soak it in water for a few hours to soften or bring up to the boil in a little water.

Improvise to make your own variations. You can bake this mixture as a bread, or cake, or in small paper cups as muffins, or make a pizza base. It really is very easy and manageable, even for the most inexperienced cooks.

Sunflower bread

1 cup organic shelled sunflower seeds
1 teaspoon salt
4-8 eggs

Cover sunflower seeds with water and soak overnight. In the morning, drain and leave to sprout in a glass jar in a light place. Make sure that the seeds stay moist, so rinse them once or twice a day. In 2–4 days little shoots will grow. At this point blend the seeds with salt and eggs in a food processor into a thick porridge-like consistency. Taste the salt and adjust to your preference. Bake in a bread tin lined with greased baking paper at 170°C (338°F) for 40–60 minutes. Check occasionally with a dry clean knife. If the knife comes out dry, then the bread is ready.

Pizza

Make a pastry following the previous recipe and adding some salt. Spread it on a baking tray covered with greased baking paper in a layer about 2 cm (¾ in) thick. Bake in the oven for about 30 minutes. Check with a dry knife to see if it is ready.

Cool down. Spread tomato purée on the top and sprinkle with salt.

On top of the tomato purée you can put your choice of filling: slices of red/yellow/green pepper, mushrooms, pieces of cooked meat or sausages, slices of tomato, chopped greens, anchovies, fish, prawns and pineapple, etc.

Put grated hard cheese (cheddar and/or parmesan) on top of your filling, if your patient is at the stage when he or she can tolerate cheese. If cheese is not tolerated, you can use homemade mayonnaise instead. Bake or grill for a few minutes to melt the cheese.

Desserts

It is beyond the purpose of this book to give you a large choice of recipes. You will find just a few suggestions here. There are a number of beautifully written recipe books with a large choice of GAPS recipes, which you will find in *Resources* on my website www.gaps.me.

Baked apples

large cooking apples
2–3 pitted dates per apple
1–2 tablespoons butter, ghee or any other animal fat per apple
a pinch of ground cinnamon per apple; other spices can be added: cardamom, allspice, nutmeg and star anise

With a sharp knife scoop out the core with the seeds, leaving the bottom of the apple intact.

To make the stuffing, soak the dates in a little hot water for 20 minutes to soften them. Blend the dates (together with the soaking water) in a food processor with the fat and cinnamon (and other spices, if desired).

Fill each apple with the stuffing. Bake in the oven at 160–180°C (320–360°F) for 20–25 minutes, or until the apples are soft (a knife goes through easily).

Crème caramel

For one person you need:
1 egg
3 tablespoons water
1 teaspoon honey
ground cinnamon

Multiply the ingredients per number of people you want to serve.

Mix all the ingredients well. Pour into shallow greased ramekin dishes (or any other small terracotta dishes): you need one ramekin dish per person. Sprinkle some cinnamon on top. Preheat the oven to 150°C (300°F). Bake for 30–40 minutes. It helps to stand the ramekin dishes in some water, if baking at higher temperature.

Apple, carrot and apricot pie

4 large cooking apples
2 eggs

carrot pulp from juicing 1 kg (2¼ lb) of carrots, or 500 g (18 oz) carrots, grated
10 dried apricots
½ cup pitted dates, soaked in some hot water
½ cup unsalted butter, ghee, tallow or another animal fat

Cut the apples into pieces and place on the bottom of your baking dish (you don't need to use baking paper). Chop dried apricots into small pieces and sprinkle over the apples. Add the soaking water from the dates.

In a food processor blend together eggs, butter, carrot pulp and dates. Spread the mixture over the apricots and apples and mix slightly. Bake in the oven at 160°C (320°F) for approximately 40 minutes.

Apple, pumpkin and blackcurrant pie

4 large cooking apples
a handful of raisins
1 cup fresh or frozen blackcurrants
2–3 cups fresh pumpkin, peeled and finely chopped
1–2 cups pitted dried dates
1 cup properly prepared nuts or seeds
2-6 eggs

Soak the dates in a cup of water for 2–3 hours or overnight. Drain the dates and put the soaking water into your baking dish. Add cored and sliced apples, pumpkin pieces, raisins and blackcurrants.

In a food processor blend the dates, eggs and properly prepared nuts. Adjust the number of eggs to make the mixture into a porridge-like consistency. Spoon this on top of the pie, spreading evenly. Bake at 150–170°C (300–350°F) for an hour.

Winter squash cake

6 eggs
2 cups grated (packed tightly) winter squash with sweet orange flesh (buttercup, butternut or other)
½ cup pitted dates, soaked in some hot water
1/3 cup butter (or ghee, coconut fat, goose fat, duck fat or any other animal fat)
3 cups properly prepared almonds
3 medium-size apples

Grease your baking dish and cover the bottom with apples, cored and cut into slices. If your patient's digestive system is sensitive, then peel the apples. Otherwise you can leave the skins on.

Blend the rest of the ingredients in your blender and put the mixture on top of the apples. Smooth the top and bake at 150-170°C (300-340°F) for 40-50 minutes.

Russian custard

for one person:
2 egg yolks
½–1 teaspoon honey
multiply the ingredients for the number of people to be served

Russian custard can be used instead of cream on fruit, or you can serve it on its own. You can sprinkle some sprouted sunflower seeds on top or pieces of fruit. It can also be used instead of cream in making cakes. Separate the egg yolks from the whites, add the honey and whip the mixture until thick and quite pale. As well as being a delicious desert, it provides very good nutrition. Buy your eggs from a source you trust. Free-range, soya-free organic eggs are the best.

Apple sauce or purée

5–6 large cooking apples
½ cup butter, ghee, coconut oil, goose fat, duck fat or any other animal fat
1–2 cups water
honey to sweeten

Peel and core the apples, cut them into pieces and cook in a pan with the water until soft. Take off the heat and add butter or any other fat. Cool down, mash and sweeten with honey to your taste.

You can make pear sauce the same way, though you may not need to add honey, as pears are naturally very sweet.

This sauce will keep well in the refrigerator and can be served with some yogurt, sprouted and chopped sunflower seeds or almonds, Russian custard or on its own.

Banana ice cream

Buy some very ripe bananas (with brown spots on the skin), peel them and put in the freezer. When you want to make the ice cream, get the frozen bananas out and leave out for about 30 minutes to slightly defrost.

Blend in a food processor. Add a little bit of water to make a good creamy consistency. You can blend some fresh or frozen berries, pieces of fruit, desiccated or fresh coconut into the mixture, plus some coarsely chopped nuts (properly prepared and dried) to make different flavours.

Dairy ice cream

You can start making this ice cream when homemade sour cream has been introduced into the diet. Mix ½ l (17 fl oz) of homemade sour cream with honey to taste. Separate 6 egg yolks from the whites and whip them separately until the whites are stiff and the yolks are pale yellow and thick. Mix the cream with the whipped yolks and add any fruit, berries, nuts or seeds (properly prepared), and spices of your choice. Mix well, then gently fold in the whipped egg whites. Put into a plastic container and freeze immediately.

Fresh coconut

When you are buying a coconut, make sure that the shell has no cracks or any other damage. Hold the nut close to your ear and shake it. If the coconut is healthy, you will hear its juice splashing inside. When a coconut is damaged and its juice has leaked out, it will be rancid and unsuitable to eat.

When you bring your coconut home, the fun bit starts. You will need a screwdriver and a hammer. At the top of the coconut there are three round dots. Push your screwdriver through two of those dots to make two holes. Drain the juice through one of the holes allowing air to get inside through the other hole. The juice is very nourishing and can be used in cooking or drunk as it is. It should have a fresh sweet taste. If the juice tastes rancid, then there is no point in cracking your coconut, as it will be unsuitable to eat. After draining the juice, crack the shell with the hammer and separate the pulp from the shell. Rinse the pulp with the water to wash off any small bits of shell. There are a number of ways to eat it:

- Cut the pulp into small pieces and eat it as it is. It has a very pleasant sweet taste.
- Grind it in your food processor to make sweets (see next recipe).
- Put the pulp through your juicer to produce a thick coconut cream, which can be diluted with water to make a delicious coconut milk. The cream and milk can be added to your cooking, used as a dressing for fruit and vegetable salads, as a cream for cakes or a replacement for custard.

- Mince the coconut pulp to use in your baking, homemade ice cream and other desserts, soups, stews, salads and sauces.

A word of caution for children and adults with diarrhoea. Coconut is very fibrous and may make the diarrhoea worse, so initially I suggest putting the coconut through a juicer, which will separate the fibre from the rest of it. This way you can enjoy the freshly made coconut milk and cream, getting all the good nutrition from them without the fibre.

Coconut sweets

1 medium-size coconut
1 cup dried fruit (any of the following: apricots, figs, dates or raisins, or a mixture). Make sure they are not sorbated or coated in starch.
1 cup desiccated coconut

Soak the dried fruit for 6–8 hours. Drain.

Make two holes in the coconut and drain the liquid. Put the liquid through a fine sieve and reserve for the recipe.

Shell the coconut and rinse the pulp to wash away small bits of shell. Cut the coconut pulp into pieces small enough to put through your grinder or juicer.

Grind the coconut pulp with the dried fruit. Mix well in your food processor or by hand. If the mixture is too dry, add some liquid from the coconut.

With your hands, roll small balls from the mixture and coat them in desiccated coconut. Place on a large plate and refrigerate or freeze.

9. EGG-FREE RECIPES

Eggs are used in baking as a binder to keep all the other ingredients together. Some people have a true allergy to eggs and have to avoid them. The following ingredients will act as a binder in your baking instead of eggs.

- Pumpkin, baked and mashed;
- Butternut squash and other winter squashes (acorn, turban, hubbard, spaghetti), baked and mashed;
- Banana, mashed;
- Apple, baked and mashed or made into an apple sauce;
- Pear, baked and mashed or made into a sauce;

- Marrow or courgettes (zucchini), baked, mashed and drained of excess liquid;
- Gelatine, well dissolved in a small amount of hot water.

Egg-free bread/cake/muffin mixture

2 cups properly prepared nuts (almonds, cashews, walnuts, hazels, etc.)
3 tablespoons butter (or coconut oil, ghee, goose fat, duck fat or another animal fat)
2 cups cooked and mashed squash (butternut, pumpkin or other less watery squashes, apple sauce, pear sauce)

Winter squashes can be very hard to cut. To minimise the labour, you can bake the squash whole or cut it into halves, remove the seeds, place on a baking tray with the cut surface down and bake in the oven until very soft (a knife should go through it very easily). Cool, scoop out all the inside (or remove the skin) and mash with a fork.

You can improvise on this recipe by adding dried fruit, coarsely chopped nuts (properly prepared and dried), shredded coconut, berries and fruit pieces.

Mix all the ingredients well. Put into a well-greased baking dish and bake in the oven at 150–175°C (300–350°F) for 45–60 minutes. Occasionally, use a dry knife to check if it is ready. If it is, the knife will come out dry.

If you add 2 tablespoons of pure tomato purée (with a single ingredient: tomato) and some salt and pepper to the same mixture, you can bake a pizza base. Just spread the mixture on baking paper, shaping it with a spoon. Experiment with your own versions, using ingredients available to you from the allowed list.

10. BEVERAGES

Nut/seed milk

You can use almonds, sunflower seeds, sesame seeds, pine nuts or a mixture to make milk. Almonds make the best milk. You can add a teaspoon of flaxseeds to make the milk thicker. Soak the nuts or seeds in water for 12–24 hours and drain. Blend with water in a food processor (for 1 cup of nuts/seeds add 2–3 cups of water). A good juicer will crush the nuts/seeds to make a paste, which you blend with water. Mix well and strain through cheesecloth or a fine strainer and you have milk. You can add some soaked dates or raisins when blending to make the milk sweet.

If you find that the milk is too rich, just add more water. You can add some freshly pressed apple juice or carrot juice to it to make a very tasty and nourishing drink.

Coconut milk

Bring to the boil 1 cup of unsweetened shredded coconut and 1 cup of water. Cool down and blend well in the food processor. Strain through cheesecloth or a fine strainer.

Ginger tea

1 tablespoon ginger root, freshly grated
some boiling water

Put the grated ginger root in your teapot and add boiling water. Cover and brew for 5 minutes. Pour through a sieve. It is a warming drink and aids digestion.

Freshly squeezed juices

Use only organic fruit and vegetables for making juices. Wash your fruit and vegetables and cut off any bad bits. Do not peel and do not remove seeds.

The most therapeutic juices do not taste very nice: green and vegetable juices. To make your juices tasty and enjoyable to drink I recommend making mixes of different fruit and vegetables. You can make all sorts of juice mixes, but generally try to have:

- 50% of highly therapeutic ingredients: carrot, small amount of beetroot (no more than 5% of the juice mixture), celery, white and red cabbage, lettuce, greens (spinach, parsley, dill, basil, fresh nettle leaves, beet tops and carrot tops).
- 50% of some tasty ingredients to disguise the taste of therapeutic ingredients: pineapple, apple, orange, grapefruit, grapes, mango, etc.

Your patient can have these juices as they are or diluted with some water. Initially start with a third of a cup of juice a day. With a small child or a very sensitive adult you may want to start with a very small amount, like 1 teaspoon a day. Increase the daily amount very gradually until your patient has 2 cups of freshly squeezed juices a day. These juices should be taken on an empty stomach, so first thing in the morning and the middle of the afternoon are good times.

With these juices you can make ice lollies (popsicles). Just fill ice lolly forms with freshly squeezed juice and freeze.

You can also make ice cubes from these juices, which can be used to make a cold drink in hot weather. Just fill the glass with these ice cubes and add mineral water (still or carbonated).

The carrot pulp left from juicing can be used in your baking mixtures, together with ground nuts or as a replacement for ground nuts. You can also use pulp left from other fruit and vegetables depending on your taste preferences.

For many people it is best to introduce juices in the form of GAPS shakes, which we talked about in the chapter *Liver and Lungs*.

GAPS shake recipe: Make a juice from 1 carrot + 2–3 apples (or an equal amount of pineapple) + 1 stick of celery + a small wedge of beetroot + a small piece of white or red cabbage. You can also add a little lemon and some greens. To this juice add 1–2 raw eggs (the yolk and the white) and 4–5 tablespoons of homemade raw sour cream. If sour cream has not been introduced yet, add a similar amount of raw butter or ghee, softened at room temperature, or raw coconut oil. You can also try any animal fat, such as tallow, pork fat, lamb fat, goose fat; olive oil can also be used. Blend in a blender or whisk with a handheld tool. This 'shake' is delicious and will provide you with wonderful raw nutrients, including raw fat and cholesterol. You can add your cod liver oil to this smoothie: it will disguise its taste very effectively. Start from a small amount of GAPS shakes, such as 1–2 tablespoons per day (1–2 teaspoons for a child). When one glass is well tolerated, gradually increase to 2 glasses per day, between meals. Drink slowly, 'chewing' every mouthful. The shakes need to be taken on an empty stomach, so first thing in the morning and the middle of the afternoon are good times. GAPS shakes have an ability to slowly remove bile stones and pancreatic stones and improve digestion of fats and other nutrients. The eggs and sour cream in the GAPS shake balance the natural sugars from the fruit and vegetables, making these juices more physiological, particularly for people with poor blood sugar control.

Fruit smoothies

Fruit smoothies are easy to make once you have freshly pressed juices. You can make all sorts of combinations. Blending in ripe avocado can turn any juice into a smoothie. Adding homemade sour cream, yogurt and kefir will increase the fat and protein content of the smoothie. If you would like to make it sweeter, you can add a ripe banana or some honey.

Vegetarianism

Look deep into Nature, and then you will understand everything better.

Albert Einstein

It is generally not wise for a GAPS person to choose a plant-based lifestyle. However, every human being is unique and requires a unique set of nutrients to thrive. There are people whose constitution demands more carbohydrates in their diet to feel well, and only plants can provide those carbohydrates. Let us try to understand this issue in more detail.

I have seen many disastrous situations when misguided vegetarianism has been the cause of mental illness and chronic degenerative diseases in people. Some of these cases I have described in my book *Vegetarianism Explained. Making an Informed Decision.*[1] Please, read this book to get a full understanding of what a plant-based lifestyle means for human health and the health of our beautiful planet.

Mother Nature took billions of years to design our bodies, while at the same time designing all the foods suitable for our bodies to use. Nature has provided us with two groups of food: *plant foods* (grains, legumes, nuts, vegetables, fruit, herbs, etc) and *animal foods* (meat, fish, eggs and dairy). These two groups work differently in the human body and it is important to consume both. Human beings are omnivores: we have evolved on this planet eating everything we could find in our immediate environment from both plant and animal kingdoms. Let us have a look at these two groups of natural foods in more detail.

All energy on our planet gets recycled, while new energy comes from the sun. In order to capture the energy of the sun and convert it into solid matter Mother Nature has designed plants. They use photosynthesis to convert the sunlight into chlorophyll, building plant matter.[2]

Herbivorous animals get energy from the sun by eating plant matter. In order for herbivorous animals to digest plants and extract nutrients Mother Nature has equipped them with a very special long digestive system, called rumen. It contains several stomachs full of special plant-breaking microbes. So, it is not the cow (or any other herbivorous animal) that digests the grass, but the microbes in her rumen.[3,4]

Predators and omnivores get energy from the sun in the form of herbivorous animals. Wolves, lions, tigers, foxes and other predators cannot digest plant matter, because they are equipped with a very different digestive system.[5]

The human digestive system is similar to the gut of predatory animals. Just like predators we have only one small stomach with virtually no microbes in it. Our human stomach is designed to produce hydrochloric acid and pepsin, which are only able to break down meat, fish, milk and eggs effectively.[6,7] After these foods have been digested in the stomach, they move down into the intestine where pancreatic juices and bile are added to the mix to complete the digestive process and where the nutrients get absorbed. Our digestive systems have been designed to extract the best nutrition for us from animal foods! People have known this for millennia. That is why all traditional cultures have always put a lot of effort into hunting, fishing and keeping domestic animals.[8]

What about plants?

There is a lot of research, published in popular nutrition books, which shows that plants are full of nourishment. Yes, when we analyse different plant foods in a laboratory, they show good amounts of vitamins, proteins, fats and minerals. This information is then published in popular nutritional literature and causes confusion. Why? Because in a laboratory we can use all sorts of methods and chemicals for extracting nutrients from plants: methods which our human digestive system does not possess. Throughout human history people learned through experience that plant foods are hard for them to digest; in their raw state plants are pretty much indigestible for the human gut.[6,8] That is why all traditional cultures have developed methods of preparing plants to extract more nutrition from them and make them more digestible – fermentation, malting, sprouting and cooking.[9] Unfortunately, in our modern world, many of these methods have been forgotten and replaced with recipes which suit the food industry's commercial agenda.

If we cook and prepare plant foods properly, can't we live on them? I am afraid the answer is a big 'No'! The human body (without water) is largely made out of protein and fat (almost half and half).[6] These are the 'bricks and mortar' from which your bones, muscles, brain, heart, lungs, liver and all other organs are made. Laboratory analysis of plants and animal foods shows that the best protein and fat for human anatomy and physiology comes from animal foods. The amino acid profile of animal protein is correct for the human body, while the amino acid profile of plant-derived proteins is incomplete and unsuitable for human physiology.[10,11] The same with fat: animal fat has the right fatty acid composition for the human body to thrive on, while plant oils are less suitable.[10–12] So, when it comes to FEEDING your body and BUILDING your body tissues and structures, animal foods are the best and the only truly suitable ones.

The human body has a wonderful process, which goes on from the moment of conception until death, called *Cell Regeneration.*[7] Cells in your body (in all your organs and tissues) constantly get old, die and are replaced by newly born cells. In this way the body maintains itself, rejuvenates itself and heals any damage. In order for your body to give birth to trillions of baby cells and replace the old ones, building materials are needed – proteins and fats. The best building materials to feed your cell regeneration process come from animal foods: meats, fish, eggs and dairy.[11] Growing children need large amounts of building materials for their bodies, not only for cell regeneration but for growth, so animal foods must be a very important part of their diet. Apart from food, animal products provide the body with energy; it is a biochemical fact that the preferred source of energy for most cells in your body is fat.[11,12,13]

One of the hungriest organs in the human body is the brain: it 'sponges up' a large percentage of all nutrition floating in your blood. Your body spends a lot of effort on feeding the brain 24 hours a day, every day.[7,12] Contrary to popular beliefs, there is much more your brain needs than just energy in the form of glucose! It is a physical organ and its cell regeneration processes require feeding with good quality protein and fat. On top of that, your brain manufactures neurotransmitters, hormones, enzymes and hundreds of other active molecules, which are largely proteins; the brain needs building materials to make them. Again, the best building materials to feed your brain come from animal foods.[7,13] The brain is a very fatty organ and its tissues are rich in cholesterol.[12] It requires a lot of good quality fat and cholesterol to be fed properly and to maintain its physical structure. The human body manufactures cholesterol, but food can also be very important in supplying this essential-to-life substance to support our bodies.[12,13] There is no cholesterol in plants; it can only come from animal foods. In clinical practice we see degeneration of the brain function in people on a purely plant-based (vegan) regimen: first the sense of humour goes and the person becomes 'black-and-white' in their thinking and behaviour, personality changes, the sharpness of the mind and cognitive ability reduce, memory suffers, depression sets in and other mental problems often follow. These are all the signs of a starving brain! The longer the person stays on the purely plant-based diet the more they are unable to perceive what is happening to them. Despite obvious signs of malnutrition, which are clearly visible to people around them (anaemia, poor stamina, digestive problems, lack or absence of libido, muscle loss, low thyroid function and other health problems), the person is often convinced that they are perfectly healthy.

The success of the No-Plant GAPS Diet is a clinical demonstration that human beings can live entirely on animal foods, without eating plants at all. On this variation of the GAPS Diet people live on meats, including organ meats, animal fats, meat stock and bone broth, fish (including shellfish and molluscs), fish stock, fresh eggs and fermented raw dairy – kefir, sour cream, ghee, butter, cheese and yogurt. We have looked at the No-Plant GAPS Diet in the previous chapter. In severe cases of ulcerative colitis and Crohn's disease, FPIES, severe mental illness and other serious disorders this is the only diet that allows people to be well, to stop all medication, to reach their normal body weight, to remove all digestive symptoms and to function to their full capacity. In some cases of bipolar disorder, schizophrenia and other psychiatric conditions this diet can be a saviour. Some of these people have lived on this diet for several years and have no desire to change their eating habits, because this diet works for them. Some of them have tried to add a little vegetable or fruit to their regimen and found that their symptoms started returning, so they had to stop. This clinical experience demonstrates that human beings can live very healthily without plant foods at all. However, we cannot live without animal foods! The physical degeneration that long-term vegans go through is clear demonstration of that.

But what about all the plant-based diets shown to help with chronic disease?[14–19] Why are cold-pressed good quality plant oils shown to be beneficial for degenerative conditions? Supplementing these oils is promoted by both mainstream and alternative medical communities. What about antioxidants, enzymes, vitamins, minerals, bioflavonoids and other substances in plants, which are shown to be beneficial to health? Not a month passes without our science discovering that broccoli has anti-cancer properties, cabbage has substances which heal the digestive system, nuts boost immunity, etc., etc.[14–18] Here we come to the real purpose of eating plants: they are largely CLEANSERS. While they are unable to sustain the physical structure of our bodies to any serious degree, they are wonderful at keeping us clean on the inside. Plants do provide energy for the body to use in the form of glucose and co-factors in the form of vitamins and minerals, but their main purpose is to keep your body clean and free of toxins! Indeed, plants are equipped with powerful detoxifying substances, which can remove various man-made chemicals, pollution and other toxins we accumulate in our bodies. Plants are particularly powerful cleansers when consumed raw.[19] Their juices absorb in the upper parts of the digestive system contributing a plethora of detoxifying substances and co-factors; juicing of raw greens, vegetables and fruit is a major part of many healing protocols, including the GAPS Nutritional Protocol.

When plant matter moves further down the gut it feeds the gut flora in the bowel.[20] The human bowel is an equivalent of the rumen of herbivorous animals; it has a rich population of microbes, which can convert some plant fibre and starch into useful nutrients for the human body, such as short-chain fatty acids. However, the problem with fibre and starch is that they feed equally the 'bad' and the 'good' microbes. If your bowel flora is healthy, the fibre and starch will do you good. If it is unhealthy, the plant matter will feed the pathogens in your gut, which will flourish, produce toxins and do a lot of damage. GAPS people have abnormal gut flora, so that is why we have to remove starch and fibre for a long enough period to alter their gut flora and heal the gut wall.

When we cook plants we reduce their cleansing ability, but make them more digestible, so they provide some building materials for the body to use. Unfortunately, these materials cannot build the body to any great degree, as they are largely carbohydrates, which the body can use for producing energy. Any surplus is stored as fat. When plants are severely processed (grains in particular), they provide the wrong building materials for the body, causing disease. Consumption of products made out of flour, vegetable oils and sugar, including high-fructose corn syrup and other plant-derived sweeteners, is a major cause of most degenerative health problems in our modern world: weight gain, diabetes, obesity, heart disease, cancer, Alzheimer's disease, psychological and neurological problems in children and adults, infertility, hormonal problems, immune abnormalities, etc.[13,21]

A cleaner body always feels better than a toxic one. That is why some people feel well on a plant-based diet in the first few weeks of it. One can read some glowing testimonies in vegan and vegetarian books to that effect. But, when the body has finished cleansing, it will indicate that you need to start feeding it with animal foods. This signal comes in the form of a strong desire for a piece of meat, a pot of cream, bacon, roast chicken or another animal food. Unfortunately, many vegans and vegetarians choose this lifestyle for emotional, religious and political reasons. They do not listen to their bodies and override its signals, forcing it to continue cleansing when it needs feeding. At that point the body starts starving and deteriorating.

Veganism is a plant-only regimen, when the person does not eat anything from the animal kingdom. This regimen does not feed the body properly but provides it with a lot of cleansing. While your digestive system is busy processing plant matter (so you don't feel hungry), the diet will provide your body with large amounts of cleansing substances. The ultimately toxic people are cancer victims; they require a lot of cleansing.[19] That is why some nutritional cancer treatment protocols are vegan. Veganism is not a diet; it is a form of fasting. One cannot fast forever, so veganism is only suitable for a period of cleansing. It must never be chosen as a permanent lifestyle! When your body has finished cleansing it will need feeding, and that is when you have to introduce animal foods. If that is not done the body starves and starts cannibalising itself, breaking down muscle and bone to feed more important organs (the heart, the brain, the liver, etc). As a result, health problems start developing.

When visiting India I met some Hindu pilgrims travelling to their sacred religious sites. Part of their pilgrimage is a 41-day fast, which they described as 'very difficult'. During this fast they are not allowed to eat any animal foods at all and live entirely on plants – vegetables, fruit, rice, lentils, nuts and beans, vegetable oils and bread – precisely the Western vegan 'diet'. So, when talking about a purely plant-based regimen the word 'diet' should not be used, instead such a regimen should be called a *Vegan Fast*.

One function that is usually lost on a long-term *vegan fast* is reproduction. A man can effectively turn himself into a eunuch by following this regimen and a woman can lose her menstrual function and ability to conceive.[22,23] In order to be able to produce children we need sex hormones, and these hormones are manufactured by the body from cholesterol. Cholesterol comes only from animal foods.[23] Your body can manufacture cholesterol, but many other nutrients we get from animal foods are needed to produce cholesterol and sex hormones (animal protein, fats, zinc, fat-soluble vitamins, B-vitamins and other). Sex hormones are produced not only in our sex glands but in some other tissues in the body.[13,24] While physical castration only removes the sex glands, the vegan fast deprives all the sex hormone-producing cells in the body of building materials to produce these hormones. Not only fertility, but often even an interest in the opposite sex disappears: the majority of long-term vegans have no partners and do not create happy families. This fact has been exploited for centuries by religious orders that do not allow nuns and monks to have contact with the opposite sex.[22] Sexual energy was a problem and they needed a way to reduce it. Through experimentation they discovered that a vegan regimen did this job very well.

Vegetarian diets which include some animal foods can be adopted as a long-term strategy. It is possible to be a healthy vegetarian as long as you continue eating some animal foods, such as eggs and full-fat dairy, to provide feeding/building substances for your body. Obviously, all processed foods must be removed, the diet needs to be natural and a lot of fermented foods must be consumed. Such vegetarian cultures exist in India. People there understand just how valuable animal foods are for them. That is why the cow is considered to be a sacred animal – she provides milk, butter, cheese and ghee. Apart from cows, people in India keep goats and value their milk very much. Vegetarians in India also keep chickens and ducks and consume plenty of fresh eggs; and many consume meat and fish when they can get it. Traditional vegetarianism in

India was born out of necessity, because of poor availability of animal food while plants grew there in abundance. Western political veganism arrived in India about a hundred years ago and took root in some places, bringing confusion in its wake. Fortunately, not many Indians took to it.[26,27]

There are many forms of traditional vegetarianism: some eat fish, some eat eggs and dairy, some allow occasional consumption of meat. People who get into trouble are those who decide to stop eating meat and live largely on processed foods. They become ill very quickly. This group of people is particularly prone to diabetes, obesity, heart disease and cancer.[22,28] Another group of people who get into trouble are those who follow low-fat vegetarianism. Human beings cannot live without fats! Mother Nature took billions of years to design our foods and everything she put into them is essential, including fat.[24,30] Every component in a natural food is balanced with all other components, they work as a whole. To remove fat from a natural food is to make it incomplete and unbalanced; the human body cannot thrive on such 'food'. Low-fat vegetarianism typically leads to degenerative diseases of the nervous system and immunity.[29,30]

Traditional vegetarianism exists only in hot climates of the world, because in hot weather the body has to do more cleansing and requires less feeding/building nutrients. The colder the climate, the more people rely on animal foods and the higher the content of fat must be in the food, because animal protein and fat are essential for us to survive cold temperatures and to thrive in them.[30,31] If people from hot climates, whose predecessors have evolved on a vegetarian diet, move to a place with a cold climate, they have to eat more animal foods to feel well. And vice versa, people from colder climates, when on holiday in a tropical country, don't feel like eating a lot of animal foods and prefer to eat more fruit and raw salads. So, the weather has a strong influence on what our bodies need. But, apart from the weather, there are many other parameters which determine our nutritional needs on a daily basis. Every human being is unique and requires different proportions of feeding foods and cleansing foods every day. Please, read the chapter *One Man's Meat Is Another Man's Poison* to understand the subject of bio-individuality and how to determine what is right for you.

Let us summarise

There are two groups of natural foods on the planet and each of them has its own role to play in the human physiology.

Animal foods – meat, fish, eggs and dairy – are largely building/feeding foods. They feed the cell regeneration in the body, allowing the body to maintain its normal physical structure and chemical composition. In other words, animal foods provide the 'bricks and mortar' your body is made from. On the GAPS Nutritional Protocol we work hard on healing and sealing the gut wall, restoring the immune function and rebuilding the whole body. Your body cannot 'save' sick cells; it can only discard them and replace them with newly born healthy cells. Cell regeneration in the gut wall and the immune system is some of the most active in the body. In order to give birth to trillions of new healthy gut and immune cells your body needs building materials, and animal foods will provide them in abundance. A GAPS person's body is often made out of poor-quality building materials, which are heavily polluted and damaged by man-made toxins. Going through the GAPS Nutritional Protocol you are practically building your body anew, so you have to provide ample amounts of high-quality building materials for your body to use. Meat stock, soups, organ meats, gelatinous meats, fish stock (made with skins, bones and heads of fresh fish), fresh eggs, fermented dairy and plenty of animal fat will allow your body to rebuild itself from quality building materials, to create a strong and robust structure – a beautiful healthy body for you to live in.

Plant foods – grains, beans, fruit, vegetables, herbs, nuts and seeds – are largely cleansing/detoxifying foods, and in their natural state do not feed the body to any serious degree. Instead they keep the body clean on the inside by helping it to remove toxins and wastes (and parasites associated with these toxins). They provide energy for the body in the form of glucose. They provide some micro-elements for the body to use: minerals, vitamins, phytonutrients and co-factors. However, plants are hard to digest, particularly for a GAPS person! We have to be very careful what plants we eat, how we cook and prepare them, and in what order we introduce them into the diet. Indigestible fibre and starch in plants will feed pathogenic microbes in the gut and challenge already damaged gut wall in a GAPS person. Plants contain many antinutrients (lectins, gluten and other plant proteins, phenols, salicylates, phytates and other) which can damage the human body quite seriously, even in a person without digestive problems, let alone in a GAPS person. So, vegetarianism is not suitable for this group of people! More than that, for the most severe end of the GAPS spectrum we have to go through a No-Plant GAPS Diet (no plant foods are consumed at all!) to allow the gut wall and the rest of the body to start healing itself. Then we move into the GAPS Introduction Diet to allow more healing to happen, and to introduce plants carefully step by step, starting from the easiest ones to digest and slowly introducing more difficult ones. We cook and ferment plants carefully to make them more digestible. During the GAPS Introduction Diet and on the Full

GAPS Diet we start using freshly pressed juices, which we make at home from organic vegetables, greens and fruit. This is when we utilise plants' cleansing ability in order to assist the body in removing toxins, while protecting the gut from fibre, as juicing removes most of the fibre.

Of course, the division of animal and plant foods into building and cleansing is not black and white. Animal foods, particularly raw, have a considerable cleansing ability, while cooked and fermented plants will provide some feeding for the body. The skill is in when and how we use them to heal and restore our bodies to full health. Every human being is unique, so you have to find your own unique proportions of animal foods to plants. Humanity is wonderfully diverse in its metabolism and nutritional needs! Some people eat very few plants and thrive largely on animal foods. Other people need to eat much less animal food and thrive on more plant matter. If your predecessors come from a vegetarian culture and you feel that you need more carbohydrates in your diet, please look at the More-Plant GAPS Diet to find your individual proportions of animal foods to plants. But, before you find those proportions, you may have to work on healing your gut wall first with the GAPS Introduction Diet.

Many people in our modern world choose vegetarianism for ethical reason, believing that they are 'saving the Planet' through their choice. It is beyond the scope of this book to focus on this question; please read my book *Vegetarianism Explained* to understand all the commercially driven misinformation about a plant-based lifestyle and what the reality is for our planet.

One man's meat is another man's poison!

A man should look for what is, and not for what he thinks should be.

Albert Einstein

We are all different; every one of us is a unique individual. Not only do we look different on the outside, but just as equally we have different metabolisms, biochemistry and even some anatomy on the inside. So, 'one size fits all' never works! That is why we have such a bewildering number of diets being proposed: high carbohydrate/low carbohydrate, high fat/low fat, high protein/low protein, all raw/all cooked, etc., etc. And the interesting thing is, that every diet suits some people and does not suit others. Why is that? Because 'it takes two to tango', which means that there is no such thing as a 'bad' diet per se or a 'good' diet per se without taking into account a very important factor: *who* is eating! And not only who is eating, but also what state that person is in.

Let us try and understand this in more detail.

We all have a different heredity and constitution. If your predecessors were Vikings or Eskimos, then chances are that you will generally need to eat lots of oily fish, red meat, full-fat dairy and animal fat.[1] But if your predecessors came from a Mediterranean culture or some tropical area of the world, then you will probably need more carbohydrates in your diet.[1] In traditional cultures, through centuries of experience, people understood this: the ancient Chinese and Ayurvedic medicines tried to classify different constitutional types of people and would not dream of applying diet or herbs without this knowledge, as different constitutional types need very different approaches.[2,3] A food, that makes one person healthy and well, can make another person ill. An herb, which works miracles with one person, can be useless with another or even have negative effects. Every human being has hereditary bio-individuality and reacts in a unique way to food, herbs, supplements and other influences.

In the Western world the concept of bio-individuality has been developing slowly over the last hundred years, starting from the work of a remarkable American dentist Weston A. Price, who at the beginning of the 20th century travelled all over the world studying indigenous cultures. In those days such cultures still existed on our planet; people who lived the way their predecessors had lived for millennia and whose lifestyles had not yet been changed by the modern industrial civilisation. Weston

A. Price found that all these isolated cultures were very healthy; they did not suffer from any of the diseases which plagued European, American and other Western populations.[1] Most importantly, he discovered that every indigenous culture ate a different diet, dictated to them by their immediate environment. People, who lived in hot environments generally consumed plenty of plant matter (grains, starchy vegetables, fruit and legumes) supplemented by local animal foods (meat, fish, eggs and dairy), while people who lived in cold environments thrived on oily fish, high-fat dairy and fatty meats and ate much less plant matter. Each one of these isolated tribes of people was unique; they evolved in harmony with their unique immediate environment, climate, availability of food and activity. They could be viewed as distinctive genetic lines, where generations of people thrived on the same diet and lifestyle.

Almost a century has passed since that research was done and things have changed. Today most of the indigenous tribes, studied by Weston A. Price, have adopted modern industrialised foods and all the diseases which come with them. Most importantly, it is almost impossible to find any distinctive genetic lines anymore; the world has become a melting pot of genetics as people move, travel and mix. Most families in our modern world can now boast a number of different genetic lines amongst their predecessors from Europe, Asia, Africa, Americas and elsewhere. Every one of those genetic lines brings its own small piece of bio-individuality, making you absolutely unique in your metabolic needs and the foods that will serve these needs properly. Even in brothers and sisters, genetics can mingle and play in very different ways. This concept was confirmed by a renowned American biochemist Roger Williams, who in 1956 wrote a book called *Biochemical Individuality*.[4] His research established that every human being is biochemically unique and has unique nutritional needs; if these needs are not satisfied by the right food the person will develop disease. He proposed that, in order to prevent and treat diseases, human beings need to be divided into 'metabolic profiles'. In the following years work on this 'profiling' was started by Dr Wiliam Donald Kelly.[5] Based on the research into the autonomic nervous system done by Dr Francis Pottenger and Royal Lee in the 1930s and 1940s, Dr Kelly developed a complex protocol of classifying people into 'sympathetic dominant' or 'parasympathetic dominant' with very specific nutritional recommendations for each group. His work was continued and expanded by his colleague, a clinical researcher William Walcott, who added to Dr Kelly's observations discoveries of other scientists, such as George Watson's research on cellular oxidation and Emanuel Revici's research on catabolic/anabolic balance. Having taken into account all the information available, William Wolcott came up with a concept of *metabolic typing*, described in detail in the book *The Metabolic Typing Diet*, published in 2000.[6] There is no doubt that this concept is incomplete; new researchers will add more pieces to this puzzle as time goes by. But let us have a look at the current understanding.

According to William Wolcott people are divided into three metabolic types: the Protein Type, the Carbo Type and the Mixed Type.

Protein Type people are described as having a strong appetite, they need to eat regular meals. They love salty and fatty foods. They have low tolerance of sugar and carbohydrates; these foods are highly addictive for this group of people and cause sugar cravings and dependency. Alcohol is also very addictive for this group of people and, together with sugar and processed carbohydrates, can cause obesity, diabetes, heart disease and other manifestations of metabolic syndrome. If not eating correctly, this group of people can have unstable energy levels, from hyperactive to lethargic, which can come with mood swings. They generally do not feel well in hot weather and do best living in colder climates.

Protein Type people are advised to eat dense animal protein rich in purines: organ meats (liver in particular), red meats, oily fish with darker flesh, shellfish, high-fat dairy and eggs. They need to eat plenty of animal fats and plenty of natural salt. Starch and sugars present a real danger for this group of people; they do well living without grains and starchy vegetables at all, or eating them occasionally. Fruit is not their friend: they can eat some berries in season and occasionally have small amounts of other local fruit in season, but always combined with some fat and protein.

Carbo Type people are characterised by low appetite (sometimes no appetite at all), food doesn't seem to be important to them and they can live on snacks and not eat for long periods of time. They appear to have good tolerance of grains, starch and even processed carbohydrates. They are usually quite lean, but if they abuse refined carbohydrates, they can become overweight and even obese. Their bodies can burn carbohydrates well, providing them with a steady energy supply, though some carbo people can have a limited stamina and use lots of caffeinated drinks and sugar to get them through the day. Generally, they do well living in hotter climates and don't like to be cold.

In the book on metabolic typing the Carbo Type people are recommended to eat more carbohydrates than anything else: whole grains, starchy vegetables and fruit. Their bodies need smaller amounts of protein, largely from low-purine sources, such as breast of chicken or turkey, white fish and some dairy. High-purine meats and fish apparently are difficult for Carbo people to digest and metabolise. Fats also have to be limited for this group of people as they find them difficult to metabolise. They can have small amounts of butter and ghee, but largely are recommended to focus on plant oils, such as coconut oil, olive oil and cold-pressed quality oils from other plants. This group of people can successfully live on a vegetarian diet, as long as some animal proteins are consumed (dairy and eggs, for example). If you identify yourself as a Carbo Type person, please look at the More Plant GAPS Diet.

The 'protein' and the 'carbo' types are two extremes; not many people fit neatly into these groups. The majority of people belong to the *Mixed Type*, which is made up of an endless continuum of variations, some closer to the Protein end, some closer to the Carbo end and some in the middle. This is where metabolic typing can become complicated. It is recommended that you fill in a long online questionnaire to identify your specific ideal ratio of nutrients.[6] A great deal of scientific knowledge has been put into designing this questionnaire but, as with any science, it is never complete and never applies to everyone. Regardless of their metabolic type, it is recommended that everyone starts their new dietary regime from the same procedure, beginning from a GAPS-type diet and then gradually trying to introduce carbohydrates, starting from non-starch vegetables.

There is no doubt that the idea of *metabolic typing* is an important concept in our nutritional science! Knowing your hereditary metabolic type would be empowering and important, particularly for those who have struggled with many diets without full success. However, as with any human sciences, there are problems and limitations. Plenty of people tried to eat according to their 'metabolic type' and still did not find success in healing from their chronic disease. And, for people who are addicted to processed carbohydrates (such as a typical GAPS person), it is easy to be led astray by their addiction into thinking that they belong to the 'carbo type'. There have been other modern attempts at classifying people into metabolic groups, such as ones based on the blood type of the person. Clinical experience shows that all of them have limitations and do not work for everyone.

But the main problem is that Nature is never static! Our body functions constantly adjust to the changes in our internal and external environments, our age, our activity, our moods, our thoughts and an endless list of other variables. Even if you have correctly identified your metabolic type, there is no perfect scientific way of fine-tuning it to adjust to the daily flux and flow, in other words, the normal human life. Let us have a look at just a few parameters which change all the time.

Throughout our lives our bodies go through *anabolic/catabolic cycles*, in other words, cycles of building up and cleansing. There is a daily building/cleansing cycle, a seasonal one and 'as-it-is-necessary' ones which can happen any time. For building itself your body needs very different nutrients from those it uses for cleansing itself (animal foods are generally building, while plant foods are generally cleansing).[7] Only your body knows what it needs at every moment of your life.

Depending on what your body is doing at the time, depending on the season of the year, on the weather and the level of stress you are under, your body can adjust between different ways of *energy production*: using more glucose for example or more fats or more protein.[8] Only your body knows what is appropriate at any particular moment of your existence, and it requires very different nutrients for different patterns of energy production.

We have already mentioned the *autonomic nervous system*, which is responsible for all the 'autopilot' functions of the body: for your heart beating, for your blood circulating, for your digestive system feeding you, etc. The autonomic nervous system is made out of two branches: sympathetic nervous system and parasympathetic nervous system. These two systems generally work in opposition to each other, providing a very complex balance in every function of the body.[9] Again, depending on an infinite number of factors (daily cycle of activity and sleep, season, weather, stress, infection, feeding/cleansing, your occupation at the time and even your emotions) you will shift from being 'sympathetic dominant' to 'parasympathetic dominant'. This shift can happen several times every day, every few days, every season, and it is different in different age groups and sexes.[9] The important thing is that these two branches of our nervous system require very different sets of nutrients: parasympathetic generally likes meat and fat, while sympathetic is thought to need more carbohydrates.[6,10] Only your body knows what proportions of protein/fat/carbohydrate it needs at any given moment of your life; no laboratory or scientist will be able to calculate this for you.

Then there is the *acid/alkaline balance* in the body, which again changes all the time and every day depending on many factors. There is a myth in nutritional circles that 'being acid is bad' and that all of us have to strive to be alkaline all the time. Different foods have been classified as 'alkalising' (such as fruit and vegetables) or 'acidifying' (such as grains and meats).[11] This simply is not true. Your body shifts from alkaline to acid states all the time depending on many factors: activity of your autonomic nervous system, the type of energy production at the time, your hormonal profile at the time, respiration and kidney function. Many of these, in turn, change according to daily cycle, season, weather and your activity.[12] Depending on all those factors, an apple, for example, which is considered to be an 'alkalising' food, can make your body acid, and vice versa, a piece of meat, which is considered to be 'acidifying' can make your body alkaline. Only your body knows how to use foods at any given moment of your life; only your body has the inner intelligence to make these impossibly complex calculations.

As if that is not enough, then there is the *water and electrolyte balance* in the body, which also shifts all the time depending on many factors.

Our mainstream medicine pronounced salt to be harmful and recommends reducing its consumption. Processed salt should not be consumed, just as all processed foods should not be consumed.[12,13] However, natural unprocessed salt from salt mines or the sea contains more than 90 minerals and trace elements. Not only is it good for us, but it is essential for maintaining the right water/electrolyte balance in our bodies. Our internal environment contains all of these minerals and trace elements in similar proportions as the oceans.[12,13] Then there is the myth that we need to drink lots of water every day. Some literature even prescribes different amounts in litres-per-day. Following that advice blindly can get you into a lot of trouble, if your body is low on electrolytes and needs salt instead of water. Next time you find yourself at a tourist destination in a hot climate, try observing groups of tourists. You will notice that many of them have swollen ankles and legs and are carrying a bottle of water. Sweating removes a lot of salt from the body, which can impair kidney function and cause water retention.[8,15] Indigenous tribes who live in hot climates (desert tribes in the Middle East, for example) traditionally limit water consumption and make sure to eat salt on a daily basis.[16] This knowledge somehow got lost in our mainstream nutritional science, which advises everybody to drink lots of water all day, making the salt deficiency even worse. Following this advice many people, when travelling to a place with a hot climate, finish up with oedema, high blood pressure and headaches because of lack of salt and water retention.

No matter how clever we think we are, our science cannot calculate how much salt or water we should consume at any given time: only your body knows that, and it has excellent ways of telling you what it needs – thirst for water, desire for salt or a particular food, which may have the right mineral composition. Make no mistake, your body knows the nutrient composition of foods on this planet!

These are just a few factors to demonstrate to you that no laboratory, no clever doctor or scientist and no clever book can calculate for you what you should be eating at 8 am, or 1 pm, or 6 pm or in between. Only your body has the unsurpassed intelligence to figure out what it needs at any given moment of your life, as your nutritional needs change all the time: every minute, every hour and every day.

So, what do we do? *How do we feed ourselves properly?* The answer is: get back in touch with your body's inner intelligence. Just think: if your body needs so much protein right now + so much fat + so much carbohydrate + so much of certain vitamins and certain minerals, how would it let you know that it needs this particular composition of nutrients? And, even if your body had a way of letting you know all this information, how would you go about providing this mix of nutrients? How are you to calculate all those factors and provide the right amounts? Well, Mother Nature is kind and it is not asking us to do anything so complicated. Instead she gave us senses of SMELL, TASTE, DESIRE for a particular food and a sense of SATISFACTION after eating it. So, when your body needs a particular mix of nutrients, it will give you a desire for a particular food which contains just that right mix; this particular food will smell divine to you and taste wonderful, and you will feel satisfied after eating it. But in an hour or two the needs of your body will change, and that particular food will not be appealing anymore; instead you will have a desire for another food, which nutritionally will serve you correctly for that particular moment of your life.

So, the only way for us to serve our bodies properly with the right food is to be fully in touch with our senses!

Let us think about it a little more.

The DESIRE for a particular food

The word 'desire' has a somewhat negative image for many people, thanks to centuries of religious and political conditioning; desire is considered to be something we have 'to resist' and must not 'succumb to'. Yet, desire for particular food is the main way your body tells you what it needs at any particular moment nutritionally. So, when you get hungry stop and think: 'What would I desire to eat right now? What is the most appealing food for me right now?' Forget about all the books you have read, forget about all the nutritional mantras about what you should eat at a particular time of day, and just ask the question. The answer will come immediately, and just the thought of that particular food will fill your mouth with saliva. Respect your desire! Desire is your inner body intelligence talking to you, letting you know what it needs to keep you healthy, energetic and happy. If you listen to your desire every time you eat, you will be able to digest that food well and it will do you only good, because you have eaten it at the right time, just when your body asked for it.

The trouble is that in our modern commercial world people's desires for food have been manipulated through the use of addictive and taste-altering chemicals in processed foods. Yes, many processed so-called 'foods' contain chemicals specifically designed to make them addictive.[17,18] Listening to your desire only applies to natural foods – foods that Mother Nature has designed. Stop eating processed foods and your normal sense of desire for food will return.

The sense of SMELL

Have you ever observed animals? They will never put anything in their mouths without smelling it thoroughly first. Why? Because wild animals are fully in touch with their instincts – their inner body intelligence. The sense of smell gives your body a lot of information about food: is it safe to eat? Has it been contaminated by chemicals or microbes? Is it fresh and, most importantly, is it appropriate for your bodily needs at that moment? So, before putting anything into your mouth, smell it: if it is the right food for you at that moment, it will smell very appealing. If it is not the right food, it will smell repulsive. Respect your sense of smell and listen to it.

The trouble is that many people in our modern world have a damaged sense of smell due to use of synthetic perfumes. All scented man-made chemicals, such as laundry detergents, domestic cleaning chemicals, so-called air fresheners and perfumes block the olfactory receptors (the smell receptors) in your nose.[19] Your nose has a set number of olfactory receptors, and once they are blocked by a chemical, new molecules of that chemical have nothing to attach to, so you can no longer smell it.[20] We have all met people who smell like a perfume factory, but they do not realise just how excessively they apply their perfume. The same happens with common laundry detergents, which use very powerful perfumes to disguise the unpleasant smell of the detergent itself. People who use detergents regularly are unable to smell them, because they are constantly exposed to this scent on their clothes, towels and bedding. They cannot smell their food properly either, as the smell receptors in the nose are permanently occupied by the laundry detergent. To restore your sense of smell, remove all perfumed chemicals from your environment: replace your laundry detergent with a non-scented natural one and do not use any perfumes, scented personal care products or air 'fresheners'. In a few weeks your olfactory receptors will clean themselves up and your sense of smell will return.

The sense of TASTE

Food is one of the greatest pleasures of life, and so it must be! If the food is not pleasurable, then it is the wrong food for you at that moment no matter how 'healthy' it is supposed to be! So, listen to your sense of taste and respect it! It is your friend, as it is one of the channels of communication between your body's inner intelligence and your conscious mind. How else would your body tell you that it needs a particular mix of nutrients, but by giving you great pleasure from consuming them in the form of food?

The trouble is that many people have an altered or dulled sense of taste due to regular consumption of processed foods. Many processed foods contain taste-altering chemicals, which are deliberately added to the 'food'.[21] These chemicals are not only toxic but can alter your perception of taste for a long time, so it is essential to stop consuming processed foods in order to restore your normal sense of taste. Some nutritional deficiencies can alter the perception of taste too (zinc and protein deficiency are particularly known for this).[22] As you start consuming a natural wholesome diet your nutritional deficiencies will diminish and your sense of taste will return. Toxins in your mouth can also alter your perception of taste.[23] Try to brush your teeth with cold-pressed olive oil (or any other cold-pressed oil) instead of toothpaste: this Ayurvedic procedure has a good record in detoxifying the mouth.[24] Working with a holistic dentist is very important, as many dental materials in the mouth can make it toxic and alter your sense of taste.[25]

The sense of SATISFACTION after eating

If you have eaten a meal appropriate for your body's nutritional needs at the time, you will feel fully satisfied. There will be no cravings for something else, only a nice comfortable feeling of satisfaction, which will allow you to focus on other things in your life and forget about food for a while.

It is important not to overeat, so you don't feel 'stuffed'. If you listen to your senses of pleasure and satisfaction from food, you will stop eating as soon as the food stops being pleasurable. Pleasure on/pleasure off are the signals your body gives you to let you know about its needs. Your sense of pleasure will keep you eating as long as your body still needs the nutrients from that particular food; as soon as your body has had enough of those nutrients, the food will stop giving you pleasure.

Cravings for sweet foods are common amongst GAPS people due to unstable blood sugar levels. It takes time to normalise blood sugar and the most effective way to deal with it is to increase your fat consumption (animal fats, olive oil, coconut oil or other quality plant oils – within your pleasure zone, of course). So, to deal with sugar cravings (and chocolate cravings) consume plenty of fats with your meals. In order to keep your blood sugar at a stable level between meals, I recommend making a mixture of raw butter (or coconut oil) with some raw honey to taste, put it into a glass jar which you can carry with you, and eat a few spoonfuls every 20–30 minutes all day. This measure can be very helpful in the initial stages of the treatment. As your blood sugar regulation normalises through the use of the GAPS Nutritional Protocol, you will gradually be able to reduce and then stop eating butter/honey mixture.

How do we apply this wisdom while on the GAPS diet?

The GAPS Diet is not set in stone; you have to adapt it for your unique body and for its unique daily needs. The GAPS diet gives you the list of foods to work with. **When** you eat these different foods and **in what proportions** is up to you. Listen to your body's needs, communicated to you through the senses of desire, smell, taste and satisfaction. For example, one day you may feel like only an apple for breakfast, but tomorrow you may enjoy a large cooked breakfast made from eggs, bacon, sausages and cooked vegetables. For example, on the first day you were very happy just to drink meat stock and eat some cooked chicken, but next day you do not feel like meat or meat stock at all and are much happier to eat vegetables and yogurt. Your body will let you know what proportions of protein, fat and carbohydrate to have at every meal. How? Through desire for particular foods. So, when you sit down to a family meal, eat only what appeals to *you* at the time, and in the amounts that appeal to you.

It is essential to listen to your body's desires when you are following the GAPS Diet. Your desires will let you know how quickly to move through the stages of the Introduction Diet, how much salt and black pepper to use in preparing your meals and in what proportions meats and vegetables should be consumed from day to day. For example, a person dealing with a lot of stress may need much more salt and fat in their meal than a person whose life is relatively calm. The difference can be quite pronounced: the amount of salt needed in the meat stock to make it enjoyable for the stressed person may make it unpalatable to another person. A 'carbo person' following the GAPS Introduction Diet may want to eat large amounts of cooked vegetables in their meat stock and let someone else eat most of the meat and the fat, while a 'protein person' is happy without vegetables at all (or a small amount) and wants to eat plenty of meat and fat with their meat stock.

It is possible that you would have to eat something not allowed on a particular stage if you *really* desire it, because that is what your body requires at that time, and you have to respect it. You are unique and nobody can prescribe the exact right sequence of food introduction for you. If you are following the first or second stages of the GAPS Introduction Diet to the letter and feel well, but then one day you get a strong desire for, let's say, raw tomatoes (which are not included in the plan), then listen to this desire! This is your body telling you that it needs particular nutrients at this particular time, and raw tomatoes will provide them (particularly, if they have just ripened in your own garden). If you deny your body that need, you may get yourself into trouble: your electrolyte balance may get upset or your hormones may not work well, or something else will not work. Yes, you would have 'cheated' on the diet by eating raw tomatoes, but once that particular need of your body has been satisfied, you can continue with your programme. Any progress goes through two steps forward then one step back, and healing is no exception. So, don't worry about 'cheating' on the diet sometimes if your body has really asked for it. This is not cheating; this is working *with* your body and respecting it. Remember, your body knows infinitely more about itself than we will ever know with all our intelligence and science! This 'cheating', of course, applies only to natural foods and not to processed man-made concoctions.

Remember also that your body's nutritional needs change all the time. So, your desire for foods will also change all the time: what felt wonderfully satisfying for breakfast may not be appealing for lunch, and what was delicious in the afternoon may feel repulsive at dinner time. All these feelings are very valid and should be listened to! You are a unique individual, so what suits one person around the table may not suit you at all. Follow your enjoyment of food and you will not go wrong!

How do we apply this to children on the GAPS Diet?

As parents we have to make decisions for our children. GAPS children have altered senses of smell, taste and desire for foods, and they may have severe cravings and addictions to the very foods that harm them. The cravings and addictions usually are to processed foods. As we start the GAPS Nutritional Protocol, we remove all processed foods, and as a result your child may go through a period of withdrawal with all sorts of symptoms (behavioural and physical). This is important for the parents to understand in order to help the child go through this difficult time: your child's body is stuck in a diseased metabolic state, so it demands particular unhealthy foods to maintain and serve that state. So, unless we want to maintain this diseased metabolic state, we cannot allow the child to have those foods. Shifting the child's body to a healthy metabolic state will take time and effort, and the GAPS Nutritional Programme will do it for you. So, stick to the list of foods allowed on the GAPS Diet. However, within that list try to provide a large enough variety of foods for the child to choose from. It is very important for your child to start using the senses of desire, smell, taste and satisfaction. Your child will need time to learn to use these senses and to discover them in the first place, as in a diseased metabolic state these senses are suppressed and perverted.

It is essential for any child (GAPS or a healthy 'normally' developing child) to develop a healthy relationship with food right from the beginning of their lives. Unfortunately, in the Western world, in many cases that does not happen. It is very upsetting to see some parents working intently on the child's table manners, while not putting any effort into preparing a decent meal for the child (serving a processed microwaved concoction). A combination of poor-quality food and heavy pressure on eating that 'food' with the best table manners can put anybody off food, let alone a small child! In order for the child to develop normal senses in relation to food, the child needs natural homemade healthy foods full of flavour and taste, and the child must be allowed to explore that food on his or her terms. Table manners can come later, when the child has developed natural senses of desire for food, smell, taste and satisfaction from food, which will serve your child very well for the rest of his or her life.

What do we need to do to help the child to connect with their inner intelligence?

Babies and small children spend the first few years of their lives learning about their environment, and food is a major part of this environment.[26] In the first few years of life, starting from the first introduction of solids, children need to develop a positive RELATIONSHIP WITH FOOD. It is extremely important to do this at this stage in their lives, because, if it is missed, then many problems can follow: not only feeding problems, but problems in behaviour, attitude, emotions and even learning![27]

When introducing first foods for your baby, remember that *all the senses of the child must be involved in the process*: touch, sight, smell, taste, etc. Our babies need to touch the food, to feel the temperature and texture of it on their fingers, the aroma and the look of it. Then they need to use the movement receptors in their muscles to transfer the food to their mouth. This must be a voluntary act, coming from the child's own decision. This is very important! Then they need to smell it and taste it. Then chew and swallow. Then their body and stomach will give them feedback on how this food is affecting their insides and their whole organism. This completes the experience! It is a very complex mixture of sensory input that their little brains are facing for the first time, and it is absolutely essential for the normal development of the child. New receptors, connections and centres are formed in the brain of the child during this process that deeply affect their emotional profile, general personality and attitude to life.[27,28]

In order to make this a healthy process *it is essential to let babies and children eat with their hands*! In fact, using cutlery and being too intent on 'keeping things clean' at this stage is harmful for the child's development. This stage is very short, and the time of 'clean' eating with manners will come soon enough. But in the first few years of life being 'messy' is the best thing for your child! By all means give them a spoon and use another spoon to feed them, but the food should be in front of the children, their hands should be in the food, and they should be deeply involved in consuming the food themselves. When the child is being fed by someone else and is not allowed to be fully involved in the process, the child's brain does not develop the way it should, because it receives a limited sensory input.[26–29] It must be a *voluntary* experience for the child, an act they are deeply involved in, for their brains to develop new receptors and wake up new centres. The same food, prepared differently, is a new experience for the child. For example, a soft-boiled egg is very different from an omelette or a fried egg; different preparations of the same food can be perceived differently. So, different recipes need to be explored and the child needs to be introduced to them gradually.

Many people don't realise just what a big part of our lives food is! And, as far as babies are concerned, it is a *huge part* of their introduction to life on this planet and their harmonious development. This developmental stage will affect the way their whole life will unfold, because it shapes their emotional profile and their personality.[27–29] If you invest in this developmental stage at a very early age, the rewards will be great for your children for the rest of their lives! Children who were allowed to develop a healthy relationship with food usually have positive and sunny personalities. Children who were not allowed to touch their food and explore it on their terms have a stifled development. They finish up with a handicapped attitude to the world and an inappropriate relationship with food, often leading to fussy eating habits, eating disorders and health problems[27–29]. Unfortunately, this applies to many older children and adults in the Western world, who were not allowed to develop a proper relationship with food in their early childhood.

To develop a proper relationship with food, for all GAPS people (children and adults alike) I strongly recommend a simple therapeutic measure: eating with your hands as often as possible, particularly in the first year of the treatment. Of course, if you are eating out in a restaurant in front of strangers, use cutlery and maintain your table manners. But, when you are at home and not 'on show', *do not use cutlery but eat everything with your hands*. If you follow this simple advice for long enough, at some point you will realise how much deeper you connect to food, how much better you perceive its effects on your body. Your hands will instinctively lead you to the best pieces of food for *you*. All the work that the food was supposed to have done for your brain development in your early childhood will be slowly happening. You will be reclaiming what you may not have received as a baby! If you are trying to heal a child of any age, it may be best for the whole family to eat with their hands in order for the child not to feel 'the odd one out'. The whole family will benefit from this therapeutic measure, because eating with our hands is far more physiological for humans than using cutlery. Cutlery is a barrier between our inner body intelligence and the food; it does not allow us to receive the full sensory input from the food we eat. If health and healing are important to us, we should not allow this barrier to interfere in the process of developing a proper relationship with food. And without this relationship there can be no full recovery from a chronic illness!

Let me emphasise again, that in order to develop normal senses in relation to food, we need natural healthy foods full of flavour and taste – rich and satisfying. The food must be homemade from fresh natural ingredients!

In conclusion: Mother Nature took billions of years to design the human body; it is an incredibly intelligent creation! As the natural foods on this planet were designed during the same time, your inner body intelligence knows their composition, and knows what foods to choose for particular needs. All we have to do is treat this intelligence with respect. Use your senses to guide you in your decisions: when to eat, what foods to eat and in what combinations. And remember you are unique, so what suits your neighbour may not suit you at all.

Nutritional supplements for GAPS people

Nature designed our bodies to receive nutrition from food, not from pills. The GAPS Diet must be the number one intervention in successful nutritional management of the GAPS child or adult. No pill in the world is going to come close to the effects of the food on your body's condition. When it comes to digestive disorders in particular, and GAP Syndrome is essentially a digestive disorder, we have to be very careful what we introduce into the gut. Why? Because a lot of supplements may irritate an already inflamed and damaged gut lining and interfere with the healing process. We do not want to put a lot of effort into implementing the diet and then spoil the whole process with a pill.

Many GAPS people have recovered from their illnesses just with the diet. However, some supplements can be beneficial and helpful. The supplementation protocol has to be individual and ideally should be worked out by a qualified practitioner. Here we are going to concentrate on the most helpful ones. The majority of people progress very well with the use of the diet and this small list of supplements without adding anything else.

The most helpful supplements for GAPS patients:

1. An effective therapeutic-strength probiotic.
2. Essential fatty acids.
3. Cod liver oil.
4. Digestive enzymes.
5. Vitamin and mineral supplements.

Let us have a good look at each of these supplements.

1. Probiotics

Probiotics are beneficial microbes in the form of a nutritional supplement or fermented food, which can be taken in an attempt to replace or supplement damaged indigenous flora. Whereas antibiotic means 'against life' probiotic means 'pro life' or 'for life'.[1]

The use of probiotic microbes in the form of fermented foods goes back a long time. For thousands of years people fermented milk, fruit and vegetables, beans, fish, meats and cereals. Fermenting food improves its taste, makes it more digestible and preserves it. Today many cultures around the world routinely consume beneficial microbes in fermented foods: sauerkraut – fermented cabbage and other fermented vegetables (Russia, Germany, Eastern Europe and Asia), table olives and salumi (Mediterranean countries), kefir (Russia), mazun (Armenia), kumiss (Russia and Asia), lassi (India), gioddu (Sardinia), yogurt and cheese (all over the world), fermented fish (Korea, Sweden, Japan, Russia), fermented grains (Africa) and fermented soya beans (Asia).[2,3]

At the beginning of the 20th century Ilia Metchnikoff, a Russian scientist, put the subject of probiotics on a scientific basis.[4] Metchnikoff noted that country people in Bulgaria regularly consumed fermented milk products and lived to an unusually great age in good health. He isolated a bacterium, which he called 'Bulgarian bacillus' and used it in his scientific trials. Today this bacterium is known as *Lactobacillus bulgaricus* and is widely used in the production of commercial probiotic supplements and yogurt. Following his discovery, the use of *Lactobacillus bulgaricus* as a health supplement became popular in European countries. When antibiotics came along probiotics were largely forgotten by the Western countries. However, after Metchnikoff's death in 1916 his research was continued in various countries around the world. In Russia, Scandinavia and Japan probiotic bacteria have been in use as a treatment for humans for decades.[1,4] In the West, for most of the 20th century, probiotics were used mainly in farm animal feed and a lot of scientific data has been collected on their health-giving properties for animals. More recently, Western science started researching the use of probiotics for humans and now we see a large number of scientific publications on this subject. The scope of disorders where probiotics have been successfully used as part of treatment is rapidly growing.

Naturally the biggest use of probiotics we have seen is in the treatment of gastro-intestinal disorders:

- viral infections of the digestive tract[5,6]
- necrotising enterocolitis in infants[7]
- intractable paediatric diarrhoea[8]
- pseudomembranous colitis[7-9]
- traveller's diarrhoea[8–13]
- *Clostridium difficile* enterocolitis[10,33]
- *Helicobacter* infection[35–37]
- enteropathogenic *E. coli* infection[9,13]
- inflammatory bowel disorders: Crohn's disease, ulcerative colitis and chronic pouchitis[12]
- irritable bowel syndrome[14,15]
- lactose intolerance [6,9.10,16]

- prevention of colonic cancer in laboratory studies [6,9,10,16]
- infantile colic[18,19]

In many cases, adding probiotics to the treatment regimen not only improved the clinical picture but also cured the condition.

Apart from digestive problems many other health problems have been shown to respond to treatment with probiotics:

- allergies, including food allergy, asthma, eczema, atopy[20–27]
- autism, schizophrenia and other psychiatric conditions[28,29]
- infections of different kinds[30–32]
- hepatitis, liver cirrhosis and biliary disease[34–36]
- meningitis[35,36]
- malignancy[41,42]
- arthritis[43]
- diabetes[38,39]
- obesity[44]
- burns of various degree[35,36]
- perioperative care and intensive care in surgical patients and patients with massive blood loss[34,40]
- autoimmune disorders[17,30]
- endocrine and neurological diseases[35,36]

These are only the conditions about which scientific papers have been published. However, if you talk to any doctor or practitioner with experience in using probiotics, this list becomes much longer.

There are two groups of probiotics on the market:

1. Laboratory-grown species of microbes, where isolated species of various microbes are grown in laboratories under controlled conditions. These species are mixed together to make a probiotic supplement and every microbe is listed on the label. The majority of probiotic supplements on the market are from this category.
2. Wild-fermentation probiotics. These are wild mixtures of microbes grown on a natural medium, then harvested, dried and put into capsules. Often, we cannot even test for all the species of microbes in the mixture, so what is listed on the label is only what we can test for. These probiotics are fairly rare and seem to appear and disappear from the market. Nevertheless, they can be very effective and helpful, sometimes much more therapeutic than laboratory-grown microbes.

So, what microbes can we typically find in commercial probiotics made from laboratory-grown species of microbes?

1. ***Lactobacilli*** This is a large family of bacteria, which produce lactic acid – hence their name. Most commonly known members of this family are *L. acidophilus, L. bulgaricus, L. rhamnosus, L. plantarum, L. salivarius, L. reuteri, L. johnsonii, L. casei* and *L. delbrueskii. Lactobacilli* are normal and essential inhabitants of the human gut, mucous membranes of the mouth, throat, nose and upper respiratory tract, vagina and genital area.[45–47] They are found in large numbers in human breast milk.[48] Babies are born with some of these bacteria already populating their digestive systems. After birth *Lactobacilli* get firmly established in the body of a newborn baby in the first few days and form a complex relationship with the host for the rest of his/her life. By producing lactic acid they maintain an acidic environment (pH 5.5–5.6) on mucous membranes, which suppresses the growth of pathogenic microbes.[45] Apart from lactic acid they produce a plethora of active substances: hydrogen peroxide – a powerful antiseptic; anti-bacterial, antiviral and antifungal agents, which do not allow pathogens to grow. *Lactobacilli* engage the immune system and stimulate activity of neutrophils, macrophages, synthesis of immunoglobulins, alpha and beta interferons, interleukin-1 and tumour necrosis factor.[46] They are involved in orchestrating the cell renewal process in the gut, keeping the gut lining healthy and intact. They are the most numerous inhabitants of the stomach and intestines and are considered to be the main protecting agents in those parts of the digestive system.[45–48] *Lactobacilli* were the first probiotic bacteria to be studied and to be used as a supplement to benefit health. Indeed, *Lactobacilli* are the most common bacteria in commercially available probiotics today.
2. ***Bifidobacteria*** The most commonly known species are *B. bifidum, B. breve, B. longum and B. infantis,* though many other species have been identified. This is a large family of probiotic bacteria, which are most numerous in the human bowel, lower intestines, vagina and genital area.[49] The majority of all bacteria living in the bowel of a healthy baby are *Bifidobacteria.*[48,49] In an adult gut they are about seven times more numerous than *Lactobacilli* and fulfil many useful functions.[49] In addition to producing different antibiotic-like substances which protect the gut from pathogens, engaging the immune system, maintaining gut integrity and health, they act as a source of nourishment for the body. *Bifidobacteria* actively synthesise amino acids, proteins, organic acids, vitamin K2, pantothenic acid, vitamin B1 (thiamine), vitamin B2 (riboflavin), vitamin B3 (niacin), folic acid, vitamin B6 (pyridoxine), vitamin B12 (cobalamin), assist absorption of Ca, iron and vitamin D.[48-52] *Bifidobacteria* are the second most numerous family of bacteria in probiotic supplements available on the market.

3. ***Physiological strains of Escherichia coli* or *E. coli*** *E. coli* is a large family of bacteria. Pathogenic members of this family can cause serious infections.[53] However, physiological strains of *E. coli* are normal and numerous inhabitants of healthy human gut.[54] They normally occupy particular areas of the digestive system: the bowel and lower parts of the intestines and should not be found anywhere else. If they are found in the mouth, stomach or duodenum, that indicates an abnormality in gut ecology – gut dysbiosis.[54] Physiological strains of *E. coli* fulfil a number of beneficial functions in the body: they digest lactose, produce vitamins (vitamin K and group B) and amino acids, produce antibiotic-like substances, called colicins, and have a powerful stimulating influence on local and systemic immunity. They are very active against various pathogenic microbes, including pathogenic members of their own family.[54,55] Indeed, having your gut populated by physiological strains of *E. coli* is the best insurance against succumbing to pathogenic strains of *E. coli*. That is what German physician Alfred Nissle found in 1917 when he was trying to find out why some soldiers in the First World War did not fall prey to typhoid, when most of their comrades were ill. He identified a particular strain of *E. coli* in the stools of these soldiers, which was named the Nissle strain.[56] He grew this bacterium and sealed it in gelatine capsules. After trying this product on himself he started manufacturing it under the name Mutaflor. Mutaflor is still available on the market.[57] Some other physiological strains of *E. coli* have been studied and are used in some commercial probiotic formulas around the world.
4. ***Enterococcus faecium* or *Streptococcus faecalis*** As the name implies, these bacteria, as with many other probiotics, were isolated from human stools. They normally live in the bowel where they control pathogens by producing hydrogen peroxide and reducing pH to 5.5. They break down proteins and ferment carbohydrates. There are a number of clinical studies showing that they are effective in treating various forms of diarrhoea.[58] These bacteria are quite common in probiotic formulas on the market.
5. ***Bacillus subtilis* and other spore-forming bacilli** *Bacillus subtilis* is a soil-based microbe. It was first discovered by German microbiologists during the Second World War, which led to the use of this microorganism in protecting German troops from dysentery and typhoid. After the war *Bacillus subtilis* was extensively studied in Germany, Russia, Italy, Finland, Eastern Europe, China and Vietnam.[59,60] A number of subspecies were identified: *B. licheniformis, B. cereus, B. brevis, B. mesentericus, B. pumilis,* etc., most of which were shown to be therapeutic in animals and then in humans. This led to the development of a range of products with *B. subtilis* for animal use. A number of products with

B. subtilis and its subspecies have been used on humans by doctors in Russia, Germany, Italy, Eastern Europe, Japan, Vietnam and China for decades. In Japan *B. subtilis* has been traditionally used for producing natto – fermented soya product, very rich in vitamins, amino acids and other nutrients.[62] *B. subtilis,* its many subspecies and other spore-forming bacilli can multiply by producing spores – tiny tough seeds resistant to stomach acid, most antibiotics, extreme temperature changes, desiccation, sterilising chemicals and other influences. In their spore form bacilli are preserved and protected, so they can weather severe changes in the environment and last for many years. For a long time we thought that *B. subtilis* comes only from soil, but recent research established that this spore-forming microbe is a normal inhabitant of the human gut flora and the rumen of herbivorous animals.[59] This microbe is highly pleomorphic, which means that it can adapt to changes in the environment by changing its shape, form and functions to the point of being unrecognisable. The beneficial effects of *B. subtilis* on human health have been studied for a while: it has strong immune-stimulating properties and is considered particularly effective with allergies and autoimmune disorders. It produces a whole host of digestive enzymes, antiviral, antifungal, antibacterial and other active substances and is a great waste recycler, keeping our gut clean.[59–61] For decades *B. subtilis* subspecies have been used in industrial waste management because they have a great ability to break down rotting matter and to suppress putrefactive microbes. By clearing out old putrefaction in the gut, spore-forming bacilli may lay the ground for re-establishment of normal gut flora. In my experience, probiotics which contain this group of microbes are some of the most effective probiotics on the market.

6. ***Saccharomyces boulardii and other beneficial fungi*** *S. boulardii* is a fungus first discovered by a French scientist, H. Boulard, in 1920.[63] He observed that people in China treated diarrhoea with an extract from lychee fruit. He found the yeast in this extract, which was named *Saccharomyces boulardii*. Supplementing this yeast has been found to be effective in treating various forms of diarrhoea in children and adults.[63,64] Recently there has been a lot of interest in using *S. boulardii* as an antagonist to a pathogenic yeast – *Candida albicans*. Other beneficial fungi have been discovered since then and now the medical community is exploring the use of larger fungi – mushrooms – in rebalancing the gut flora.[65] They stimulate our immune system, maintain epithelial layers in the gut, produce enzymes, vitamins and amino acids and do many other good jobs for us. Fungi are the basis of every microbial community in Nature, they form the mycelial network/matrix for smaller microbes to live on. Research into probiotic microbes is in its

infancy and so far bacteria have received the most attention. Time will come when fungi will receive better attention and we will discover just how important they are for us.

The most potent probiotics we use in the GAPS Nutritional Protocol come in the form of homemade fermented foods. Please, look in *the chapter What we shall eat and why, with some recipes* for how to make fermented vegetables, dairy products and other fermented foods. By making these foods a regular part of your diet you will be receiving a diverse community of alive and active beneficial microbes at a very low cost. Many people around the world have recovered from chronic illnesses by using homemade fermented foods and never taking commercial probiotics. Some people use both, and there are people who need commercial probiotics because they cannot tolerate fermented foods for different reasons.

Let us have a look at the commercial probiotic supplements. The market offers a wide range of probiotic products from probiotic drinks to powder, tablet and capsule forms. Unfortunately, many of them are not strong enough or do not contain strong enough species of bacteria to be of therapeutic benefit. So, how do we choose a good probiotic?

It always makes sense to work with a qualified practitioner with experience in using probiotics who will help you to choose good quality supplements. If you are trying to choose a probiotic yourself, then there are some general guidelines to follow.

1. A good probiotic should have as many different species of beneficial microbes as possible. A human gut contains uncountable numbers of species of different bacteria, fungi and other microbes. We should try to get as close to that as we can. Different species of probiotic microbes have different strengths and weaknesses. If we have a mixture of them, then we have a better chance of deriving maximum benefit.
2. A mixture of strains from different groups of probiotic bacteria is more beneficial than just one group. For example, many probiotics on the market contain just *Lactobacilli.* A combination of representatives from the three main groups: *Lactobacilli, Bifidobacteria* and spore-forming bacilli usually works best. Addition of beneficial fungi makes the product even more effective.
3. The manufacturer of the probiotic should test every batch for strength and microbial composition and should be prepared to publish the results of testing.
4. A good probiotic should have concentrated amounts of bacteria: at least 8 billion bacterial cells per gram. You need to provide probiotic bacteria in large enough doses to see an improvement. However, probiotic formulas with the highest bacterial count are not always the

best, because probiotics can cause 'die-off' reactions. Let us talk in more detail about it.

A good therapeutic strength probiotic will always produce a so-called **'die-off reaction'**. What is it? As you introduce probiotic bacteria into a digestive system, they start destroying pathogenic bacteria, viruses and fungi. When these pathogens die they release toxins. These are the toxins which give you or your patient their individual symptoms. So, whatever characteristic symptoms the patient has may temporarily get worse. Your patient may also feel more tired than usual, be generally 'off-colour', develop a headache, a skin rash, a backache, a bout of cystitis, emotional instability or sleep problems. It is a temporary reaction and usually lasts from a few days to a few weeks in different individuals. To make this reaction as mild as possible, build the dose of your probiotic slowly. Start with a very small amount. Observe the patient for any 'die-off' symptoms. If there are none, then increase the dose. When you see a reaction, let your patient settle on this dose until the 'die-off' symptoms disappear. Then increase the dose again and let the patient settle on it. In this manner keep on increasing the dose until a therapeutic level is reached. This period of building up the dose can take from a few weeks to a few months in different patients. It is very individual and depends on how much overgrowth of pathogenic microbes the person has in the gut. There is no need to fear the die-off reaction! It is good news: it means that the microbes, which caused your disease, are leaving. So, some die-off symptoms have to be tolerated as part of the treatment, but it is a good idea to control their intensity to make sure that the person does not get debilitated.

The therapeutic dose of probiotic is individual and your health practitioner should be able to help you with that. There are no standard doses for wild fermentation probiotics; we have to follow the manufacturer's recommendations. For laboratory-grown species of microbes we can suggest standard therapeutic doses, which apply to the majority of probiotic supplements on the market. However, there may be probiotics which do not fit this standard, so please check with the manufacturer or your health practitioner.

Here are general guidelines for a probiotic made out of laboratory-grown microbes:

An adult should have around 15–20 billion bacterial cells per day.
An infant up to 12 months of age can have 1–2 billion bacterial cells per day.
A toddler from 1 to 2 years of age can have 2–4 billion bacterial cells per day.

A child from 2 to 4 years of age can handle 4–8 billion bacterial cells per day.
A child from 4 to 10 years of age can have 8–12 billion bacterial cells per day.
From the age of 12 to 16 we can increase the dose to 12–15 billion per day.

Once the patient has reached the therapeutic dose level, it should be maintained for around six months on average. It takes at least this length of time to remove the pathogenic flora and start re-establishing normal gut flora. Adhering to the diet is absolutely essential in this period. If you carry on feeding your pathogens in the gut with sugar and processed carbohydrates, then the probiotic will not have much chance of helping you.

After the therapeutic period is over the dose of the probiotic can be reduced to a maintenance dose level, which the patient has to adhere to for some years. It is important to reduce the dose as gradually as you have been increasing it. Observe any reactions in this period. The maintenance dose is very individual. Usually it is half of the therapeutic dose. In some cases, the patient's maintenance dose is the same as the therapeutic.

Why do we have to carry on taking probiotic microbes? The reason is this: we have been designed by Nature to have these microbes every day with every mouthful of food or drink. We have changed our environment, water and food to such a degree that we are depriving our bodies of these vital microbes. For people who have good, healthy resident gut flora it may not present a big problem. However, for patients with GAP Syndrome it is a big problem. For GAPS people it is particularly vital to consume probiotic microbes every day of their lives, because they do not possess their own. Their gut has been populated by pathogens instead of beneficial microbes, and these pathogens are extremely difficult to drive out. Unfortunately, most supplemental probiotics do not settle or colonise on the gut wall. They do their work in the lumen of the gut and then come out of the system. We have not yet found a way to replace the pathogens on the gut wall with beneficial microbes. So, patients with GAP syndrome need to carry on consuming probiotic microbes indefinitely, and the best way to do it is by consuming homemade fermented foods daily. To maintain the probiotic you do not have to carry on taking commercial preparations. You can supplement your diet with fermented foods in the form of homemade yogurt, kefir, sauerkraut and other homemade fermented foods.

One of the concerns about probiotic bacteria is that many of them do not survive the stomach acid. Patients with GAP Syndrome usually have low stomach acidity, so this is not a big problem for them. But, to make sure that your probiotic survives the stomach acid, the general rule is to take it with food or after food, when most stomach acid is bound to food particles. Some manufacturers put an enteric coating on their probiotic capsules to protect them from stomach acid. I do not support this practice for two reasons. First, the stomach needs probiotic bacteria just as much as any other part of your digestive system. In a stomach with low acidity all sorts of pathogens grow on the stomach walls. We need probiotics to deal with these pathogens. Second, patients with digestive abnormalities are often not able to break down the enteric coating on capsules. These capsules can go in and out almost unchanged without doing any good.

Perhaps not all microbial species in your probiotic will survive the stomach acid. But, an important point to make here is that, even dead, the probiotic microbes will do a lot of good in your gut.[66] Their cell walls contain substances to stimulate immune response, and they will also absorb toxins removing them from the body. Some food manufacturers have picked up on this fact and are adding dead probiotic bacteria into various foods.

In conclusion, probiotic supplementation is absolutely vital for treating any of the GAPS conditions. These microbes should be supplemented in the form of homemade fermented foods first and foremost. Many people do very well just with fermented foods, without adding any commercial probiotics. For other people commercial probiotics have been very helpful in combination with fermented foods. In our modern world the probiotic market has become intensely competitive. Part of this competition is a well-publicised idea in mainstream medicine that 'probiotics don't work'. Clinical experience and thousands of published studies tell us otherwise.

2. Fats: the Good and the Bad

Unthinking respect for authority is the greatest enemy of truth.
Albert Einstein

About half of the dry weight of the human body is fat.[1] Whether you are slim or overweight, a large part of the physical structure of your body is made out of fats, and this physical structure is being constantly renewed. In order for our bodies to maintain their physical structure, let alone renew it, building materials are required, a large percentage of which must be fats. That is why Mother Nature put fats into every food on this planet. A human brain is about 60% fat (dry weight).[1,2] Every membrane of every cell in the human body and every organelle inside those cells is largely made of fats. Many hormones, neurotransmitters and other active substances in the body are made out of fats. Some 70% of our bone marrow is fat; that is where our blood cells, immune cells, bone cells and many other vital cells are born.[1,2] Our internal organs are sitting in their own fat stores, which insulate them, protect them and provide them with energy. Our whole body is wrapped in a blanket of under-skin fat, fulfilling multiple functions for us.[1,2]

There has been a great deal of conflicting information and misinformation about fats in the Western world. In our modern society fats have been pronounced evil, and a food industry has sprung up to produce an abundance of low-fat and no-fat products. Animal fats, including those in meats, butter and eggs, have been blamed for all sorts of ills, so industry again has been quick to provide us with synthetic substitutes, butter replacements and spreads. Generations of people were told that vegetable oils are healthy, so a variety of different vegetable oils have become cooking oils instead of traditionally used pork fat, goose or duck fat, lamb fat, beef fat or clarified butter. What the public has not been told is how all these processed oils and fats are made, what exactly they contain and what effect they have on human health.

Processed fats

Vegetable oils, cooking oils, margarines, butter replacements, spreadable butter, hydrogenated oils, shortenings and all other artificial fats are processed; they are alien to human physiology and must not be consumed by anybody, let alone GAPS patients.[2–8] You can find processed fats and oils in most processed foods: breads and pastries, pre-prepared meals, crisps, snacks, chocolates, ice cream, biscuits, cakes, takeaway meals, condiments, mayonnaise, etc. The basis of most processed fats is vegetable oils, extracted from seeds and plant matter (corn, soya, sunflower seeds, rapeseed, etc.). They are cheap to produce and are very profitable for the food industry.[3] In their natural state these oils have very unstable unsaturated fatty acids, which are easily damaged by heat, oxygen, pressure and light. In the process of extraction very high temperatures, pressure and various chemicals are employed. These change the chemical structure of fragile fatty acids in the natural seeds and plants creating a plethora of unnatural harmful fatty acids.[2,3] The oils are then sold as cooking oils in supermarkets. Due to decades of relentless advertising and propaganda these oils have replaced the natural animal fats which people have used in cooking for millennia.

To make vegetable oils solid and to increase their shelf life they are hydrogenated.[3] Hydrogenation is a process of adding hydrogen molecules to the chemical structure of oils under high pressure at a high temperature in the presence of toxic metals. Remnants of these metals stay in the hydrogenated oils (nickel, aluminium and other). Nickel and aluminium are both toxic metals, adding to the general toxic load which the body has to work hard to get rid of. Toxic metals have been linked to many degenerative conditions, including mental illness, autoimmune illness and other chronic disease.[2,5]

Processing changes the chemical structure of the natural oils, producing a whole host of very harmful fats. Many of these changed fats have not been studied very well yet and so we don't know what havoc they can wreck in the body. But a group called trans fats have received a great deal of attention.[2,6] These are unsaturated fatty acids, beneficial for us in a natural state, whose chemical structure has been changed through processing. Trans fatty acids are very similar in their structure to their natural counterparts, but they are somewhat 'back to front'. Because of their similarity they occupy the place of essential fats in the body while being unable to do their jobs, thus making cells disabled. All organs and tissues in the body get affected. For example, trans fats have great immune-suppressing ability, playing a detrimental role in many different functions of the immune system.[5–8] They have been implicated in diabetes, atherosclerosis, cancer, neurological and psychiatric conditions.[2,4,8] They interfere with pregnancy, normal production of hormones, ability of insulin to respond to glucose and ability of enzymes and other active substances to do their jobs, and they have damaging effects on liver and kidneys.[2,5] A breastfeeding mother will have trans fats in her milk fairly quickly after ingesting a helping of a 'healthy' butter replacement.[2,6] A baby's brain has a high percentage of unsaturated fatty acids.[2] Trans fats can replace them and interfere with the brain development. Trans fats are so harmful that there is simply no safe limit for them established. And yet a packet of crisps (potato chips) will provide you with about 6 grams of trans fats, a snack packet of processed cheese or cheese biscuits will provide 8 grams, a tablespoon of a common margarine will give you 4–6 grams, a portion of French fries, cooked in vegetable oil, will serve you with 8-9 grams.[2–8] It is estimated that an average intake of trans fatty acids in the Western diet can be as high as 50 g (2 oz) a day. Given their ability to impair bodily functions on the most basic biochemical levels, there is no doubt that the role of trans fats in our modern epidemics of degenerative disease is greatly underestimated. Trans fats are only one problem with processed vegetable oils, there are many others, making them some of the unhealthiest substances in food.

I would like to repeat that no processed fats are allowed on the GAPS diet. That means all common cooking and vegetable oils, hydrogenated oils, margarines, spreads, vegetarian fats and shortenings, butter replacements and spreadable butter. In turn this means that all processed foods are out, as processed fats are one of the main ingredients of processed foods.

What fats are good for GAPS patients? First things first!

The most important fats for GAPS patients, which should be consumed daily and which should constitute the bulk of all fat consumption, are animal fats: fats in fresh meats, fats rendered from meats, dairy fats (butter, cream and ghee) and fats in egg yolks.

I almost hear you asking a number of very common questions: What about the 'deadly' saturated fats? Don't they cause heart disease? Aren't animal fats all saturated? These questions are the result of the relentless efforts made by the food industry to fight their competition. What is their competition? The natural fats, of course. There is not much profit to be made from the natural fats, while processed oils and fats bring very good profits. So, it is in the food industry's interest to convince everybody that natural fats are harmful for health, while their processed fats, hydrogenated and cooking oils are good for us. We have been subjected to this propaganda for almost a century now; no wonder that many of us have succumbed to it.

Saturated fats in particular were singled out by the food industry. How did that happen? The late Dr Mary Enig, an international expert in lipid biochemistry, explained: 'In the late 1950s, an American researcher Ancel Keys announced that the heart disease epidemic was being caused by the hydrogenated vegetable fats; previously this same person had introduced the idea that saturated fat was the culprit. The edible oil industry quickly responded to this perceived threat to their products by mounting a public relations campaign to promote the belief that it was only the saturated fatty acid component in the hydrogenated oils that was causing the problem... From that time on, the edible fats and oils industry promoted the twin idea that saturates (namely animal and dairy fats) were troublesome, and polyunsaturates (mainly corn oil and later soybean oil) were health-giving.'[2]

The wealthy food giants spend billions on employing an army of 'scientists' to provide them with 'scientific proof' of their claims. In the meantime, the real science was, and is, providing us with the truth. However, it is the food giants who have the money to advertise their 'science' in all the popular media. Real science is too poor to spend money on that. As a result, the population hears only what the commercial powers want them to hear.

So, what is the truth? What does the real science tell us?

1. Processed fats, hydrogenated fats and cooking vegetable oils cause atherosclerosis, heart disease and cancer.[5,9] This is a fact, proven overwhelmingly by real, honest science.

2. Fresh unprocessed animal fats do not cause heart disease, atherosclerosis and cancer, in fact they prevent them. Our human physiology needs these fats; they are important for us to eat on a daily basis.[9]
3. Saturated fats are heart protective: they lower the Lp(a) in the blood, (Lp(a) is a very harmful substance which initiates atherosclerosis in blood vessels.), reduce calcium deposition in the arteries and are the preferred source of energy for the heart muscle.[10] Saturated fats enhance our immune system, protect us from infections and are essential for the body to be able to utilise the unsaturated omega-3 and omega-6 fatty acids.[9,10] One of the most saturated fats that Nature has provided is coconut oil. It has been shown to be wonderfully healthy and therapeutic in most degenerative conditions.
4. Animal fats contain a variety of different fatty acids, not just saturated ones (M.G. Enig, 2000).[10] Pork fat is 45% monounsaturated, 11% polyunsaturated and 44% saturated. Lamb fat is 38% monounsaturated, 2% polyunsaturated and 58% saturated. Beef fat is 47% monounsaturated, 4% polyunsaturated and 49% saturated. Butter is 30% monounsaturated, 4% polyunsaturated and 52% saturated. This is the natural composition of animal fats and our bodies use every bit, including the saturated part. If you want to understand how important every bit of the animal fat is for us, let us have a look at the composition of human breast milk. The fat portion of the breast milk is 48% saturated, 33% monounsaturated and 16% polyunsaturated.[10] Our babies thrive beautifully on this composition of fats, and the largest part of it is saturated.
5. We need all of the natural fats in natural foods, and saturated and monounsaturated fats need to be the largest part of our fat intake.
6. The simplistic idea that eating fat makes you fat is completely wrong. Consuming processed carbohydrates causes obesity.[11,12] Dietary fats go into the structure of your body: your brain, bones, muscles, immune system, etc. – every cell in the body is made out of fats to a large degree.[13]

These are the facts which honest science has provided. Unfortunately, as already mentioned, most of us do not hear about the discoveries of honest science. Spreading any information in this world costs money. So, the population at large mostly gets information that serves somebody with a fat wallet. In order to get the real, true information on any subject, we have to search for it, rather than relying on the 'news' and 'scientific breakthroughs' unleashed on us by the popular media.

I would like to draw your attention to the fat composition of human breast milk again: it is 48% saturated, 33% monounsaturated and 16% polyunsaturated.[10] Mother Nature does not do anything without good reason! Human breast milk is the best and the only suitable food for a human baby, and there have been historical accounts of its healing powers for adults and the elderly. Human physiology does not fundamentally change as we grow, mature and age; our requirements for a particular fat composition in food stay about the same throughout our lives.[13] The only dietary foods that provide us with this composition of fats are animal products: meats, eggs and dairy; and these are the foods that should provide us with the bulk of all fats we consume.

What about plant oils? All plants contain fats, and these fats have a very different fatty acid composition, they are largely polyunsaturated. Polyunsaturated fatty acids are very fragile, they are easily damaged by heat, light and oxygen.[5,10,13] That is why Mother Nature has locked them up and protected them very well in the complex cellular structure of the plant. When we eat fresh plants in their whole natural state, we get those fatty acids in their natural state, unchanged and beneficial to health. When we extract oils from plant matter in our big factories, we damage fragile polyunsaturated fatty acids and make them harmful to health. But the most important point is this: when we consume whole natural plants, we get their polyunsaturated oils *in small amounts* which are compatible with our human physiology.[10] Our bodies do not need a lot of polyunsaturated fats, the bulk of our fat consumption should be saturated and monounsaturated fatty acids. When we consume factory-made vegetable and cooking oils, we consume their polyunsaturated fatty acids in excess, far too much for healthy human physiology. Consumption of excessive amounts of omega-6 polyunsaturated fatty acids from vegetable and cooking oils is, to a large degree, responsible for our epidemic of inflammatory degenerative conditions, from heart disease, mental illness, various autoimmune problems to cancer.[4–11]

What about cholesterol?

When we talk about animal fats, a question about cholesterol invariably comes up, because everybody has heard about cholesterol 'clogging up your arteries' and 'causing heart disease'. This idea came from **the diet-heart hypothesis**, first proposed in 1953.[9] Since then this hypothesis has been proven to be completely wrong by hundreds of scientific studies. George Mann, eminent American physician and scientist, called the diet-heart hypothesis 'the greatest scientific deception of this century, perhaps of any century'.[9,15] Why? Because while science was still working on proving the hypothesis wrong, the medical, political and scientific establishments fully committed to it. To admit that they were wrong would do too much damage to their reputation, so they are not in a hurry to do that. In the meantime, their closed ranks give complete freedom to the commercial companies to exploit the diet-heart hypothesis to their advantage. Their relentless propaganda through the popular media ensures long life for the faulty diet-heart hypothesis. Please, read about it in detail in my book *Put your heart in your mouth. What really causes heart disease and how to prevent and even reverse it.*[14]

Thanks to the promoters of the diet-heart hypothesis, everybody 'knows' that cholesterol is 'evil' and has to be fought at every turn. If you believe the popular media, you would think that there is simply no level of cholesterol low enough. And, of course, the profession which has been subjected to this propaganda most thoroughly, is the medical profession. Fighting cholesterol has become the modern dogma and religion of the mainstream medicine.

The truth is that we humans cannot live without cholesterol. Let us see why?

Every cell of every organ in our bodies has cholesterol as a part of its structure. Cholesterol is an integral and very important part of our cell membranes; the membranes that make the cell wall and the walls of all organelles inside the cells.[16] And we are not talking about a few molecules of cholesterol here and there. In many cells, almost half of the cell wall is made from cholesterol.[16,17] Different kinds of cells in the body need different amounts of cholesterol, depending on their function and purpose.[17] The human brain is the most cholesterol-rich organ in the body: around 25% of total body cholesterol is in the brain.[18.19] Every cell and every structure in the brain and the rest of our nervous system needs cholesterol, not only to build itself but also to accomplish its many functions. The developing brain and eyes of the foetus and a newborn infant require large amounts of cholesterol.[18,20] If the foetus doesn't get enough cholesterol during development the child may be born with a congenital abnormality called a cyclopean eye.[20] Human breast milk provides a lot of cholesterol.[19] Not only that, mother's milk provides a specific enzyme to allow the baby's digestive tract to absorb almost 100% of that cholesterol, because the developing brain and eyes of an infant require large amounts of it, as do all other organs and systems. Children deprived of enough cholesterol in infancy end up with poor eyesight and brain function.[21,22] Manufacturers of infant formulas are aware of this fact but, following the anti-cholesterol dogma, they produce formulas with virtually no cholesterol in them.

One of the most abundant materials in the brain and the rest of our nervous system is a fatty substance called myelin. Myelin coats every nerve cell and every nerve fibre like an insulating cover around electric wires.[19,21] Apart from insulation, it provides nourishment and protection for every tiny structure in our brain and the rest of the nervous system. Well, about 20% of myelin is cholesterol.[19] If you start interfering with the supply of cholesterol in the body, you put the very structure of the brain and the rest of the nervous system under threat. The synthesis of myelin in the brain is tightly connected with the synthesis of cholesterol.[21] People who start losing their myelin develop a demyelinating disorder, such as multiple sclerosis. GAPS people often test positive for the same antibodies against myelin, as do people with multiple sclerosis. Due to these antibodies both groups of patients have ongoing damage to their myelin in the brain and the rest of the nervous system. In order to rebuild myelin their bodies require a lot of cholesterol. In my clinical experience, foods with high cholesterol and high animal fat content are an essential medicine for people with multiple sclerosis or any other myelin disorder.

One of the most wonderful abilities we humans are blessed with is an ability to remember things – our human memory. How do we form memories? By our brain cells establishing connections with each other, called synapses.[23] The more healthy synapses a person's brain can make, the more mentally able and intelligent that person is. Scientists have discovered that synapse formation is almost entirely dependant on cholesterol, which is produced by the brain cells in a form of apolipoprotein E. Without the presence of this factor we cannot form synapses, and hence we would not be able to learn or remember anything.[24] Memory loss is one of the major side effects of cholesterol-lowering drugs.[25–27] Dr Duane Graveline, MD, former NASA scientist and astronaut, suffered memory loss while taking his 'cholesterol pill'. He managed to save his memory by stopping the pill and eating lots of cholesterol-rich foods. Since then he has described his experience in his book, *Lipitor – Thief of Memory, Statin Drugs and the Misguided War on Cholesterol.*[25] Dietary cholesterol in fresh eggs and other cholesterol-rich foods has been shown in scientific trials to improve memory in the elderly.[26–28] In my clinical experience, any person with memory loss or learning problems needs to have plenty of these foods every single day in order to recover.

Let us see which foods are rich in cholesterol.

1. Animal brains can provide 1–3 grams of cholesterol per 100 g.[29,30] The human brain is not much different in its cholesterol content! Most traditional cultures around the world prized dishes made out of animal brains as a delicacy beneficial to health, particularly mental health.
2. Organ meats are rich in cholesterol. Veal kidney can provide 791mg per 100g while chicken liver can provide 563mg per 100g. Other organ meats – livers and kidneys of other animals, heart, tongue, tripe, pancreas and poultry giblets will all provide good amounts of cholesterol.[26,27,29] Organ meats have always been considered to be health foods and sacred foods in traditional cultures all over the world.[31]

3. Caviar (fish eggs) is the next richest source; it provides 588 mg of cholesterol per 100 g.[29,30]
4. Cod liver oil follows closely with 570 mg of cholesterol per 100 g. There is no doubt that the cholesterol element of cod liver oil plays an important role in all the well-known health benefits of this time-honoured health food.[31]
5. Fresh egg yolk takes the next place, with 424 mg of cholesterol per 100 g.[27–31] I would like to repeat – fresh egg yolk, not chemically mutilated egg powders (which contain chemically mutilated cholesterol)! Practically all animal research on the 'harmful' effects of cholesterol were done by feeding animals chemically mutilated cholesterol, which makes these studies absolutely untrustworthy.[27]
6. Butter provides a good 218 mg of cholesterol per 100 g. We are talking about natural butter, not butter substitutes.[27–31]
7. Fresh coldwater fish and shellfish, such as salmon, sardines, mackerel and shrimps, provide good amounts of cholesterol, ranging from 173 mg to 81 mg per 100 g.[27] The proponents of low-cholesterol diets tell you to replace meats with fish. Obviously, they are not aware of the fact that fish can be almost twice as rich in cholesterol as meats.
8. Lard provides 94 mg of cholesterol per 100 g.[27–31] Other animal fats follow.

These foods help the body by supplying cholesterol, so it does not have to work as hard to produce its own.

What a lot of people don't realise is that most cholesterol in the body does not come from food![26,27] The healthy human body produces cholesterol as it is needed. Cholesterol is such an essential part of our human physiology that the body has very efficient mechanisms to keep blood cholesterol at a necessary level at every moment of your life. When we eat more cholesterol, the body produces less; when we eat less cholesterol, the body produces more.[26] However, cholesterol-lowering drugs are a completely different matter! They interfere with the body's ability to produce cholesterol, and hence they do reduce the amount of cholesterol available for the body to use.[25,26,28] If we do not take cholesterol-lowering drugs, most of us don't have to worry about cholesterol. However, many GAPS patients are different: due to toxicity and nutritional deficiencies their bodies are unable to produce enough cholesterol.[26,32] Research shows that people who are unable to produce enough cholesterol are prone to emotional instability and behavioural problems. Low blood cholesterol has been routinely recorded in criminals who have committed murder and other violent crimes, people with aggressive and violent personalities, people prone to suicide and people with aggressive social behaviour and low self-control.[33–35] The late Oxford professor

David Horrobin, in his criticism of statins (anti-cholesterol pills) has stated: 'reducing cholesterol in the population on a large scale could lead to a general shift to more violent patterns of behaviour. Most of this increased violence would not result in death but in more aggression at work and in the family, more child abuse, more wife-beating and generally more unhappiness.'[33] People whose bodies are unable to produce enough cholesterol do need to have plenty of foods rich in cholesterol in order to provide their organs with this essential-to-life substance.

What else do our bodies need cholesterol for?

After the brain the organs hungriest for cholesterol are our endocrine glands: adrenals and sex glands. They produce steroid hormones. Steroid hormones in the body are made from cholesterol: testosterone, progesterone, pregnenolone, androsterone, estrone, estradiol, corticosterone, aldosterone, cortisol and other.[36,37] These hormones accomplish a myriad of functions in the body, from regulation of our metabolism, energy production, mineral assimilation, brain, muscle and bone formation to behaviour, emotions and reproduction. Lack of cholesterol in the diet or inability to produce cholesterol will lead to problems in all of these vital functions. Infertility is a big problem in the Western world and lack of cholesterol in people's bodies is one of its causes (due to statin prescriptions and low-cholesterol diets).[26,37,38] Our stressful modern lives consume a lot of stress hormones, leading to a condition called 'adrenal exhaustion'. This condition is diagnosed a lot by naturopaths and other health practitioners and is common amongst GAPS patients. There are some herbal preparations on the market for adrenal exhaustion. However, the most important therapeutic measure is to provide your adrenal glands with plenty of dietary cholesterol, so it can manufacture plenty of steroid hormones to deal with stress.[38,39] Infertility and adrenal exhaustion are only two manifestations of the body's inability to manufacture steroid hormones, there are many others.

Cholesterol is essential for our immune system to function properly. Animal experiments and human studies have demonstrated that immune cells rely on cholesterol in fighting infections and repairing themselves after the fight.[40] It has been recorded that people with *high* levels of cholesterol are protected from infections: they are four times less likely to contract AIDS, they rarely get common colds, and they recover from infections more quickly than people with 'normal' or low blood cholesterol.[40–47] On the other side of the spectrum, people with *low* blood cholesterol are prone to various infections, suffer from them longer and are more likely to die from an infection.[40,42] A diet rich in cholesterol has been demonstrated to improve these people's ability to recover from infections. So, any person suffering from an acute or chronic infection needs to eat high-cholesterol foods to recover.[40–47] Cod liver oil, one of the richest sources of cholesterol, has long been prized as one of the best remedies for the immune system.[31] Those familiar with old medical literature will tell you that, until the discovery of antibiotics, a common cure for tuberculosis was a daily mixture of raw egg yolks and fresh cream (rich in cholesterol).[48] Ubiquitous prescriptions of statins (anti-cholesterol medications) in our hospitals are an important cause of our hospital infections! Statins supress patients' immune systems making them susceptible to infections.[40–47]

We have talked about a few functions of cholesterol in the body. But one of the most important functions for GAPS people is the fact that no healing in the body can happen without large amounts of cholesterol![38,39] A GAPS person is trying to heal from a chronic disease. The body needs building materials to create new healthy cells and tissues in order to heal. Cholesterol is one of those building materials.

In conclusion: cholesterol is one of the most essential substances in the body. We cannot live without it, let alone function well. GAPS patients are in particular need of cholesterol; that is why the GAPS diet provides plenty of it.

Essential fatty acids

Our bodies can make many fatty acids. But, according to research, there is a group of fatty acids which our bodies cannot make; we have to get them from food. These are called essential fatty acids and the most researched amongst them are omega-3 and omega-6 fats.[49] We need them in very small amounts and, when we eat natural unprocessed foods, we get plenty of these essential fats. Unfortunately, many people in the modern world live on processed foods and, as a result, don't get enough essential fats in their diets, particularly omega-3, but instead get plenty of harmful trans fats and other chemically mutilated fatty acids. The GAPS Diet provides the right proportions of fatty acids, including the essential fats. However, some GAPS people find it helpful to supplement essential fatty acids at the beginning of the protocol. So, let us have a look at this subject in detail.

There are two essential fatty acids, from which all others are made:

omega-3: Alpha-Linolenic Acid or **LNA** for short and

omega-6: Linoleic Acid or **LA** for short.

The richest sources of LNA (omega-3) are flaxseed oil (linseed oil), hemp oil and some exotic oils from kukui (candlenut) and chia. In smaller amounts this fatty acid is present in walnuts, pumpkin seeds, dark green leafy vegetables, egg yolk, animal fats (particularly from grass-fed and wild animals), raw animal milk and in human breast milk.[49]

The richest sources of LA (omega-6) are evening primrose oil, safflower, sunflower, walnut, hemp oil and pretty much all fresh unprocessed seeds and nuts. In smaller amounts it is found in egg yolks, milk and human breast milk.[49]

LNA and LA are called 'the parent fatty acids'. From these two fatty acids the healthy human body can make other fats.

Omega-3 fats

From LNA (Alpha-Linolenic Acid) two very important omega-3 fatty acids are formed: **EPA** (Eicosapentaenoic Acid) and **DHA** (Docosahexaenoic Acid). EPA and DHA are vital for many functions of the body. They are found in abundance in brain cells, nerve synapses, visual receptors, adrenal and sex glands.[49,50] However, to make them from LNA the body needs a good supply of some nutrients: vitamins C, B3 and B6, magnesium, zinc and some enzymes. Environmental toxins can block conversion of the parent fatty acids into EPA and DHA.[50] GAPS patients are almost routinely deficient in these nutrients and accumulate toxic substances, so their bodies are often unable to convert parent omega-3 (LNA), from flax oil for example, into EPA and DHA. So, just supplementing LNA with flax seed or any other plant oil is not enough for these patients. They need EPA and DHA ready made. The best sources of these two oils are coldwater fish: salmon, sardines, mackerel, trout and eel.[49,50] The GAPS Diet encourages the person to eat plenty of oily fish. The oil from these fish can be found as supplements. Seawater and freshwater algae and phytoplankton are rich in these oils as well; that is where the coldwater fish get their supply of omega-3 fats. Smaller amounts of EPA and DHA are found in seal fat, whale blubber, pike, carp, herring and haddock.[50] Cod liver oil is a good source of DHA and EPA and one of the oldest ways of supplementing these essential fats. But apart from that, it is a good source of natural vitamins A and D and cholesterol.[49] What about just eating fish? Eating fresh oily fish at least twice a week is the best way of getting EPA and DHA for healthy individuals and for many GAPS people. However, for some GAPS children and adults that may not be enough, due to their inability to digest foods properly. Until their digestion improves it can be helpful for them to take supplements of EPA and DHA in the form of cod liver oil and natural fish oils.[51] There are supplements of synthetically made EPA and DHA on the market, which I do not recommend.

Omega-6 fats

LA (Linoleic Acid) is a parent fatty acid for **GLA** (Gamma-Linolenic Acid), **DGLA** (Dihomogamma-Linolenic Acid) and **AA** (Arachidonic Acid). These fatty acids are essential for the structure and function of the brain, the immune system, hormone metabolism, inflammation, blood clotting and many other functions in the body.[50] Omega-6 oils can be very efficiently supplied through regular consumption of nuts (walnuts, hazelnuts, pecans, pine nuts, Brazil nuts, etc.) and oily seeds (sunflower, sesame and pumpkin), particularly when properly prepared. The GAPS Diet provides plenty of these foods, so for the majority of GAPS people taking supplements of these oils may not be necessary. However, some people benefit from them, particularly at the beginning of the programme, so let us discuss them in more detail.

Just as with omega-3 oils, to convert the parent LA into its derivatives GLA, DGLA and AA the body needs magnesium, zinc, vitamins B3, B6, C and other nutrients, which a GAPS person may be deficient in. Many toxins from the environment can block this conversion.[49] So, this conversion may also be a problem for GAPS patients, which means that derivatives have to be supplied as well as the parent LA. The first two derivatives GLA and DGLA are found in evening primrose oil (9%), borage oil (24%), blackcurrant seed oil (18%), hemp oil (2%) and some other oils. The third derivative deserves particular attention as far as the GAPS conditions are concerned – **Arachidonic Acid (AA)**. It is an essential part of every cell membrane in the body and fulfils many vital functions, such cell growth and proliferation, immune functions, detoxification and many other. It is particularly abundant in the brain, liver and muscles.[49,53,54] GAPS patients often have a deficiency in this essential fatty acid. There are enzymes which release AA from cell membranes and in GAPS patients they can be overactive (PLA2, PLC and other) because of ongoing inflammation in their bodies and accumulated toxicity. Due to this factor GAPS patients actively lose AA from their tissues in the body, and so it is vital to keep replenishing this essential fatty acid. Where do we get AA from? AA comes from fresh meat, eggs and dairy products.[49,53,54] You cannot find it anywhere else! The GAPS diet is rich in these foods and provides large amounts of AA, so vital for GAPS patients to have. There are supplements of AA available on the market, but they will never compare favourably to natural foods rich in this essential fatty acid.

All foods on our planet contain fats! All raw plants provide us with omega-3 and omega-6 oils, as well as other omega oils (7, 9, etc) – vegetables, fruit, berries, nuts, oily seeds and other. As long as we eat these plants in their natural raw form, we can get enough essential fatty acids from them. Most animal foods, particularly from pasture-fed animals, also contain these fats.[49] So, for many GAPS people just following the GAPS Diet provides the right proportions of all necessary fats, including essential fatty acids. Please remember, we need essential fatty acids in *tiny* amounts and the bulk of fat consumption should come from animal fats for all of us!

However, a proportion of patients do benefit from supplementing essential fatty acids, particularly at the beginning of the protocol, to undo many years of damage caused by consumption of processed fats. It is estimated that humans should have more omega-3 oils than omega-6 in their diet. The ideal ratio is disputed, as it is probably very individual, but generally it is accepted that 2:1 of omega-3 to omega-6 is the correct ratio in oil blends.[52] A good supplementation protocol should provide not only parent essential oils (LNA and LA) but also their derivatives (EPA, DHA and GLA). That is why it is important to supply not only seed and nut oils, but fish oils as well.

There are good blends of seed/nut oils available on the market, where flax oil is the main source of parent omega-3 LNA and evening primrose oil is the main source of omega-6 LA and GLA. Look for the brands with more omega-3 fatty acids than omega-6. Look for high quality blended oils which have not been refined, deodorised or adulterated in any way.[55] Heat, light and oxygen destroy seed/nut oils very quickly, so they have to be cold extracted, supplied in dark glass bottles and refrigerated at all times. Never use them for cooking. They can be mixed with cold or warm food to give to the GAPS child or adult as supplements.

People who benefit from taking seed/nut oil blends also benefit from supplementing EPA and DHA through good quality cod liver oil and fish oil. These oils are highly perishable and should be refrigerated and protected from light and oxygen.

For people who suffer from epilepsy I do not recommend any oil supplements (plant oils or fish oils) for the first year of treatment at least. Oil supplements have been known to trigger epileptic seizures in a proportion of these patients, and we don't know why. This group of patients need to focus on consuming plenty of animal fats as part of their GAPS Diet. When epileptic seizures have stopped for at least six months or longer, a person who is prone to common colds could consider a supplement of cod liver oil as an immune system support during the cold season. Always start from a tiny dose and gradually build up to avoid any reactions.

To summarise: The majority of GAPS people don't need supplementing with plant or fish oils, as they get them from their diet. However, some GAPS people benefit from supplementing essential fatty acids in small amounts, particularly at the beginning of the treatment.

1. **A good seed/nut oil blend** in approximate ratio of 2:1 of omega-3 to omega-6 fatty acids. Make sure that the oil is high quality, in dark glass and refrigerated. For GAPS adults start with a teaspoon a day and slowly increase to 4–5 tablespoons a day. From the age of 12 months, children should start from a drop per day (with food) and gradually get up to 1–2 teaspoons a day. The dose can be higher for older children. I recommend introducing these oils gradually to avoid any reactions, which are quite possible in individuals with severe fatty acids deficiency.
2. **Cod liver oil**, which will supply EPA, DHA, vitamin A and vitamin D. Please, read the next chapter for more information on cod liver oil.
3. **Fish oil**. Start with a small amount added to your food (not hot) and slowly build the dose to 1–3 teaspoons a day for a child (up to 1 teaspoon for children under the age of 24 months). An adult should start with a small amount and build the dose up to 3–4 teaspoons a day. Fish oil does not provide vitamins A and D, only EPA and DHA. That is why we need to supplement cod liver oil as well as the fish oil.

There are some oils which patients ask about the most, as they contain both omega-3 and omega-6 fats in considerable amounts. These are hemp oil and flax seed oil.

Hemp oil contains both omega-3 and omega-6 fatty acids in the ratio of 1:3. It is too heavy on omega-6 fatty acids to be supplemented on its own.

Flax seed oil is too heavy on omega-3 LNA; it contains four times as much omega-3 as omega-6 fatty acids, and also should not be supplemented on its own.

Cold-pressed olive oil is a time-proven health-giving food, used by Mediterranean cultures for centuries. The long list of benefits include lowered risk of heart diseases, healing and anti-inflammatory effects, stimulation of bile flow, activation of liver enzymes, antioxidant activity, stimulation of pancreatic enzymes, anti-cancer effects, antibacterial and antiviral activity, membrane development, cell formation and cell differentiation. Virgin cold-pressed olive oil has been shown to improve brain cell maturation and function.[56] And yet it doesn't have much in the way of essential fatty acids, which shows us that we need much more than just omega-3 and omega-6 oils (though it does contain more omega-6 than omega-3).[49] It is a rich source of oleic acid (omega-9) – a monounsaturated fatty acid, which has an ability to strengthen the Th1 arm of the immune system. But the most important elements in olive oil are its minor components: beta carotene, vitamin E, chlorophyll, squalene, phytosterols, triterpenic substances, polyphenols and many others. Many health-giving properties of olive oil are probably due to these minor components. However, heat, deodorisation, refining, degumming and other processing destroys and removes these vital substances. That is why it is very important to buy unrefined extra virgin cold-pressed olive oil. 'Virgin' means that the oil has been extracted from whole, undamaged olives without refining. If it does not say 'virgin' on the bottle, then the oil is refined. There is no international standard for cold pressing of oils, so different manufacturers mean different things when they say that their oil is 'cold-pressed'. However, there is a distinct difference in taste between cold-pressed virgin olive oil and plain virgin olive oil, so I recommend buying cold-pressed virgin oil to use on ready served meals and salads. It is not a good idea to cook with it, as the heat will destroy the minor components and change unsaturated fatty acids into harmful trans fatty acids. Cooking should be done with stable fats: ghee (clarified butter), butter, coconut oil, goose and duck fat, pork fat, lamb fat and beef fat, because they do not alter their chemical structure when heated and are beneficial to health.

Coconut oil is a rich source of saturated fats.[49] That is why coconut and products made out of it (coconut oil and butter, coconut milk, coconut cream, etc.) have been out of favour in the West for decades. In more recent times these products have become very popular. About 50% of fatty acids in coconut is lauric acid. Research shows that in the body lauric acid gets converted into a highly potent antiviral, antibacterial and antifungal substance, called monolaurin.[57] Such pathogens as *candida albicans*, *helicobacter pylori*, HIV virus, measles virus, herpes virus, cytomegalovirus, Epstein-Barr virus, influenza and many others are susceptible to monolaurin. Lauric acid is also one of the natural ingredients of human breast milk, protecting the baby from infections.[49] Other fatty acids found in coconut are caprylic and myristic acids, which also have pronounced antiviral, antibacterial and antifungal properties. For example, caprylic acid has been in use as an antifungal, anti-candida supplement for decades in the form of capsules and tablets.

It is a good idea for GAPS patients to have coconut on a regular basis. Coconut can provide a natural source of antifungal, antibacterial and antiviral substances for these patients as well as many other nutritional factors. The question is: in what form?

People in the tropics use coconut in its natural state. The nut and juice inside are very rich in saturated fats, fibre, vitamins, minerals, vitamin E, tocotrienols, carotene and many other micronutrients.[50] Fresh virgin coconut oil, full of flavour, contains many of these useful substances and is used extensively in tropical countries for cooking. It is stable when heated. It is important to make sure to get good quality coconut oil in its natural virgin state, not hydrogenated or processed with solvents or other chemicals.

As usual, the best thing is to follow Nature and have coconut in its natural form. You can get fresh coconuts in most supermarkets. Many companies now produce good quality virgin coconut oil, coconut milk and cream. Dried coconut and coconut flour can also be used for GAPS patients. Make sure that these products are pure, without any additives. You will find some recipes with coconut in the chapter *What we shall eat and why, with some recipes*.

In conclusion

We should consume **natural** fats in their **natural** state. It is processed foods, which contain masses of unnatural adulterated fats, that should be blamed for our modern health problems: the crisps (potato chips) and chips (French fries), margarines and butter replacements, breads and pastries, biscuits (cookies) and cakes, sweets (candy) and chocolates, our TV dinners and other pre-prepared lazy meals, takeaway meals, our cooking oils and spreads, our salad dressings and mayonnaise, our snacks and condiments, etc, etc. Eat fats in the form that Nature provided us with, and you will not go wrong.

The most important fats to consume for GAPS patients are animal fats from pork, goose, lamb, beef, duck, chicken, ghee, butter, etc. These fats have the best physiological profile of fatty acids for the human body and are the most natural fats for us to eat. They should constitute the bulk of all the fats your patient consumes. Apart from eating meats with good fat covering, render these fats at home and use them for all your cooking, baking and frying in generous amounts. You will find instructions on how to render fat in the chapter *What we shall eat and why, with some recipes*.

I would like to emphasise that GAPS children and adults need plenty of natural fats. Let them eat the fat on the meats, the skin on the poultry and the skin on oily fish, pour plenty of cold-pressed virgin olive oil on their served meals and use good quality coconut oil in baking and cooking. For some GAPS people it is helpful to supplement their diet with good quality cod liver oil and fish oil on a daily basis, and with small amounts of good quality blends of cold-pressed nut/seed oils with 2:1 ratio of omega-3:omega-6 fatty acids (LNA, LA, GLA). As well as olive oil, you can use these oils as a dressing on salads and ready served meals.

Contrary to popular beliefs, fat is a preferred source of energy in the human body. Remember, fat is a major structural element of our bodies and getting this element right lays a solid foundation for good health and healing from any disease.

There are some added benefits in supplying your GAPS patient with good amounts of natural unprocessed fats. The more natural fats the GAPS person has with his/her meals the less he/she will crave sweet and processed carbohydrates, which will make it easier to remove these harmful foods from the diet. And, as you remove processed foods from the diet, you will automatically remove the bulk of harmful processed fats and trans fats as well.

A good supply of natural dietary fats has another benefit, important for GAPS patients. It stimulates bile production. Secreting bile is the natural way for the liver to rid itself of toxins. GAPS children and adults are toxic people. The bulk of detoxification in the body happens in the liver. Allowing the liver to drain itself on a regular basis will help the patient to detoxify quicker.

We live in a world of fat phobia, created by commercial interests and funded by them. Fats constitute a large part of our bodily structure and functions. That is why every health problem can be linked to abnormalities in fat consumption: lots of unnatural fats and deficiencies in natural fats. Stick to the natural fats and make sure that your GAPS patient gets plenty of them. You will see the results for yourself!

3. Cod Liver Oil

Cod liver oil has been around for a very long time. For centuries the northern populations of Russia, Scandinavia, Iceland, Scotland, Greenland and Canada have fermented fish livers and guts, and consumed the oil rendered by the fermentation process.[1,2] In the Roman Empire a product called *garam* was produced by fermenting fish livers and fish guts and used as food and medicine. From the 18th century European doctors started to use cod liver oil as medicine, a practice which continued well into the 20th century. Many people of older generations remember how their parents gave them a spoon of this oil every day to keep them strong and healthy. Oil collected from fermenting shark livers is still used as medicine in Tahiti and other islands in the southern hemisphere.[3]

Amongst its health-giving properties cod liver oil provides omega-3 essential fatty acids (DHA and EPA), cholesterol, vitamin A and vitamin D. We have discussed the omega-3 fatty acids and cholesterol in the previous chapter. Let us have a look at vitamins A and D.

Vitamin A

Vitamin A is a fat-soluble vitamin, which exists in many biochemical forms. The fully functional vitamin A is called retinol. Common dietary sources are organ meats, such as liver and kidneys, dairy products, eggs and oily fish. The richest sources are liver oils from marine fish, such as cod, halibut and shark and from marine mammals.[2,4] The most accessible liver oil available to us is cod liver oil.

Cod liver oil contains vitamin A in its natural preformed biochemical shape. Due to digestive problems GAPS children and adults usually cannot absorb or use other forms of vitamin A, commonly found in supplements: retinyl palmitate, retinyl acetate and others. A natural form of vitamin A found in animal foods, oily fish and cod liver oil is the best form for these patients.

But why do GAPS patients need supplementation with vitamin A?

Vitamin A deficiency is a big problem in the less developed world. But in Western countries deficiency in this vitamin is considered to be rare, because of widespread consumption of dairy, eggs and meats. Also, the body has a good ability to store enough vitamin A, mainly in the liver, to last for at least three months.[4,2] On top of that, theoretically, vitamin A can be manufactured in the body from a large group of plant-based substances, called carotenoids. There are approximately 600 different carotenoids in nature (in green, leafy and brightly coloured vegetables and fruit), 50 of which theoretically can be converted to vitamin A. Based on this, the general advice in the West is not to supplement vitamin A, as sufficient quantities can be obtained from the carotenoids in fruit and vegetables.[2] This may indeed apply to some people with a very healthy digestive system and metabolism, but for the majority of the Western population this conversion is very problematic. In people with digestive problems, such as GAPS children and adults, it is virtually impossible to obtain vitamin A from fruit and vegetables. The absorption rate of carotenoids can be less than 5%, which makes them largely useless as a source of vitamin A.[1,4] Also, in order to convert carotenoids into vitamin A, the body needs magnesium, zinc, many amino-acids and other vital nutrients, which are always in short supply in a person with a poor digestion. Various toxins have an ability to block the conversion of carotenoids into vitamin A, and GAPS patients are very toxic people.[5] To absorb retinol (the preformed vitamin A) from dairy, liver, eggs and other foods a good supply of bile and pancreatic enzymes is needed.[2,5] Many GAPS patients have whitish pale stools indicating that their bile production and fat digestion are very poor. In clinical practice, people who cannot digest fats always present with vitamin A deficiency.[5]

Digestive problems and vitamin A deficiency are in a 'chicken and egg' relationship. As we have already discovered, poor digestion causes vitamin A deficiency. But vitamin A deficiency can cause digestive problems.[6,7] In fact, gut disease is one of the symptoms of vitamin A deficiency, because the gut lining is one of the most active sites of cell production, growth and differentiation. Neither of these processes can happen properly without a good supply of vitamin A. Leaky gut and malabsorption are the typical results of vitamin A deficiency.

According to WHO, in Western countries lactating women and infants are two groups at high risk of being deficient in vitamin A.[8] Lactating mothers need to have much more of this vitamin in their diet than the rest of us.[1,2,4,5] In our modern society women may have poor reserves of vitamin A, which means that many infants do not get a good supply of this vitamin in the first months of life.[9] This makes their digestive system prone to developing problems later on. As always, the health of the baby starts from the health of the mother.

It isn't just the digestive system that suffers from an inadequate supply of vitamin A. Its functions in the body are multiple, involving pretty much every aspect of health.[5-7] It is essential in immune function, brain development, vision, cell differentiation, embryogenesis, reproduction, growth and many other processes.

One of the functions of vitamin A is its role in immunity. In fact, the earliest name for vitamin A was 'anti-infective vitamin'.[2,5] In vitamin A deficiency both specific and non-specific immunity are impaired: the humoral response to bacterial, parasitic and viral infections, cell-mediated immunity, mucosal immunity, natural killer cell activity and phagocytosis. Supplementation of vitamin A in children shows proliferation of normal B and T cells and better response to antigens.[10] Acute deficiency of vitamin A with night blindness and xerophthalmia is indeed rare in the West, but vitamin A inadequacy is not rare at all. People with vitamin A inadequacy do not have any visual problems, typical for deficiency. Instead they are very prone to infections, because their immune system does not function properly. Infections, particularly with a high fever, destroy a lot of vitamin A in the body. In clinical practice patients with febrile conditions require supplementation with this vitamin.[10,11] GAPS children and adults have inflammation in their digestive systems and elsewhere in the body, which reduces their vitamin A reserves and predisposes them to infections.

Obviously, the best way to establish whether the patient has a vitamin A deficiency is to test for it. But simply by analysing the clinical picture and health history, I would say that most GAPS people need supplementation with a **natural** form of vitamin A, the best source of which is cod liver oil. As always, Nature knows best. Clinical experience shows that synthetic forms of supplemental vitamin A (retinyl palmitate, retinyl acetate, etretinate, accutane and others) do not work well for these patients.[5]

Many people are concerned about overdosing on vitamin A. Indeed, in excess, this vitamin can be toxic.[11] However, to reach toxic levels you have to have more than 10 times the recommended daily allowance for a period of weeks to years. For an adult, that is 20 teaspoons of cod liver oil every day for weeks or years. For a small child it is 10 teaspoons a day. I cannot imagine anybody taking that amount of cod liver oil once, let alone on a regular basis. To cause an acute toxicity an adult has to have 100 times more than the recommended dose and a child 20 times more,[11] which translates into 20 teaspoons of cod liver oil for a child of 3 years of age. So, taking a teaspoon of cod liver oil per day is not going to cause an overdose of vitamin A. It is synthetic forms of this vitamin, which are often added to processed foods, that can cause an overdose.

In the last few decades many processed foods in the Western world have been fortified with synthetic vitamin A, an excess of which can cause health problems in people.[11,12] It is particularly dangerous in pregnancy, because it can cause damage to a developing foetus.[13] Unfortunately, instead of advising pregnant women to stop eating processed foods, our mainstream medicine tells them not to eat natural foods rich in vitamin A, liver and cod liver oil in particular. Liver provides *natural* vitamin A (which cannot be compared to the synthetic one) in combination with other fat-soluble vitamins, the full spectrum of B vitamins, vitamin C, protein and a myriad of other nutrients, all of which are absolutely essential for a growing foetus. Eating liver on a daily basis used to be a duty of all pregnant women in most traditional cultures around the world![14,15] It was not optional for a pregnant mother, because people knew through experience that eating liver would make sure that her baby was born healthy. Deficiency in real natural vitamin A, found in liver, high-fat meats, eggs, high-fat dairy and oily fish, can lead to many problems in the baby's body, including the proper development of bones, eyes, nervous system, immune system and connective tissue.[7,11]

Vitamin D

Cholesterol is the major building block of vitamin D: vitamin D is made from cholesterol in our skin when it is exposed to sunlight.[16] Our recent misguided fear of the sun and avoidance of cholesterol-rich foods have created an epidemic of vitamin D deficiency in the Western world.[17]

Sunlight is by far the most important source of this vital vitamin for us, as the typical diet can only be considered as a minor source of vitamin D.[11] So, sunbathing is not only good for us, it is essential! The skin cancer, blamed on sunshine, is not caused by the sun.[19–31,33] It is beyond the scope of this book to go into this subject in detail, but it is a fact that skin cancer (just like any other cancer) is caused by our modern processed foods and our modern toxic lifestyles.[17,19] Trans fats from vegetable oils and margarine and other toxins stored in the skin are particular culprits.[16] In addition, some sunscreens contain chemicals which have been proven to cause skin cancer.[29,30] Just as with cholesterol, someone's misguided idea (about sunlight causing skin cancer) has been picked up by commercial powers and made 'the common knowledge'. We, humans, have spent our lives outdoors in the sunlight for millions of years, before we started hiding from the sun. When we are exposed to sunlight, even in cold weather, we produce vitamin D. In those times of the year when there isn't much sunlight, vitamin D production drops. So, these are the times when we have to pay particular attention to our diet, making sure we consume plenty of foods with a good amount of this vitamin: cod liver oil, oily fish, eggs, butter and liver.

The recommended daily allowance for vitamin D in Western countries is minimal, set only to avoid developing rickets or osteomalacia.[11,34] To have optimal health, the majority of people need more vitamin D per day than the recommended allowance.[16,17] GAPS patients, due to poor digestive function and toxicity in the body, require much larger amounts of vitamin D than the recommended allowances. Spending time outdoors in sunlight and sunbathing are the best ways of getting vitamin D.[33,34] In winter, when there is less sunlight, eating plenty of oily fish and supplementing cod liver oil is a good way to get some vitamin D. That is why, when we look at the traditional diets of people around the world, the further from the equator we move, the more people prized and consumed oily fish, fish livers and polar animal livers, particularly in the winter.[15,16]

What does it mean for our bodies to be deficient in vitamin D?

A long list of suffering:[31–35]

- Diabetes, as vitamin D is essential for blood sugar control[36]
- Heart disease[37,38]
- Mental illness[39]
- Auto-immune illness, such as rheumatoid arthritis, lupus, inflammatory bowel disease, multiple sclerosis and other[40]
- Obesity[41]
- Osteoarthritis[42]
- Rickets and osteomalacia[43]
- Muscle weakness and poor neuro-muscular co-ordination[44]
- High blood pressure[45]
- Cancer[46-48]
- Chronic pain[49]

- Poor immunity and susceptibility to infections[50]
- Hyperparathyroidism, which manifests itself as osteoporosis, kidney stones, depression, aches and pains, chronic fatigue, muscle weakness and digestive abnormalities[51]

Unfortunately, apart from sunlight and cholesterol-rich foods, there is no other appropriate way to get vitamin D. Of course, there are supplements, but clinical experience shows that no supplement can compare with natural food. The synthesised vitamin is not the same as the natural vitamin.[35] It does not work as effectively, and it is easy to get a toxic level. It is impossible to get toxicity from natural vitamin D obtained from sunlight or cholesterol-rich foods, because the body knows how to deal with it.

Vitamins A and D are partners!

Vitamin D has been designed to work as a team with vitamin A.[34–36] They do not work properly without each other and a deficiency in one creates an excess in the other (to the point of making it toxic). In the last decades many Western processed foods have been fortified with synthetic vitamin A (without any thought of supplying vitamin D).[52] Because of the widespread deficiency in vitamin D, this synthetic vitamin A becomes toxic in the body, causing various health problems. This is just another example of how much risk we put ourselves in when we consume processed foods!

Recent testing revealed that a large proportion of the Western population has 'too much' vitamin A stored in their bodies, thanks to fortification of processed foods.[53,54] When both A and D vitamins are present in the body in the right amounts, they do not allow each other to get out of control. If the person has stored too much vitamin A, it means that this person is deficient in vitamin D. And indeed, that is the case for the majority of the Western population – vitamin D deficiency is rampant.[41,53] As a result of these findings cod liver oil has come under attack, as it provides more vitamin A than D. As often happens in nutritional science, the immediate 'knee-jerk' reaction was that we must not consume cod liver oil! As the authorities still tell the population to stay away from the sun and avoid cholesterol-rich foods, they have no alternative but to recommend synthetic Vitamin D supplements.

Vitamin A and vitamin D are partners – they have been designed to work together. Who designed it that way? Mother Nature! That is why natural foods rich in one are usually rich in the other. By taking cod liver oil we can obtain both vitamins at the same time.

How much cod liver oil should we supplement?

Before talking about doses we have to think about quality. Unfortunately, today's mass-produced cod liver oil is very different from the oil our grandparents used to consume. The industrial process of oil extraction involves heat, pressure, solvents, alkali refining, bleaching, deodorisation, etc.[55] Apart from small traditional cultures around the world and a couple of pioneering manufacturers in the West, nobody uses traditional fermentation or any of the other traditional ways of producing cod liver oil.[55] Industrial production destroys most of the vitamins A and D in the oil, so their synthetic counterparts are then added in different amounts. Some manufacturers add natural vitamins A and D to the oil, but this practice is becoming increasingly rare because synthetic counterparts are less expensive. It is important to find good quality cod liver oil to use as a supplement for your GAPS patient, and the best oil is produced using traditional methods. If it is not possible to find this quality of cod liver oil, try to find a brand of oil with natural vitamins A and D added. I do not recommend consuming synthetic vitamins.

It is difficult to assess the exact amounts of vitamins A and D in naturally produced cod liver oil, as these vitamins exist in many different forms in nature.[55] Testing methods are being improved all the time, but we cannot fully rely on them at present. The cod liver oil in your local pharmacy or supermarket has exact amounts of A and D listed on the label, because the manufacturers know how much they added to the oil after it was refined and deodorised. The trouble is that these vitamins are likely to be synthetic, which makes it difficult to predict how much good they are going to do in the body. Add to that the fact that we are all different. Every one of us, humans, has a unique metabolism and a unique set of circumstances, which would dictate unique requirements for various nutrients. On top of that our nutritional needs change all the time: from day to night, from winter to summer, from being stressed and overworked to being relaxed, etc. So, working out individual doses of any nutrient, including cod liver oil is more of an art than a precise science.

Generally, I recommend about a teaspoon per day of cod liver oil for adults, double that dose for pregnant and lactating women, and half that dose for children. In my clinical experience, it is safe to double these doses for a few weeks at the beginning of the programme, as GAPS patients are in particular need of all the nutrients the fermented cod liver oil will provide. For babies and very small children it works to rub cod liver oil into their skin (the nappy area is suitable), as the skin only absorbs what the body needs.

If ordinary cod liver oil is used (with natural vitamins added), then it is generally recommended to look for oil with a ratio of vitamin A to vitamin D of around 10 to 1. As all manufacturers add different doses of vitamins to their oil, it is a good idea to consult the manufacturer about dosages. The typical recommended daily doses are: one teaspoon for adults, half that dose for children and a third of a teaspoon for babies and very small children. Lactating mothers and pregnant women can have 1.5-2 teaspoons per day.

These amounts of cod liver oil on a regular basis over time would gently help to correct A and D deficiency. And let us not get too focused on the exact ratios of these vitamins in the oil, as cod liver oil is *not* the only source of these vitamins for a GAPS patient. The GAPS diet is going to be the main source of vitamin A and a good source of vitamin D. Sunlight exposure is going to provide the remaining vitamin D for you, so make sure to spend a good amount of time outdoors every day. Keep in mind that we supplement cod liver oil only to remove the tip of the deficiency iceberg; diet and lifestyle are the most important changes to make. I find supplementing cod liver oil in the cold season helpful, but in the summer the majority of people don't need to supplement it, as long as you allow the sun to do its work for you.

4. Digestive Enzymes

1. Stomach acid booster

People with abnormal gut flora, almost without exception, have abnormal stomach acid production. Toxins produced by overgrowth of pathogenic microbes in the gut have a strong ability to reduce secretion of stomach acid; the condition is called *hypochlorhydria* (low stomach acid).[1] Unfortunately, it is also routine for mainstream medicine to prescribe drugs aimed at reducing stomach acid production (in gastritis and many other stomach problems). These drugs (PPIs or other) are typically taken for long periods of time, causing serious chronic hypochlorhydria.[2]

What does it mean to have low stomach acid production and why is it important?

The stomach is the place where protein digestion begins. Hydrochloric acid produced by the stomach walls activates protein-digesting enzymes (such as pepsin), which start breaking down the very complex structure of dietary proteins into peptides and amino acids. To do its work properly pepsin needs the pH of the stomach to be 3 or below. In hypochlorhydria not enough acid is produced, so the pH in the stomach is not low enough for pepsin to do its job properly. The most studied proteins in this situation are gluten and casein. In GAPS patients the digestive system converts them into opiate-like substances, called casomorphin and gliadomorphin, which are thought to find their way to the patient's nervous system and interfere in its normal activity.[3] In *hypochlorhydria* not only does casein and gluten leave the stomach improperly digested, but all other proteins absorb in a partially digested state causing many problems in the body.[1–3]

As a result of low stomach acid production, the whole process of protein digestion in the body goes wrong from the very beginning (in the stomach). The maldigested protein then passes through into the small intestine. The intestinal wall and pancreatic enzymes, which accomplish further steps in the protein digestion, expect the protein to arrive from the stomach in a particular form in order to do their job properly. It is like a conveyer belt or an assembly line in a factory. If the first person does a poor job, then no matter how well the rest of the people in the line may work, the end product is likely to be of a poor quality. However, what happens in the body is even worse. The problem is that in the body 'the rest of the line' cannot work properly either, because it is regulated by the 'first person'. This 'first person' is the stomach acid. Stomach acidity is the major regulator of pancreatic and liver ability to respond to arriving food.[4] In a normal situation, food coming from the stomach into the duodenum has to have a pH of 2 or below to stimulate production of two very important players in the whole digestive process. These players are two hormones, produced by the walls of the duodenum, which get absorbed into the blood and carried to the pancreas, liver, stomach and many other organs in the body. These hormones are **secretin** and **cholecystokinin.**[4] The first hormone, secretin, gives the stomach a command to stop producing its juices, stimulates the liver to produce bile and lets the intestinal lining know that food is coming, so it makes enough mucus to protect itself. But the most important thing that it does is to stimulate the pancreas to produce alkalising bicarbonate solution. This solution neutralises the acid in the food which has just arrived from the stomach. This is vital, because the duodenum and the rest of the small intestine need to have a far more alkaline pH to allow the pancreatic enzymes and bile to do their job of digesting proteins, fats and carbohydrates.[5]

To produce its digestive enzymes the pancreas needs the command of the second hormone – cholecystokinin. If cholecystokinin is not made by the walls of the duodenum (because of too little acid coming from the stomach with the food), then the pancreas will not produce its alkaline juice effectively to deal with that food. In addition, cholecystokinin tells the stomach to stop its activity, makes the gallbladder empty its bile into the duodenum, ready to digest fats, and opens the gates for pancreatic juices to flow and start digesting arriving food. [4]

These two hormones are so important in normal food digestion that without them this digestion simply cannot happen. Unfortunately, in a person with low stomach acidity that is exactly what happens. The food coming from the stomach is not acid enough to trigger the production of secretin and cholecystokinin. So, the pancreas does not produce its juices and bile is not secreted to work on the fats. Maldigestion and malabsorption follow. Partially digested proteins, like casomorphin and gliadomorphin and many others, get produced and absorbed through the damaged leaky intestinal wall, acting as opiates in the body. Other maldigested proteins cause allergies and autoimmune reactions. A lot of essential vitamins, amino acids and minerals do not get absorbed, causing nutritional deficiencies. Maldigested carbohydrates get consumed by abnormal microbial flora, which converts them into alcohol, acetaldehyde and a whole host of other toxins.[6] Fats do not get digested, which makes the person deficient in extremely important fat-soluble vitamins A, D, E and K and essential fatty acids, and results in pale floating stool or diarrhoea (steatorrhea). Undigested food simply rots in the digestive tract, poisoning the whole body.

In the chapter *The Liver and the Lungs* we talked about the formation of bile stones; insufficient stomach acidity plays a role in this problem. In addition, when stomach acidity is low, stones also form in the pancreas. The lack of secretin and cholecystokinin leads to low production of alkaline solution in the pancreas, so proteins in its juice precipitate and form plugs.[7] These plugs calcify over time and form pancreatic stones, which obstruct the flow of the pancreatic juices. The build-up of pancreatic enzymes behind the obstruction damages the pancreas, leading to *pancreatitis* (acute or chronic) or a milder condition, called *pancreatic insufficiency*.[8] These are usually painful conditions, because the pancreas is located close to the solar plexus (one of the largest nerve centres in the abdomen). If the process lasts long enough, the pancreas can get damaged quite seriously, leading to diabetes mellitus and/or pancreatic cancer. Lack of bicarbonate solution in the pancreatic juice creates a favourable environment for various microbes and intestinal worms to make a home in the pancreas itself. These creatures add their own damage and can cause an infection in the pancreas or cancer.[9]

Apart from literally ruining the whole digestive process and leading to accumulation of pancreatic and bile stones, lack of acid in the stomach has other serious implications. Stomach acid is the first barrier for huge numbers of microbes that arrive with every bit of food or drink we put into our mouths. If the stomach is not acid enough, these microbes have a good chance of getting into the intestines, which they will colonise and then cause trouble (such as SIBO – small intestinal bacterial overgrowth). They even start growing in the stomach itself.[10] Normally the stomach is the least-populated area of the digestive system due to its extremely acid environment. However, in a person with hypochlorhydria all sorts of pathogenic and opportunistic bacteria and fungi can grow on the stomach wall, such as *Helicobacter pylori, Campylobacter pylori, Enterobacteria, Candida, Salmonella, E. coli, Streptococci* and other. The most research in this area has been done in stomach cancer patients, the majority of which show low levels of stomach acid production.[10,11] Microbes, which populate low acid stomach, play a very important role in causing stomach cancer, ulcers and gastritis. To understand this subject in more detail, please read the section *Stomach Problems* in the *Chapter A–Z*.

Of course, most of these microbes love to eat carbohydrates, particularly the processed kind. The digestion of carbohydrates starts in the mouth with the action of saliva. Stomach acid normally stops this digestion, so carbohydrates have to wait until the duodenum to be digested. In the stomach with low acidity, overgrowing microbes start fermenting dietary carbohydrates, often with the production of various toxins and gases.[11] Accumulating gases cause excessive belching and burping. And pathogens grow around the sphincter muscle at the top of the stomach. This round muscle normally separates the stomach from the oesophagus and does not allow food to go back up. Pathogens growing in that area, and the toxins they produce, partially paralyse the sphincter muscle, which causes reflux: regurgitation of food back up into the oesophagus.[12] Even with low stomach acid production there is some acid in the regurgitated food, which burns the walls of the oesophagus, giving the person typical symptoms of 'acid indigestion'. Antacids are usually prescribed for acid indigestion and reflux. They may alleviate the immediate symptoms, but in the long run make the whole situation worse as they reduce stomach acid production even further.

So, what do we do?

I believe that many GAPS patients need supplementation with stomach acid. The most physiological preparation available on the market is Betaine HCl with added Pepsin. One capsule typically provides 200–300 mg of Betaine HCl and 100 mg of Pepsin. It should be taken at the beginning of each meal. The capsules usually contain an adult dose. However, I find that children as young as eight can take this dose without any trouble. A lot of patients report improvements in their reflux, bloating and stool in just a few days from starting Betaine HCl with pepsin. Make sure that you do not take supplements of probiotics together with Betaine HCl as the acid is likely to damage the probiotic bacteria. Take the probiotic first thing in the morning, between food or after food, when the stomach acid is at its lowest. This does not apply to fermented foods which you eat with your meals, as the probiotic microbes are protected inside particles of the food. If you forget to take your supplement of Betaine HCl at the beginning of the meal and develop indigestion after the meal, there are supplements of pure hydrochloric acid (not buffered as a Betaine HCl) with or without pepsin on the market. These supplements work faster and will help you to increase acidity in your stomach quite quickly, so your meal digests well.

Apart from supplementing stomach acid, there are natural things we can do to stimulate the body to produce its own stomach acid. Cabbage juice (fresh and fermented) is one of the strongest stimulants. Having a few spoonfuls of cabbage juice or a small cabbage salad before a meal will help to digest that meal. Sauerkraut and its juice are even stronger: a small helping of sauerkraut or a few tablespoons of its juice will prepare the stomach for the arriving food. It is good to mix some sauerkraut into your fresh cabbage salad and any other salad. Having a cup of homemade meat stock with your meal will also help to increase stomach acidity. With children the easiest thing is to give them a cup of homemade meat stock with a few spoonfuls of sauerkraut juice or cabbage juice mixed in it. Bitter herbs (such as artichoke, dandelion, gentian, blessed thistle and other) have a good ability to stimulate stomach acid production and have been used for centuries in traditional *digestive bitters* all over the world. Today there are a number of digestive bitters available on the market; a few drops of these supplements in some water or meat stock will help to prepare your stomach for the arrival of food. It is important to experience the bitter taste of these herbs in order for them to work, so they cannot be taken in capsules or tablets.

2. Pancreatic Enzymes

These are the enzymes that people are talking about when they say 'digestive enzymes'. They usually include a mixture of proteases, peptidases, lipases, amylase, lactase and cellulase, which normally would break down your food in the small intestine. In a healthy digestive tract most of these enzymes are produced by the pancreas. If we can restore normal stomach acidity then this stage in digestion should be problem free, because the stomach acid will trigger the pancreas to produce its own enzymes. That is why I consider restoring the stomach acid level far more important than supplementing pancreatic enzymes.

Some people try to take pancreatic enzymes instead of changing their diet, hoping that the enzymes will handle the processed foods they want to continue eating. Not surprisingly, this approach does not work for the majority of people, because supplements can never replace proper diet. The diet, which we describe in this book, is designed to heal the gut and to re-establish normal gut flora. No enzyme can do that!

Generally, in my clinical experience, I see a lot of improvement from supplementing stomach acid or stimulating its production. However, sometimes I do not see much happening from supplementing pancreatic enzymes. If the patient feels that they really help, then there is no reason why he or she should not take them, providing the supplement does not contain fillers, binders and other ingredients, which may interfere with the healing processes in the gut. In my experience, the majority of patients do very well with just supplementing stomach acid, because it will trigger production of their own pancreatic enzymes through secretin and cholecystokinin, as well as triggering bile secretion and many other important players in the digestive process, making it far more natural.

Digestive enzymes do not need to be taken permanently. As the gut starts healing, the person can slowly withdraw the stomach acid supplementation and/or pancreatic enzymes, taking them only with heavy meals, or if something not allowed on the diet has been eaten. Long term, it is far more natural and practical to use fermented foods, particularly containing fermented cabbage, and digestive bitters to stimulate production of normal amounts of digestive enzymes in your gut. For children in particular, I recommend focussing on cabbage juice and bitters first before considering stomach acid boosters.

5. Vitamin and Mineral Supplementation

GAPS patients have many nutritional deficiencies, so it is a natural desire to get rid of them. The question is: how?

Is it a matter of simply testing how much magnesium, for example, a person is missing and then supplementing that amount? Or is it a matter of taking a supplement 'specifically designed' for your health condition? Maybe we should just give megadoses of all the nutrients which the person is deficient in, hoping that the body will sort it all out?

Many health practitioners turn to testing for nutritional deficiencies. For every nutrient there are optimal tests, which are considered to give the most accurate information about that particular nutrient, and there are less optimal tests, which may be quite misleading. Trying to use the most optimal test for every nutrient is impractical and can be very expensive. Usually one or two tests are performed for all the nutrients at once, which does not represent the true picture. So, trying to work out a nutritional supplementation protocol based on these tests is shaky from the start.

On top of that, many supplements on the market have a very low absorption rate, some only about 9%, so the amount the patient's body actually gets can be way below what it says on the bottle.[1] Of course, the majority of manufacturers would not tell you on the bottle how low the absorption rate of their supplement is, even if they knew. So, choosing a supplement can be quite difficult.

Absorption of supplements is a complicated process which, quite apart from the quality of the supplement, also depends on the state of the patient's digestive system. Two different people may absorb different amounts of nutrients from the same supplement. The GAPS digestive system is generally not in good shape and may not absorb any of those nutrients particularly well.

To complicate the whole matter even further, many nutrients compete for absorption sites in the gut. So, if we supplement too much calcium, for example, it may impair absorption of other nutrients: magnesium, zinc, copper, iron, some amino acids and others, creating deficiencies in those nutrients.[2]

Indeed, this is a very confusing area of nutrition. The truth is, nobody knows how to prescribe vitamins and minerals, because we do not have enough research or knowledge on this subject. Every nutritionist or medical practitioner has his/her own collection of favourite supplements and most of them are used on a trial-and-error basis.

Taking vitamin and mineral supplements has become very common, not only because many of us take 'health pills', but because a lot of foods are fortified with vitamins and minerals to compensate for the loss of those nutrients in the food processing. And many foods are grown using intensive farming techniques, which makes them nutrient poor from the start. Unfortunately, a lot of these supplemented nutrients are synthetic. The body has been designed to use natural forms of these nutrients and often does not recognise the synthetic forms or know what to do with them. There is a growing suspicion that a lot of cases of kidney stones, for example, are caused by supplementing synthetic forms of vitamin C.[3]

There is a highly publicised opinion that in our modern world we cannot be healthy without taking nutritional supplements, because our diet cannot provide us with optimal amounts of nutrients. Indeed, if you live on cereal and toast for breakfast, sandwiches for lunch and a standard dinner, you will not provide your body with optimal amounts of nutrition and you will have to take supplements. The diet, described in this book, will provide you with concentrated amounts of nutrition in a natural form, which the body recognises and knows what to do with. Juicing will add more concentrated amounts of vitamins, minerals and other useful substances. A good probiotic, on average, increases the absorption rate of nutrients from food by 50% or more.[4] On top of that, probiotic microbes in the gut flora are supposed to be the main source of vitamins group B, K2, biotin, biological amines and many other substances in the body.[5] Usually that is the first group of nutritional deficiencies to disappear when the patient starts eating fermented foods and taking therapeutic doses of a strong probiotic. The diet and probiotic will start healing the digestive system, so the patient will start absorbing the nutrients from the food properly.

Another important point we have to consider, when it comes to our GAPS patients, is that their digestive system is inflamed and damaged. A lot of synthetic supplements, fillers and binders in tablets and capsules will aggravate and irritate already sensitive GAPS gut lining and interfere with the healing process. I have seen many patients who put a lot of effort into implementing the diet, but did not achieve the best results until they removed most of their supplements.

That is why I normally do not recommend any vitamin or mineral supplementation at the beginning of the programme. I recommend putting most effort into implementing the diet first and starting the healing process in the gut. Once the digestive system starts working properly, nutritional deficiencies may disappear without any supplementation! They disappear the natural way, as the body starts working properly.

Of course, all patients are different and some of them require targeted supplementation. But that is a matter for a qualified practitioner to decide. Here are some important points to keep in mind.

- Choose supplements without any ingredients which may aggravate the gut condition. Supplements in a liquid form are better than in powder, tablet or capsule. Substances, which are not allowed on the diet, should also be out.
- Choose supplements with a high absorption rate, for example, vitamin and mineral supplements with added *fulvic acid*. Fulvic acid (not to be confused with folic acid) is produced by microbes in soil. It can ensure a higher absorption rate for a supplement the natural way. It also has good chelating properties for toxic metals.[6] Soil bacteria in your probiotic will provide your gut with this acid.
- Keep supplements to an absolute minimum!

Detoxification for People with Gut and Physiology Syndrome

All chronic and degenerative diseases are caused by two and only two major problems: toxicity and deficiency.

Charlotte Gerson

We live in a polluted world.[1,2] Every day we breathe in car fumes and industrial wastes. We eat foods containing pesticides, herbicides and other agricultural chemicals. We drink milk and eat meat and eggs from animals which are routinely given antibiotics, steroids and other drugs. We eat a countless number of chemicals in processed foods. We use personal care products full of chemicals shown to be carcinogenic and generally toxic for humans.[1] Our modern energy-conserving homes and offices have become toxic places. Modern building materials, insulation, paints, domestic cleaning chemicals and fire retardants all outgas toxic substances which we breathe day in and day out. Hospitals and shopping centres have very high amounts of toxic substances in the air, which is why many people feel so tired and drained after a shopping trip or a long visit to a hospital. We live in a world increasingly filled with electromagnetic pollution from electronic devices, and this pollution is getting more and more intense.[3] Our mobile phones, wireless technologies and other electronic inventions fill our homes, offices and other spaces with invisible radiation, which has now been proven to cause cancer, infertility, neurological and endocrine damage and heart problems.[3,4] And as if all that is not enough, we routinely take prescription drugs, drink alcohol and smoke tobacco.

So, how do we survive? How do we manage to live our lives, go to work and have children, without just dropping dead after our first breath of traffic-jam air in the morning?

We survive thanks to a very important system in our bodies. A system which, until recently, we did not know much about – a DETOXIFICATION SYSTEM.[5,6] This system is like a cleaner in the body. It constantly cleans out all the toxins produced as a result of normal body metabolism, as well as toxins arriving from the outside. Its headquarters is in the liver and it has departments in every cell of the body. The sophistication and complexity of this system is staggering to even the most knowledgeable biochemists, and there is a lot we still don't know about how it works so efficiently.[6] But what we do know is that this system, in order to function well, has to have a constant supply of nutrients: high-quality protein and fats, fat-soluble vitamins, minerals and trace elements, enzymes, vitamins, etc – all the substances, which our GAPS children and adults are usually deficient in. Due to these deficiencies the detoxification system cannot function at an optimum level in a GAPS person. At the same time this system is overloaded with work, because GAPS patients are very toxic people. Imagine a worker who is being starved of food and drink, and at the same time is being given more and more work to do. How is he going to cope? He is going to put most of this work into a backlog, hoping for easier times when he will be able to attend to it. That is exactly what the detoxification system does in a GAPS patient – it stores various toxic substances in different tissues in the body in order to deal with them later. That is why, when these patients are tested for toxic metals, petrochemicals and other toxins they always test positive.[7] Unfortunately, a lot of these chemicals have an affinity for fats and therefore get stored in body fats.[8] The brain and the rest of the nervous system, endocrine system, bone marrow and many other vital organs have a high proportion of fats in their tissues and become storage sites for these toxins. Organs clogged with toxicity cannot function well. In a more severe situation the detoxification system breaks down, so the person's body is unable to handle toxicity anymore. We see this very clearly in GAPS patients with chronic fatigue syndrome, multiple chemical sensitivity, fibromyalgia, myalgic encephalomyelitis, severe mental illness, neurological and endocrine illnesses, chronic infections (such as Lime disease and chronic viral infections) and many other.[5-7]

So, what do we do? How do we lift this toxic load off the bodies of our GAPS patients to allow them to function properly? How do we restore their damaged detoxification system? This mighty system has ways of removing toxicity out of our bodies that our science hasn't even discovered yet! No man-made 'detox' measures can ever match the abilities of our own natural detoxification system, when it is working properly. It is absolutely essential to restore this system back to life in order to heal from any disease.

No matter how many toxins a GAPS person is exposed to from the environment, the major source of toxicity in the body is the bowel. The first and most obvious thing to do is to remove this main source of toxicity, which means cleaning up and healing the digestive system. So, the GAPS Nutritional Protocol is the main treatment! For many people just following the GAPS Diet solves the problem, but in others removing the major source of toxicity may not be enough. What do we do with all the toxins stored over the years in these patients' bodies? What do we do with toxic metals and man-made chemicals? This accumulated toxicity creates a perfect ground for breeding parasites in tissues and organs. The parasites produce their own toxins for our bodies to deal with and drain an already overburdened immune system.

There are a number of natural things we need to do as part of the GAPS Nutritional Protocol to help the body to unload toxicity and heal. Let us look at them in detail, starting from the most basic considerations.

1. Reduce your general toxic load

The GAPS Diet is the main method for restoring our detoxification system. It is a hungry organ and requires high-quality nutrition. However, while we are trying to feed this organ properly and restore it back to life, it is important *not* to present it with extra work. So, a reduction in the general toxic load on the patient's detoxification system is an important part of the treatment.

What is general toxic load?

Anything toxic we eat, breathe, touch or apply on our skin absorbs very quickly and puts a heavy workload on our detoxification system.[1,2] The GAPS patient's detoxification system is already damaged, and it is not sensible to add more to its workload by exposing the person to toxic substances from the environment. What substances are we talking about?

Tap water in most modern houses contains chlorine, agrochemicals, pharmaceutical drugs, fluoride and other contaminants. It is important to filter this water before drinking it or cooking with it. There are many water filters available on the market. I do not recommend reverse osmosis filters or distilled water, because these methods of purification damage the energetic bio-physical properties of water.[9] They create 'dead' water which is not healthy for us to consume. Natural water has a hexagonal physical structure where molecules of water connect with one another in a particular pattern, and it is important for us to consume water in this state.[10] I recommend using a simple carbon filter to remove most of the man-made contamination. This kind of filter is affordable for the majority of people and should not damage the bio-physical structure of water. In my clinical experience it is not necessary to buy a lot of expensive equipment to have an acceptable quality of water in your house. For example, there are various devices for energising water on the market which I don't consider to be essential. Just adding fresh lemon, organic cider vinegar, vegetable medley liquid or a tablespoon of kombucha to your glass of water will change its energetic pattern and make it more health-giving.

Dishwashing soaps, particularly those used in the dishwashing machine, stay on the dishes and cutlery to make them look shiny. When we rub dishes by hand, using a sponge or a brush, they are cleaned properly with no chemical residue left on them. The dishwasher cannot rub the dishes, it uses sprays of water to wash them, so strong detergents have to be used and they do not get washed off completely. We eat these toxic chemicals at every meal and for a GAPS person this toxicity is unacceptable. That is why, particularly at the beginning of the programme, I recommend that dishes are washed by hand using hot water, mustard powder, vinegar or bicarbonate of soda. Mustard powder used to be the main dishwashing 'detergent' before the chemical industry replaced it with more lucrative alternatives.[11] Mustard powder is inexpensive and removes grease and food very effectively, leaving nothing toxic or unnatural on your dishes and cutlery. Dissolve 3–4 tablespoons of mustard powder in 2 l (3½ pt) of hot water, wash your dishes in it by hand and rinse with clean water.

The *patient's house* should be kept as chemical free as possible by using no domestic cleaning chemicals, paints, carpet cleaners or pesticides, air 'fresheners' and other man-made chemicals. All widely available domestic chemicals are toxic. Bathroom detergents, floor cleaners, polishes, etc. all stay in the air and on the surfaces, contributing to the general toxic load on the patient's detox system. Toxic domestic chemicals can be replaced with safer biodegradable alternatives from various conscientious companies. However, generally try to use as little as possible. A lot of cleaning around the house can be done with water. Add a bit of vinegar or lemon juice, bicarbonate of soda and olive oil. You can clean your wood floors with strong tea. You can polish your furniture with a mixture of 1 cup olive oil and ¼ cup white vinegar. You can pour white wine on red wine spills on your carpet to remove the stain. You can wash glass with vinegar. There are many natural ways of cleaning the house. Look online or for books dedicated to this subject.

It is wise *not* to redecorate or renovate the house or install new carpets or furniture while the patient is trying to detoxify and heal. Paints, modern building materials, new carpets, curtains and new furniture outgas a plethora of extremely toxic chemicals, which we absorb through our lungs, skin and mucous membranes.[1,2] New carpet can outgas considerable amounts of highly carcinogenic formaldehyde for a few years. New furniture is full of fire retardants, which are great contributors of toxic metals and other poisons in our systems. Fresh household paints outgas dozens of extremely toxic chemicals into the air of the house for at least six months. It takes at least a year for a person's detoxification system to recover fully, so I recommend that no redecorating or refurnishing is done for that period of time, minimum.

Laundry detergents are large contributors of powerful toxins in many modern households.[1,2] Washing powders and liquids stay in the fabric of our clothes, bedding and towels; we absorb them through skin and lungs 24 hours a day, placing another heavy burden on our detoxification system. It is important to remove this source of toxicity! Try to look for safer ecologically friendly alternatives. Avoid anything with a smell; modern fragrances and synthetic perfumes added to laundry detergents and other domestic chemicals are toxic in themselves and have been proven to cause cancer and other illnesses.[12]

Air your house regularly by opening the windows. There should be no artificial smells in the house: so-called air-fresheners are toxic chemicals pumped into your house. If you live in a polluted area, consider moving, but in the meantime, you may have to use an air purifier.

Houseplants are our great friends when it comes to keeping our houses toxin free. They consume the toxic gases and replace them with oxygen and other beneficial substances. Fill your house with geraniums, ivies, spider plants, Aloe vera, ficus and other varieties of houseplants. The more the merrier, particularly in your bedrooms! Keep your houseplants healthy. Don't let them become mouldy, as some GAPS people may react to moulds. If you water your houseplants with the dregs of coffee and tea, or water which you used to wash raw meats (liver in particular!), they will thank you with vigorous growth and beauty.

Very important contributors to the general toxic overload in the body are cosmetics, toiletries, perfumes, make-up, hair dyes and other *personal care products*.[12–14] The personal care products industry is self-regulated. Thousands of carcinogenic and toxic chemicals are widely used in the formulation of shampoos, soaps, toothpaste, cosmetics, perfumes, creams, deodorants, etc. The old opinion, that our skin is a barrier and does not let toxins in, has proven to be completely wrong. Toxins which go into the body through the digestive system have to pass through the liver, where most of them get broken down and rendered benign. Human skin, however, absorbs most things from the environment very efficiently. That is why the pharmaceutical industry has started producing more and more drugs which are applied to the skin as patches, because the skin absorbs them better than the digestive system and they get straight into the bloodstream without passing the test of the liver.[15]

The wide use of personal care products is a major contributor to our cancer epidemic.[13] Children, women and men are unknowingly exposing themselves to huge amounts of carcinogenic substances, which they apply to their skin. A good example is breast cancer. Cells removed from a cancerous breast in many cases contain a lot of aluminium (aluminum) – a toxic metal.[13,16] Where does this aluminium come from? From deodorants, which are absorbed through the skin in the woman's armpits.[17] Recent research into toxic metals showed that, when a pregnant animal is exposed to these metals, they accumulate in large amounts in the foetus.[13,14,18] That is why it is particularly important for a pregnant or breastfeeding mother to be careful about personal care products and the cosmetics she puts on her skin, face and hair. In this book we cannot go into details of all the toxins present in our toiletries and cosmetics. But let us list some of the most common ones.[19.20]

- Talc or talcum powder can cause ovarian cancer. Do not use it, particularly on babies!
- Sodium Lauryl (Laureth) Sulfate (SLS) – a highly toxic detergent that is present in most shampoos, soaps and toothpaste.
- Fluoride – a terrible poison for every system in the body. Widespread in toothpaste and other dental care products, it is also added to some water supplies and given to babies as drops. If you are not familiar with its toxicity, I would strongly advise you to learn more about it and avoid it like the plague.
- Titanium dioxide – carcinogenic.
- Triethanolamine (TEA) and Diethanolamine (DEA) form carcinogenic nitrosamines.
- Lanolin, itself a non-toxic natural substance, is often contaminated with DDT and other carcinogenic pesticides.
- Dioxanes are inhaled and absorbed through skin – highly carcinogenic.
- Saccharin – carcinogenic.
- Formaldehyde – a toxic and carcinogenic substance.
- Propylene glycol – carcinogenic.
- Lead, aluminium and other toxic metals are present in many personal care products, particularly in deodorants and make-up.

In patients with GAP Syndrome the use of personal care products should be reduced to an absolute minimum or removed altogether. The more severe the health condition of the person, the more stringent we must be. The general rule is: *if you cannot eat it, you cannot put it on your skin, scalp or teeth*! Only edible things can be used! We can brush our teeth with olive oil; this Ayurvedic procedure has a good record of cleansing the mouth, improving the condition of the gums and the teeth and reducing the general toxic load in the body (please, research *oil pulling*). Dip your toothbrush into some zeolite powder or bentonite clay and brush your teeth: this will provide another cleansing for your mouth and leave your teeth sparkling white. Occasionally we can use activated charcoal or bicarbonate of soda for brushing our teeth to whiten them. We can wash our hair with raw egg yolks: separate the egg yolk from the white and use as you would a shampoo (if you have long hair, use several egg yolks). This is how people used to wash their hair for centuries before shampoos were invented. As a moisturiser for the skin we can use any edible fat: coconut oil, olive oil, another cold-pressed natural oil. But a real medicine for dry skin and any form of dermatitis is tallow (please, see how to render tallow and make a skin cream from it in the chapter *What we shall eat and why, with some recipes*). Our bodes do not need washing with soaps, shower gels or bubble baths. These chemical concoctions not only contribute to the general toxic overload, but also wash off important oils, which protect the skin from infections and drying out and provide habitat for the microbial skin flora. Washing with water and a sponge is quite enough for a human being, particularly for babies and children! The best deodorant is a small amount of juice squeezed from a fresh lemon: it will remove any possibility of smell but will not stop you from sweating. Sweating is a very important cleansing function: our bodies remove many toxins through sweat.[21] Chemical deodorants stop production of sweat, increasing your general toxic load in the body while adding more toxic chemicals to this load.

There are a number of companies today which produce safe personal care products without harmful substances. Typically, these companies are small and have been started by people with allergies and skin problems, who were looking for solutions and found, that only natural unprocessed ingredients can be used on the human body.

Reducing our exposure to man-made chemicals should be an important part of any healing protocol. Human beings lived on this planet for eons without using any of these toxic chemicals. We do not need them! More than that, they damage our bodies and cause disease.

We, modern humans, have filled our lives with hazardous man-made things, which can damage our health and destroy our bodies. Many of these things are unavoidable, we are exposed to them no matter what we do. Air pollution, water pollution, toxic building materials, toxic chemicals, electromagnetic pollution and other hazards are everywhere. However, the fact that they are everywhere doesn't mean that we should expose ourselves to them recklessly. We can take steps to reduce our exposure and to make sure that our bodies are well nourished and strong enough to survive this onslaught.

Modern vaccinations for children and adults are amongst these hazards. Whether you are pro-vaccinations or against them, it is a fact that they damage and destroy the health of many people in the world.[22-26] Many Western countries are making vaccinations mandatory. If you or your child have to be vaccinated, it makes sense to take steps to protect your body from any damage.

Here are a few simple steps to take:

1. Make sure that you or your child are absolutely healthy and well at the time of vaccination – no cold, runny nose or inflammation anywhere

in the body, no medications taken, no particular stress or strain or sleep deprivation. It is essential to have no nutritional deficiencies, particularly in animal protein, animal fat and fat-soluble vitamins (A, D, E and K). So, prior to vaccination and after it, make sure to eat plenty of good quality high-fat animal foods, including gelatinous meat stock.
2. Insist on having single vaccines! Injecting several serious infections in one needle is convenient for the vaccine manufacturers and medical profession, but most definitely is not in your interest or your tiny baby's interest. Single vaccines do exist; any doctor can obtain them on your request; and you have the right to insist on it.[27]
3. Space vaccinations as widely as you can, giving your body or the body of your child time to recover from the previous vaccine before attacking it with the next one. Spacing will also give you a chance to observe your child or your body for any damage after the previous vaccine. Changes in small children in particular can be subtle, and only by spacing the vaccines can parents see what is going on. Is your child's development progressing normally? Is eye contact still good? Is the child still eating well, growing well and looking well?
4. For babies it is essential to be breastfed during vaccinations. If the mother cannot breastfeed, it is important to find a local wet nurse. There is no synthetic baby formula in the world that will ever come close to the quality of fresh breast milk from a healthy woman. Please, read more about this in *Wet Nursing* in *A–Z*.

2. Daily baths at bedtime

Taking baths in natural mineral waters is a very old healing tradition. In Europe, Asia, Americas and other areas of the world people bathed in natural spas and hot springs in order to recover from chronic illnesses and prevent health problems.[28] I highly recommend visiting such places when you have a chance, but in the meantime, we can benefit from bathing at home. To assist elimination of toxins, I recommend making it a daily bedtime routine to have a warm therapeutic bath with one of the following substances dissolved in the water:

- a cup of Epsom salt
- a cup of cider vinegar
- a cup of seaweed powder
- a cup of natural salt
- a cup of bicarbonate of soda

These baths have a gentle but considerable ability to remove toxins out through the skin, while your body can absorb some useful minerals when you are in the bath. The detoxifying ability of these baths can be quite powerful: in a toxic person these baths can cause a so-called 'detox reaction', when the person may get a headache, feel faint, dizzy or get heart palpitations. To minimise any possibility of such a reaction, I recommend that we start from a more diluted solution (just a tablespoon of any of the above substances in the bath), make the bathwater cooler and spend only a few minutes in it. Depending on how your body responds to the first few baths, you will be able to make these baths gradually hotter, more concentrated and spend a longer time enjoying them. These baths will help your body to detoxify gently over time, while relaxing you and preparing your body for a good night's sleep.

3. Swimming and barefoot walking

Swimming pools are very toxic places.[20,29] Some people believe that going to the swimming pool is a healthy exercise. This cannot be further from the truth. Apart from a few rare pools sterilised with ozone, the rest of them use chlorine-based chemicals for sterilising the water. Chlorine is a poison, which affects every system in the body, particularly the immune system and the liver. It absorbs quite well through the skin. In addition, a thick layer of chlorine gas floats above the swimming pool water, which we inhale while swimming. Inhaled chlorine absorbs extremely well through the lungs into the bloodstream. GAPS patients are already very toxic. Swimming in a chlorinated pool would add to that toxicity.

All people (and GAPS people in particular) should swim in the natural waters of lakes, rivers, seas and oceans only! Natural waters are full of life, biological energy from plants and different creatures, minerals, enzymes and many other beneficial substances. Swimming in natural living waters has been prized as a therapy for many health problems for centuries. Obviously, you have to make sure that the water, you swim in, is as far as possible from any source of industrial pollution.

It is important for human beings to walk barefoot as often as possible! Our bodies can be seen as electromagnetic machines, which must connect to the biggest magnet – our planet Earth. Research in this area shows that when we walk barefoot, we rebalance our electromagnetic properties, which are essential for good health.[30] Obviously, it is important to make sure that the ground we walk on has not been contaminated by industrial pollution (make sure to get out of the city to a natural environment). The soles of our feet are an important detoxification organ in the body: when we walk on grass, sand or soil there is an exchange of toxins and beneficial substances through the soles of our feet. It is particularly beneficial to walk on the beach or paddle in clean shallow waters of the sea, lakes or rivers. Based on this, there are some therapeutic detoxification remedies on the market, such as foot patches and foot baths, which many people find helpful.

4. Sunbathing

It is wonderful what one ray of sunlight can do for your soul!
Fyodor Dostoyevsky

We, human beings, have evolved on this beautiful planet living outdoors for most of our existence and wearing minimal clothing. So, daily exposure to sunlight and sunbathing is programmed into our bodies, they are not optional for us! We have talked about vitamin D production in the skin under sunlight (in the chapter on cod liver oil). We need to expose our whole body to the sun in order to produce good amounts of this vital vitamin, which is made from molecules of cholesterol in the skin. We now know that something even more amazing happens during sunbathing: newly formed vitamin D and cholesterol in the skin get sulphated, which makes them water-soluble![31] Why is this important? Because cholesterol and vitamin D are not water-soluble; the body has to package them appropriately to deliver to places where they are needed, which takes time. Sulphated vitamin D and cholesterol go into your blood in seconds and get around the body easily because they are water-soluble. Recent research has discovered that these molecules are some of the most powerful detoxifying and cancer-destroying substances known to science.[31] So, when we sunbathe we detoxify and remove cancer cells from our bodies!

Recent misguided fear of sun has caused an epidemic of vitamin D deficiency in the Western world. This deficiency is now one of the recognised causes of many chronic diseases. There is no connection between skin cancer and sun exposure, as far as solid science is concerned.[32-43] However, commercial powers that profit from sunscreen lotion sales have launched a multibillion propaganda campaign, which unfortunately has influenced the medical profession as well.[42] This propaganda has created sun phobia in the population. Incidentally, many sunscreen lotions contain chemicals that have been proven to cause skin cancer.[42,43] I do not recommend using any of them! In order not to burn, it is important to build sunbathing time gradually while developing the brown pigment in your skin (suntan). When your skin turns brown you are better protected from burning. Obviously, it is important to sunbathe sensibly, particularly in tropical and other hot areas of the world. In such places we should sunbathe in the early morning and late afternoon, but stay in the shade in the middle of the day when the sun is at its strongest. (This is usually what the local people do!). In cooler counties we need to sunbathe in the middle of the day to get any tan at all and to produce vitamin D in the skin. If you get sunburnt apply sour cream, live yogurt or kefir, homemade tallow, coconut oil and essential oil of lavender to the skin and stay out of the sun for a couple of days.

Sensible sunbathing is not only natural for us, humans, but absolutely essential. Lack of sun exposure, and hence vitamin D deficiency, is the explanation for the fact that people with darker skin, who move to colder countries, are particularly prone to heart disease, diabetes, cancer and other health problems.[44] The pigmentation in dark-skinned people does not allow enough sunlight through, essential for vitamin D production. When dark-skinned people live in countries with lots of strong sunlight, they do not have this problem. So, in colder countries, taking any opportunity to sunbathe is particularly important for dark-skinned people.

A growing proportion of people in the Western world develop a health problem called photosensitivity; they get an itchy skin rash if they sunbathe.[45] Our skin is a major site for storing pharmaceutical drugs and other toxins, particularly chemically mutilated fatty acids from vegetable and cooking oils (trans fats). Sunbathing initiates removal of toxic chemicals out of the skin and the rest of the body, which causes the itchy rash in toxic people.[45] For these people I recommend taking steps to detoxify their skin prior to the sunbathing season. A natural detoxifying substance, called beta-carotene, targets the skin and can prepare you for sunbathing in a matter of months. Drinking freshly pressed carrot juice daily (and green juices) and taking supplements of beta-carotene has a good record in removing photosensitivity.[46] The GAPS Nutritional Protocol will gradually cleanse the skin and the rest of the body and remove photosensitivity permanently.

Intolerance of the sun is also common amongst people with ginger hair, freckles and light-coloured skin (the so-called Viking descendants). These people evolved eating salmon and other oily fish daily, high-fat milk from northern breeds of cows (Highland cow, Shetland cow and other rare breeds) and fatty lamb. Today most of these Viking descendants live on bread, sugar, vegetable oils and other modern 'foods' and do not consume their ancestral diets. I have had clinical experience with a few such people, who could not spend any time in the sun at all before commencing the GAPS Nutritional Protocol. After about a year on the programme, they discovered that they could sunbathe without burning and could develop a nice tan.

Many wonderful things happen when we spend time outside in the sun, even if the weather is cold and we have to be warmly dressed. For example, it is important for us to receive enough sunlight during the day in order to have a good sleep at night. Melatonin is a hormone essential for good sleep and many other vital functions in the body. It can only be produced by your brain if it has received enough sunlight during the day through your eyes.[47] If you spend your days indoors in artificial light, particularly in front of computer or TV screens, then your melatonin production may become abnormal. This can lead to many health problems, such as poor sleep, poor immune function, poor brain function and a propensity for developing autoimmune disease and cancer.[48] Wearing sunglasses on a regular basis is a major cause of melatonin deficiency in our modern world – a very unhealthy habit![49] People who habitually use sunglasses can develop sensitivity to daylight: they cannot tolerate any amount of sunlight without dark glasses, even on a cloudy day. This can also happen to people with vitamin A deficiency. The GAPS Diet will remove vitamin A deficiency quite quickly. In the meantime, for people with this problem, I recommend making it a daily routine to sit facing the sun with your eyes closed (without any glasses!). Start from any amount of time you can tolerate per day, then gradually increase to at least one hour per day. The sunlight will shine through your closed eyelids, and gradually train your eyes to accumulate enough vitamin A and other nutrients to tolerate bright daylight without any problems. This measure can also improve your eyesight and, in combination with the GAPS Diet, in my clinical experience, has removed many chronic eye problems in children and adults.

Sunbathing is not optional for humans! When you sunbathe (expose your whole body to the sunlight without clothes) different parts of the sunlight spectrum go through your body, reducing the growth of pathogenic microbes and parasites, removing cancer cells and rebalancing your physiology on a bio-physical level (on the level of electromagnetic properties of atoms and molecules).[50] The physical properties of water inside your body change when you are exposed to the sun. Your immune system gets rebalanced and strengthened, your hormonal balance normalises, your nervous system improves its functions; the whole body gets into harmony with the environment and within itself. Good health is harmony! The sun is our friend, it always has been our friend. It is a source of all life on the planet and there can be no good health without it! GAPS people need to spend as much time as possible outdoors in the sunlight in order to recover from any chronic illness.

5. Juicing

Juicing is a time-proven way of detoxifying, taking out various poisons without side effects or harmful complications.[51] And a very tasty way too.

Children in particular love it! Thousands of people all over the world free themselves from deadly diseases with juicing. Dozens of books have been published on this subject full of testimonies and hundreds of wonderful recipes. Some very big names in natural medicine have strongly advocated juicing and used it actively in the treatment of their patients – Dr Gerson and Dr Norman Walker, for example. Hundreds of scientific studies have been published on the health benefits of fresh raw fruit and vegetables. Juices provide all the goodness from these fruit and vegetables in a concentrated form and in large amounts. For example, to make a glass of carrot juice you need a pound of carrots. Nobody can eat a pound of carrots at once, but you can get all the cleansing and nutrition from them by drinking the juice. On top of that, juicing removes the fibre, which impairs absorption of many nutrients in fruit and vegetables and aggravates the condition in the already sensitive digestive system of a GAPS patient. The digestive system has virtually no work to do in digesting juices, they get absorbed in 20–25 minutes.[51] Drinking two glasses a day of freshly extracted juice will provide your patient with many cleansing substances and useful nutrients. A combination of pineapple, cabbage, carrot and a little bit of beetroot in the morning will prepare the digestive system for the coming meals, stimulating stomach acid production and pancreatic enzymes production. A mixture of carrot, apple, celery, greens and beetroot has a wonderful liver-cleansing ability. Green juices from leafy vegetables (spinach, lettuce, parsley, dill, carrot and beet tops) with some tomato and lemon are great sources of magnesium. Cabbage, apple and celery juice stimulates digestive enzyme production and is a great kidney cleanser. There is an endless number of healthy and tasty variations you can make from whatever fruit and vegetables you have available at home. To make the juice taste nice, particularly for children, generally try to have 50% of less tasty but highly therapeutic ingredients: carrot, small amount of beetroot (no more than 5% of the juice mixture), celery, cabbage, lettuce, greens – spinach, parsley, dill, basil, fresh nettle leaves, fresh dandelion leaves, beet tops, carrot tops, white and red cabbage – and 50% of some tasty ingredients to soften the taste of the other ingredients: pineapple, apple, orange, grapefruit, grapes, mango, etc. (for more details look in the chapter *What we shall eat and why, with some recipes*).

It is important to use only chemical-free vegetables, fruit and greens for juicing. Organic standards have been compromised, but it is still safer to buy organic than not. But the best source of vegetables and fruit is your own garden or someone else's chemical-free garden.

What about fibre? Drinking juices doesn't mean that the patient stops eating fresh fruit and vegetables, providing there is no diarrhoea and the person is ready for consuming fibre. Treat the juices like a supplement of concentrated amounts of nutrients in a glass. They should be taken on an empty stomach 20–25 minutes before food and 2–2 ½ hours after a meal.

But can't we just buy juices in the shops? The answer is a big NO! Juices in the shops have been processed and pasteurised, which destroys all the enzymes and most vitamins and phytonutrients. They are a source of processed sugar, which will feed unhealthy bacteria and fungi in the gut. In freshly extracted juice the natural sugars are balanced with active enzymes and other substances, which allow the body to use the juice in a healthy manner. When you make your juice at home you know what you put into it, you know that it is fresh without any contamination and oxidation, and you can have great fun mixing different fruit and vegetables together, making different tasty combinations. There are a large number of books on juicing with wonderful recipes for every health problem and every occasion.

In the GAPS Nutritional Protocol we often turn juices into ***GAPS shakes*** by whisking 1–2 raw eggs and 1–4 tablespoons of homemade raw sour cream or coconut oil into a glass of freshly pressed juice. This turns the juice into a milkshake consistency, which most people find delicious. Juices have a high content of natural sugars; adding fat in the form of sour cream or coconut oil and protein in the form of raw eggs balances the sugars in the juice, providing a complete mixture of nutrients necessary for cleansing and feeding the body. On top of that, regular consumption of the GAPS shakes is effective at removing bile stones from the liver (read more about this in the chapter *Liver And Lungs*). Some people replace their breakfast with the GAPS shake, particularly if they have limited time in the morning.

The eggs need to be fresh from pastured chickens and we use both the yolk and the white, unless the person has an anaphylactic reaction to egg. The majority of people with egg allergy are sensitive to egg white and not to egg yolk (though it is possible to be allergic to both). If a person cannot tolerate the egg white, use raw egg yolks only in this recipe (carefully separated from the whites). Raw egg whites have been used in traditional cultures for removing toxic metals and other poisons from the body; cooking the egg is thought to reduce or remove this ability. Remember, that in the GAPS Nutritional Protocol we pay attention only to anaphylactic type allergies (the dangerous type). Non-anaphylactic reactions are due to the damaged gut wall and we work on healing and sealing the gut wall with the GAPS Diet in order to deal with these allergies. If, in your case, the reaction to egg is serious and immediate, then initially avoid eggs and follow the GAPS Introduction Diet. When enough healing has happened in your digestive system, you may be able to introduce raw eggs slowly and gradually.

Like any other detoxifying procedure, juicing and consuming GAPS shakes should be introduced when the person is ready for it. Start from a few tablespoons of the juice per day, diluted with water, and see how you tolerate it. As your tolerance improves you will be able to increase the amounts of juices and GAPS shakes to two glasses per day, gradually and slowly.

Juicing as part of the GAPS Nutritional Protocol works as a gentle way of detoxifying. I would like to emphasise that at other times of the day the person needs to follow the GAPS Diet. The animal protein and fats in the diet will make sure that the body handles sugars from juices appropriately. People who try to live entirely on juices for long periods of time can develop an unhealthy condition called fatty liver (non-alcoholic fatty liver disease), where sugars from juices can get stored in the liver as fat.[52] The major causes of this problem are processed carbohydrates, sugar and soft drinks with high-fructose corn syrup, but a prolonged period of only drinking fruit juices can do it too.

To turn your juice into a powerful immune remedy, consider adding *black elderberries* to it. Black elderberry is a small tree, which grows pretty much everywhere from cold to very warm climates. In spring it bears large clusters of tiny whitish flowers, which at the end of the summer turn into small juicy black berries. The medicinal properties of this plant have been appreciated for centuries. Its flowers, berries, leaves and bark were traditionally used for treating colds, pneumonia, flu, sore throat, hay fever, wounds, eye infections and many other ailments. In England the berries are still used for making elderberry wine, in Scandinavia the flowers are used for making elderflower cordial. Black elderberry has strong immune-stimulating properties and it is one of the most powerful antiviral remedies.[53] You do not have to be an experienced herbalist to use this plant. Many people have this tree in their gardens as it is quite decorative. At the end of the summer collect clusters of berries. Make sure that you collect ripe berries – ripe berries are very black and squashy. At home separate the berries from their twigs using a fork. Put the berries into small plastic bags or small containers and freeze them. When you start juicing, particularly in the cold season, make it your bedtime routine to take 1–2 tablespoons of berries out of the freezer and leave them at room temperature to defrost overnight. In the morning juice them together with any fruit and vegetables you planned to use. During the cold season, together with the GAPS Diet, these berries will help you to minimise any possibility of colds for your family.

You can also collect elderberry flowers in spring and freeze them. During the winter they make a very pleasant aromatic tea, or you can just crush them, while frozen, with your hand and add them to your salads. The flowers also have strong immune-stimulating properties. Use them as a tea to remedy colds, flu and fever. The same tea can be used topically on wounds and grazes, sunburn, frostbites and sore eyes. It is also a traditional remedy for hay fever.[54]

In conclusion: reducing exposure to environmental toxins and natural methods of removing toxins from the body are an important part of the GAPS Nutritional Protocol. The human body is part of Nature! The closer we can get to Nature and all its wonders, the healthier our bodies will be. Normalising gut flora, appropriate nourishing diet, sunbathing, swimming in natural waters, walking barefoot, juicing and avoiding exposure to toxins are natural measures which work well and without any side effects. They will allow your detoxification system to recover and start working again! This system is very powerful and is perfectly designed to take care of your daily exposures to toxicity.

In the majority of GAPS people, the simple measures described in this chapter are enough. However, for some people with particularly severe illnesses they may not be enough. Let us have a look at a specific problem, which many people have to face today: our body burden of toxic metals.

Toxic metals

Our environment is exposing us to many toxic metals in increasing amounts.[55–58] Some of these metals are called heavy metals because of their high molecular weight and density – mercury (Hg), lead (Pb), arsenic (As), cadmium (Cd), chromium (Cr), thallium (Tl) – while some are light, for example aluminium (Al). So, it is more appropriate to call them toxic metals, rather than heavy metals. Their toxicity for all life on our planet has been well established.[55] Many chronic degenerative diseases have been linked to the accumulation of toxic metals in the body: learning disabilities and mental illness, autoimmune diseases, neurological illnesses, endocrine problems, allergies, chronic fatigue and fibromyalgia, multiple chemical sensitivity and mould allergy, Lime disease and other chronic infections, and cancer.[59] Awareness about mercury toxicity from dental amalgam fillings has brought this subject to the attention of the public and the medical profession in the last few decades. Mainstream dentistry has been under heavy pressure to stop using these poisonous fillings, and they have been banned in some countries. Dental amalgam fillings are just one example of toxic metal exposure in our modern world, but the environment exposes us to many other sources of toxic metals, which accumulate in the body and undermine its health and resilience.[55–59]

Many people try to remove toxic metals in an attempt to recover from their illness.[60] Removing toxic metals out of the body is called *chelation* (from the Greek word for a crab's claw). Various chelating chemicals (chelators) have been invented over the years; this group of drugs was initially used by the military for treating acute exposure to heavy metals and other toxic substances. Since the advent of an autism epidemic in the Western world many doctors have experimented with using these drugs on children with learning disabilities. Some doctors have started using them for treating heart disease, multiple sclerosis and other maladies. Successful testimonies are published, but it is not clear how many people improve and how many see no improvement or even get worse.[60] When chelation is used in acute exposure to toxic metals, the results can be quite positive. However, in chronic exposure it is less clear how positive the results are.[61]

Many protocols and methods of chelating toxic metals have been invented and used over the years, in many cases raising grave concerns amongst the medical profession. Chelating drugs are drugs. Like any drug they come with side effects and complications. These are not benign substances. Let's have a look at some known problems.

1. Chelating drugs cause dose-related bone marrow suppression, which manifests as neutropenia and thrombocytopenia, which can affect blood clotting and blood immune response to infections and other toxins.[61,62] Patients who are on a chelation programme must have their blood composition monitored on a regular basis. In some children and adults this reaction can be very serious.
2. Chelating drugs cause an explosion of pathological fungal and bacterial growth in the gut and other places in the body.[61,62] That is why doctors who practise chelation advise their patients to deal with their gut dysbiosis first before trying to chelate. Anybody who has any experience with treating gut dysbiosis knows how difficult it is to 'deal with it'. GAPS patients have gut dysbiosis as their most basic and primary pathology and, despite all the experience of treating it, we still cannot say whether you can completely get rid of it.
3. In addition to taking out toxic metals, chelating drugs bind essential minerals and also take them out of the body. That is why most chelation protocols include very heavy supplementation with a large number of different nutrients.[60–62]
4. Patients on chelating drugs show high amounts of enzymes called transaminases in their blood, which is an indication of liver damage.[63]
5. Chelating drugs are contraindicated in people with renal problems because they have a damaging effect on kidneys. Kidney function and liver function have to be regularly monitored during chelation.[62–64]
6. During chelation a long list of side effects are reported: regression in mental symptoms, anorexia, fatigue, irritability, nausea, sleep disturbances, diarrhoea, flatulence and a skin rash. In some cases doctors

have observed serious complications, such as Stevens–Johnson Syndrome (severe toxic reaction with high fever, diarrhoea, polyarthritis, erosive skin rash, myalgia, pneumonitis – usually treated with steroid medication), haemolysis (red blood cell destruction), serious neutropenia (low count of blood cells, called neutrophils, which are involved in immune response) and thrombocytopenia (low count of thrombocytes, which are blood cells mainly responsible for blood clotting).[62,63]

7. Many people improve while taking standard chelation drugs, but they regress back to their previous state as soon as chelation stops.[64-66] One explanation for this phenomenon may be that these patients reaccumulate toxic metals from the environment, because their own detoxification system is unable to deal with these metals.

For years my clinical experience made me very cautious about chelation of toxic metals. One major concern is that chelating chemicals can redistribute toxic metals around the body, taking them out of fairly safe storage places (such as under-skin fat) and moving them into the brain and other vital organs.[61,62,64] This phenomenon is partially addressed by the *Andrew Cutler Protocol*.[61,64] The late Andrew Hall Cutler was a chemist educated in pharmaceutical kinetics (the knowledge about how drugs behave in the human body, how they interact with each other and our organs and how they leave the body). Having developed severe mercury poisoning from dental amalgam fillings, Andrew Cutler used his professional knowledge to try and develop a safe protocol for chelation of toxic metals for himself. He helped many other people to do the same. He wrote two books on the subject: *Amalgam Illness: Diagnosis and Treatment* and *Hair Test Interpretation: Finding Hidden Toxicities*.[61] Andrew Cutler added a major piece to the puzzle of chelation – working with chelating substances based on their half-life. The half-life of a chemical is how long it takes to lose half of its initial strength and ability. When we take a chelating substance, it binds to mercury or another toxic metal and starts moving it around the body. When the half-life of this chemical is reached, it gets weaker and is no longer able to hold on to that molecule of mercury, dropping it wherever in the body this happens. When we accumulate mercury, lead or any other toxic metal over a prolonged period of time, the body will work hard to store these poisons in safe places, tucking them away in fat cells or somewhere else, where they will not do too much harm. Chelating chemicals remove toxic metals out of those safe storage places and carry them around the body. When its half-life is reached, the chelator may drop the toxic metal in vital organs and tissues, where they will do much more harm compared to where they were stored before. Chelating drugs are known to redeposit mercury and other toxic metals in the brain, the rest of the nervous system, bone marrow and other vital organs, which can cause many symptoms and even trigger a new illness.[61.62,64] That is why, according to Andrew Culter, it is very important to take a new dose of any chelating chemical as soon as its half-life is reached, in the hope that this new dose will pick up the mercury and other toxic metals, which were dropped by the previous dose.

Andrew Cutler used three chelators: ALA (*alpha lipoic acid*), based on its half-life of three hours, DMSA (*dimercaptosuccinic acid*) with a half-life of four hours and DMPS (*dimercaptopropanesulfonate sodium*) with a half-life of eight hours. Based on his knowledge of chemistry he did not recommend any other chelators and specifically warned against using many of the common ones, including natural chelators, such as cilantro and chlorella.

He explained that ALA (*alpha lipoic acid*), which is often prescribed as an antioxidant by the medical profession without any knowledge that it is a powerful chelator, will redeposit toxic metals from safe places into vital organs in the body after three hours (its half-life). Unfortunately, the mainstream medical profession often recommends that ALA is taken once or twice a day in quite a large dose. According to Andrew Cutler, chelating chemicals must be taken in very small doses and for a short period of time: usually three days. The person must then take a rest of at least four days before taking chelators for another three days ('a round of chelation'). During those three days the person uses an alarm clock to make sure that he/she takes ALA every three hours day and night, DMSA every four hours and DMPS every eight hours. This protocol is followed for two years or longer in an attempt to remove toxic metals slowly and gently.[64]

ALA (*alpha lipoic acid*) is produced by the human body naturally. It is available as a nutritional supplement without prescription and, perhaps, is the safest chelator used in the Cutler Protocol. It is fat-soluble and gets into all organs and tissues. DMSA (dimercaptosuccinic acid) and DMPS (dimercaptopropanesulfonate sodium), however, are not fat-soluble and cannot get inside cells and many organs. They are synthetic drugs available only through prescription in the Western world; they have many side effects and negative influences on the body. They raise serious concerns amongst experienced biochemists, who consider them to be only partially effective at holding on to toxic metals.[66] Perhaps for all these reasons many people who follow the Andrew Cutler Protocol use only ALA.

There are successful testimonies about the Andrew Cutler Protocol online, but no scientific research has been done. It is beyond the scope of this book to go into this protocol in detail. If you would like to know more, I recommend reading a useful book, written by Rebecca Rust Lee and Andrew Hall Cutler, *The Mercury Detoxification Manual. A Guide to Mercury Chelation.*[64]

I have limited clinical experience with the use of alpha lipoic acid (ALA) according to the Andrew Cutler Protocol. Based on this experience I would like to make a few suggestions. The problematic time is when you stop taking the chelating substance: as the last dose of the chelator gets washed out of the body, the toxic metals which it was holding onto will be dropped in your body wherever they happen to be. It is essential to keep your body in a peak state to handle that amount of toxic metals appropriately. And it is important to assist your body in removing them as soon as possible. So, here is what I recommend:

1. In order to keep your body strong and able to handle toxic metals, follow the second or third stages of the GAPS Introduction Diet for 2–3 days after stopping the round of chelation. Avoid all fruit, nuts and cold salads. Focus on rich hot soups, stews and vegetables cooked in plenty of animal fat. Don't challenge your digestive system with any cold drinks or food, as cold can arrest digestion. It is essential to have fermented foods during this time, particularly from fermented raw dairy (sour cream, kefir, yogurt and whey). Fermented vegetables can also be added to your meals. Probiotic microbes are some of the most powerful chelators known to man; they will bind loose toxic metals in your digestive system and take them out in your stool.[67–69] It is natural for your body to remove toxic metals through the gut, so you need to assist your digestive system to do that work as best as it can.
2. During chelation and when the round of chelation stops, your body will be using the bowel for removing toxic metals in the stool. Allowing this toxic stool to linger in your bowel for any period of time may let some toxic metals reabsorb back into your blood stream. Microbes in your bowel can convert toxic metals into their organic forms, which are very poisonous for the human body (for example, methylmercury).[69] Reabsorption of these metals will force the body to protect itself by growing large colonies of fungi to bind these poisons. The fungal overgrowth can make you feel quite ill, with fatigue, a headache, inability to focus ('foggy brain'), memory lapses, aching muscles and joints, eczema, thrush and other unpleasant symptoms. So, I strongly recommend using daily enemas during the round of chelation and for a day or two after stopping the chelator. The enemas will flush toxicity out as soon as it accumulates in your stool. It is important to keep your bowel empty most of the time, so do an enema as soon as you sense your lower bowel filling up; typically, first thing in the morning. It is essential to add probiotics into every enema to

bind loose toxic metals and not allow them to absorb into your blood stream. The best probiotic to add to the enema is homemade raw whey, kefir, yogurt or sour cream. If there is anaphylactic type allergy to dairy, then you have to use commercially available dairy-free probiotic powders. *An adult* will do well using coffee with a teaspoon of natural salt dissolved in it (please, refer to the chapter *Bowel Management* for the coffee enema procedure). Always add a cup of whey per 1 l (2.1 pt) of coffee or 1/3 cup sour cream, kefir or yogurt. The coffee can be diluted with water to any concentration and should not be held in the bowel for any period of time; we are using it to flush the bowel. Coffee stimulates the bowel to empty quickly, and some of the cleansing substances in the coffee do absorb in a short period of time to stimulate the liver to cleanse. If you have to use a commercial probiotic powder, try to add 40–50 billion live cells per 1 l (2.1 pt) of coffee. *For a child* we can use warm water or chamomile tea with some natural salt in it (1 teaspoon per 1 l/2.1 pt of water). Always add a cup of whey per 1 l of water (or 1/3 cup sour cream, kefir or yogurt). If there is an anaphylactic dairy allergy, add 40-50 billion live cells of any commercial dairy-free probiotic per 1 l of the enema water. This solution will work for a child of any age, but for children older than 14 years we can use diluted coffee the same way as for an adult. For detailed explanation about enemas please look in the chapter *Bowel Management*.

3. The Andrew Cutler Protocol includes using many nutritional supplements during chelation, as the majority of people using this protocol live on a standard Western diet and may have nutritional deficiencies. The GAPS Diet is nutrient dense and will provide all the necessary nutrients for your body in abundance. So, in my experience, there is no need to add nutritional supplements, unless there is a specific individual requirement.

If you have had chronic exposure to toxic metals over a long period of time, I recommend not rushing with chelation. In chronic exposure, before following any chelation protocol, I recommend that GAPS people work on healing their gut for about a year. When the body uses the digestive system to remove toxic metals, they damage its integrity and the composition of the gut flora. So, it is important to make your gut strong enough to handle chelation. To make chelation effective we also need a fully functioning detoxification system. It may take a year of following the GAPS Nutritional Protocol to restore this vital system in a GAPS person. In chronic exposure your body has taken steps to store toxic metals in safer places. Your detoxification system and your gut need to be ready to handle the metals when the chelating substances start moving them around the body, so that these poisons do not reaccumulate in vital organs.

If you have had an acute exposure to toxic metals (from newly placed or recently removed dental amalgam filling, for example), then you may need to consider implementing the Andrew Cutler Protocol as soon as possible. Indeed, it is in acute exposure that people find chelation of toxic metals most helpful. Just make sure to stay strictly on the GAPS Diet and use enemas to remove toxic metals from your bowel before they do damage.

Our own detoxification system is very powerful and able to remove all kinds of toxicity out of the body. Unfortunately, in GAPS people this system is often broken down or does not work very well, that is why their bodies accumulate toxic metals and other poisons. The GAPS Nutritional Protocol will restore your detoxification system, so it starts working again. It is important to get it working first before trying to remove chronic accumulation of toxic metals. I have had children in my clinic who tested very high in mercury and lead before starting the GAPS Nutritional Protocol. After following it for a year, retesting found that these metals had gone without having to do anything special about them. It appears that the child's own detoxification system had recovered and handled the metals naturally. This may happen to anyone, adult or child. However, some people with severe chronic illnesses may still have to consider chelation later on in the programme, particularly people with multiple sclerosis, amyotrophic lateral sclerosis, Parkinson's disease, chronic fatigue syndrome and other severe chronic degenerative conditions. Many toxic metals are fat-soluble and often accumulate in high-fat tissues, such as the nervous system.[66] Some years ago, the dental industry changed the composition of amalgam fillings, increasing the amounts of copper in it. Unfortunately, these new high-copper amalgam fillings released more mercury per day into the person's body than the previous amalgams. As this new amalgam became the industry standard, a rapid increase in the numbers of people developing multiple sclerosis has been recorded.[70] In my experience most (if not all) patients with this terrible disease (and many other degenerative neurological diseases) have an accumulation of toxic metals in the brain and the rest of the nervous system. I still recommend to all these patients to follow the GAPS Nutritional Protocol for a year or even longer before considering chelation of toxic metals. It is essential to heal the gut, improve the composition of the gut flora and restore the detoxification system of the person before trying to chelate metals.

In our modern world it is impossible to have a completely clean body; we are all contaminated by man-made chemicals, including toxic metals. However, some people react to them while others don't. Many clinicians will tell you, that some patients show high levels of contamination on testing and yet show no clinical signs of poisoning, while other patients may have more or less clear tests, while being 'sick all over'. Sometimes we meet older people with 7–10 amalgam fillings in their teeth, which have been there for decades, and yet show no signs of mercury toxicity. Why does this happen? Because a healthy human body has a good ability to bind toxic metals, making them neutral and then imprisoning them – storing them somewhere in fat tissue, so they do no harm. In our toxic modern world, we probably all have these toxic stores, which stay with us for most of our lives. As long as our detoxification and immune systems work well, they can keep these stores under control. In GAPS people these systems don't work well, and the detoxification system is usually broken down. As a result, incoming toxins are not properly bound and neutralised; they cause many symptoms and can make the person very ill. On standard testing we may find that the person doesn't have large stores of toxic metals (or other toxins); the tests may look quite 'good' while the person is suffering greatly. A good example is *Hair Mineral Analysis*: it may show very few toxic metals stored in the hair, but this means very little. Based on his knowledge and experience, Andrew Cutler wrote a book on how to interpret hair mineral analysis in relation to metal toxicity, and the interpretation can be quite complicated.[71] According to his interpretation a 'good-looking' test may actually mean severe metal toxicity going on in the body.

So, the real question is not *how much* toxicity is accumulated in someone's body, but does the body have a problem with these toxins, has the body handled them appropriately and made them harmless or allowed them to do damage? So, before considering any chelating protocol, it is helpful to find out if the body has a problem with metals. The MELISA test (*Memory Lymphocyte Immunostimulation Assay*) is fairly expensive and you usually have to travel to the laboratory to do it.[72] However, it is a good way to find out if your body reacts to toxic metals in a pathological way. The test produces two results: an allergy to metals and a toxic reaction. An allergy to a metal means that your body responds to the metal in an over-exaggerated way, making you ill. Toxic reaction, however, is even worse: it means that your white blood cells drop dead on contact with the metal in question. People who have a toxic reaction to metals typically have consistently low white blood count.[73] The MELISA test is widely used by holistic doctors and dentists before deciding what materials can be put in the person's teeth.

I would have liked to be able to give the reader clear recommendations on how to deal with metal toxicity. But the truth is, we are still learning about chelation and we do not really have fully safe and effective methods of removing toxic metals from the body. Andrew Culter has added an important piece to this puzzle, but many pieces are still missing. We need more research in chelation of toxic metals and removal of other man-made chemicals. The vast majority of the Western population is contaminated with these poisons. Humanity's love affair with mercury is not over; it is still present in many pharmaceutical drugs, including some vaccines, in personal care products, in dental materials, domestic chemicals and other man-made preparations.[74,75] Lead is present in personal care products, paints and dyes, processed foods and many chemical preparations used industrially and in people's homes.[74] Most rice grown in the world is heavily contaminated with arsenic from agricultural chemicals.[76] These are just a few examples, but there are other toxic metals finding their way into our bodies regularly. The man unloads these poisons into the woman's body through semen.[77] The mother's body unloads these poisons into the body of her baby during pregnancy. In our modern world the majority of babies are born with a considerable load of toxic chemicals already in their little bodies.

The kind of environment we humans have created on our planet makes it impossible for any of us to stay 'free' of these chemicals; we are all contaminated. The only way for our bodies to cope with this situation is through proper nutrition and natural lifestyle, which keeps the detoxification system strong and able to deal with toxicity on a daily basis. If this system cannot remove the toxin from your body, it has unsurpassed intelligence to make it benign by 'imprisoning' it in some safe place, where this toxin can stay for the rest of your life doing you no harm, as long as you don't disturb it by inappropriate chelation or man-made 'detox' methods. The GAPS Nutritional Protocol is natural, we work according to Mother Nature's rules. As a result, this protocol has proven again and again its ability to recover a person's detoxification system and maintain it at peak performance. Mother Nature has equipped our bodies with every tool to stay strong and healthy. All we need to do is not stray away from Nature thinking that we are 'cleverer'. The more natural your lifestyle and your diet, the more chance you will have to stay healthy and feel well, no matter how much toxicity your body has accumulated.

To demonstrate this point, let us have a look at two clinical examples.

Case study 1. Melanie (the name has been changed), 48 years old, has had three large amalgam fillings removed from her teeth in one day. The procedure was done by a conventional dentist without any special preparation or protection. She has been following the GAPS Nutritional Protocol for many years prior to this procedure and was quite healthy and strong at the time. In the weeks after amalgam removal Melanie developed severe belching. Large amounts of gas were generated in her upper digestive system day and night, forcing her to release this gas every few minutes. This disrupted her sleep, as she had to wake up several times during the night to release the gas from her stomach. On top of that she developed loose stools and, when her bowel was full, she had cramps in the muscles of her legs and feet. Emptying the bowel always stopped the cramps. Apart from some inflammation in her stomach mainstream medical investigations found nothing wrong in Melanie's body.

Let us discuss what happened to Melanie. The amalgam removal released a large amount of mercury into her mouth, which finished up in her stomach. In order to defend itself from this mercury onslaught, the stomach grew a large colony of fungi to absorb the mercury and protect Melanie's body from its poisonous effects. This overgrowth of fungi produced abnormal amounts of gas in her stomach, causing the belching. The body tried to remove mercury and fungi through the stool in the amounts it could manage. When this toxic stool spent any time in her lower bowel, she got muscle cramps, because our lower bowel absorbs water out of the stool and substances dissolved in it. Enough mercury was absorbing from her stool to cause the cramps until she emptied her bowel. Mercury affects the peripheral nervous system, which often manifests with muscle cramps, sensory abnormalities and other neurological symptoms.

Thankfully, Melanie continued to follow strict GAPS Diet, so the only problems she got from her amalgam removal were belching and occasional muscle cramps. Overall, she remained healthy and well, had plenty of energy and continued living her life unimpeded.

The next case study will show you, what can happen when a conventional dentist removes amalgams in a person, whose body is not as strong as Melanie's.

Case study 2. Debra (the name has been changed), 40 years old, had two amalgam fillings removed by a conventional dentist without any proper protection or preparation. In the following weeks she developed severe depression, serious memory decline and panic attacks. She could not focus on anything for more than a few seconds, she kept forgetting things and soon became unable to work or look after her family. She had severe muscle cramps all over her body, to the point of not being able to sleep at night. On top of that, she started developing abnormalities in her muscle tone, loss of sensitivity in her limbs and other neurological problems. Debra had average health most of her life and was not on any special diet at the time. Her situation declined to the point of being hospitalised into a psychiatric facility and put on medication. At the same time, she was referred to a neurologist who diagnosed her with multiple sclerosis and put her on more medications.

What happened to Debra? Mercury released from her amalgams got into her brain and caused mental illness. Mercury got into the rest of her nervous system and caused neurological illness. Her body was unable to handle this mercury onslaught and allowed it to get into her vital organs.

Amalgam fillings, placed and removed by conventional dentists, are a major cause of acute mercury poisoning in our world.[78] Holistic dentists will never use amalgam fillings and are specifically trained on how to remove them safely. However, it is difficult to find a holistic dentist and their services are expensive. So, the vast majority of amalgam removals are done by conventional dentists, who are not trained on how to do it safely. As you can see, Debra developed a much more severe illness as a result of acute mercury poisoning than Melanie did. This is because Melanie had been on the GAPS Nutritional Protocol for years before the amalgam removal and continued to follow the protocol afterwards. Her detoxification system was working properly. Her body was strong and found a way to cope with the situation without allowing mercury into her nervous system or any other vital organs. Some species of fungi naturally live in a healthy human stomach and Melanie's body used these fungi to handle mercury, allowing fungal proliferation in her upper digestive system. Fungi are masters at producing gas. It is not comfortable to have belching, but it is much easier to live with it than to have the mental and neurological illnesses which poor Debra developed!

To conclude this chapter on toxic metals, I would like to encourage the reader to trust their body. The human body is a wonderful creation, it knows what it is doing at any moment of our existence! Whatever circumstances we create for ourselves, the body will find the best way to deal with the situation. We all have toxic metals in our bodies! If you had a recent event, which caused acute metal poisoning, then you need to take steps to help your body to deal with that situation; chelation may be imperative and should be done as soon as possible. But, if your exposure was chronic or happened a long time ago, then there is no need to rush with chelation. Prepare your body first for such intervention by following the GAPS Nutritional Protocol. For some people the good news is, that after a year on this protocol, they find that metals are not an issue for them anymore! For other people with more severe health problems, chelation can be done later in the programme, when the body is stronger.

The goal for all of us is to reach a point where we are strong, healthy and feel well enough to live our lives without worrying about how many toxins may be stored in our bodies. We can delegate that work to the body and trust that it will take care of toxicity in the best possible way for us, as long as we feed it well and look after it with kindness and respect.

Bowel Management

Well-functioning balanced gut flora is essential for forming normal stools and moving the bowel comfortably and regularly. GAPS people have abnormal gut flora. As a result, they often have abnormal stools. Some suffer from chronic diarrhoea or loose stools, some are constipated, others have various combinations of diarrhoea and constipation. Let us have a look at some of the most common scenarios.

Diarrhoea

Diarrhoea is a natural cleansing reaction in the body and should not be feared. Many toxins are removed from the body through the bowel, and diarrhoea is the natural way for the bowel to flush these toxins out. Short term diarrhoea, when we have food poisoning or pick up a 'tummy bug', is an essential part of healing from these afflictions. However, when diarrhoea becomes chronic, it can be a problem in itself, draining nutrients from the body and making the person malnourished and weak. Many GAPS children and adults suffer from chronic diarrhoea.

The main treatment for diarrhoea, whether acute or chronic, is to stay on the first and second stages of the GAPS Introduction Diet. In cases of long term profuse watery diarrhoea, we have to exclude all plant foods for a while: the person has to stay on the GAPS No-Plant Diet. Once the stools improve, well-cooked vegetables can be slowly introduced. Fermented dairy products with high protein content – homemade yogurt, kefir and whey – are very effective at removing diarrhoea in the majority of cases. They should be introduced quite rapidly right from the beginning of the programme in fairly large amounts per day; as much as the patient is comfortable to consume. Adding them to meat stock and consuming a cup of this mixture every hour will deal with diarrhoea, and any damage it may cause, quite quickly.

If the person has an anaphylactic-type allergy to dairy then, of course, it has to be avoided. In this case I recommend introducing juices of fermented vegetables and the liquid of the vegetable medley (p. 235). A non-anaphylactic type of dairy allergy or intolerance can be ignored in this situation. For people with non-anaphylactic dairy allergy I recommend starting from one teaspoon of whey (dripped from homemade raw yogurt or kefir) with every meal, and then increasing the daily amount as fast as possible. Once whey is tolerated, try to replace it with kefir or yogurt. Using goat's milk, ewe's milk, camel milk or any other less-common milk for making yogurt or kefir is often better tolerated by sensitive individuals. Unfortunately, cow's milk production in the Western world is the most commercialised, hence it produces more reactions in people than milk from other less commercialised animals.

People with ulcerative colitis, Crohn's disease and other inflammatory digestive problems, where diarrhoea is chronic and may have blood in it, should consider staying on the No-Plant GAPS Diet for as long as it takes for the diarrhoea to subside. Once the stools become more normal and the inflammatory markers reduce or disappear, then the person can try to move into the first stage of the GAPS Introduction Diet. Your doctor will be able to test your inflammatory markers for you. Doing GAPS Liquid Fast, when no solids are consumed, can also be helpful for this group of people.

Once diarrhoea fully subsides on the first and second stages of the GAPS Introduction Diet, the person can move through the rest of the Introduction Diet stage by stage.

Faecal compaction with an over-spill syndrome

In some GAPS patients, chronic loose stools and even chronic diarrhoea are the result of *faecal compaction*.[1,2] What is it? It is a situation when the bowel is full of old hard masses 'glued' to the gut wall, so the stool squeezes past these masses and comes out as diarrhoea, an over-spill. The stool can also be loose or soft, coming out in strange shapes due to squeezing past the hard masses. Sometimes, the stool can leak out in small amounts and soil the person's underwear during the day.[3] This situation can be seen as a combination of constipation and diarrhoea and is the basis for many chronic degenerative conditions, from autism, schizophrenia and other psychiatric problems to autoimmune disease, neurological illness and fibromyalgia. The compacted old faeces produce powerful toxins, which absorb into the blood stream causing serious symptoms all over the body. Passing stool typically does not shift the compacted masses and does not empty the bowel. Children and adults with this problem often spend a long time on the toilet, because they feel that something remains in the bowel and that the evacuation was not complete. Following the GAPS Nutritional Protocol resolves this situation over time. Using daily enemas (in combination with the GAPS Diet) helps to remove compaction from the bowel more quickly and more fully. That is why I strongly recommend enemas for people with faecal compaction.

Constipation

Many GAPS people suffer from constipation, which can be chronic or periodic. Abnormal gut flora does not allow the bowel to form normal stools and to pass them comfortably. Many chronically constipated people take large amounts of fibre to pass any stool at all. For these people I recommend starting from the Full GAPS Diet and eating plenty of fibrous vegetables and greens. It is not a good idea for a chronically constipated person addicted to fibre to start from the GAPS Introduction Diet, because it is low in fibre and is likely to make the person even more constipated. Once constipation is resolved, the Introduction Diet can be implemented when the person is ready for it and if there is a need for it.

Constipation is always a sign of deficient gut flora. The beneficial microbes that normally populate the bowel play a crucial role in proper stool formation and elimination. These microbes produce a whole host of enzymes and other active substances whose action is essential in proper stool formation. They stimulate the wall of the bowel to produce mucus for lubricating the stool and for passing it out as soon as it is ready. A healthy person should have 1–2 stools a day. The GAPS Nutritional Protocol will re-establish normal microbial population in the gut and normalise the stool. However, this work takes time and no child or adult should be left constipated. Chronic constipation is extremely harmful for the whole body. It lays the ground for all sorts of digestive disorders, including bowel cancer, and it produces a huge amount of various toxins, which poison the whole body.[4] As an immediate remedy for constipation there is nothing more effective than an enema. A patient with persistent constipation should have a daily enema every night before bed, followed by a warm bath with one of the following: ½–1 cup of Epsom salt, seaweed powder, cider vinegar, bicarbonate of soda or sea salt. After the bath, rub some Udo's oil, hemp oil, cold-pressed sunflower oil, castor oil or cold-pressed virgin olive oil on the skin of the abdominal area. These oils absorb quite well through skin and will help to relieve constipation in the long run. The whole procedure should be repeated every bedtime, until the patient starts producing a regular stool on his/her own.

Enemas provide instant relief from constipation and reduce the toxic load in the body quickly and effectively. Long-term resolution of constipation can be more difficult. In many people just following the GAPS Diet and taking probiotics does the trick, but other people may need more help. Every person is different, and long-term resolution of constipation can take different amounts of time. Here are measures which work, in my experience, for cases of stubborn constipation.

1. Impaired bile production is a major cause of constipation. When not enough bile is excreted by the liver into the duodenum, the fats do not get digested properly; instead they combine with alkaline salts and turn into a form of sticky 'soap' in the intestine, binding food together and making the person constipated. The most common reason for poor bile production is gallstones. Please, read the chapter *Liver and Lungs* on this subject, where a full explanation about gallstones is given and methods of dealing with that situation are described. Regular consumption of GAPS shakes is one of those methods. They provide a balanced mixture of freshly pressed juices with raw protein and fat, which stimulates bile production, cleanses the liver and allows it to flush the bile and gallstones out. Many people add their daily dose of cod liver oil or other supplements to the GAPS shakes, as it disguises their taste quite well, particularly for children. I recommend gradual introduction of GAPS shakes for every chronically constipated person from the beginning of the programme. Coffee enemas also help to unblock the biliary ducts in the liver and allow the bile to flow better, helping to resolve chronic constipation. Please, read about coffee enemas further down.
2. Removing dairy products from the diet can be helpful, as it is the dairy protein that seems to be constipating for some people. This does not apply to ghee and butter, which are almost pure fat and help to resolve constipation. For many people just replacing yogurt and kefir (high-protein dairy) with sour cream (high-fat dairy) does the trick. It is important to make the sour cream at home by fermenting fresh organic cream (preferably raw). Consuming sour cream on a daily basis will also assist in removing gallstones and improving bile flow.
3. Drinking more water per day helps in some cases. Drinking homemade kvass helps even more, as it provides not only water but probiotics and enzymes to digest the food better and to stimulate normal production of digestive juices. Kvass can be made from beetroot, cabbage and other vegetables, as well as fruit and berries. Please look in the chapter *What we shall eat and why, with some recipes* for ideas on how to make kvass.
4. For some people muscle fibres from meats can aggravate constipation. So, it is important for them to reduce muscle meats (particularly lean!) in the diet and replace them with gelatinous meats instead: soft tissues around joints, bones, skin of poultry or pork, bone marrow, tongue and feet. These foods are a staple of the GAPS Diet and should be consumed on a daily basis.
5. Increasing animal fat consumption with every meal helps in many cases (due to improvement in the bile flow, as one mechanism). If

you find it difficult to digest fats, introduce them gradually and take supplements of ox bile with every meal to help you in fat digestion.

6. Supplementing magnesium may help: use amino acid chelates of magnesium (magnesium glycinate, malate and other) as a daily supplement. As a laxative the person can use magnesium oxide occasionally to provide a quick relief. But it is not a good idea to take magnesium oxide regularly, as it can be irritating for the gut lining and interfere with healing.
7. Supplements of spirulina, blue-green algae, chlorella or dunaliella can be used as laxatives, particularly in children. Follow the manufacturer's instructions for doses. Low thyroid function can lead to constipation and iodine can help in improving thyroid function. Use iodine paint to see if your body needs more iodine. Please, read more about this in the chapter *Hormones*.
8. Castor oil applications help with constipation, particularly with children. At bedtime apply a handful of castor oil on the abdomen and massage it well with gentle clockwise movements (moving along the natural peristalsis of the bowel from the right hip up, across the belly and down to the left hip). Cover the abdomen with a tea towel, put a hot-water bottle on it and let the patient go to sleep. The oil absorbs through the skin overnight and helps to loosen the bowel in the morning. Other cold-pressed oils may also be used: olive oil, coconut oil, avocado oil, hemp oil or a mixture of oils.
9. As an occasional remedy, castor oil can be taken internally as a laxative to provide a quick relief.
10. In order to empty your bowel comfortably, it is important to make sure that your position on the toilet is correct. For most of our existence on the planet humans emptied their bowel by squatting on the ground; this is the right position for emptying the bowel. Modern toilets have been invented fairly recently and do not allow the body to get into the right position. Although they work for many people, for a constipated person a modern toilet can be an impediment. It is important to bring your body as close as possible to the position of squatting on the ground: the distance between your abdomen and your knees needs to be as small as possible. You can put your feet on a small stool or simply lean forward, bringing your chest close to your knees. This makes sure that all the organs inside you are in the right position to empty your bowel easily.

For a chronically constipated person it is a good idea to use all of these approaches, or most of them, at the same time. I do not recommend any mainstream laxatives, drug or herbal, as they can be harsh on the gut and many of them feed pathogenic microbes.

While we are resolving the physical causes of constipation, it is important to remember that involvement of the conscious mind in emptying the bowel can be an important cause of chronic constipation. In order to pass the stool normally and comfortably it is essential to take your conscious mind *off* the bowel function. Obviously, you have to use your conscious mind to get yourself to the place where it is socially acceptable to empty your bowel. But, as soon as you are sitting comfortably on the toilet, make sure to occupy your mind with something else, taking it away from the bowel function. The act of emptying your bowel has to be largely an unconscious act ruled entirely by the autonomic nervous system. Straining and thinking about it can interfere with this function. The autonomic system of your body will do the job for you nicely, if it is allowed to get on with it without any interference from above. So, tell yourself that your bowel knows what it is doing and will empty itself comfortably and perfectly, and after that occupy your mind with something completely unrelated to the bowel. Reading an interesting book helps, or watching comedy on a portable electronic device, or doing anything else that can keep your mind busy with something pleasant and relaxing. And it is important that the distraction is pleasant and relaxing! Do not attempt to do work or anything that can make you tense or stressed, because that will stimulate the parts of your nervous system which may not allow your bowel to open. In order for your bowel to empty comfortably your body must be in a parasympathetic state, happy and relaxed.

ENEMAS

A lot of people in the West find the subject of enemas repulsive. And yet this safe and very effective procedure is probably as old as humans. There is a whole chapter in *Manual of Discipline,* which was recorded two thousand years ago in the *Dead Sea Scrolls,* describing in detail how to perform an enema and how beneficial it is for health.[5,6] Another third-century manuscript, found in the archives of the Vatican, called *The Essene Gospel of Peace,* gives a full procedure for performing an enema and strongly advises doing it as the 'holy baptizing by the angel of water'.[5,6] The famous 11th-century Arabian physician, Ibn Sina Avicenna, in his timeless work *Canon Medicinae* advocated regular enemas to 'clear the body and soul'.[5] Regular enemas are an integral part of many natural treatment programmes for such serious health afflictions as cancer, psychiatric problems and autoimmunity. The enema kit is a common tool found in family bathrooms in many Eastern countries, performed without any medical assistance or prescription on children and adults alike.

I do not recommend enemas for patients who have diarrhoea with blood and mucous in the stool! These are people with ulcerative colitis, Crohn's disease and other inflammatory bowel conditions. The diarrhoea in these people is often accompanied by abdominal pain and other symptoms of severe inflammation in the digestive system. We have to work on healing and soothing the gut wall first, using the GAPS Introduction Diet or even the No-Plant GAPS Diet and GAPS Liquid Fast. For this group of people, after about a year of following the diet, and only when enough healing has happened in the gut wall, enemas can be considered.

For other GAPS people, including babies and small children, enemas are safe and can be very helpful for reducing general toxic load in the body, relieving constipation, removing faecal compaction, introducing probiotics directly into the bowel, cleansing the liver, healing haemorrhoids and dealing with many other issues. If the person is not prepared to try enemas, they can be referred to a local colonic irrigation clinic. Colonic irrigation can be very helpful, but quite costly. An enema kit is inexpensive and will serve you for many years. Home enemas allow you to be in control of the procedure and, after the first few sessions, people find that they feel quite comfortable with it. If you feel uncomfortable about performing the enema yourself for the first time, you can employ a nurse or a trained colonic therapist to help you.

You can get an enema kit from various health shops and health companies online. There are bucket enema kits for your bathroom and compact enema kits for travel. Any GAPS person who is travelling for longer than a couple of days should take an enema travel kit with them. It will allow you to deal with constipation, food poisoning, migraine headaches, haemorrhoids and other issues which may arise during travel.

What is the right temperature for the enema solution? If you are using the enema to clear the bowel, the temperature of the solution should be slightly lower than the body temperature. If you would like to hold the solution inside for a while, then make the temperature slightly warmer than the body temperature.

Enemas can be performed on babies, children and adults.

Enemas for children

For babies and small children (up to two years of age) use enemas in cases of constipation only: if the child has not passed a stool for two days or more.

Exclusively breastfed babies can be an exception from this rule: sometimes they may pass no stool for a few days without any apparent ill effect. Mother's milk is the most suitable food for a baby; it requires very little digestion and may absorb fully without leaving much waste. It is important to observe a baby in this case, making sure that she is in no discomfort and is completely well. Mother's diet is an important factor in the baby's digestive function, because everything the mother eats and digests finishes up in her blood and her milk in some form. A breastfeeding mother should stay on the Full GAPS Diet, making sure to eat plenty of animal fats and liver.

For children in this age group we use a *bulb syringe enema kit*; the usual sizes of bulb syringes available are 50 ml (about 2 oz) or 100 ml (about 4 oz). Boil some water and cool it down to body temperature. Dissolve a pinch of natural salt in it to bring the water closer to a physiological solution. Fill the bulb syringe enema kit with this water, lubricate the nozzle and the anus of the baby with homemade sour cream, coconut oil, olive oil, ghee, butter or any other animal fat, insert the nozzle into the anus and gently squeeze the bulb letting the water into the bowel. Remove the nozzle, hold the bottom of the child closed while gently massaging the tummy for a minute or two, and then put a nappy on and let the baby empty the bowel. Use only filtered or bottled water (not from the tap). For this age group I do not recommend adding anything else to the water apart from a pinch of natural salt. If your bulb syringe kit is new, rinse it well with hot water first before using.

For children from three to five years of age we can use a bulb syringe or an adult enema bucket. For this age group we can add some probiotic to the enema water: about 1–2 billion live cells per enema, preferably from Bifidobacteria group, but Lactobacilli can also be added. A few teaspoons of homemade whey can be used instead of commercial probiotics. It is important to add some natural salt to the water to bring it closer to the physiological solution: generally, 1 level teaspoon per 1 l (2.1 pt) of water is enough.

For children older than five we need to use an enema bucket as the syringe bulb will not provide enough water. We can add a probiotic to the enema water: some homemade whey or a commercial probiotic (about 3–4 billion live cells per enema), preferably from Bifidobacteria group, but Lactobacilli can also be added. We can also add 1 level teaspoon of natural salt per litre of water used.

The first enema is crucial to making the child comfortable with the procedure, so it is essential to make it as relaxed and pleasant as possible.

If the first enema went well, then your child will accept it next time without any apprehension.

If no one in the family has ever had enemas, then it is important for the mother or the father to do a couple of enemas on themselves first before doing it on their child! This will allow you to gain experience and make sure that you are not nervous when performing the first enema on your child. Children always know when a parent is nervous and will become nervous themselves; they may even refuse the enema, depriving themselves of this valuable help. Make sure that you have an adult helper, either to perform the enema or distract the child. You need to make this procedure as comfortable for the child as possible. Make a nice soft place for him/her to lie down – underneath the enema bucket and not far from the toilet, or have a potty ready. Have some favourite toys, books or a video handy to occupy him/her. Lie your child on the right side with bent knees close to his/her chest or hold the child in your arms. Apply olive oil, sour cream, coconut oil or any other edible fat as a lubricant on the nozzle of the enema and on the anal area of your child. It is a good idea to warm up the nozzle before doing the enema by placing it in warm water. Insert the nozzle into the anus of your child 1–2 cm (½–¾ in) deep and open the tap of the enema. Because you positioned the enema bucket at least 1 m (3 ft) higher than the child, the water will flow by gravity through the enema pipe into the rectum. Initially 100 ml (3½ fl oz) of water in the enema bucket may be enough, later on you may use more water (up to 1l/2.1 pt). The more water you can comfortably get in, the better the cleaning that will take place. The child will let you know when enough water has gone in. At that point close the enema tap and take the nozzle out. Try to encourage your child to hold the water in for as long as he/she feels comfortable. The longer your child keeps the water inside, the better the cleaning. Your child will let you know when he/she is ready to go on the toilet or a potty. Let your child sit on the toilet for at least 10-15 minutes to empty his/her bowel completely. Occupy him/her with toys, books, videos or anything that works to keep the whole experience pleasant. The relief of chronic symptoms that your child may get from the first enema will encourage your child to ask for it again. Children with chronic constipation and compacted bowel often love the enema procedure and ask for it when they feel they need it.

Enemas for adults

For adults we use a *basic enema solution* (1 l/2.1 pt of warm water with 1 teaspoon of natural salt and 1 teaspoon of bicarbonate of soda dissolved in it). This solution can also be used for children from the age of 5 years. Use only filtered or bottled water for enemas, not tap water. Bring some water to boil (1 cup is enough). Put bicarbonate of soda into a glass jug or bowl and pour this boiling water over it. This will release gas from the soda. Then add salt and enough cold water to bring the solution to body temperature. The salt will bring the mineral content of the water to a more natural balance for the human body. The bicarbonate of soda will provide alkaline pH, which is natural for the bowel and can help to bring yeast overgrowth down. This is the basic enema solution which should be used with adults and older children.

For adults, apart from cleansing enemas with the basic enema solution, I recommend using coffee enemas. If an enema is used by an adult as a constipation relief, I recommend emptying the bowel with the basic enema solution first and then finishing with a coffee enema. I do not recommend coffee enemas for children, though for older children (14 and above) they are safe to use and can be helpful in cases of haemorrhoids, headaches and chronic constipation.

Coffee enemas have been used as a healing remedy for some 100 years; they are particularly well known as part of the Gerson Protocol for treating cancer.[6] Coffee enemas are considered to be one of the best ways of cleansing the liver and speeding up detoxification processes in the body. They can be very effective as an immediate remedy for haemorrhoids (please, read more on this subject in the *Chapter A–Z*). Many people report that coffee enema gives a good pain relief as well.

The mechanism of its function is not clear, but it is thought that various substances in the coffee absorb through the rich capillary bed of the rectum into the portal veins, which lead directly to the liver. These substances dramatically enhance the liver functions and bring symptomatic relief for many people.[6,7] People with hyperactive thyroid function, particularly Graves disease, should not have coffee in any form, and that includes the coffee enemas. The same may go for people with high blood pressure, transitory ischaemic attacks, anaphylactic allergy to coffee and other life-threatening situations. If in doubt, please seek medical advice before considering coffee enemas.

In the Gerson Protocol four coffee enemas are performed every day.[7] A GAPS person does not have to do that; I recommend doing a coffee enema whenever there is a need, which can be once a day, once every few days or once in a while. Here is what my patients report after using coffee enemas: migraine headaches disappear; feel better, more clear-headed and more energetic; nausea goes away or greatly reduced; pain relief (anywhere in the body); better mood; acne clears up; other skin problems clear up; less reflux; better sleep; feel 'less toxic' and haemorrhoids disappear. Once a person has experienced the coffee enema, they usually know when they need another one.

In order for the coffee enema to have a full effect one has to hold the coffee in the bowel for about 15 minutes. In the Gerson Protocol people do four enemas per day, so their bowels are kept more or less empty all the time. For a person who does enemas occasionally, holding coffee in for 15 minutes can be very difficult or impossible because the bowel is full. That is why I recommend clearing the bowel out first with a few cleansing enemas before getting the coffee in.

Coffee enema recipe

Bring to the boil 1 l (2.1 pt) of water, add 3 heaped tablespoons of organic ground coffee (medium roast), boil for 2 minutes, then reduce the heat to a minimum, cover the pan with a tight lid and simmer for another 10 minutes. Cool down to 40–42° C (104–108°F) and strain. The coffee needs to be comfortably warm when it goes into the bowel. Make sure to plan the whole procedure, so the coffee is the right temperature for when you are ready for it. It is a good idea to add some homemade sour cream or homemade whey to the coffee just before using it (usually a quarter of a cup is enough for one coffee enema). This will introduce probiotic microbes directly into the bowel, as well as useful nutrients for healing the bowel wall. If there is an anaphylactic reaction to dairy, commercial probiotics can be added to the coffee instead (approximately 10 billion of live cells).

Coffee enema procedure

Before doing the coffee enema, it is important to have a good cleansing enema with the basic enema solution.

Lie down on the right side with knees brought up to the tummy (or the left side, if it is more comfortable), or assume a knee and elbow position (so the exit of the bowel is higher than other parts of the bowel, allowing the water to flow in). Let 0.5–1.5 l (17 fl oz–2½ pt) of the basic enema solution into the bowel, take the nozzle out, gently massage the abdomen for a few seconds and then empty the bowel. This procedure should be repeated 2–4 times until the water starts coming out looking fairly clean (no more solids). This indicates that the bowel is more or less empty. After that, lie down on the back for a few minutes and relax. This will allow the remaining faecal masses (further up in the bowel) to move along the bowel to be expelled (a so-called 'ileal flush').

When the bowel is empty, slowly get the coffee in. It is recommended that you lie on your left side, but it will work in any position that is comfortable for you. It is desirable to keep the coffee inside for 15 minutes to allow it to absorb into the portal system. In order to hold the coffee for that long, I recommend keeping the pipe in the rectum (after the coffee has gone in) to allow gases to escape. There is always some gas in the bowel and, when a bubble of gas arrives at the rectal area, it can cause an urge to empty too quickly. Changing position also helps to keep the coffee in longer. So, when there is an urge to empty too soon, try to turn onto another side, or onto the back, or assume a knee and elbow position. Don't worry if you were not able to hold the coffee in for 15 minutes; the procedure will still work if you had to empty your bowel earlier.

The whole procedure takes about two hours, so allocate plenty of time and have a good book to read.

As mentioned before, after the enema it is helpful to have a nice warm bath with sea salt dissolved in it, or Epsom salt, or seaweed powder or bicarbonate of soda (½-1 cup of any of those per bath). If you are planning to wash your hair in the bath, I recommend adding ½ cup of cider vinegar instead.

Enemas for common worms

A child or an adult with an infestation of pinworms or other common worms may have itchy anus, particularly at night, and grind their teeth during sleep. Sometimes parents find tiny white worms on the child's underwear. The mature female (of pinworms and other worms) comes out through the anus to lay eggs in the groin, which causes severe itching. The person scratches the itchy area getting microscopic eggs under their fingernails, and in the morning many of these eggs get swallowed with food. This is how the clever worm makes sure that its babies finish up in your upper digestive system again. It is easy to deal with this infestation with a simple garlic enema. Worms activate during full moon and coming up to it. That is why it is helpful to take the moon cycle into account when planning enemas for removing worms.

The garlic enema recipe for adults and children. Crush 1–2 cloves of fresh garlic and add to 1 l (2.1 pt) of warm water (40–45°C/104–113°F). Mix, leave for a few minutes and then strain. Use this water for doing an enema. Repeat this procedure every bedtime for 4–5 days until the itching stops. Repeat the whole course during the next full moon. Garlic solution can be irritating for the rectum, so I recommend applying homemade sour cream to the anus after the enema.

For a small child who tolerates milk well, there is a *traditional milk and garlic enema,* which is less irritating for the rectum. Put a medium head of garlic into 1 l (2.1 pt) of fresh milk, bring to boil and simmer for 5 minutes. Strain, and cool down to body temperature. Use as an enema. Repeat this procedure every bedtime for 4-5 days until the itching stops. Repeat the whole course during the next full moon.

The basic enema solution for adults (water with some salt and bicarbonate of soda) is a good remedy for removing many worms, because they find this solution uncomfortable. Worms in the bowel are always associated with fungi, such as candida, which grow around the worm, insulating it from the surrounding environment. Bicarbonate of soda is deadly to fungi; it exposes the worm to the salty and alkaline solution, making it let go of the gut wall. The basic enema solution sweeps it away and out of the bowel. I have fascinating photos of various creatures, which my patients have removed from their bowels during enemas.

There are other recipes for removing worms and parasites with the use of enemas. It is beyond the scope of this book to look at all of them. Please, research this subject deeper if your personal situation calls for it.

Enemas can be used for all sorts of ailments.

- Warm meat stock with sour cream, or whey and kefir with warm water can be used to sooth and heal an irritated and inflamed lower bowel. Fresh homemade whey is particularly soothing and healing for a sore gut wall; it is an effective remedy for chronic diarrhoea when used as an enema and consumed as food.
- People who cannot eat for some reason (after dental treatment or facial surgery, for example) can provide nourishment for their body through meat stock enemas. Make sure always to add plenty of animal fat to the stock, plus some whey, kefir or sour cream. Raw egg yolks can also be added to the stock, which will provide valuable nutrition for a malnourished person. Make sure to clear the bowel with the basic enema solution first, then get the stock in slowly and hold it inside for as long as possible. The warmer the stock, the more nourishment will be absorbed from it (it should be warmer than the body temperature).
- Dehydration and lack of electrolytes can be remedied very quickly by a warm enema with natural salt and a little bicarbonate of soda in it. This can be particularly useful during severe vomiting, when the person can lose a lot of water and salt. If the vomiting is accompanied by diarrhoea, use 1 l (2.1 pt) of warm meat stock with a cup of whey in it. Repeat these enemas every 30 minutes until dehydration is over. The meat stock should be made with gelatinous meats and salt should always be added at the beginning of cooking.
- The basic enema solution can work wonders for metabolic acidosis. This serious condition can develop due to kidney and liver problems, alcoholism, poisoning with drugs and chemicals, food poisoning, excessive sweating or vomiting, excessive exercise, in cancer patients and during shock.[8] An enema with warm basic enema solution can bring the person to a much better physical state quite quickly. Very high temperature can also be brought down safely by using the basic enema solution (make the solution slightly cooler than the normal body temperature).

To conclude this chapter, I would like to emphasise that the bowel can be the biggest source of toxicity in the body. It is important to be aware of this fact and manage your bowel in order to protect your body from toxins. In our busy world people often don't have time to pay attention to the signals from the bowel, which can lead to chronic constipation, compaction, bouts of diarrhoea, low energy levels, headaches and other problems. It is important to establish a daily routine, where emptying your bowel takes an important place.

Healing

The healer you have been looking for
is your own courage
to know and love yourself completely.

Yung Pueblo

Healing goes through stages. It is like peeling an onion: the body peels off the outer layer of disease and you start feeling better than before. Then the body accumulates enough resources to start peeling the next layer of the disease, and you start feeling ill again. Once that layer of the disease is removed you feel better again; until the body decides to peel the next layer off. Please understand that it is your own body that heals itself; not the doctor, not the diet, not the medicine or the supplements!

The bodies of people in the Western world today accumulate countless numbers or man-made poisons, all of which cause damage, manifesting as a long list of diseases.[1] When you start the GAPS Nutritional Protocol, your body will start removing toxins and healing the damage. But it cannot deal with all of it at once, because that would take a lot of resources which your body may not have. In order to deal with *all* the damage, your body has to prioritise: what part of the illness must be dealt with first and what has to wait for a while. Once the first part is dealt with, then the body will start on the second priority. Depending on how ill you are and how much healing your body has to accomplish, the list of priorities for your body to deal with can be quite long. So, don't be disheartened if a particular symptom does not disappear for a year or two; pay attention to symptoms that *are* going or have already *gone*.

For example, an overweight person starts the protocol and after two years they still have not lost weight. However, their migraines have gone, the psoriasis and polycystic ovaries have gone, the ulcerative colitis has gone and so has the depression. The body saw those health conditions as more important than the excess weight. Give your body time and it will get to that particular layer of the 'onion' when it is ready. Excess body fat holds many toxins. The body needs to be ready to face these toxins and deal with them appropriately.

A common feature of this 'onion peeling' is so-called histamine intolerance, mast cell disorder and other 'allergic-type' conditions (discussed in detail in the *Immune System* chapter). After a fairly long period of feeling better on the GAPS Nutritional Protocol people may start to feel as if their whole body is inflamed, and they start reacting to various foods, chemicals and even emotions. Very often these people are diagnosed with a health condition, which signifies that their immune system has launched a full-body inflammation. As uncomfortable as it is, we need to understand that inflammation is our friend! It is the best way the body has for killing infections and neutralising and removing toxins. If you have felt well on the diet for quite a long time and then suddenly develop systemic inflammation, it means your body has made a decision that now it has enough strength to start a new level of healing. It has enough resources to attack and remove pathogenic microbes and toxins, which it wasn't strong enough to deal with before; your body has got to the 'next layer of the onion'. Inflammation floods the body with histamine, prostaglandins, leukotrienes, complement, kinins and many other powerful molecules, all of which make us feel very unwell. We start reacting to various foods, which we could tolerate before, we start getting pain in our muscles and joints, headaches, nausea, skin rashes and various other unpleasant symptoms. Very often this is interpreted as histamine intolerance, because that is what our science has discovered so far and that is the information people find. Histamine is part and parcel of the inflammatory response, but it is not acting alone. That is why many people find that removing 'histamine-rich foods' doesn't solve the situation. This is because, when systemic inflammation is launched, many other powerful molecules will be active together with histamine. Why would the body launch systemic inflammation? Because that is the best tool for dealing with a particular lot of toxins in your body (and parasites associated with these toxins). These toxins and parasites are systemic (they are everywhere in your tissues and organs). Trust your body! It knows what it is doing at any time of your life.

There is a place for all forms of healing in this world! When something goes wrong with our health, the majority of people first go to a mainstream doctor. Mainstream medicine is very well equipped to deal with emergencies and life-and-death situations. However, when it comes to chronic diseases, mainstream medicine is unable to deal with the root of the problem. It may be able to make you a bit more comfortable by suppressing pain, inflammation and other symptoms. But it has no idea how to work *with* your body to help it heal. The symptoms are the way your body communicates to you that something is wrong and that you need to change your lifestyle, because it is that very lifestyle that is damaging the body and causing the disease. Symptoms are your body's way to call for help. Suppressing symptoms with mainstream medication is telling your body to stop calling for help and suffer in silence, while you continue destroying it. So, when you get a chronic disease, a mainstream doctor may be the last person you should go to for help. You need a health practitioner who understands how to work *with* the body and assist it in healing itself. There are many alternative health professions that may be able to help you: naturopathy, acupuncture, osteopathy, homeopathy, energy healing, herbalism, mind-and-body practitioners, meditation and other. But first you must address nutrition! We eat at least three times a day, sometimes more often than that. Every morsel of food you put into your mouth alters your metabolism, hormonal balance, energy production, immune system function and a myriad of other health parameters. Food is immensely powerful when it comes to health! Making a few changes in your diet can bring improvements in your health, which you would never have thought possible.

Apart from diet, what else has to change? Stress is a major influence on health and healing, so let us have a good look at it.

What level of stress do you experience?

Every one of us lives at a certain stress level, which has a profound effect on the body's ability to heal. Since Canadian researcher Hans Selye (1907–1982) discovered the concept of *stress*, generations of researchers have studied it. Selye defined stress as a *'nonspecific response of the body to any demand'*.[2] Any demand! Even positive things in life can be stressful. Healing is no exception.

Humanity has been learning about stress for more than a century now, so let us examine what we have learned.[3,4] Imagine that your body has a building, which we can call *The Stress House*. This building has four levels and every one of us spends some time on one level or another. This is the 'house' we live in all of our lives, so we need to know it.

The Ground Floor of Your Stress House

This is the level where we have no duties or obligations, we are at peace. Small healthy children live on this level and we all sometimes visit it when we are on holiday and are happy, carefree and resting. You wake up in the morning and there is nothing you 'must' do or 'have' to do today! On this level your body is eating, digesting and assimilating food nicely. It is healing itself, cleaning out any damage and rebuilding. The body is in an anabolic state, when it builds its physical structure and can lay down some healthy fat stores for a 'rainy day'. Your immune system is strong and deals with any threats quickly and efficiently. You are relaxed, you learn new information slowly and deeply, led by your interests, and life is calm. This is how you may feel when you have just graduated from school and have already been accepted by a college or university. Studies will not start till September and you have the whole summer for yourself, when you can do whatever your heart desires. This is how the Ground Floor feels.

The First Floor of Your Stress House

This level is more active and purposeful. Imagine that the summer is over and your studies at the college have begun! You still don't have any particular duties or obligations. You had a good rest during the summer and you are now enjoying your new student life very much. You are learning and achieving, making new friends and life is good. Your body is in a good balance, neither in anabolic (building itself) or catabolic (breaking down) state, so your weight is stable. You are active and purposeful, making good progress in whatever you are doing, while your body is eating, digesting and assimilating food well, and keeping on top of healing and building itself. You sleep well, you have plenty of energy to work and play, and your learning is focussed and much faster than on the Ground Floor.

The Second Floor of Your Stress House

You had a fun year at college, but now exams are looming; you have just a little time left to prepare. The stress level is growing and your body now has a specific short-term goal to achieve (to pass the exams). To achieve this goal the body uses its resources in a focussed manner, which is 'expensive' for your body. All your energy now goes towards preparing for the exams, while the functions of healing, repair, food assimilation and balance maintenance are put on hold. Your immune system is suppressed for a while, because you have no time for fighting infections, and your digestion is not efficient. Your body moves closer to a catabolic state (breaking down materials to produce energy), so you may lose some weight. Stress hormones are high, but within normal limits. Your mental state is on a high alert, so you can be short-tempered, impatient and aggressive. Your sleep is light and your focus is sharp.

This state is healthy as long as it is *short*! It is like a sprint where an athlete can put all he's got into running as fast as he can to the finishing line, but then he must stop and rest. Imagine that the finishing line never comes? This state becomes very unhealthy and destructive if it is long or becomes the general lifestyle of the person. Unfortunately, many people in our modern world live in this state most of their lives. They work hard, holding onto a stressful job, anxious that they have many debts to pay, they stay in stressful relationships and drive their children into the stress-filled life of a high achiever. When they have a break, they fill it with loud music, disturbing TV shows and partying in the belief that they are 'relaxing'. In this state the body is not able to heal itself, repair damage, digest or assimilate food well, protect itself from infections or maintain any balance. If you spend too long on this Second Floor of your Stress House you are on the road to illness. If you are already ill with a chronic health condition, staying on this floor will not allow you to heal. No matter what you do, what forms of treatment or medicine you employ, living on the second floor of your stress house will not allow you to recover from an illness. Instead the illness becomes chronic and new symptoms keep developing.

The Top Floor of Your Stress House

This is the floor Hans Selye described in 1936 in his definition of STRESS.[2] He subjected animals to damaging influences (extreme temperatures, pain, loud noise and negative emotions) and measured their body's response to them. This floor exists for life-and-death situations, for survival when the body has to mobilise all its resources. Being on this floor for any period of time is very damaging for your body. Hans Selye described stomach ulcers, enlargement of the adrenal glands and shrinking of the lymphoid tissue (suppressed immune system) in his experimental animals as a typical response to a *short* stay on this floor. If the stressful influence continued over a longer period of time, the animals suffered strokes, heart attacks, autoimmune illness and death. After Selye generations of researchers have described the body's reaction to stress in greater detail: the immune system and digestion are shut down, healing and repair stop, sleep and ability to learn or work are severely disrupted and the body is in a catabolic state (tearing apart valuable tissues for energy production in order to survive).[3,4] Occasionally life may present us with situations when we have to go up to the top floor of our stress house to survive, but it is not possible to live there permanently and it is not a good idea to visit that floor too often.

Behind our response to stressful events are stress hormones, which are largely produced by the adrenal glands, but also by our gut. The hormone that is considered to be the main problem in chronic stress is *cortisol*. It is a very important hormone fulfilling many essential functions in the body, such as regulation of blood sugar level, immune function, mental function, blood pressure and other. However, on the second and top floors of the stress house its release can become excessive and dysregulated. Hormones are the rulers of our metabolism, they affect everything in the body, so *abnormal levels of cortisol have endless consequences* for us.[2,4,5]

- High blood pressure, high pulse and extra work for your heart. At the same time your blood clotting increases. This creates a situation in the body which can easily lead to a stroke or a heart attack.[2,4,5]
- Cortisol changes the way we breath: your breathing becomes shallow and fast (panting like a dog), which removes too much carbon dioxide from the body, causing hyperventilation. This situation creates many unpleasant symptoms: heart palpitations, anxiety, dizziness, abdominal distress and nausea, headaches, asthma, blurred vision, muscle tension and many more.[2,4,5]
- Cortisol increases your blood sugar level on a chronic basis. This creates metabolic syndrome in the body, laying the ground for development of type two diabetes, obesity, heart disease, Alzheimer's disease and cancer.[1,2,4,5]
- Abnormal cortisol production dysregulates your immune system, leading to susceptibility to infections, chronic inflammation, allergies and autoimmunity.[4]
- Dysregulated production of cortisol affects the function and production of other hormones in the body (thyroid hormones, sex hormones and all other).[2,4,5] Cortisol reduces thyroid function and slows down your metabolism, which can lead to gaining weight and inability to lose it, depression and many other problems, but most importantly slow and inefficient healing. Sex hormone production is usually low and unbalanced when cortisol is high, leading to many abnormalities in that area. Our adrenal gland produces another hormone, called aldosterone, responsible for normal mineral metabolism and blood pressure. High cortisol gets production of aldosterone dysregulated. As a result, you may lose excessive minerals through sweat and urine and your blood pressure can become abnormal. Does your dog lick your feet or hands excessively? If the answer is 'yes', then you are losing too much sodium, magnesium, potassium and other minerals in sweat.
- Cortisol increases the blood flow to your muscles (to allow you to run away from danger), while reducing the blood supply to many other organs and tissues in the body: your digestive system, your immune system, kidneys and other organs which are not involved in a fight-and-flight situation. As a result, your digestion is not very good! You can be eating the best food in the world, but your digestive system cannot digest it properly or absorb it. By suppressing your kidney function and urine production cortisol can create predisposition to frequent urinary infections.[4,5]
- Cortisol is a catabolic hormone – it breaks down your muscle tissues to produce energy, converting proteins into glucose.[2,4,5] Normally your body prefers to use fat for producing energy; fat is

a very efficient source of energy and sustainable long term. Cortisol diverts energy production from using fat to using mostly glucose. As a result, you start losing your muscle mass, which can cause increasing physical weakness. A large percentage of glucose produced from the muscle proteins cannot be used for energy and is promptly converted into fat. This particular fat is stored around your abdomen. People, who are constantly under stress often have slim arms and legs (loss of muscle mass) and are large around the middle. For a person, who permanently lives on the second or top floor of their stress house, it is very difficult or can even be impossible to lose weight.

- Poor sleep.[3,5,6] Normal production of cortisol in healthy humans follows the sun: it reduces around sunset to allow us to relax and fall asleep. As the sun starts rising in the early hours, so our cortisol production starts rising to reach a peak in the morning, enabling us to wake up and face the day. This process follows the seasons: the day is shorter in the winter and longer in the summer. So, in the winter we need to sleep more and go to bed earlier than in the summer. In order to have a deep restful sleep, we need to have a low cortisol level. People, who stimulate themselves in the evening with a cup of coffee, television, loud music or doing stressful jobs, force their bodies to produce more cortisol than normal and at an abnormal time. Not only do they miss the window of opportunity to have a proper sleep, but they put themselves into a state of chronic stress. In order to heal from any illness healthy sleep is essential! It is during deep sleep that our bodies repair damaged tissues, remove toxins, rebalance the nervous and immune systems, rejuvenate and do a myriad of other vital jobs. Sleep is not a 'useless' time taken away from 'productive' daily activity, but just the opposite! For example, during sleep our brains are busy doing the very important work of processing information acquired during the day. If this process has not been completed by morning, your ability to put more information into your brain may suffer. Long term this situation leads to poor ability to learn, problems with short-term memory and depression.[6]

Our bodily flora is affected by stress profoundly and quite quickly. Starting from the 1960s, animal research has discovered that stressful situations alter skin flora. When the animal is under severe stress, healthy microbes which normally live on the skin disappear and are quickly replaced by pathogenic species, which appear 'almost out of nowhere'.[3] Similar changes were observed in the blood of animals. Normally blood plasma is bactericidal, but under severe stress it loses this ability and becomes a perfect food for pathogenic microbes.[3] Recent research has not only confirmed these findings but expanded on them. We now know that gut flora is severely affected by stress, losing its normal balance and composition and developing various pathogenic species of microbes.[7] The changes are usually very individual – different in different people.

So, daily stress has to be taken very seriously, because it has a profound effect on our ability to heal from any illness. Coming back to our analogy of the Stress House, *HEALING ONLY HAPPENS ON THE FIRST TWO FLOORS*! If you have a chronic illness and you are trying to heal yourself, you must stay on those two floors all the time and not allow yourself to climb any higher. For some people this involves difficult decisions – changing their job, breaking away from a destructive relationship or moving house. Your daily duties and responsibilities need to be re-evaluated: what is less important should be dropped, leaving only essential things for you to do. If you need help, then ways of getting that help should be explored. Mental attitudes need to be looked at (please, read about this in the chapter *Mind Over Matter*).

GAPS Nutritional Protocol will help you to become stronger physically and mentally and more able to deal with stressful events without 'climbing up to the next floor of your stress house'. Food is powerful medicine! Apart from food, there are many other methods for reducing your cortisol level and coming down to the two first floors of your stress house. People use meditation, *EFM* (*Emotional Freedom Technique*), breathing exercises, yoga, homeopathy, Bach flower remedies, massage, energy medicine, prayer, affirmations and spiritual development. There are natural remedies (herbs and mushrooms), called adaptogens, which can help us normalise our response to stress: ashwagandha, astragalus, bacopa moniera, ginseng, rhodiola rosea, reishi, chaga, codyceps and other.[3,8] We can make tea from these plants or take them as supplements. *It is important to take the first dose of an adaptogen first thing in the morning, before getting out of bed*! So, prepare your morning dose of adaptogens in the evening, and have them on your bedside table with a glass of water, so you can take the first dose while still in bed under your blanket. This will allow your body to start the day on the right level of your stress house.

Most importantly, we need to change our lifestyle! Make as much time for silence in your life as you can: every day put aside some time when you avoid music, TV, computers and other mainstream media and just listen to Nature or to your own thoughts! Contact with Nature and animals does wonders for our health. Stroking a fluffy pet for a few minutes has been proven to reduce cortisol level and high blood pressure.[9] Use only gentle comfortable exercise such as walking in Nature (without headphones!), as strenuous exercise is a source of stress in itself and will raise your cortisol level.[5] Make sure to go to bed no later than

9 pm to get a really good sleep and, perhaps, even have a nap in the afternoon. And, of course, our relationships with other people are very important! Loving caring relationships help us to produce hormones which oppose cortisol and reduce its effects on the body (oxytocin, progesterone, dopamine, endorphins and other).[10]

The good news is that stress is your body's *response* to a stressful stimulus, it is not the stimulus itself! That is why different people can respond to the same stressful situation very differently: one person is hardly affected by it, while another can fall apart. This depends on how the person perceives the threat. So, every floor of your stress house is very individual, uniquely yours. Life can be unpredictable and it is not possible to avoid stressful situations. The fact that stress is not the situation itself, but our reaction to it is good news! We cannot always control life events, but we *can* control our reactions to them.

To conclude this chapter, I cannot repeat often enough that it is your own body that does the healing. Mother Nature took billions of years designing the human body; it is an amazing creation! All the healing, repair and maintenance of healthy balance is programmed into your body. Allowing your body to do the work, listening to it, respecting what it is doing and assisting it correctly is the *only* way to heal from a chronic illness! Nature has no quick fixes, only humans indulge in such foolish ideas. Healing takes time, it takes a change in consciousness and in attitude to life as a whole. If you really want to heal from a chronic illness, *you* have to change!

Changing your attitude to life as a whole is a major part of healing. Taking time to think about your priorities and what is *really important to you* is vital. Some will say, that there is nothing accidental in life and the illness, you have, has a purpose. Maybe you lost your way in life and need to change your direction? Maybe there are some unhealthy attitudes that need to be changed? A serious illness may force you to re-evaluate your life, your attitudes, habits and relationships and make the right changes; the changes which may bring you true happiness. Healing is a journey of discovery, wonderful changes, huge learning curves and proud achievements. It is a journey of growth of the person inside you, which makes it a journey for life!

Mind over matter

The greatest mistake physicians make is that they attempt to cure the body without attempting to cure the mind; yet the mind and body are one and should not be treated separately!

Plato, 428–348 BC

I will never forget a patient of mine, when I was a young neurologist in one of the largest hospitals in Moscow – a handsome young man of 22 years of age from Ukraine, who was visiting his relatives in Moscow. All his life he had been fit and healthy. Just before his flight home he suddenly became paralysed from the waist down and was brought to our hospital by an ambulance. We conducted various tests, scans and examinations and could not find any physical reason for this young man's predicament. I spoke to a colleague in the psycho-somatic department and he recommended trying a particular medication. This medication temporarily disconnects the upper parts of the brain from the deeper more ancient parts of the brain. These deeper parts operate our autopilot, which makes sure that all organs work without our conscious involvement: the heart beats without us having to think about it, our liver and kidneys do their very complicated work without us being any the wiser, and our muscles know how to work and accomplish every movement precisely, without us having to think about what every muscle fibre should be doing. The upper parts of the brain represent our conscious mind. So, in effect, this medication could temporarily remove the influence of the mind from the body. The patient had an injection of this drug, and in twenty minutes he stood up from his wheelchair and walked briskly upstairs from the first floor to the fourth. His paralysis completely disappeared while the drug was in his system. Next morning, we had an explanation: the patient's relatives came to visit, and it transpired that this young man had been involved in a group crime back in Ukraine. Fearing retribution, he had fled to Moscow to stay with his relatives. The night before his flight, he had a phone conversation with one of his friends back home, who told him that the police were looking for him. He could not stay with his relatives any longer and had no money to go anywhere else. Naturally he was in fear of going back home. His mind could find no other way out of this situation than to cause a drastic illness in his body, which would delay his return home. This patient was not pretending, one cannot imitate a paralysis. The paralysis was created by his subconscious mind. Once the influence of the mind was removed by a drug, his paralysis disappeared. Over the next few weeks this patient recovered fully, once he understood what had happened to him. He had to go back home to Ukraine to face his responsibility.

This example shows just how powerful our mind is! Our beliefs, attitudes and emotions have a profound effect on our physical state.[1-3] Fear, worry, anxiety, despair, frustration, hatred, jealousy, resentment, selfishness are all capable of causing most serious physical problems. Research in this area shows that positive emotions flood the body with hormones and other active chemicals, which promote healing and recovery, while negative emotions do just the opposite: they flood the body with destructive hormones and chemicals, which induce inflammation and promote disease.[3]

Negative emotions, beliefs and attitudes can cause serious disease in the healthiest of people. For a person who is already ill, negative frames of mind are simply incompatible with recovery; they can and will undermine every effort you make to get better. So, if you have a chronic health problem and want to recover, you simply have no choice but to replace negative attitudes with positive emotions. I am afraid it is not optional; it is a must!

Of course, fear, worry, anxiety, frustration, hatred, envy and resentment are all very human and getting rid of them is easier said than done. I would agree that it is not easy, but we live in a world of abundant and easily available information, so you can always find help if you look for it. There are excellent books which will start you on this road, such as those by good old Dale Carnegie and Louise Hay.[4,5] Once you have read them, they will lead you to many more resources which will widen your knowledge in this area and help you further. If you have some particularly difficult emotional issues to deal with, you may find it helpful to work with a hypnotherapist, a psychologist, an energy healer or a spiritual healer. Various relaxation techniques, meditation, yoga, EFT (emotional freedom technique) and gentle physical exercise, particularly in the fresh air, will also help. But simply talking to a good friend can be wonderfully healing and will cost you nothing. Pets can be very helpful in keeping you in a positive frame of mind; their unconditional love can be a real comfort in difficult times. There are published studies which have shown that simply stroking a cat or a dog for 10-15 minutes can reduce high blood pressure, normalise pulse and reduce anxiety.[6] Contact with Nature is absolutely essential to healing from any disease! That is why, traditionally, all places of healing were set in a pristine natural environment.

The human mind has immense power, acknowledged through the ages by philosophers, scientists and doctors. If you do not *believe* in your recovery, then you will not recover no matter what you do![7] As simple as that! Seek any and all help you can find in order to plant a solid belief in your mind that you will be healthy again. Seek the company of people who will help you to develop that belief and avoid like the plague people who try to dispel it. If you believe in God, use prayer for recovery; there have been instances where people have recovered from 'incurable' diseases through prayer alone. Seek the company of people who make you laugh and help you to be positive. Avoid people, who are negative and who make you feel inadequate or hopeless. Every one of us, human beings on this planet, probably has about equal proportions of 'good' and 'bad' in us. If you absolutely refuse to see the bad in a person and focus only on his or her good side, then that is the side this person is likely to show *you*. Use this tool with people whose company you cannot avoid, such as members of your family. You may just discover how wonderful your family really is! Watch only comedy films and 'feel-good' films, avoid thrillers, horrors and films about crime. The same goes for books and radio programmes. Avoid reading newspapers and watching news on TV, as the news is largely negative, creating negative emotions with destructive biochemistry in the body, and will undermine your recovery. Every day, when you wake up, say to yourself: *What a wonderful day it is and I am going to get the best out of it!* Then live your day with this frame of mind. If it is raining outside, think of all the plants in your garden being nourished by this rain, think about the fact that every droplet picks up pollution from the air, so you can breathe clean air. Keep your thoughts under control all the time: positive, joyful, happy and grateful! Don't let your mind go lazy and slide down into anything negative. Remember that negativity will undermine your recovery.

If you are trying to heal a child, it is imperative that you do your best to keep your child in a positive frame of mind. Criticising, scolding, blaming, punishing and neglecting to praise can undermine your child's physical recovery. Unconditional love, approval of your child just the way he or she is and acknowledging every little success and achievement with sincere praise can do wonders. It is a known psychological phenomenon that a person can make themselves ill and maintain illness simply to get attention and unconditional love.[3] This phenomenon can be true in both adults and children. Give your child no reason to develop attention-seeking behaviour, give him or her plenty of good positive attention with laughter and fun, actively look for things to praise and approve, playing down all faults and mistakes. For example, if your child breaks something, instead of saying: "*You* broke it!" try to say: "It broke!"; this subtle change in phrasing will spell the difference between blame and simply stating a fact.

Involve your children in household chores: this will make them feel useful and worthwhile, give them self-respect and good reasons to recover. Even a bed-ridden person can do some useful chores. Don't forget to praise a job well done; a child needs to feel a useful member of the family and a much needed one. We, parents, are like gods to our children; our words and actions have a profound effect on their minds, and the younger the child the more profound is the effect. So, we have to be careful how we phrase our thoughts when we speak to them. Apart from not giving your child any psychological reasons to maintain an illness, constantly give your child many reasons for full recovery and motivation to get better. Keep telling them things like: 'When you are healthy, you will: ride a bicycle, play on a trampoline, have a party with friends, go paintball shooting, go skiing, go snorkelling, go diving, etc', depending on your child's age and interests. Engage in dreaming together about future fun. Keep your child's mind occupied by positive plans so they can forget the illness. Be very careful not to plant into your child's mind an idea that they are incurably ill, and do not allow anybody else to do that, including your doctor. No matter how grave the diagnosis may be, do not deprive your child from hope of recovery. In our litigious medical industry, there is a new phenomenon called 'not to give false hope'. Some doctors have even lost their licence to practice through being accused of 'giving false hope'. How can hope be false? Hope is not a science; it cannot be defined by a formula! People recover from terminal cancers, from the most horrendous traumas and injuries simply because they have hope. Never allow anybody to deprive you or your child of hope! The fact that your mainstream doctor doesn't know how to help you doesn't mean that the knowledge doesn't exist elsewhere! Just thank that doctor and move on. Keep looking for a solution which is right for you or your child.

Talking about positive frames of mind, it is important to mention one very old habit of humanity – complaining. Observe yourself and note how much of your day you have spent complaining about something. People complain about weather, politics, neighbours, family members, their health, doctors, their life and anything else. Every time we complain we are focussing on the negative. Worse than that, we make victims out of ourselves. When we complain, we put ourselves into the position of a victim of whatever it is we complain about. No matter how seductive it may feel to moan about being 'hard done by' and 'poor unfortunate me', being a victim is a very dangerous thing! The energy of a victim always attracts an opposite energy, that of an abuser. By choosing to be a victim, you attract people and events into your life which will bring you harm. At the same time your subconscious mind, which is ever present and listening, will do its best to really make you a victim. The illness you are complaining about can be made much worse by your subconscious mind, no matter how bad it already is.[1-3] If you really want to recover from a chronic illness, you have to stop complaining! It is a difficult habit to break, but it is a must.

Whatever we focus upon we give our energy to, so it grows and becomes bigger and more effective in our lives. When Mother Teresa was asked to take part in an anti-war demonstration, she refused. But she said that if someone organised a demonstration *for peace*, she would gladly take part in it. Can you see the difference between the two? The more we focus on the war, even if we demonstrate against it, the more energy we give to the war and the more war we create. If we want peace, that is what we need to focus upon. The more we fight disease the more disease we get. Instead of that, why don't we focus on *creating health* in our bodies? Our mainstream medicine is focused on 'fighting disease'. As a result, it is estimated to be one of the leading causes of disease in the modern world.[8,9] If you want to be healthy then HEALTH is what you have to focus on, all the time. Give very little thought to your disease and your symptoms. Instead focus on the overall health of your body (whatever good health you have at the moment), good things in your life, on new exciting plans and projects, living your life to the full and on being happy and fulfilled. Be conscious of *what* you are giving your energy to on a daily basis, *what* you are focusing upon, *what* you are making bigger and stronger in your life!

You have a powerful mind: if you keep it in positive mode, it can do wonders for you! It is beyond the scope of this book to go into detail about the many methods of altering your attitude to life to make it more positive. There are hundreds of excellent books written on this subject by very knowledgeable people. There are audio courses, video courses and electronic books. There are practitioners who will teach you one to one. Keep learning! Everything in our lives happens for a reason: maybe you got ill in order to learn something very important?

I would like to finish this chapter with a wonderful quote from Mahatma Gandhi:

> "Keep your thoughts positive, because your thoughts become your words.
> Keep your words positive, because your words become your behaviours.
> Keep your behaviours positive, because your behaviour becomes your habits.
> Keep your habits positive, because your habits become your values.
> Keep your values positive, because your values become your destiny."[10]

A few last notes

Everything is connected to everything else by a Presence whose power is infinite, exquisitely gentle, yet rock-solid.

David R Hawkins

Dear reader! I hope this book has been helpful to you. The GAPS Nutritional Protocol has existed for almost 20 years and has helped many people around the world. It is not an easy programme to follow, but for people with severe chronic illnesses it is easier to follow it than not. It will change your life and it will change you, as it has done for so many. To conclude this book, I would like to make a few last suggestions.

Healing from a chronic disease must involve spiritual work!

Have you ever wondered why every human creation is perishable? No matter how shiny and beautiful at the moment of manufacture, everything we humans make decays and eventually falls apart. The clothes you buy become old, worn out and turn into rags. Your new car starts slowly deteriorating from the moment it leaves the factory, and you have to repair it constantly. Our houses, furniture, tools, electronics, machinery, roads, boats, planes, bridges, cities and villages all break up or fall into ruin unless we constantly maintain them. There is wear and tear, of course, but human inventions fall apart even if we don't use them. Why? Because of a universal phenomenon, called ENTROPY. According to the second law of thermodynamics, every particle, molecule and atom keeps moving, spinning and jittering. This movement creates heat, which cannot be harnessed and gets wasted.[1] This loss of energy has been called *entropy*, and in our physical world it is ever present, leading all our technological creations into disorder and destruction. This law of physics applies to *non-living* objects only; they cannot resist entropy. *Living things* not only resist entropy, they actually harness and use it to their advantage.[2] So what is the difference between living things and non-living things? Scientists have been pondering this question for a long time, and so far have not come up with any answers. This is the most fundamental question of all: WHAT IS LIFE? What is it in microbes, plants, insects, fish, animals and humans that makes them alive, different from non-living objects?

To understand that, perhaps we need to examine death. Let us contemplate what happens to the bodies of humans, animals, fish, plants and all other living creatures when they die. A minute before death an animal's body is warm with an active metabolism and there is no entropy present. A minute after death it is still the same body (it looks the same, it is still warm and is the same biochemically), but the force of entropy has moved in and decay starts. Depending on the temperature, the body can decay in a matter of days. What was keeping entropy out before death? What was maintaining the body in its alive functional state? Why can a tree live for hundreds of years, growing larger and more magnificent but showing no signs of entropy? From the moment this tree dies, entropy moves in and the tree quickly decays. What force left that tree at the moment of death? What force was protecting its living body from entropy? Through millennia humans have made up many names for this force: God, spirit, soul, life force and other. No matter what name we give it, there is no doubt that this force exists, and it is the only force in the world that can resist entropy! As long as a body is inhabited by this living force, it thrives, grows, develops, loves, procreates, breathes, eats, feels and shows no signs of falling apart. This should not be confused with ageing, which has nothing to do with entropy. From the moment of conception a human body follows a complex hormonal programme: evolving from an egg into a baby, from a baby to a growing child, from a child to a mature adult capable of procreation, moving into old age when procreation is done, and living as an elderly adult for as long as the life force is there. No matter how old, as long as the life force is still present in the body, the person will live and resist entropy.

When the living force leaves, the body dies and immediately succumbs to entropy. But what happens when the living force has not left, but is weakened? The weaker the life force, the more chance there is for entropy to start creeping in. Perhaps this is the cause of chronic disease? What can weaken the living force, or spirit, or soul or God within you?

To understand that, please, observe Nature. Pick up any leaf or any piece of grass, observe a bird, an insect or a mammal, and you will realise how perfect they are! How infinitely complex their structure and functions are, how sensible, how well-thought out and how beautiful! Matter equals energy, according to the fundamental laws of physics; energy solidifies into matter. What energy could possibly have created the perfection of Nature? There is only one energy that could have solidified to create life on Earth – the energy of LOVE. This is obvious to anyone capable of seeing, thinking and feeling. The human body is part of Nature and has been created from the same energy, and is maintained by the same energy in its perfect state. Indeed, rare people who have this energy only, who do not allow any other energy into their being, are beautiful, healthy and well.

Every one of us can feel the energy of other people; this ability seems to have been programmed into us. Years of clinical experience has led me to an understanding, that full recovery from any illness is not possible without addressing the following questions: what is the person's prevailing energy? What kind of soul is within?

- Is it the energy of victimisation? Being a victim seems to be a favourite occupation of humanity; whole nations engage in it joyfully. How we love to complain about being hard-done-by! How sweet is the attention and pity of others when we complain! I have seen enough people who get ill just to receive this attention. If the person cannot get attention any other way, then what is their chance of recovery from a chronic illness? Very slim! Maintaining an illness is far more important for this person, than recovery. No matter what we do, the person will remain ill until they make a conscious decision to stop being a victim.
- Fear is another popular energy in humanity. Some people seem to want to be afraid of something, actively looking for something to fear all day long. They bounce fear off each other, getting more of it from the news on TV, newspapers, governments, neighbours, etc. Fear is nobody's friend! It creates disease, and it is not possible to recover from a disease while living in fear.
- Shame and guilt have very low vibrations. People whose conscience is not clear are in a self-destructive mode. If the person is serious about recovering from an illness, they have to face their actions and do their best to correct them. Apology is the minimum. Only then is forgiving yourself possible. And only after that can a search for the energy of LOVE begin. Without it there is no healing from a chronic illness.
- Living in resentment, pride, grief, apathy, dishonesty, greed or other negative attitudes creates disease and prevents healing.

We are talking here about the *prevailing energy* of the person, not the passing emotions, which all of us experience now and then. This energy determines every aspect of our lives, not only health, but relationships, work, hobbies and behaviour – the very essence of the person. Healing must involve spiritual work, connecting to your real essence, examining it, understanding it and moving its energy closer to the energy of LOVE. It is beyond the scope of this book to go into this subject in detail. Thankfully there is a lot of help available: good books, meditation and teachings from spiritual leaders. Everyone can find information that resonates with their personal situation.

Chronic disease comes to us when we need to learn something important on a spiritual level, when we need to evolve spiritually! Disease is your spiritual lesson; denying and avoiding this lesson not only prevents full healing of your body, but also the spiritual growth this lesson brings. Your spirit wants to grow, but your ego and mind may have another agenda. The lesson is painful, going through it fully is very hard work, so your ego and mind may offer you an easier path. Everybody has to make choices about how to live their life. You may decide to go the mainstream route and take medications to suppress the symptoms. This will make you more comfortable physically, while your body will continue to deteriorate. Changing your diet is not easy: you have to face your food addictions, go through die-off and detox reactions, not to mention all the cooking, shopping and cleaning involved. Going through this process requires the support and help of your family and friends, which may not be forthcoming. And recovery from a chronic disease may deprive you of that extra attention and compassion from these people, which may be very important for your ego. Life often presents us with hard choices, and it is important for you to think carefully about what you want to do: do you want to recover fully from your disease (with all the hard work involved) or live with this disease for the rest of your life? Do you want to take the spiritual lesson this disease brings, or are you not interested in that opportunity? Nobody can make this decision for you; this is your life and your choice. And nobody has the right to judge you for your choices.

If you choose full recovery from your disease, then you are making the first step on an exciting journey, on an adventure of a lifetime – a journey of spiritual growth through healing your body! It is a quest for something every human being craves – universal unconditional love. Every person with a chronic disease has to do some soul searching to try and understand what is preventing them from reaching the energy of LOVE – love for oneself and love for every living thing around.

Some people ask: how does one love oneself? The following points may help to make a good start.

Changing your diet to home-cooked best-quality food is showing yourself love.
Protecting yourself from man-made toxins is showing yourself love.
Being open and honest with yourself and others is showing yourself love.
Treating other people with love is showing yourself love.
And treating our wonderful Planet with love is showing yourself love.

Following the GAPS Nutritional Protocol will take you on a journey of healing and learning, where you will meet many good people and make lifelong friends. It will transform you as a person and transform your life completely! Your priorities and choices will change. Some people around you may leave, because their life path will become incompatible with yours. But other people will be drawn to you – people, who are on a similar journey and who will bring you real companionship and joy. There will be ups and downs, there will be tears and laughter and there will be growth of the person within you, growth of your spiritual essence. And, of course, there will be lots of delicious cooking and eating, sunbathing, gardening, swimming in lakes, rivers and sea, walking barefoot and communing with Nature!

Healing from a chronic disease must involve reconnecting to our Planet!

Our planet Earth is alive and we, humans, have a deep connection to it. Our bodies are an integral part of the planet's ecosystem: we build our bodies from the planet's resources, which are returned back to the planet when the body dies. During our lives the planet provides the perfect environment for us to live in. The Earth is our home, our source of everything we need to thrive; it is like a loving parent who gives and gives without asking for anything in return! Humanity understood its connection to Planet Earth until recent times, when modern humans started distancing themselves from Nature. The more we remove ourselves from Mother Nature, the more dysfunctional and unhealthy we become, and the more callous and predatory our attitude towards our Planet. The most harmonious and healthy societies have always lived in close proximity to Nature and had a deep reverence for it. In order to recover from a chronic illness, it is essential to get back in touch with this source of life, beauty and divinity. Gardening, planting and growing, and looking after animals are wonderful, joyful activities, because they get us back in touch with our planet's prevailing energy – the energy of LOVE. They get us into the fresh air and sunshine, raise our spirit and heal us on every level: physical, mental and spiritual. Many of my former patients, who went through the GAPS Nutritional Protocol, bought some land and created small holdings. City dwellers became farmers, and they couldn't be happier! Some people keep chickens, some have milking goats, some even have a house cow, and all create gardens and orchards. Producing your own natural, chemical-free food is a joy and very satisfying: this is food which you can trust completely, because you grew it yourself. I myself am one of those farmers and practice *regenerative agriculture*. The aim of this kind of agriculture is not only to produce best quality food, but to regenerate our Planet.

One of the most destructive human activities has always been arable agriculture. Ploughing, tilling, digging and other traditional methods of growing crops destroy topsoil and, over time, create deserts. The soil under your feet is the most precious part of Nature: all life begins and ends in the soil. Healthy soil is a complex microbial community and it is the biggest reservoir of carbon on Earth. This carbon is stored in the form of humus – a stable carbon polymer, which can hold carbon in the soil for hundreds of years. Humus also absorbs very large amounts of water, maintaining the moisture in the soil and preventing flooding. Arable agriculture destroys humus and kills the microbial community in the soil, and this process has intensified since the introduction of agricultural chemicals. A large percentage of the carbon accumulating in our atmosphere (causing global warming) is destroyed humus, released from the soils of arable fields around the planet in the form of carbon dioxide. Dead soil cannot feed plants and cannot hold water. Rain runs off these fields and floods villages downstream, carrying dead soil with it. According to science, all the world's deserts have been created by human activity.[7] Today, staggering amounts of topsoil are being turned into desert in the developed world thanks to industrial arable agriculture, growing grains, soya, sugar beet, cotton, maize and other commodity crops. It has been estimated that every year 24 billion tonnes of fertile soil are lost globally, which is 3.4 tonnes per person on the planet.[3]

Not many people know that our industrial agriculture overproduces grain.[4,5,6] In order to have a market for that grain and make a profit, animals have been locked in prisons – CAFOs (Confined Animal Factory Operations), where they are fed this overproduced grain. Grain is not an appropriate food for farm animals; they get sick from eating too much grain. Mother Nature designed them to live on pasture. Cows, goats and sheep should live on natural pasture, eating grass and other vegetation only. Chickens, turkeys and other birds eat a lot of grass and herbs and find their own meat on pasture (worms, insects and grubs). Pigs should live in a forest, where they find their own food, and they too eat a lot of grass and vegetation. This is how Mother Nature designed farm animals and this is the only way for them to be healthy and happy! But our industrial agriculture makes its profit on overproducing grain and soy. Once they are overproduced, they need to be sold, so the animals and birds are subjected to imprisonment and fed these grain and soy, which make them sick.

The manure produced from CAFOs washes into local waterways, poisoning all life in them and producing greenhouse gases. Manure from animals on pasture is a precious fertiliser for the soil, but our industrial agriculture has turned it into a problem. Industrial agriculture has been created with one aim only – profit! It is an abomination which is destroying our planet and producing disease-causing 'food', which fills the shelves in our supermarkets. If we are to regenerate our planet back to health, and if we are to be healthy ourselves, this model of agriculture must be abolished.

Regenerative agriculture recreates healthy soil, and animals are a key part of this process. Their excrements and activities on the land produce the rich microbial community of the soil, which is the essence and basis of all life on the planet. The more natural regenerative farms we have, no matter how small, the more chance our beautiful planet has to survive and to return to being the garden of Eden it once was. We already have a lot of knowledge on how to regenerate the planet, while producing plenty of *good* food for humanity. The problem is that the commercial and the political powers of the world are not interested. So, it is up to individuals to make a decision to do this work themselves, wherever they can. No scale is too small!

We, humans, have inflicted untold damage to our planet. There is a naïve thinking that, if we remove humans from a damaged area and 'return it back to Nature', the land will regenerate itself. Research in this area shows that this is not the right thing to do at all.[7] It shows that, if we work with damaged lands with love, using the knowledge we already have, we can do much better. The *Allan Savory Institute* has demonstrated this with millions of hectares of grasslands all over the world.[8] Grazed by large herds of animals *in the right way*, vast expanses of damaged land can be transformed into rich pastures! There are amazing projects turning deserts into lush gardens and forests.[9,10,11,12,13] These projects require large amounts of biomass from dead vegetation. Instead of allowing the appalling deforestation that is happening in the Amazonian rainforest right now, we could give the local people a business opportunity to harvest sustainably dead vegetation from their local area. This biomass can be shipped to deserts to regenerate them, while stopping the slash-and-burn deforestation of Amazonia, and giving a decent living to the local people. Rainforests are easy to destroy; they are fragile and delicately balanced ecosystems. Once destroyed, they may be impossible to restore. There is a way to preserve them, while regenerating other damaged lands on the planet! These are just a few examples of what is possible, there are many others.

By following the GAPS Nutritional Protocol, we stop supporting industrial agriculture, because we don't use their commodity crops: grains, soya, sugar beet, sugar cane, rape seed and maize. Their production on an industrial scale is a major destructive force on the planet. We do our best to buy food from natural organic farmers, who treat their land, soil and animals with love and care. We support proper animal husbandry, where animals live on natural pasture and have a healthy happy life. We do our best to grow our own vegetables, fruit and herbs. And we do not waste food, because we connect to it on every level – from the soil to the table. By eating this way, we help to regenerate our planet one meal at a time.

Healing from a chronic disease involves being cautious with science!

I strongly recommend to my patients not to be too scientific. Clinical experience has taught me a hard lesson: if you want to lose your way, follow the science! Let us not confuse technology with natural sciences. Technology – dealing with non-living objects – has achieved great heights and transformed our lives. However, when it comes to living things, our science has no ability to perceive them and even less ability to interfere without doing damage. Why? Because it tries to treat LIFE as non-living objects, employing the same methods used in technology.

Mother Nature took billions of years to design life on Earth, including our bodies. Our science has tinkered in its laboratories for a few decades only. For every study telling us something in medicine or nutrition, there is an equal number of studies telling us exactly the opposite. Why is our science so inept? Because it denies the spiritual aspect of life on Earth and has no ability to study it. Modern science is purely materialistic: it really believes that there is nothing more in the world than the physical reality our senses can perceive. The physical realm plus the human mind are the two dimensions a mainstream scientist understands. The third dimension – spiritual – is aggressively denied. Anybody, who tries to introduce this third dimension into science, is labelled 'a vitalist' and promptly dismissed. As long as our science stubbornly remains materialistic, it will be unable to explain or even understand the infinite complexity of life on Earth. Thankfully, this applies to mainstream science only. Outside it, research into the spiritual side of life has been going on for decades and is already producing interesting results. Please, look in the *Recommended Reading* section for some fascinating books on this subject. Every truly great scientist in history has accepted and emphasised the spiritual aspect of life on Earth, including Isaac Newton and Albert Einstein. There is no doubt that one day our mainstream science is going to do the same, because without accepting and studying the spiritual side of everything living, there is no future for that science.[14] In the meantime, we cannot take any mainstream scientific paper at face value, let alone try to use it in clinical practice, no matter how clever it looks. Please, read more on this subject in my first GAPS book *Gut and Psychology Syndrome,* chapter *Genetics*.

Your own body, mind and spirit are your healers. Trust them! Assist them! Love them!

This point has been brought to your attention several times in this book, dear reader. I would like to emphasise it again. The power of healing yourself is programmed into you. Don't give this power away to anyone! In emergencies you have to trust others to help you to repair your body but, after the basic repairs are done, the healing of your whole being is your work and only yours. You can seek help and advice, and there is plenty of help and wonderful information available. The GAPS Nutritional Protocol will help you to lay a solid foundation for healing from any chronic disease, because it will allow you to rebuild your body from quality materials, making it strong, robust and able to resist any damage. But, every human being is unique and needs a unique approach to their mind and soul. In those realms you need to follow your intuition and feelings to find the right way. There are many ways to connect to those intangible parts of us, such as various forms of meditation, prayer, psychotherapy and simply talking to a friend. But, perhaps, the best way is talking to ourselves. When I was a young doctor, I was fortunate enough to work alongside a brilliant professor of neurology, who was quite elderly. She was always muttering something to herself, and one day another colleague asked her who she was talking to. She replied: 'I am talking to a very clever person and getting all the right answers!'

You are the cleverest person in your life! Talk to this person as often as you can, spend quality time with this person alone and listen to what comes up. Be brutally honest with this person! Keep asking this person questions; you are likely to get the right answers! The good news is that we are not alone: other people have been down that road before us and are happy to share what they've learned. Keep reading, keep learning. The right people and the right books will come to you at the right moment, just be ready to accept them and pay attention to them. And keep talking to the biggest authority in your life – yourself!

In conclusion, I would like to say that healing from a chronic disease is a wonderful journey full of revelations, big lessons and proud achievements. It is an opportunity to grow as a HUMAN BEING, to get wiser, kinder, deeper and more loving. Before you know it, you will be helping others to heal, which will bring you even more joy. By helping others you will make new discoveries, which in turn will help you on your healing journey. In any journey, the harder the adversity you have to overcome, the sweeter the victory, and the more worthwhile the journey.

Bon voyage!

A–Z: GAPS conditions in alphabetic order

It is impossible to cover all the health problems which can be treated with the GAPS Nutritional Protocol. Here is a small sample of the most common chronic health conditions where people find this protocol helpful. Many other health problems have already been covered in other chapters.

Contents

Alcoholism

Please, read the chapter *Food Addictions*. Alcoholism begins in childhood from addiction to sugar and other processed carbohydrates. To treat the disease, start by changing the person's diet! All other methods of helping alcoholics (including medical, psychological and spiritual treatments) are secondary, and will work much better and more quickly when the gut is healed and food addictions are a thing of the past. It can be dangerous for an alcoholic to stop drinking abruptly. Instead, work on changing the diet, while gradually reducing alcohol consumption. Alcohol and sugar addictions are two sides of the same coin. In order to overcome an addiction to both sugar and alcohol we need fat, lots of fat! Breakfast, lunch and dinner should include a large helping of animal fats. An alcoholic may have difficulties digesting fats, so we need to work on improving their bile flow (please, see the chapter *Liver and Lungs*), while healing the gut with the GAPS Nutritional Protocol. Once the diet is fully implemented, in my clinical experience, stopping alcohol consumption is almost easy! Once the person has 'dried out', they need to stay on the GAPS Diet for the rest of their life. It is vital to understand that, because their body will always be ready to get back into addictions to sugar, other processed carbohydrates and alcohol if these things are reintroduced.

Alopecia areata

Every hair grows from a root with its own blood and nerve supply and lymphatic system. Our hair is a storage site for vital nutrients, such as minerals and trace elements; it is also a storage site for toxins.[1] When toxins accumulate in the hair root, they attract the attention of the immune system, which will try to clean the area using inflammation and autoimmunity. Alopecia – loss of hair – is caused by damage to the hair roots. It is considered to be an autoimmune condition, and is associated with other autoimmune diseases, such as rheumatoid arthritis, coeliac disease and type one diabetes.[2] All autoimmunity is born in the gut, and the GAPS Nutritional Protocol has a good record of helping people to recover from alopecia. Please, read about autoimmunity in detail in the chapter on the immune system. It takes time to heal from any autoimmune disease; we need to restore the gut flora, heal the gut and rebalance our immune system. In the meantime, it is essential to avoid skin and scalp contact with all man-made chemicals. No shampoo, shower gel or soap, hair conditioner or any other chemical concoction is to be used. Only edible natural things can be used on the skin and the scalp. You can wash your hair with raw egg yolks, herbal teas or plain water. Washing your hair in a natural lake or river is therapeutic (using only water), as is seawater. Regular applications of homemade kefir all over the scalp (or any other skin area with alopecia) will populate the skin with beneficial microbes and help to remove toxicity. Try to rub the kefir into your scalp for 10–15 minutes prior to washing your hair with raw egg yolks. Rinse with some black or green tea, or any homemade herbal tea. There are some herbal remedies with a good record of helping people with hair loss, such as oils and tea of sandalwood, lavender, rosemary and thyme.[2] When toxicity is removed and the autoimmune attack subsides, many of your hair roots will recover and the hair will grow again.

Amyotrophic lateral sclerosis (Lou Gehrig's disease), other motor neuron diseases (MNDs)

I do not have clinical experience in treating this group of disorders. However, from my experience of using the GAPS Nutritional Protocol successfully with many other very serious and 'incurable' illnesses, I would give it a try. The person will need to go through the GAPS Introduction Diet several times, with periods of the Full GAPS Diet in between. There are indications that toxic metals (lead in particular) may be implicated in this group of disorders.[3] So, after a year on the diet, it may be sensible to do chelation of toxic metals according to the Andy Cutler Protocol for two years at least, while continuing with the GAPS Diet. Agricultural chemicals, pharmaceutical drugs, radiation and electronic pollution are also implicated in this group of disorders, so it is important to work on reducing the toxic load in the body.[2,4] The GAPS Nutritional Protocol will heal the gut, rebalance the immune system and switch the detoxification system back on. Once these things happen, people recover from all sorts of illnesses.

Ankylosing spondylitis

People with this chronic condition develop inflammation and structural changes in the joints, particularly joints of the spine. The sad thing about this disease is that it may begin quite early in life – in the 20s and 30s. I believe that ankylosing spondylitis is a GAPS condition. To understand it fully, please read about collagen disorders in this chapter, and about autoimmunity in the chapter *Immune System*. People with this condition have abnormal gut flora and damaged gut wall, allowing partially digested foods and other toxins to absorb. These toxins trigger chronic inflammation, autoimmunity and sclerotic changes in the joints. Recent research has confirmed that these patients have a damaged gut wall allowing toxins and bacteria to absorb into the body.[5] A common microbe, which lives in the human gut, called *Klebsiella pneumonie,* has been found to overgrow in the digestive system of people with ankylosing spondylitis, triggering an active immune response.[6,7] Based on this finding, antibiotic treatments have been proposed for this disease. During antibiotic treatment an improvement in the symptoms has been observed in some people.[6,7] However, when the treatment stops ankylosing spondylitis comes back. It is never a good idea to take antibiotics for long periods of time. While you are trying to attack one microbe, a myriad of beneficial microbes in your body get destroyed, causing unpredictable damage to the most fundamental part of your physiology – your microbial flora.

There are no quick fixes for this disease. I believe that people with ankylosing spondylitis need to stay on the GAPS Diet more or less for the rest of their lives. You may start from the Full GAPS Diet initially. The Full GAPS Diet will give you a wider choice of foods and an ability to eat out sometimes, while you are reorganising your kitchen, learning new recipes, finding permanent suppliers of organic or biodynamic food and generally getting used to a new lifestyle. After a few months, or possibly even a year, you will be ready to go through the GAPS Introduction Diet. This diet will achieve deeper healing in your body. Don't rush through the Introduction Diet, give it time. It is very individual how long a person has to stay on the Introduction Diet; please study it and find your own pace. This diet will allow you to stop mainstream medication. It is sensible to remove the drugs slowly by reducing the daily dose gradually; remove one medication at a time. After the pain and inflammation are gone, I recommend that you follow the Full GAPS Diet most of the time for the rest of your life. If you go through a particularly stressful period or have an infection, some symptoms of ankylosing spondylitis may come back, and you may need to go through the GAPS Introduction Diet again. This time you will find that healing happens more quickly and you will be back to normal before you know it. From then on continue on the Full GAPS Diet.

Asthma and other lung conditions

Please look at the chapter *Liver and Lungs* to understand how and why lung disease develops. You may start from the Full GAPS Diet, but at some point it will be very helpful to go through the GAPS Introduction Diet. It will achieve deeper healing in the gut wall and the lungs. People, who are ready to do the Introduction Diet from the beginning, should start from it. Once the Introduction Diet is completed, move into the Full GAPS Diet and follow it for many years. When fully recovered, you may find that you can eat foods not allowed on the diet occasionally, without bringing asthma or any other lung disease back. Lungs love animal fats, particularly raw fat! So, if you suffer from a cough or any chronic lung condition, make sure to consume *salo* (*lardo*) daily and add plenty of animal fats to your meals. You will find the recipe for making salo in the chapter *What we shall eat and why, with some recipes.*

Back pain, chronic

Chronic back pain is common in people with abnormal gut flora. Let us understand why. Every spinal nerve is connected to its own segment of the body, where it collects information and provides nerve supply.[8] The lumbar and sacral regions of the spine collect sensory information from the intestines and the bowel, while the lower chest region is involved in collecting information from the stomach. When there is inflammation, toxicity, faecal compaction and other problems in the gut, that information is passed to the related segment of the spinal cord, where sensory signals are converted into motor signals. These motor signals are like 'decisions' made by your spinal cord, based on the information received from the gut. These 'decisions' are conveyed to the muscles, fascia, ligaments, skin and other structures in your back connected to that particular part of the spinal cord. All these structures respond, they get tense and slightly displaced, causing chronic aching back pain. If the situation continues for a long time, the tense muscles pulling in the wrong direction will displace discs in your spinal column, causing disc damage. This is when X-rays will show that you have a collapsed or damaged disc. People are often offered surgical operations at this point, but typically they don't bring a permanent solution, because the gut flora is still abnormal and the gut is still unhealthy. Manual treatment and chiropractic adjustments can bring temporary relief, but to deal with the root of the problem we need to heal the gut. Follow the *GAPS Diet*. It is very helpful for people with chronic back pain to start from the *GAPS Introduction Diet*, while clearing their bowel with enemas every 1–2 days. A cleansing enema with the basic enema solution, followed by a coffee enema (with some whey or sour cream added to the coffee), can bring immediate relief from acute back pain, making you much more comfortable. It is helpful to have daily baths with Epsom salt; the magnesium from the bath water absorbs through the skin quite well, bringing relief from back pain.

Magnesium supplements or magnesium oil can also be helpful (make sure to get supplements with amino acid chelates of magnesium, such as malate, bisglycinate and other).

Bed-wetting, cystitis and other urinary problems

Please read the chapter *Problems Down Below*. Urine is one of the ways toxins leave the body. Abnormal gut flora produces a lot of toxins, which are excreted in urine. This toxic urine irritates the lining of the bladder and causes a low-grade inflammation, so the person gets symptoms of chronic cystitis. The bladder gets irritated by small amounts of toxic urine, so the person has to empty it frequently. If a child (or an adult) with this condition is fast asleep, then the bladder may empty without waking the person up, hence bed-wetting. Die-off increases levels of toxins in the body, so the urine will become more toxic, exacerbating the problem.

The GAPS Programme will eliminate this problem long term, as it will remove its cause. In the meantime, do what works to help the situation: drink plenty of water and use supplements of cranberry and mannose to reduce inflammation in the bladder. Apply homemade kefir or yogurt to the groin daily to populate the urethra with beneficial flora. To train the child to go to the toilet during the night you can use various mechanical alarms and devices developed for enuresis. But simply waking your child up a few times during the night and taking him or her to the bathroom can achieve good results in a matter of weeks, combined with the GAPS Diet.

Body odour and breath odour

Pathogenic microbes in your digestive system produce toxins, many of which leave the body in the form of gasses. These gasses are called Microbial Volatile Organic Compounds (MVOCs) and have an unpleasant smell.[9] They include alcohols, aldehydes, ketones, amines, aromatic and chlorinated hydrocarbons, terpenes and sulphur-based compounds. Many MVOCs have been researched and it has been demonstrated that they are produced by a large group of bacteria and fungi. Having absorbed into your blood and lymph from the digestive system, they get distributed around the body, causing damage. Your body tries to get rid of them, and many of these toxins are eliminated through sweat and breath, giving them a powerful and often unpleasant smell. This can be a feature of the die-off period at the beginning of the GAPS Nutritional Protocol, as well as the die-off later on in the programme. Die-off is a temporary situation, but while it is taking place, you may have an unpleasant body or/and breath odour (no matter how often you wash yourself or brush your teeth). Sometimes you may be aware of it, but sometimes not. Unfortunately, people nearby will always notice it, and so it can cause social problems. Using deodorants usually does not help, plus they contain toxic chemicals that add to the already high level of toxicity in your body. What you need to do is to change your gut flora. You need to take those pathogens under control, and the GAPS Diet will do that for you. Introduce kefir as soon as possible (made from raw organic milk, using live kefir grains). From my clinical experience, kefir is particularly powerful in removing body odour. It takes under control the very microbes which produce those smelly chemicals. Drinking kefir first thing in the morning (when your stomach is empty) or adding it to your GAPS 'shakes' can stop the body odour in a matter of days in some people! Kombucha can also be helpful, as well as other fermented foods. But the most important thing is to remove processed foods, which feed the pathogens in your gut and get converted into those 'smelly' chemicals.

Instead of conventional deodorants use fresh lemon juice: cut a lemon in half, squeeze the juice into your hand and apply to your armpits daily. The lemon juice suppresses growth of fungi and other microbes on your skin. To deal with breath odour, brush your teeth with olive oil several times a day and a little bicarbonate of soda once a day. Doing *oil pull* with olive oil or any other cold-pressed good quality oil also helps: take some oil into your mouth and swish it around for 15–20 minutes, spit it out and rinse your mouth. This ayurvedic procedure is known to detoxify the mouth.[10]

Cerebral palsy

Cerebral palsy is due to damage to the brain, which can happen during pregnancy, delivery and early childhood. I recommend putting the child on the GAPS Diet permanently, staying on the second stage of the GAPS Introduction Diet for long periods of time. Of course, the condition is not going to disappear, but the person will be healthier physically and easier to look after. The seizure frequency usually goes down, muscle tone becomes more comfortable, mood and behaviour become stable and, in many patients, learning ability improves. I believe that this approach gives the child or the adult with cerebral palsy the best quality of life they can achieve.

Coeliac (celiac) disease

Coeliac (celiac) disease is an autoimmune condition of the intestines and has similar symptoms to SIBO (small intestinal bacterial overgrowth).

Blood tests and an intestinal biopsy are done to make the diagnosis. It is considered to be caused by gluten – a protein found in wheat, barley, rye and other grains. However, it is not just gluten that is the culprit. Just about all other proteins found in grains (serpins, purinins, amylase/ protease inhibitors, globulins, farinins, lectins, etc) can trigger an allergic IgG and IgA mediated immune response.[11,12] Plant proteins in all seeds, including beans, lentils, nuts, vegetables and fruit, can cause cross-reactions, triggering the same symptoms as gluten.[12] Just removing gluten from the diet is typically a waste of time; some symptoms may improve, but the disease will still be there. The GAPS Diet will address the root cause of the problem – the abnormal gut flora and damaged intestinal wall. Following the GAPS Introduction Diet for a long enough time is important. In severe cases with stubborn diarrhoea we have to go further to the No-Plant GAPS Diet for a period of time, and then return to the Introduction Diet. It is important not to rush and to give your body plenty of time to heal. It is possible to heal from a coeliac disease! There are people with this diagnosis, who have recovered to the point of being able to eat ordinary pasta and sourdough bread occasionally without any problems. But, before reaching that point, the GAPS Diet needs to be followed strictly for at least 4–5 years.

Collagen disorders (any arthritis, rheumatoid arthritis, systemic lupus erythematosus, systemic sclerosis, EDL – Ehlers Danlos syndrome, Alport syndrome and other)

Please, read about collagen disorders in the chapter *Immune System*. People with these disorders need to be prepared to stay on the Full GAPS Diet for the rest of their lives, more or less. You can start from the Full GAPS Diet, but at some point it is very beneficial to do the GAPS Introduction Diet. Many people with collagen disorders have to go through the Introduction Diet several times, depending on their symptoms and the severity of the illness. It is vital to provide plenty of building blocks for your body to build new collagen, which means building new healthy connective tissue. This tissue is the major part of your joints, bones, muscles, blood vessels, peripheral nervous system, fascia and other organs, which are affected by your collagen disease. The joints, skin, heads, tails, internal organs and feet of animals are made from very similar molecules as our own – they are rich in collagen and other vital proteins. So, focusing on foods, prepared from those parts of animals, is vital for a person with any collagen disorder. Gelatinous meat stock, soups, stews, organ meats and animal fats are the real medicine for this group of people.

Crohn's disease and ulcerative colitis

The GAPS Nutritional Protocol has a good record of helping people to recover from these illnesses. Please, study the *No-Plant GAPS Diet* and the *GAPS Introduction Diet*. Following these protocols is vital for recovery. Progress may be slow, and it is important to be ready for that. Most people with these problems take mainstream medications, which we cannot remove abruptly; they need to be removed gradually when the symptoms start improving. It is important for the patient to understand that they will need to stay on the GAPS Diet all their life. There may be particularly good periods when they can cheat a little, but most of the time they need to be strict. So, spend the time to implement the diet properly, learning to cook the right way. There are many people around the world who have recovered fully from Crohn's disease and ulcerative colitis and are leading healthy lives. You will find a few testimonies in the *GAPS Stories* book and online.[13]

Diabetes, type one

Type one diabetes is considered to be an autoimmune disorder, where the body attacks and destroys insulin-producing cells in the pancreas. However, our pancreas has a great ability to regenerate, to rebuild itself, as long as the attack on it stops. All autoimmunity is born in the gut. Following the GAPS Programme will heal the gut and rebalance the immune system. In my experience, as the patient progresses through the treatment, some of them are able to slowly reduce the dose of insulin and in some cases to stop the injections altogether. It takes time and patience to heal from type one diabetes. Before the body can attend to insulin production it has to heal the gut lining first, which can take considerable time. It is important for the patient not to expect any changes in the blood sugar regulation or the insulin doses for a while, and just keep working on healing the gut. Only when the gut wall has sealed itself, and food starts digesting properly before absorbing, can the immune system downregulate its autoimmune activity in the pancreas. It's only then that the pancreas can regenerate and start producing its own insulin.

Some patients find that removing all dairy products for a while helps to recover from type one diabetes. This is not the case for everybody, but it is worth giving it a try at the beginning of the protocol.

Diabetes, type two

Type two diabetes is caused by the body becoming insulin resistant because of long-term consumption of processed carbohydrates. Please, read the section on *Metabolic Syndrome*. The GAPS Diet removes all processed carbohydrates, so the body can heal the damage and remove diabetes. The progress depends on how long the person has been suffering from this disease and the amount of damage diabetes has inflicted on the body. Once better, as long as the person continues to stick to the GAPS Diet for the rest of his or her life, the diabetes should never return.

The GAPS Diet is very beneficial for people with type two diabetes, obesity, and other forms of insulin resistance (metabolic syndrome), as it cuts out complex carbohydrates. People with this problem need to limit their carbohydrate consumption, so don't go heavy on honey or desserts. It is essential to have plenty of animal fats in order to keep blood sugar at the right level. For people with unstable blood sugar I recommend having a few tablespoons of coconut oil, raw butter or homemade sour cream every half hour throughout the day. Freshly pressed juices have many sugars in them, so I do not recommend them for people with diabetes. When your blood sugar is normal and stable, you can try to have GAPS shakes, where we balance the sugars with fat and protein by blending into the juice 1–2 raw eggs and 1–2 tablespoons of homemade sour cream or raw butter or coconut oil (per person). Once your juice is mixed with eggs and fat, you do not need to worry about getting too much sugar from the juice.

Sugar cravings and chocolate cravings are common amongst people with diabetes and can be quite a barrier for implementing any diet. It is a good idea to mix raw butter or coconut oil with a little raw honey to taste; make the mixture in advance and keep eating it throughout the day. This mixture will help you to overcome cravings for carbohydrates and to come through the initial stages of treatment. When sugar cravings are gone, you will be able to maintain your blood sugar at a normal level between meals, without having to eat anything. For more details on this approach please look at *Sugar cravings, chocolate cravings* in this chapter.

Duodenum, problems

The first part of the intestines – the duodenum – is about 25-38 cm (10–15 in) in length, and is the place where bile and pancreatic enzymes are added to the food to continue its digestion. This is a primary place where many parasites live – worms and flukes. We all have them and, as long as they are balanced with the rest of the gut flora and our immune system, there is no need to worry about them. Unfortunately, in a person with abnormal gut flora these creatures overgrow. Some of them live outside the intestines in the liver, the pancreas, the spleen and abdominal cavity, but come into the duodenum in the middle of the night to feed. This can disrupt the person's sleep, causing belching, hot flushes and night sweats, abdominal cramps and nightmares. It is impossible to eradicate these creatures completely, but reducing their numbers is very important. Mainstream drugs developed for parasites are often toxic, don't work in everybody, and it is easy to get reinfected after using the drug. It is best to use herbal remedies, garlic, essential oils, diatomaceous earth and other natural approaches. Please, read more about this in the section *Parasites and worms*. These approaches have to be applied for many months. Following the GAPS Diet strictly during this time will allow the gut to heal itself, while the parasites are being removed. As your gut flora gets more balanced and the immune system in the gut wall gets stronger, the parasites will not be able to overgrow again once treatment has stopped.

Ear infections

This subject has been covered in great detail in the first GAPS book (*Gut and Psychology Syndrome*) in the chapter *Ear Infections and Glue Ear*.[14] The middle ear is connected to the back of the nose through a tiny tube, called the Eustachian tube. A GAPS person has abnormal microbial flora living in the nose and the throat, causing chronic inflammation in the tube, which closes up. Quite quickly after that, the middle ear fills with mucous, impairing hearing. An infection can arrive at any point, giving the person earache and a high temperature. In order to remedy the situation long term, we need to follow the GAPS Nutritional Protocol. In the meantime, we populate the throat with beneficial flora by using homemade kefir or a commercial probiotic. Finish every meal with some kefir, so its microbes can work on the flora in the back of your throat between meals. Every bedtime we use kefir again or pour some probiotic powder on the tongue, giving it a chance to work on healing the mucous membranes in the area during the night.

Eczema

Eczema and many other skin rashes are GAPS conditions. The child or adult has abnormal gut flora, which produces many toxins. At the same time, the gut wall is damaged and porous, letting undigested foods through and creating food allergies and intolerances. Our skin is a major detoxification organ: many toxins leave the body through sweat. When these toxins go through the skin, they cause damage on the way. Our skin is populated by a community of microbes, which interact with toxins in the sweat, often adding more damage. The immune system deals with that damage using inflammation. It is the inflammation that shows up as a rash, often itchy. So, to remedy eczema or any other rash *long term* we need to reduce the level of toxicity in the body. As most toxicity comes from the gut, that is the place we need to heal with the GAPS Nutritional Protocol.

Short term we can use baths with bicarbonate of soda (1/2 a cup per bath) or oatmeal (put uncooked oatmeal in a cotton bag and run the water to fill the bath through this bag). These baths have a soothing effect on inflamed skin. As a moisturiser apply any cold-pressed edible oil onto the patches of eczema. You can also use raw butter, sour cream, tallow or mashed ripe avocado.

Very severe eczema patches (wet and cracked skin) will get a lot better with *applications of raw honey or seaweed* overnight. Try to alternate the two: one night apply honey, the next night seaweed. Use local raw honey, preferably organic. To use seaweed powder, add some hot water and mix to make a paste. After applying the honey or the seaweed paste to the eczema patches, cover the area with some fresh leaves of burdock, cabbage, sage, plantain or lettuce. Natural leaves are healing in their own right. If leaves are not available, use cling film (Saran wrap) or parchment paper. Wrap the area in cotton cloth. In the morning rinse off the honey or seaweed and apply any edible oil or animal fat.

Remember *the general rule about skin*: IF YOU CANNOT EAT IT, DO NOT APPLY IT TO THE SKIN! The skin absorbs most things applied to it. So, never use any soaps, shampoo, moisturisers or other man-made chemicals on the skin of a person with eczema or any other skin problem. Wash the skin with plain water. Use only edible oils and animal fats as moisturisers: coconut oil, olive oil, hemp oil, mashed ripe avocado, ghee, butter, any other animal fat and tallow. Tallow is particularly healing for the skin! You will find a recipe on how to make a skin cream from tallow in the chapter *What we shall eat and why, with some recipes*.

Research shows that clothes made from superfine merino wool are healing for people with eczema.[15] The wool doesn't let the skin lose moisture and is very gentle on the skin. The key to this is the processing. Standard industry processing of wool uses many toxic chemicals, which remain in the final product. It is these chemicals that cause a reaction, not the wool itself or the lanolin in it. Because of these chemicals, wool has the reputation of being irritating to the skin. In reality, wool is one of the most natural and healthy fabrics to have close to your skin. There are companies which use more natural processing of wool and their products are wonderful, from clothing to mattresses, duvets and pillows. It is important for people with any skin conditions to avoid all synthetic materials and even conventional cotton (which is often genetically modified and treated with toxic chemicals).

Failure to thrive

There is a detailed chapter on this subject in the first GAPS book (*Gut and Psychology Syndrome*).[14] Please, also look in the section *FPIES* in this chapter.

Fatigue. Chronic Fatigue Syndrome, Fibromyalgia, Myalgic Encephalomyelitis (ME) and other conditions with severe fatigue

Many GAPS people have fatigue to some degree. This means that your mitochondria are not working well. Mitochondria are our energy factories. These tiny organelles inside our cells are very efficient at producing energy, but are vulnerable to toxins, antibiotics, chronic inflammation and autoimmune attack.[16] In a GAPS person the body is filled with toxins. Our bodies are equipped with a powerful detoxification system designed to deal with toxicity. In a GAPS person this system is overloaded with work and often breaks down, so toxins accumulate in the body damaging mitochondria. The immune system adds more damage through inflammation and autoimmunity (many GAPS people test positive for anti-mitochondrial antibodies).[17] These people develop severe fatigue, which is the main symptom of chronic fatigue syndrome, fibromyalgia and ME. The detox system needs energy to function, so the person is trapped in a vicious cycle of not being able to produce energy or detoxify.

As the detoxification system is disabled, any amount of die-off is poorly tolerated. Die-off increases toxicity in the body, and there is nothing to handle it. That is why people with these problems have to go slowly with increasing probiotics or fermented foods. Coconut oil has antimicrobial substances and also causes some die-off. Try to modify your GAPS Diet according to your personal needs: move through the stages of the *GAPS Introduction Diet* slower or faster, sometimes take a day or two following the *GAPS Liquid Fast* to 'unload' your system or follow the *No-Plant GAPS Diet* for a while. It may be helpful for you to take digestive enzymes with your meals: stomach acid booster at the beginning of the meal and pancreatic enzymes at the end. It is really important to work on introducing animal fats; the more fat is consumed with every meal, the quicker you will recover.

A large percentage of people with chronic fatigue syndrome, fibromyalgia and ME have Lyme disease or MSIDS (Multiple Systemic Infectious Diseases Syndrome). Please, read about these in more detail later in this chapter.

It may take many years for a person with chronic fatigue syndrome, fibromyalgia and ME to recover fully, as their bodies have accumulated many layers of damage. After recovery it is important to stay on the GAPS Diet for the rest of your life.

Food poisoning

Food poisoning happens most often when we travel and eat unfamiliar food. Typically, it starts with a headache, followed by diarrhoea and vomiting. The headache is a sign of toxicity produced by the infection. Diarrhoea and vomiting are the remedies which your body uses to expel the infection and its toxins; they should be welcomed and assisted. How do we assist the body in cleansing itself during food poisoning? For example, sometimes there is severe nausea but no vomiting, which means that toxins have accumulated in the upper digestive system. It is a good idea to drink a large glass of cool water and then induce vomiting to expel that toxicity. To induce vomiting, put a couple of fingers deep into your throat and tickle the back of the throat to stimulate the vomiting reflex. When the stomach has emptied itself, try to drink more water and vomit it out. Usually two or three glasses of water are enough to empty the stomach of the remnants of the food that caused the problem. After clearing the stomach, a cup of hot, strong tea can be very helpful (black or green tea with nothing added). Sip it slowly. The tea will help to stop the vomiting reflex and calm the irritated stomach lining, which will remove nausea. Diarrhoea can last for a day or two and is a powerful mechanism the body uses for cleansing itself. During the second or third day of food poisoning we can give the body some assistance by performing a cleansing enema. Use the basic enema solution (1 l (2.1 pt) of warm water + 1 teaspoon of natural salt + 1 teaspoon of bicarbonate of soda) to remove any remnants of infected food and its toxins. If the headache persists, it is very helpful to perform a coffee enema (for adults) after emptying the bowel with the basic enema solution. Often it is necessary to do enemas for a couple of days to deal with food poisoning completely.

Food poisoning is as old as humans and should not be feared. Usually, there is no need for any medication. Food poisoning gives the body a chance to clean up old accumulation of toxicity in the digestive system and elsewhere. It is vital not to eat anything, apart from home-made meat stock, on the first day after the food poisoning. If you are travelling, find a place where you can have some freshly made hot soup with clear meat or fish stock (no starch or any other thickener added to the stock). Eat the liquid in the soup but leave the solids. Continue drinking hot strong tea (black or green) without adding anything to the tea. On the second day you will be able to have cooked eggs, meat, fish, cooked vegetables, fermented dairy and, of course, meat or fish stock (the first two stages of the GAPS Introduction Diet). Avoid raw plant matter for a few days. Avoid nuts and other seeds for a week or two after full recovery.

FPIES (Food Protein Induced Enterocolitis Syndrome)

Please, read about this condition in the chapter *No-Plant GAPS Diet.* This is a fairly new diagnosis, which is rapidly becoming more and more common.[18] Typically it is diagnosed in babies and small children, but recently adults are starting to get this diagnosis too.[19] Please, follow the *No-Plant GAPS Diet* slowly and patiently. There is a growing group of children in the world recovering from this disease fully with the use of this form of the GAPS Diet. And there are parent groups online providing help and support.

Gout

Gout is a very painful condition when crystals of uric acid accumulate in the joints, causing acute inflammation. Typically, the joints of the big toes or thumbs are affected, but any joint can suffer. I am convinced, that gout is caused by particular microbes living in the gut of the person, and recent research into microbiome agrees with this idea.[20] People with gout have been found to have distinctly different gut flora to people without this disease; certain species of bacteria are prevalent in their gut (*Bacteroides cacao* and *Bacteroides xylanisolvens,* for example).[20] These microbes produce toxins which interfere in the normal purine metabolism in the body, causing formation of uric acid crystals. The GAPS Nutritional Protocol works very well for these patients! It changes the person's gut flora, taking under control gout-causing microbes, and as a result prevents gout attacks long term.

Because uric acid is formed from purines in the body, mainstream thinking blames them for gout, advising people not to eat meat. The majority of purines come from our normal body metabolism, not from food. The real culprits are processed carbohydrates, sugar, high-fructose corn syrup and beer. Beer consumption is a particular problem for people with gout! If you are prone to gout, you have to say 'goodbye' to beer for the rest of your life. Beer causes gout in two ways. First, beer is very starchy and has other carbohydrates in it, which feed gout-causing pathogens and let them produce their toxins. Second, the alcohol occupies the liver and stops it from attending to other toxins. Over-consuming any alcohol (including wine) can start a gout attack, because the liver is too busy dealing with alcohol and cannot clear the toxins out.

During a gout attack it is best to eat nothing and drink only water. Clearing your bowel with several water enemas will remove a large amount of toxicity from your body and speed up your recovery. Make sure that there are no solids left in your bowel at the end of the enema. Do the enemas twice a day, as more solids will reach your bowel to feed the gout-causing microbes. Having removed the solids, it may be a good idea to follow with a coffee enema, because it has a good record of cleansing the liver and improving its function. A painkiller *indometacin* is typically prescribed for gout attacks as it helps to reduce the pain. However, for people with a sensitive digestive system it can be a problem, as it damages the stomach wall. Try to chew the tablet and mix it well with saliva before swallowing. Never take aspirin during a gout attack; it will make the whole problem worse! I do not recommend long-term medication for gout; it is best to deal with the root problem – abnormal gut flora.

Haemorrhoids

Haemorrhoids are the visible signs of high blood pressure in the portal system. What is a portal system? It is all the veins which collect blood from your digestive system – your intestines and the bowel in particular, which includes the rectum. Having collected the blood from those organs, the portal system of veins then brings it into the liver to be filtered. In the GAPS person the liver is overloaded with toxins and cannot process the blood quickly enough. As a result, the pressure in the portal system increases and can be quite high, despite the fact that the general blood pressure in your body can be normal. The high blood pressure in the portal veins stretches them and makes them protrude into the wall of the rectum. These are the haemorrhoids – the bulging veins covered by the mucous membrane of the rectum. The mucous membranes above these veins can get stretched and damaged causing ulcerations, bleeding, obstruction and other unpleasant symptoms.

The best remedy for immediate relief is a coffee enema. It will unload your liver and allow it to start processing the portal blood much faster. As a result, the blood pressure in the portal system will reduce to normal and you may find that your haemorrhoids disappear after a good coffee enema. After a couple of days, they may start filling up again, so you will need to do another coffee enema. Please study the coffee enema procedure in the chapter *Bowel Management.* I would like to emphasise that it is essential to clear your bowel well with several enemas using the basic enema solution before you try a coffee enema. When you put the coffee into an empty bowel it will have maximum effect. I recommend using homemade sour cream as a lubricant on the enema nozzle and applying it to your rectum afterwards to sooth and heal that area.

In order to eliminate haemorrhoids long term, you need to follow the GAPS Nutritional Protocol to change the gut flora and heal the gut. As the flow of toxins from the gut to the liver drops, your liver will be able to process the portal blood more quickly, and it will stop backing up to cause haemorrhoids.

Hay fever

Please, read the chapter *Immune System* first to understand how hay fever develops. As with any atopic condition, hay fever will disappear as you heal your gut and change your gut flora. The immune system gets rebalanced and all atopic conditions gradually disappear. In people with mild hay fever this problem disappears quite quickly, while other people have to go through the GAPS Introduction Diet slowly and patiently to achieve this result.

Headaches (migraines, tension headaches and other)

It is an interesting fact that our brain tissue cannot feel pain; it has no pain receptors. When we have a headache, it is not the brain that hurts but all the surrounding tissues outside and inside the skull. Muscles, tendons, blood vessels, the bone and other tissues have many pain receptors. The brain is wrapped with three layers of protective tissue. The outermost layer is tough and fairly thick and is attached to the inside of our skull. It is called dura mater ('hard mother' in Latin) and can be extremely painful. When we have headaches, dura mater is usually involved.

There are many varieties of headaches with different causes. Infections, tumours, vascular malformations, intracranial bleeding and trauma can cause severe headaches. Sinus infections, pharmaceutical drugs and allergies can cause headaches. But the most common headaches are migraines and so-called tension headaches, which often overlap. The majority of sufferers of both types are women of reproductive age, and the menstrual cycle is very much involved: headaches typically happen around menstruations or during an ovulation. In men they can happen at any time.

During the *tension headache* the whole head hurts, often feeling like a tight ring around the head with pressure behind the eyes and forehead. These headaches are usually not too severe; they are unpleasant, but the person can function and painkillers usually help. *Migraines* typically happen in one side of the head (focussed in the temple and the eye), when the pain can be pulsating and severe. A migraine can be accompanied by nausea, vomiting, other digestive symptoms and sensitivity to light and smell. In about a third of people an aura of flashing lights and other visual disturbances may appear just before the headache. Migraines can be debilitating, last for days and painkillers often don't help.

Tension headaches and migraines are very common amongst GAPS people. I have no doubt that toxicity coming out of the gut is responsible for the problem. These toxins come to the liver first, and in GAPS people the liver is usually overloaded with work and cannot cope. So, the toxins finish up in the bloodstream and get carried to the head. The blood comes to the head through a large artery, called the *carotid artery*. In the neck this artery divides into two large branches – internal and external. The *internal carotid artery* goes inside the skull to feed the brain. This artery is long and has a few twists and turns before reaching the brain. It plays no part in common headaches because the brain has no pain receptors and, if the blood-brain barrier is intact and working well, then the brain will be protected from the toxicity. Common headaches typically happen in the *external carotid artery*'s domain. This artery is fairly short and straight (giving toxins quite a direct route); at the end it divides into branches, which feed all the places where the pain of migraine is located: the temple, the eye socket and the brow, the upper jaw and teeth and the temporal area of the head. A large part of the very painful dura mater on the side of the head is fed by the *external carotid artery* through one of its branches, which goes inside the skull – the *middle meningeal artery*.[21]

As always, we have to marvel at how Mother Nature designed our bodies. It gave us headaches in order to protect the brain! The headache lets us know that there is toxicity coming to the head which may damage the brain. It is important to pay attention to headaches and not just suppress them with painkillers. The headache is a warning that your brain is in peril, so it is important to slow down, rest, sleep and take steps to reduce the toxic load in the body. The brain has protection in the form of a blood-brain barrier. However, this protection can be damaged and breached by toxicity, inflammation and autoimmunity, and in many GAPS people it is already damaged to a degree. In these patients the brain responds to the toxins with various symptoms (mood alterations, memory problems, sensory problems and other psychological and neurological signs). So, headaches need to be taken seriously. If you ignore them, far more severe problems may follow. Instead of viewing headaches as a nuisance, I think we should see them as a blessing!

How do the toxins in the blood cause a migraine? We don't know the precise mechanism yet, but from the clinical perspective there is no doubt that the cause of the symptoms is inflammation of the whole area. Toxins in the blood damage the walls of the arteries making them porous. This leaches a whole stream of substances (including the toxins) out of the blood into the surrounding tissues and launches inflammation in the area. Inflammation causes swelling of the tissues leading to pain and a feeling of pressure. As the blood pounds through the blood vessels of the area, the pain becomes pulsating (like a vehicle driving through a field flooded with water, it causes waves). Inflammation in the dura mater always causes the muscles and fascia of the head and the neck to tense and stiffen to provide more support, which we see in meningitis for example. Meningitis is caused by an infection, but toxicity can cause the same symptoms without any infection. The tense fascia and muscles will give the person all the symptoms of a tension headache (heavy pressure with the 'ring around the head'), which we should really call a toxic headache.

When we remove toxicity from the blood, headaches disappear. To remove the source of toxicity *long term* we must heal the gut, and the *GAPS Nutritional Protocol* will do that for you very effectively. The *GAPS Introduction Diet* in particular removes the headaches fairly quickly in the majority of people. In those people where headaches persist, we need to take steps to cleanse and support the liver. Toxicity from the bowel hits the liver first. If the liver of the person is overburdened and unable to cleanse the blood, the headaches will continue. Please read more about the liver in the chapter *Liver and Lungs*.

As an immediate remedy for any headache I recommend a good cleansing enema, followed by a coffee enema. From clinical observation I have no doubt that the vast majority of toxins, which cause common headaches, come out of the bowel. Cleansing the bowel thoroughly removes this source of toxicity. This means putting water (or basic enema solution) inside the bowel several times until no solids come out. For some people just emptying the bowel stops the headache, but for many it is necessary to follow with a coffee enema. For detailed explanation about enemas please look in the chapter *Bowel Management*.

IBS (Irritable Bowel Syndrome)

Irritable Bowel Syndrome should be renamed gut dysbiosis. The person has abnormal gut flora, which causes all sorts of digestive symptoms. The GAPS Nutritional Protocol has a very good record of removing this condition. It is important to work on normalising stomach acid production and healing the whole digestive system.

Infertility

Infertility is already a big problem in the industrialised world and is getting worse every year.[22] The reasons for this epidemic are all man-made: EMF (electromagnetic pollution), modern low-cholesterol and low-fat diets, hormone-disrupting chemicals in the environment and having children later in life. Mobile phones are a serious culprit: our reproductive organs are particularly vulnerable to their powerful microwave radiation, and many young people carry their phones in their trouser pockets, subjecting their gonads (ovaries in women and testes in men) to concentrated radiation. Sperm count is falling dramatically in young men of reproductive age, and mobile phones are likely to be an important cause of this problem.[23] Unhealthy gut flora can play a serious role in hormonal abnormalities. Please, read more about it in the chapter *Hormones*. The GAPS Nutritional Protocol has helped many couples to conceive and produce a healthy baby.

Kidney problems

The most common reason for damaged kidney function is improperly digested proteins being filtered through the kidneys. Where do they come from? From the gut! When the gut wall is damaged and porous, proteins in food are not broken down properly before they absorb. When the body tries to eliminate these proteins through urine, they block up the kidneys causing nephropathy and kidney failure. The immune system uses inflammation and autoimmunity in order to 'unblock' the kidneys, which can add more damage. Mainstream medicine knows that it is protein that is damaging the kidneys, so the recommendation is to reduce protein-rich foods. However, that does not address the real problem – the damaged gut wall. Also, we need to understand that the most damaging and undigestible proteins come from plants! Animal proteins are much easier for us to digest and they are far more compatible with our human physiology.

The GAPS Introduction Diet will heal the gut wall. As a result, protein in food will start digesting properly. So, when it is absorbed, it will do no damage to kidneys or any other tissue in the body. In the initial stages, focus on gelatinous meats rather than muscle meats, as they heal the gut lining quicker. Once the Introduction Diet has been completed, stay on the Full GAPS Diet for several years at least. It is possible that you will have to stay on this diet for most of your life, because your kidneys may remain vulnerable. You do not need to remove salt, but what you absolutely must do is to use only NATURAL UNPROCESSED salt, such as Himalayan Crystal salt or Celtic salt. This means that you can never have processed foods as they are full of processed salt, which is unhealthy for anybody, particularly for a person with sensitive kidneys. Kidneys have a good ability to regenerate and heal as long as they are not bombarded with undigested proteins and toxins.

Kidney stones. Kidney stone disease is due to the body's inability to handle minerals properly. The first and most important reasons are lack of animal fats in the diet and fat-soluble vitamin deficiencies, particularly vitamins K2, D and A.[24] Without these vitamins the body cannot use calcium as it should: instead of going into bones and teeth calcium settles in soft tissues. So, the person develops osteoporosis and tooth decay, while calcium is causing stone formation in the kidneys and liver, calcification of blood vessels and brain structures and damage in other places.

To prevent stone formation it is important to consume plenty of animal fats in your meals. The major source of vitamin K2 for us is our own gut flora; the microbial community in the gut produces this vitamin.[25] People with abnormal gut flora typically have a deficiency in this vitamin. The best food sources of K2 are fermented foods, such as high-fat fermented dairy (aged traditional cheese in particular) and natto (traditional fermented soya). Vitamin D is a sunshine vitamin, we produce it in our skin when sunbathing. It also comes from oily fish and other animal foods (eggs, meat and milk), if the animals have been raised on pasture under direct sunlight. Vitamin A comes from the organs and fat of animals. Many people in the world follow low-fat diets and become prone to kidney stones. Many people also have abnormal gut flora producing many toxins, which impair proper processing of nitrogen and uric acid. The most common stones are made from calcium oxalate and calcium phosphate, but there are some less common stones made from uric acid, cysteine and other substances. Every stone is covered by a coat made from proteins, fats and other organic materials.[24]

Passing a kidney stone is very painful: the pain is usually located in the back or side of the body. The person may feel nauseous and feverish and have anxiety. Taking a magnesium supplement, drinking a solution of Epsom salt (1 teaspoon dissolved in a cup of warm water) or having a bath with Epsom salt can be helpful. These remedies act as antispasmodics, and your doctor may give an antispasmodic medication. Drinking plenty of water and herbal teas will help to flush the stone out. Freshly pressed juices can also be very helpful during an acute phase. Long term it is important to normalise mineral metabolism in your body, and that involves a plentiful supply of fat-soluble vitamins and animal fats. There are some rare causes of kidney stone disease, but in the majority of people staying on the GAPS Diet permanently removes any possibility of kidney stones or any other kidney problems. The body is properly nourished, minerals are properly processed and foods are properly digested. The very basis of stone formation gets removed and the kidneys function well.

Lyme disease, MSIDS (Multiple Systemic Infectious Diseases Syndrome) and other chronic infections

Please, read about this subject in the chapter *Toxins and Parasites*. More than 300 chronic degenerative conditions have already been associated with Lyme disease and the list is growing: chronic fatigue syndrome, fibromyalgia, ME, MS, ALS, dementia, Parkinson's disease, arrhythmia and many other chronic degenerative conditions. A bacterium called *Borrelia burgdorfery* (Bb) has been blamed for Lyme disease. However, research is finding that borrelia doesn't act alone, but in the company of a growing list of other pathogens: rickettsia, babesia, bartonella, ehrlichia / anaplasma, chlamydia, mycoplasma, prions, fungi, worms, flukes and a whole host of viruses (coxackie virus, herpes family of viruses, CMV, EBV, VZV, etc.).[26] All these creatures can exist in many pleomorphic forms: spiral, straight, granular, cist, spore, mycelia, cell-wall deficient and other. And now a new diagnosis has been created for this situation: *MSIDS* (Multiple Systemic Infectious Diseases Syndrome).[27]

The plethora of microbes living in the body form mixed biofilms in various tissues, hiding the microbes from the immune system. Standard mainstream testing for Lyme and other chronic infections is quite ineffective and gives many false negatives and false positives. Alternative tests have been developed and are somewhat more effective (EliSpot or enzyme-linked immunospot assay, for example), but none of them give a 100% accurate result.[27] The mainstream approach of treating Lyme disease with powerful antibiotics (often administered for two or more years!) is only partially helpful in a proportion of patients. In the majority, antibiotics do not clear the infection; instead they cause the rise of cell-wall deficient microbes, systemic fungal infections and a host of other debilitating problems in the body. At the end of the treatment, testing may not detect any more *Borrelia burgdorfery*, but the patient feels worse than before. Alternative approaches show better results (such as Cowden protocol for Lyme disease), but they are very expensive and out of reach for many people.[28]

There are many other chronic infections in the world, where people don't get satisfactory results from antibiotics, antiviral medication or other mainstream treatments: Gulf War syndrome, Chronic Fatigue syndrome, chronic viral infections (Epstein Barr and other viruses in the herpes family, hepatitis B and C, retroviruses and other viral infections), mycoplasma, HIV/AIDS, chronic respiratory infections and infections of the digestive system, persistent low-grade fever, chronic painful joint and muscle swelling, mental illness, etc. The more we study chronic degenerative conditions, the more we find chronic infections behind them: Alzheimer's disease, Parkinson's disease, autism, schizophrenia, epilepsy and the full spectrum of autoimmune diseases. In most cases we find a community of microbes acting together, just like in Lyme disease. And in most cases, worms and parasites are involved as well, large and small. Mainstream medicine tries to kill any identified creatures, but the results are not good: the microbial community just changes and adjusts to the new environment, making the person even more unwell. In acute infections antibiotics can be lifesaving. But it is time for us to understand, that in chronic infections we cannot get health by killing anything! A vast proportion of the human body contains microbes; if we go to war with them, we are going to lose! We can only create health and well-being by rebuilding our bodies from quality clean materials, without man-made pollution, and rebalancing our inner microbial community.

The GAPS Nutritional Protocol will allow your body to cleanse and rebuild itself, and rebalance its microbiome. It will allow you to build a strong immune system and a powerful detoxification system. Both of these systems are essential for the body to cleanse itself and to deal with infections. In many people just doing the protocol helps them to get Lyme disease and other chronic infections under control, enabling them to have a good quality of life, without having to take antibiotics or doing any other treatments.

Here is a letter from the mother of 23-year-old Emili, diagnosed with Lyme disease, who not only regained her health with the GAPS Diet, but got pregnant and delivered a healthy beautiful baby.

> ***Emili had many antibiotics in her life. At home she was eating the GAPS Diet and feeling well. After getting married at 23 she moved away from home and was not careful with her diet. She began to complain of depression, lack of energy, inability to control negative thoughts, stopped studying and felt sick most of the time. Lyme disease was discovered and confirmed by a laboratory test. Emili got very ill and moved back in with her parents, where her mother implemented the GAPS Diet again. 'I cooked all day and night! My daughter stayed with me for almost six weeks. Her husband came to spend weekends with us, and it broke my heart to see him leaving without his wife, such a young boy, at the beginning of their married life. But, I think, he was happy to see her getting better day by day. I could hardly believe that in little more than a month she gained weight, had energy and her disposition improved, colour had come back to her cheeks and glitter to her eyes! She was able to go home with her husband and resume their married life. She continued with her GAPS Diet at home. I was very proud of her and everything was going great! In December Emili gave me one of the best Christmas gifts possible: she was pregnant! We decided to continue with what was already working – the GAPS Diet. We followed the instructions in the chapter, 'Having a New Baby in the GAPS Family' in the book Gut and Psychology Syndrome. In addition to the GAPS Diet, she started taking bovine liver capsules, since she could not handle the taste of liver, and fermented cod liver oil. Emili had a great pregnancy and came to visit us every month.' A few times during pregnancy Emili had to stay with her mother again because she was too tired to cook for herself and started losing weight. 'I was cooking day and night and Emili eating everything as fast as I cooked it! There wasn't anything I put on her plate that she did not devour in a few minutes and then***

ask for more! It was clear to us that Emili needs FOOD and rest. That's really what every pregnant woman should have! It's amazing how her body reacted so well and seemed to 'wake up' with only food. She moved with energy, slept well, and was happy to prepare to receive the baby. Her body was working as it should, and at 38 weeks and 5 days Emili gave birth to a perfectly healthy baby girl! The delivery was normal, quiet and fast. Her body was strong and did what it was supposed to do. After birth Emili stayed with me for another two weeks and guess what: I spent another couple of weeks cooking non-stop and Emili eating non-stop. I would leave soup ready for her at night, and she would eat it during the early morning hours when she woke up to breastfeed. By taking care of my pregnant daughter and seeing her give birth to a completely healthy baby, even with Lyme disease, and knowing that the only thing she needed was an appropriate diet, I just wanted to scream at the world, 'Hey! Our bodies need food! Food properly prepared! Real food!' Today my granddaughter is almost three months old and she continues to grow normally. She breastfeeds and already takes kefir, sauerkraut juice, fermented garlic water, beet kvass and a purchased probiotic. She sleeps well, is very alert and smiles! I feel immensely grateful to have participated in the development of my granddaughter! I graduated as a Nutritional Therapist recently, along with my 20-year-old daughter Carolina. Emili was my client during my course, and now she is also taking the Nutritional Therapist course and thinking of becoming a GAPS Practitioner! We came from being a GAPS family, and now we are going to be a family of GAPS Practitioners!' Liliane Widmer, November 2017

Metabolic syndrome: obesity, diabetes, heart disease, hypertension, cancer, Alzheimer's disease and more

Metabolic syndrome has been described in detail in my book *Put your heart in your mouth. What really is heart disease and what can we do to prevent and even reverse it.*[31] Please, read this book to understand the concept in detail. Here I can only give a short explanation of what metabolic syndrome is: it is when your blood insulin level is always high. Insulin is a powerful hormone; it has an effect on every tissue and organ in the body, and when its level is abnormally high, everything in the body goes wrong. Insulin is a master fat-storage hormone, so the person starts gaining weight, which can go all the way to obesity. As long as your insulin level is high, you will store everything you eat as fat. Metabolic syndrome is the cause of our obesity epidemic.[29] Insulin is a master pro-inflammatory hormone. As long as you have too much insulin in your blood, your body will have chronic ongoing systemic inflammation and nothing will be able to stop it. We now know that chronic inflammation is the basis for developing heart disease, cancer, diabetes, obesity, Alzheimer's disease and autoimmune illnesses.[30] Constantly high blood level of insulin is the major cause of these health problems, all of which continue gaining epidemic proportions in the modern world. Many other metabolic parameters go wrong in the body if your insulin level is constantly high.

Why and how do people develop a chronically high level of insulin? And why did metabolic syndrome virtually not exist until fairly recent times? Because of the change in the way we eat. With the advent of the food industry, humanity started consuming growing amounts of processed carbohydrates (sugars). We have talked about these 'foods' in other chapters. Sugar and flour, breakfast cereals and snacks, soft drinks and high-fructose corn syrup, desserts, sweets and condiments force your body to overproduce insulin. It is the primary role of insulin to handle carbohydrates. A modern person starts their day with breakfast cereal or porridge, toast, bread, cakes and sugar with cordial, coffee or tea. A sandwich, made with highly processed bread, follows at lunch, and pasta, potatoes and other processed starchy carbohydrates at dinner. In between people snack on sweets (candy), chocolate bars, potato crisps and other processed carbohydrates. A real disaster for our bodies was the development of the soft drink industry! These bottles with colourful liquids provide concentrated amounts of sugar, high-fructose corn syrup and other processed carbohydrates, in combination with chemicals harmful to health. As a result of this diet of sugars upon sugars the population developed metabolic syndrome. The process usually begins in early childhood and we have an obesity epidemic amongst our children. All overweight and obese individuals have chronic inflammation in the body, which lays the ground for many chronic illnesses.[31]

Processed carbohydrates cause chronic magnesium deficiency. In order to contract, our blood vessels need calcium, and we always have plenty of this mineral. But in order to relax, our blood vessels need magnesium, which is in short supply in the majority of modern humans. So, blood pressure goes up. Daily consumption of processed carbohydrates is *the cause* of our hypertension epidemic (high blood pressure)![32] The medical profession prescribes powerful drugs to interfere in immensely complex mechanisms of blood pressure regulation in the human body. These drugs can reduce the blood pressure for a while, but the real cause of the problem has not been addressed: the person continues eating processed carbohydrates and causing magnesium deficiency in their body. At some point the drugs don't work anymore, other drugs have to be tried and added, with many side effects and problems of their own. The only way to free yourself from hypertension is to stop eating processed carbohydrates! Apart from high blood pressure, magnesium deficiency causes many other problems in the body: mood swings, hyperactivity and inability to focus in children and adults, memory problems and other neurological and psychiatric problems, abnormal mineral balance, headaches, muscle cramps and restless legs, sudden death in athletes, pre-eclampsia and eclampsia in pregnancy, allergies, heart disease, etc. [31,32]

Our gut flora responds to food very quickly. Processed carbohydrates reduce the numbers of beneficial microbes and encourage growth of pathogens in the gut and other places in our bodily microbial community (the microbiome).[33] Indeed, science is discovering that people with obesity, heart disease, diabetes, cancer, hypertension and all other metabolic syndrome manifestations have abnormal gut flora. These microbes add their own damage to the body, causing allergies, autoimmunity, systemic toxicity, nutritional deficiencies, etc.

In my clinical experience, many people with metabolic syndrome may not have severe digestive problems. So, they don't have to start from the GAPS Introduction Diet and can just follow the Full GAPS Diet. This diet eliminates all processed carbohydrates, thus removing the cause of metabolic syndrome. At the same time, it will normalise the gut flora and nourish the body properly. Treating metabolic syndrome with the GAPS Nutritional Protocol is very rewarding, as these people improve very quickly: blood pressure normalises, excess weight melts away and all other health problems disappear one by one. It is important to make the Full GAPS Diet your permanent diet. You can never go back to eating sugar and wheat flour, as your body has no tolerance of these substances; it has already been primed for developing problems from these 'foods'. If, on top of metabolic syndrome, you have serious digestive problems, then you will need to go through the GAPS Introduction Diet at some point. As metabolic syndrome comes with magnesium deficiency, it can be helpful to take a good quality magnesium supplement for a few weeks at the beginning of the protocol (amino acid chelates of magnesium).

Mouth problems

Our digestive system begins in the mouth, which has a very rich microbial flora. It is interesting that the composition of this flora is very similar to the flora in the stool of the person.[34] People with abnormal flora in the mouth often have mouth ulcers, an unpleasant taste in the mouth and can have a breath odour. The tongue can tell us a lot.[35] Maybe that is why it is instinctive for many of us to look at it in the morning? A white coating on the tongue is typically an overgrowth of candida and other fungi. A brown coating usually indicates gastritis and liver congestion. A swollen tongue is a typical indication of low thyroid function; the tongue will have indents on its sides left by the teeth. Red and sore tongue is a typical symptom of B-vitamin deficiencies. It is often accompanied by cracks in the corners of the mouth.[35] Dental health has a profound effect on the health of your mouth.[36] Most dental materials are toxic and change the environment in your mouth, promoting growth of pathogenic microbes. It is important to work with a holistic dentist to keep your mouth healthy. If there are mouth ulcers or breath odour, I recommend brushing your teeth with olive oil and bicarbonate of soda once or twice a day. Dip your toothbrush into the oil, then into the bicarbonate of soda, brush as usual and rinse well. To populate your mouth with beneficial flora, finish all your meals with a little homemade kefir, yoghurt or any fermented vegetable. Drinking kombucha will also help. If fermented foods are not tolerated yet, you can open a capsule of a multi-strain probiotic onto your tongue and let the powder dissolve in your mouth. Following the GAPS Diet will remove the root causes of any mouth problems, such as nutritional deficiencies, autoimmunity, systemic inflammation, allergies and other.

Mould sensitivity/allergy. Multiple chemical sensitivity

People with these disorders have abnormal gut flora, overgrowth of fungi in the body and a damaged detoxification system. So, the immune system is dealing with many assaults at the same time and it is using chronic inflammation, allergic reactions and autoimmune mechanisms in different combinations. The activity of the immune system produces many unpleasant symptoms in these people, from mild to quite debilitating. Reducing your exposure to moulds and man-made chemicals is very important, and patients with these disorders put a lot of effort into this aspect. However, it is not enough! The GAPS Nutritional Protocol will lay a solid foundation for removing the root causes of these problems. The person needs to be patient and stay on the diet for many years, doing the GAPS Introduction Diet periodically at least once a year. The Full GAPS Diet has to become the permanent diet for the rest of their life. Working with an allergy specialist who is trained in methods of *neutralisation* can be helpful. Sauna, GAPS baths, sunbathing, swimming in the sea and ocean, walking barefoot and other cleansing procedures are essential. You may remain sensitive, but all these measures will make you well, feel healthy and enable you to lead a normal productive life.

Myelin and demyelinating disease (multiple sclerosis (MS), neuropathies, leukodystrophies, myelopathies, Charcot-Marie-Tooth disease, Guillain-Barre syndrome and other)

Myelin is a layer of fatty insulation around the nerve fibres in the nervous system.[37] Myelin is made by very specialised cells, called oligodendrocytes. These cells stretch out long 'arms', which wrap themselves many times around the bare nerve fibre, 'hugging' it and creating many layers of myelin sheath. These 'arms' are basically made out of two layers of the cell's wall (cell membrane) with a little bit of the cell's cytoplasm in between. So, in effect, myelin is made out of many layers of cell membrane. What is the cell membrane made out of? Largely fat and cholesterol, so fat-soluble things get into it easily. Unfortunately, many toxins produced by abnormal gut flora and toxins from the modern environment (toxic metals, dental materials, agricultural chemicals and pharmaceutical drugs) are fat-soluble and can accumulate in the myelin. Studies in fluorescent microscopy show patches of accumulated toxic metals in the cell membranes of oligodendrocytes.[38] These change the position and shape of proteins in the myelin making them look 'foreign' to the immune system. The immune system tries to clean contaminated parts of myelin using inflammation, autoimmunity and possibly other methods. Myelin provides the nervous system with protection, insulation and nourishment. As myelin gets damaged, the unprotected nerve fibres and cells get damaged as well, leading to paralysis of different severity, lack of sensitivity or abnormal sensitivity, impaired muscle function and co-ordination, vision and eye movement problems, hearing and speech problems, incontinence, fatigue and mental degeneration.[39]

Our nervous system works on electricity and electricity is temperature-dependant. When the body temperature rises, the nerve fibres with a damaged myelin cover start short-circuiting, while normal electrical conduction along these nerves slows down or can even shut down altogether. That is why patients with demyelinating disorders usually feel worse in hot weather and are better able to function in colder conditions.[40] In my experience, people with autism, schizophrenia, other severe mental illness and many autoimmune disorders have the same heat sensitivity, indicating that their myelin sheath is under attack.

More and more evidence is being accumulated showing that toxic metals play an important part in the development of demyelinating disorders (multiple sclerosis (MS) in particular): mercury, gold, palladium, lead, titanium, nickel, aluminium and other.[41] A major source of toxic metals in the body is dental work, and MS patients are found, on average, to have more tooth decay, and hence more dental work, than the general population.[42] Not only mercury can get into the system from amalgams and other dental materials but many other toxins. Careful removal of dental amalgam fillings by a holistic dentist has been recorded to cure some cases of MS.[36,42] Unfortunately, the majority of amalgam removals are done by conventional dentists, who are not trained to remove them safely, so large amounts of mercury are released into the body of the person during the procedure. As a result, conventional amalgam removal is one of the major causes of demyelinating disorders.[43] Another major source of toxic metals in our bodies are cosmetics, hair dyes and make-up.[44] It is quite possible that this explains why women are two to three times more likely to get MS than men. Personal care products are also full of many other toxic chemicals, which absorb through skin, scalp and mucous membranes quite effectively, are circulated around the body and stored in fatty tissues. MS and other demyelinating disorders are becoming more common amongst children.[45] Many of these children are born with a large toxic load, acquired from the mother during pregnancy, and accumulate toxins from vaccines (aluminium in particular) and the environment. Processed foods are another major source of damaging chemicals in the body. One of these toxic chemicals comes from sugar-free soft drinks where sugar has been replaced with an artificial sweetener aspartame (acesulfame). This has been linked with MS and other degenerative diseases for at least a decade now.[46]

It has been found that people with MS have abnormal gut flora with an overgrowth of bacteria *Acinetobacter* and *Akkermansia*, leading researchers to a conclude that MS comes from the gut.[47] Systemic chronic infections have been found in people with MS and other demyelinating disorders: *Clostridium perfringens* type B; Epstein-Barr virus; Human herpes virus 6; Human endogenous retroviruses; Lyme *Borrelia* complex; *Chlamydophila pneumoniae*; heat shock protein 60 (prions) and worm larva.[48] In 2016 American pathologist Alan MacDonald and his team found migrating worms in the spinal fluid of MS patients.[49] As they 'have not found one case of MS without worms in the brain', they are convinced that these worms are instrumental in the development of multiple sclerosis. Where there is contamination with man-made toxins, there will always be microbes and parasites. Please, read more about this subject in the chapter *Toxins and Parasites*.

MS and other demyelinating disorders are GAPS conditions. The gut wall is always damaged in these patients, leading to absorption of undigested foods and toxins. The immune system is out of balance leading to systemic inflammation and autoimmunity (please read about it in the chapter *Immune System*). The detoxification system is broken down and is unable to process toxins, leading to their accumulation in the body. Following the GAPS Nutritional Protocol should be the baseline treatment for these patients. For the majority, I recommend starting with the Full GAPS Diet and considering doing the Introduction Diet sometime later. As the gut wall heals, the flow of toxicity into the body reduces dramatically. The immune system gets rebalanced and the detoxification system starts working again. As a result, the body is able to cleanse itself and start rebuilding myelin, and the person starts recovering.

Myelin is especially rich in cholesterol: it comprises 22% of normal human myelin and amongst its many functions provides the myelin sheath with stiffness, so it can retain its shape. [50] Cholesterol and saturated fatty acids not only make the structure of myelin, they are essential in all healing and scar formation in the body.[51] When it comes to dietary recommendations for demyelinating disorders, these are the substances that should be provided in unlimited amounts in order to rebuild the person's damaged myelin. So, eggs, fatty meats, fresh fish and fermented raw organic milk products are the foods of choice. The easiest to assimilate are *raw* fats and cholesterol from foods which have never been cooked; these nutrients are rich in enzymes, easy to digest, and go directly to build damaged tissues. Real myelin resuscitation can be provided by raw fats from raw butter, raw egg yolks, raw sour cream, raw cream, raw coconut oil, raw animal fats (raw bone marrow and raw-cured pork fat) and raw or fermented oily fish.

I recommend introducing GAPS 'shakes' as soon as the diarrhoea has cleared in order to improve fat digestion. If the person is not prone to diarrhoea, introduce the shakes from the beginning. It is important to introduce good quality cod liver oil from the beginning of the programme: start from 2 tablespoons per day for 1-2 months, and then gradually reduce to 1 teaspoon per day. Cod liver oil will provide you with much needed vitamins A and D. Sunbathing is essential, introduced gradually as the person's heat tolerance improves.

Some MS sufferers lose weight on the GAPS Diet, but some gain weight. It is likely that the body is not yet able to remove fat-soluble toxins. So, it moves them from the brain and the rest of the nervous tissue into a less critical place – the under-skin fat. When the body is ready to move them out, the excessive weight is usually lost easily. Some people have to wait for a few years for this to happen, but in the meantime the symptoms of MS or another demyelinating disorder slowly disappear.

Some patients have to consider chelation of toxic metals to make a full recovery. I recommend using chelation later in the programme, when the gut is healed, because naturally toxic metals leave the body through the bowel and your digestive system needs to be robust enough to withstand that. Please, read more on this subject in the chapter *Detoxification*.

It is essential for this group of patients to work with a holistic dentist. The dental work, which you have had throughout your life, may have caused your condition in the first place! All amalgam fillings and root canals have to be removed carefully and slowly, and only a holistic dentist is trained to remove them without doing more damage.[36,42]

As the person gets stronger on the GAPS Nutritional Protocol, at some point it can be helpful to address worms and parasites using herbal remedies, diatomaceous earth, bentonite clay and other natural substances.

MS and other demyelinating disorders can be frightening, and mainstream opinions about them don't help. But, like all autoimmunity, they are reversible. It may take a few years to heal completely, but the effort is worth it. With all autoimmunity we have to start from healing the gut!

Here is a case study of recovery from multiple sclerosis:

When Eda was 13, her parent divorced, which was very traumatic for her. She started smoking heavily and eating processed foods. After food poisoning, she became quite ill, developing severe fatigue, depression and aggressive tendencies. Her sleep become abnormal: she was up all night and then asleep all day. She remembers that, around the same time, she had a tick bite, which was never investigated. At the age of 16 she developed pain all over her body. She was addicted to smoking, Coca-Cola and Red Bull soft drinks. Some inflammation was found in her lungs and she took antibiotics.

Starting from the age of 20, Eda had four children. During pregnancies she seemed to feel better, but between pregnancies her symptoms got worse. She developed weakness in her legs with a heavy feeling, severe fatigue, lethargy and dizziness. Her hands became weak and she kept dropping things. She was given painkillers, antidepressants, antibiotics and other medications, none of which helped. After her third pregnancy she had temporary paralysis in her right arm and the right side of her face. After the fourth pregnancy all her symptoms got worse and her vision became blurry. At this stage she was diagnosed with multiple sclerosis (MS). She was still addicted to cigarettes and caffeinated soft drinks. Her marriage ended in divorce.

Having found out that there is no effective mainstream treatment for her condition, Eda stopped smoking and started researching natural treatments for MS. She came across the GAPS Nutritional Protocol and decided to give it a try, though she was sceptical at the beginning. This is what she wrote about her experience: 'Two weeks on GAPS Intro, I got my energy back! No more brain fog. One month later I was thinking so clear and all the pain was gone. For the first time in 15 years!! My legs were like feathers. I got my life back! Finally, I found that little girl in me that I lost a long time ago. I was always going to sleep early, and had to sleep during daytime, but now I can stay up. In the morning I am not in pain anymore and I am not frozen. I had a lot of mental issues; I was really insecure and they even thought I had a borderline personality disorder. Now I am perfect! My children have changed on the GAPS Diet – their behaviour is perfect now. My

second son had learning problems and now he is one of the best at school. I don't give them processed food anymore and I cook now, like the ancient people did, with meat stock, bone broth and lard. I really can't explain what you did for me and my family, Dr Natasha, even my grandchildren in the future will know your name! My mother was on many drugs for her rheumatoid arthritis, atherosclerosis and other health problems. She stopped everything and changed her diet after reading your book and she never felt better. God bless the MS, the so-called MS, which made me a strong person. I'm now on my way to being a holistic doctor.'

Apart from following the GAPS Diet, Eda used low-dose naltrexone and supplements of vitamin D3, Curcumin, Milk Thistle and Nigella Sativa oil.

Oesophagus problems

The oesophagus is a pipe that passes food from the mouth down into the stomach. Its lining has a similar flora as in the mouth and normally it is well protected by extensive mucous production. However, if the food passing through the oesophagus is full of toxins, its lining can get damaged and many problems can develop. Processed foods, tap water, agricultural chemicals and pharmaceuticals provide many toxins which can damage the oesophagus. Dental materials, amalgam fillings in particular, are very common sources of this damage.[42,43] Mercury never stops leaching from amalgam fillings. It contaminates the mucous membranes of the oesophagus leading to chronic inflammation – *oesophagitis*.[52] In this situation many microbes overgrow in the oesophagus, and its lining becomes inflamed and sore. This condition can make swallowing uncomfortable and difficult, cause nausea, vomiting and heartburn. If it continues for many years, it can lead to cancer of the oesophagus. Some people can develop an allergic condition, when the oesophagus closes up on contact with a particular food, particularly seafood (which may contain mercury) or 'smoked' meats and fish (which were not smoked traditionally, but smeared with a special chemical). When this happens, the person gets pain or discomfort behind their sternum and cannot swallow food, water or even their own saliva. This situation can last from a few minutes to a few hours. Other processed foods containing artificial chemicals can also trigger this reaction. Regular regurgitation of food from the stomach (reflux) can damage the oesophagus and cause inflammation and even ulcers in its lower part.[52] This condition is called GORD (gastroesophageal reflux disease) or GERD (gastroesophageal reflux disease) and is due to the overgrowth of pathogenic microbes in the stomach (please look in the *Stomach Problems*).

The GAPS Nutritional Protocol has a good record in healing the oesophagus, as well as the rest of the digestive system. I recommend finishing every meal with ½ cup of kefir, a few spoons of sour cream or some probiotic powder dissolved in a little water, so the good microbes can work on healing the mucous membranes in the throat and the oesophagus between meals. Working with a holistic dentist is essential in order to deal with amalgam fillings and other dental materials, which are a common source of oesophageal problems.

Pancreatic problems

The pancreas is a major digestive organ.[53] It produces about 1.5 l (3.1 pt) of alkaline pancreatic juice per day, full of enzymes necessary for us to break down food. Pancreatic enzymes are released into the duodenum in an inactive form (called zymogens or proenzymes). The cells lining the duodenal wall produce brush-border enzymes. One of these enzymes is called enteropeptidase (or enterokinase); this enzyme activates the pancreatic juices, allowing them to start digesting food.[53] In a person with abnormal gut flora the duodenal wall is usually not able to produce enough brush-border enzymes, including enteropeptidase. As a result, the pancreatic juices may not be fully activated.

In the chapter *Digestive Enzymes* we talked about pancreatic stones. These stones form as a result of low stomach acidity in many GAPS people. If the stomach is not producing enough acid, then the pancreas does not produce enough alkaline solution. This leads to precipitation of proteins in pancreatic ducts and formation of pancreatic stones, obstructing the ducts.[54] Powerful enzymes, building up behind the obstruction, damage the pancreas, which can lead to acute or chronic *pancreatitis*, *pancreatic insufficiency* and *pancreatic cancer*.[55] As the tissue of the pancreas gets damaged, the person can develop diabetes (both type one and two), because the pancreas is not able to produce enough insulin.

The pancreas has its own microbial community living in the ducts.[56] The alkaline juices make sure that this community has a certain composition. When the pancreas is not producing enough bicarbonate liquid, this microbial community changes. All sorts of pathogenic microbes, parasites and intestinal worms get inside the pancreas and can cause an infection or even cancer in this organ. It is essential to heal the whole digestive system in order to heal the pancreas, and stomach acidity is the first issue that has to be addressed. This acidity is essential for the pancreas to produce enough bicarbonate to make a normal healthy pancreatic juice. Without this juice the pancreas is not able to keep itself free of parasites, infection, stones or any other disease-causing elements: the organ stagnates, which is never a healthy situation! Because of lack of bicarbonate the pH in the pancreas can become more acidic, which encourages growth of fungi, such as candida. Growth of fungi is a major factor in cancer formation, including cancer of the pancreas. On top of that, the tissues of the pancreas get damaged by pancreatic enzymes, when the ducts are blocked and this organ cannot flush them out. Any damaged tissue will have growth of microbes in it, so it is inevitable that fungi will be there.

The pancreas is hidden deep inside our abdomen close to the solar plexus – a very complex formation of peripheral nerves. That is why any unhealthy situation in the pancreas is painful, and the pain can radiate into the back and spread to other parts of the abdomen. The pain can be quite severe and is usually made worse by eating. If the process is acute, the person may develop nausea and vomiting, have high fever and feel quite unwell. In chronic pancreatitis, diarrhoea with fat in the stool (steatorrhea) is common, because the fats are not being digested properly.[55]

Alkaline juice from the pancreas is essential for appropriate digestion of food in the small intestine. In a person with low stomach acidity the pancreatic juices don't flow very well. This means that the digestive system has to digest food without the help of the pancreas, which is not possible. People with this condition develop malabsorption and deficiencies in nutrients, including weight loss, anaemia and failure to thrive. Many celiac patients have this problem to various degrees, as do people with other digestive disorders. Undigested food, travelling through the intestines, feeds microbes, leading to an overgrowth of pathogenic microbial community in the intestine.

In the chapter *Liver and Lungs* we have talked about gall stones and how to remove them gently and safely. In my clinical experience, the same procedure helps to remove stones from the pancreas and improve the flow of pancreatic juice. GAPS shakes and coffee enemas work, though it may take time to deal with the problem fully. The GAPS Diet is essential to follow for any pancreatic problem. If the problem is acute, follow the first and second stages of the *GAPS Introduction Diet.* During the days with the worst symptoms some people find it helpful to follow the *GAPS Liquid Fast,* before commencing the Introduction Diet. On the GAPS Fast the person drinks only homemade meat stock, whey, juices and brine from fermented vegetables, warm water and herbal teas. When the pain subsides, these people can start the Introduction Diet. Try to use coffee enemas daily for pain relief and removal of stones. I do not recommend using stomach acid boosting supplements during acute pancreatitis! Instead, use small amounts of sauerkraut juice, vegetable medley, brine from fermented vegetables and fresh cabbage juice for stimulating stomach acid production. Natural herbal bitters can also be used. When the acute phase is over, you can follow the remaining stages of the Introduction Diet and then move into the *Full GAPS Diet*. When on the *Full GAPS Diet*, it will be possible to start using stomach acid boosting supplements, if necessary.

There is an Interesting fact: the highest concentration of vitamin K2 in the human body has been found in the pancreas![57] Nature doesn't do anything without good reason! Obviously, the pancreas needs high amounts of vitamin K2. So, supplementing fermented cod liver oil, quality emu oil and butter oil (rich in vitamin K2, as well as other fat-soluble vitamins, D and A in particular) can be very helpful for people with pancreatic problems, acute or chronic. These are the only supplements I would recommend in acute pancreatitis. If, initially, no amount of fat is tolerated orally, you can rub these oils on your abdomen, cover the skin with a towel and put a hot-water bottle on it. Doing this procedure daily can provide your body with some amounts of fat-soluble vitamins, essential for the pancreas to heal. Another effective way to supplement these oils is through enemas.

The good news is that the pancreas has an amazing ability to regenerate! Understanding what is going on is vital in order to take the right steps in helping the pancreas to heal. The pancreas is a team player: it is part of the whole digestive system. One cannot heal the pancreas without healing the whole gut!

PANDAS (*Paediatric Autoimmune Neuropsychiatric Disorders Associated with Streptococcal Infections*)

It is likely that this disease is caused by a cell-wall-deficient form of streptococcus, created by penicillin-type antibiotics.[59] These stealth forms of bacteria are very difficult to detect and to treat; they are resistant to all mainstream antibiotics. However, the body knows how to deal with them, as long as we help the body to become strong, healthy and able. GAPS Nutritional Protocol has a good record of helping patients with PANDAS/PANS (Paediatric Autoimmune Neuropsychiatric Syndrome). It is a very distressing disorder, but the recovery can be quite quick and full. There are several case studies of recovery from PANDAS in the book *GAPS Stories*.[58] The following case study will demonstrate what it is like to have this disease.

Case study of recovery from PANDAS from the clinic of Dr Shantih Coro, a Certified GAPS Practitioner.

Giacomo was 10 years old when he came to see Dr Coro with his parents. He had a diagnosis of PANDAS and had been taking antibi-

otics and antipsychotic medications. Medical history revealed that the boy had been a GAPS child from the start of his life. He was born through a C-Section, breastfed only for 1 month and brought up on formula milk. He had recurrent ear and chest infections, which led to heavy use of antibiotics since infancy.

At 1½ years of age Giacomo had an episode of febrile seizures, became hyperactive, irritable and fussy with food. He started suffering from absences, hypersensitivity to noises and odours, phobia of insects and his eye contact become poor. Later on, he developed tics involving his eyes and tongue. These symptoms were dismissed and the parents were told that they would go away with age. But, around the age of five, Giacomo woke up one morning making absurd requests and screaming, as if someone was torturing him. He was making so much noise that the neighbours called the police!

Having had several disappointing experiences with doctors, the parents diagnosed their son with PANDAS through an internet search and went to a doctor who specialised in this disease. The diagnosis was confirmed and Giacomo started antibiotic therapy. Antibiotics brought some improvements in eye contact, tics and an ability to draw, but Giacomo still had fears, attention deficit, uncontrollable anger and aggressiveness. He was diagnosed with OCD. He was having screaming and crying episodes and was terrified of everything. Antipsychotic medication was added to the antibiotics, which Giacomo had to take permanently. Gradually he could not tolerate clothes anymore and went around the house naked. He could not go to school, had anxiety and apathy, was extremely fussy with food and did not want to leave the house. Out of desperation, the parents decided to try nutrition and went to Dr Shantih Coro.

The boy's diet consisted of pizza, pasta, bread and pastries, with little fat or protein, no vegetables or fruit, and lots of sweets. Giacomo had severe digestive problems with abdominal pain, bloating, constipation and abnormal stools (pale with rotten egg odour). He had trouble falling asleep and had nightmares.

The GAPS Diet was suggested, which was not received well by the parents. A traditionally Italian family could not imagine life without pasta and bread. They did not remove these foods, but tried to reduce their amounts and saw some improvements in Giacomo's attention, bowel movements and sleep. Then Dr Coro had a serious conversation with Giacomo alone, and for the next 30 days the boy followed his recommendations strictly. As a result, after those 30 days he had no more tics and all his symptoms were improved immensely. The parents were shocked to see such change in their son; they could not believe

that food could have such an effect! Giacomo stayed on the GAPS Introduction Diet for six months, after which he followed the Full GAPS Diet. By then all his symptoms had improved by 60%. He started wearing clothes and went to school (after staying at home for three years). His behaviour and life become practically normal for his age.

Then, after nine months on the GAPS Diet, Giacomo started expelling parasites. This went on for three months and brought back some of his symptoms. The parents collected a sample of Giacomo's stool, where they could clearly see parasites moving. This sample was sent to a lab, but 'nothing was found'. By the end of parasite removal Giacomo had improved even more; his bloating, abdominal pain, smelly stools and hyperactivity were gone completely. His tics, fears and anxiety disappeared. And his focus and concentration had improved to such an extent that the parents moved Giacomo to a mainstream school.

After 18 months on the GAPS Diet, Giacomo had no symptoms at all, the diagnosis of PANDAS was removed and all medications stopped. Giacomo was able to slowly introduce other foods into his diet. He had a healthy childhood, and today Giacomo is a healthy young man. He is preparing for his exams to enter the University of Medicine in Rome. His dream is to become a neurologist and open a multidisciplinary centre to help children with PANDAS.

Parasites and worms

Worms and parasites are inevitable, we all have them. Please, read the chapter *Toxins and Parasites* about their role in Nature. Common worms have an interesting life cycle. After eggs hatch in the digestive system, larvae burrow through the gut wall and travel all over the body, fulfilling different stages of their development in different organs.[60] When a larva is mature enough to become an adult, it burrows through the back of the throat or travels up from the lungs into the throat, to be swallowed again. Once in the upper digestive system, mating occurs and new eggs are laid. There is a limited research to show that, while they travel around our organs, these creatures accumulate large amounts of toxins from the surrounding tissues.[61] They keep the toxins inside themselves and, when they have completed their life cycle, they leave in the stool taking the toxins with them. So, these larvae and adult worms can be seen as little vacuum cleaners, hoovering tissues and organs in our bodies to keep them clean. When the body is healthy and strong, the number of parasites is small and in balance with the rest of the microbial community. But in a toxic body their numbers can be too high. Unfortunately, many people in our modern world have a large toxic load in their bodies and, as a result, a large parasitic load.

When worms and parasites overgrow, they can produce unpleasant symptoms:

- Abdominal pain in the upper gut, particularly at night. During the day many worms and parasites spend time outside the digestive system. In the middle of the night they crawl back inside the gut to feed on the remnants of your dinner.[60] This can cause crampy abdominal pain. This pain may be worse coming up to the full moon and during the full moon, because this is the time when common worms procreate inside your digestive system.
- Diarrhoea, excessive gas production in the upper and lower gut, nausea, periodic vomiting and, sometimes, constipation. Again, the symptoms may be worse during the full moon.
- They can keep the gut wall porous and leaky, because too many larvae constantly migrate through it. It is difficult to heal a damaged gut wall during a parasite infestation.[62] This would perpetuate allergies and food intolerances.
- They manufacture toxins of their own, which can cause many unpleasant symptoms, from headaches, periodic fever, joint aches, skin rash, teeth grinding, recurrent vomiting to mental problems.[63]
- Low body weight and difficulty putting on weight. An overgrowth of worms can consume all the food inside your gut, leaving you malnourished.[63]
- When the larvae are mature enough to mate, they travel from the lungs up your breathing passages or burrow through the back of your throat in order to be swallowed again.[60] This process can lead to irritating dry cough and a sore pharynx. The ENT specialists will see that the back of your throat has a 'bumpy' surface with some inflammation.
- Getting into different organs, worms and parasites can produce organ-specific symptoms. They can take part in chronic inflammation in these organs and formation of tumours, both malignant and benign.[63]

GAPS people often have an overgrowth of worms and parasites, which needs to be addressed in order for the person to recover from their illness. But, before attacking parasites, we need to understand that the whole procedure will bring a lot of disturbance into the body, extra toxicity and inflammation. So, it is important to prepare properly for parasite cleansing! First, we need to heal the gut to a considerable degree in order for it to cope! Second, we need to restore the detoxification system. When this system starts working and removing toxins naturally, the body will let go of many worms and parasites more easily (because it will not need their services anymore). The immune system needs to be rebalanced and strengthened as well, so it can cope with parasitic die-off and release of toxicity. So, in the GAPS Nutritional Protocol we do not focus on these lodgers at the beginning of the programme but wait for at least six months, preferably a year. In many people, just healing the gut and rebalancing the microbiome takes worms and parasites under control. In other people, after initial considerable improvements in their health, they may come to a point when their healing slows down and some symptoms stubbornly will not go away. This may be the time to address worms and parasites and can be a year or more after the beginning of the GAPS Nutritional Protocol.

There are some important considerations to take into account in order to deal with these creatures effectively.

1. It is best to use natural methods rather than pharmaceuticals (with a few exceptions). The reason for this is that worms and parasites have hooks, claws and suckers to attach themselves to your gut lining or any other tissue in your body. A pharmaceutical drug is usually designed to kill the parasite (an adult or a particular stage of larvae). These dead bodies can hang in your tissues and organs for a long time, decaying and producing large amounts of toxins, as well as releasing back into your system the man-made toxicity they 'hoovered up' from your tissues. This toxin release can lead to many unpleasant symptoms and worsening of the main disease. There are a few drugs which can be useful in an acute infestation of some microscopic parasites (for example *ivermectin, metronidazole* and *praziquantel*). But, for chronic infestations of worms and parasites, it is best to use natural herbal remedies. Why? Because, herbs and other natural methods are not designed to kill the parasite, but to make it uncomfortable, so it leaves the body voluntarily taking its cargo of toxins with it. In order to achieve this, we need to take the herbs for a few months.
2. Many herbal protocols recommend taking herbal remedies for two months, having a break for a month, and then repeating the treatment for another two months. Why? Because no remedy in the world can kill all the life stages of a parasite (whether natural herbs or mainstream drugs). All of the remedies address only a few life stages, so there will always be some larvae left somewhere in your body. When the treatment is over, these larvae will continue maturing. Giving the treatment a break for a month will allow these larvae to mature to the point when the herbs may be effective. So, the full course of herbal treatment may take 5-6 months. For some GAPS patients we have to do this treatment

once a year. And we need to keep repeating the course for a few years in order to keep the parasitic load down. With every course people typically see larger improvements in their health, as stubborn chronic symptoms start disappearing. We continue following the GAPS Diet strictly throughout this period. At some point, your body becomes strong enough to keep worms and parasites in balance with the rest of the microbiome, so you can stop repeating the antiparasitic courses.

3. All life forms on our beautiful planet respond to the moon cycle. Why? Because most of our bodies consists of water, and water follows the pull of the moon. The tides in the seas and oceans show just how powerful this phenomenon is! Worms and parasites activate coming up to the full moon and during the full moon. This is the time when adults congregate inside the gut, mate and lay eggs. So, this is the time to catch the majority of them! Start your herbal course coming up to the full moon and finish it two months later, taking a few more days to finish after the next full moon. Take a break for a month, then start again coming up to the full moon, finishing two months later after the next full moon. There are some anti-parasitic enemas for adults and children, which we have discussed in the chapter *Bowel Managment.* These enemas should also be done coming up to the full moon and during the full moon.

What herbs can be used for driving worms and parasites out of your body? The list is very long. Every country and region of the world has its own collection of herbs, which people have found effective through experience over hundreds of years. Most commonly used are black walnut hulls, tansy, cloves, artemisia, pumpkin seed, thyme, neem, anise, salvia, epazote, basil, goldenseal, berberine, barberry, papaya seed, fennel seed, garlic, onions, oregano, cayenne and chilli peppers, ginger, cucumber seed, mimosa pudica, tribulus, grapefruit seed, passion flower, vidanga and olive leaf. This list is not complete by any means. Please, research your local herbal remedies in your part of the world and use them. Every part of the world has its own parasites. Local people, through experience, are likely to have found local remedies which work best for these parasites.

Apart from herbs, traditionally people used clay (many different varieties), diatomaceous earth, ash of lime trees (or other trees) and other natural remedies. Some antiparasitic formulas on the market include these ingredients.

Enemas are important during any antiparasitic course. It is a good idea not to let weakened or dead parasites linger in your bowel, but flush them out regularly. Some enemas are specifically designed to drive out common worms. For example, use garlic enemas and eucalyptus and lemon enemas for rope worms. Please, see more information on enemas in the chapter *Bowel Management.*

Overall, there is no need to fear worms and parasites. They are normal parts of our microbial community in the gut and elsewhere in the body. No matter how much we may fight them, they will always come back! They are impossible to eradicate fully and we don't want to do that, as they fulfil many useful roles in our body. All we need to do is to bring them into balance with the rest of our microbiome, our immune system and our detoxification system.

Psoriasis

Psoriasis is a full body disease and it has an autoimmune component. It is associated with other autoimmune conditions, as well as with diabetes, heart disease and other manifestations of metabolic syndrome.[64] About 30% of patients develop psoriatic arthritis as well as psoriatic skin patches. All autoimmunity is born in the gut, and that is where the treatment has to start. The GAPS Nutritional Protocol has a good record of helping people with this disease. It takes time to recover, because it takes time to heal the gut and rebalance the immune system. In the meantime, use topical preparations described in the *Eczema* entry in this chapter to soothe and heal the skin. You will find a recipe for tallow cream in the chapter *What we shall eat and why, with some recipes*; this topical cream can be really helpful in psoriasis. There is a nice testimony of recovery from severe psoriasis with psoriatic arthritis in the *GAPS Stories* book.[65]

SIBO (Small Intestinal Bacterial Overgrowth)

SIBO (small intestinal bacterial overgrowth) is becoming a common condition.[66] It is not just bacteria that overgrow in the intestines but many other microbes and larger creatures (flukes and worms). Healthy intestines have their own microbial flora, which is protected by normal stomach acidity. The stomach acid is a barrier, which stops harmful microbes and parasites in food and water. When the stomach acid is low, these creatures get through and settle in the stomach, as well as lower down in the intestines. Our intestines are the place where absorption of food happens. When the intestinal wall gets populated by pathogenic flora, it becomes inflamed and sore and is unable to fulfil its functions. The person develops many unpleasant symptoms: bloating, abdominal pain or discomfort, diarrhoea or constipation. Food digestion and absorption become abnormal and the person develops malnutrition and multiple nutritional deficiencies. The gut wall gets damaged and becomes porous and leaky, leading to food intolerances and allergies. Many pathogens in the intestine produce histamine and other biogenic amines, leading to symptoms of HIT (histamine intolerance). In some people, toxins produced by pathogenic microbes paralyse the muscles in the intestinal wall, making them sluggish and slowing down the food transit, which leads to chronic constipation. In other people, the muscles become hyperactive, so the food transit becomes too fast, leading to diarrhoea and malnutrition.

The mainstream approach to SIBO (as usual) is to try and kill the microbes, so antibiotics are prescribed. Alternative practitioners try to replace antibiotics with natural antimicrobial substances, essentially following the same idea. But the key is to improve stomach acid production and provide healing for the gut lining. It is essential to follow the GAPS Introduction Diet in this condition and eat plenty of fermented foods. While the stomach is being healed, it is a good idea to supplement stomach acid before meals (Betaine HCl or HCL & Pepsin).

Sinusitis, chronic

Chronic sinusitis is due to two factors: abnormal microbial flora populating the sinuses and systemic toxicity coming from unhealthy diet and abnormal gut flora. Sinuses are lined by mucous membranes, which produce mucous to clean and protect themselves. Mucous production is part of our immune function, and it is very efficient in dealing with all problems on our mucous membranes.[67] Unfortunately, many pharmaceutical drugs and man-made toxins reduce or impair mucous production in the body, making the mucous membranes dry and unable to look after themselves. Abnormal microbial flora, living in the sinuses, cause chronic inflammation and a runny nose.[68] This clear liquid is a sign of abnormal mucous production. Narrow face and narrow nasal passages can contribute to the whole problem (please, read about this in detail in the chapter *Bones and Teeth*). The GAPS Nutritional Protocol will remove systemic reasons for chronic sinusitis. In the meantime, it is important to populate that area with beneficial microbes. To cleanse the sinuses, rinse them daily with warm salty solution (1 teaspoon of natural salt dissolved in half a cup of warm water). To populate them with beneficial microbes, you can use a commercial probiotic or homemade whey, kefir, sour cream or yoghurt. You can use a pipette to put the solution into your nose. People find all sorts of positions to reach places in their sinuses: tilting your head back or lying on your back is usually helpful. Every night it is important to put some probiotic microbes onto your tongue as the last procedure before going to bed, so eat some kefir or dissolve some commercial probiotic powder in your mouth. The microbes will be working on your mouth and throat flora overnight and will travel to the back of your nose.

Stomach problems

Your stomach is the first place in your digestive system where anything you swallow gets to stay for a while – for a few hours or even days sometimes. So, if there is anything damaging in what you swallow, your stomach lining is the first place to pay the price. If it gets damaged, inflammation sets in – gastritis. There are many different influences that can start this process, but pharmaceutical drugs are by far the most common cause of gastritis.[69] Painkillers, taken for headaches, toothaches, aching joints or any other painful condition, are the most common culprits. Other drugs, if taken frequently and for prolonged periods of time, will also start the process: antibiotics, antidepressants, cholesterol-reducing drugs, blood pressure drugs, etc. It is not just the active ingredients in the drug that can damage your stomach, but the many other ingredients (just look at the list on the packaging). Many of these toxins accumulate in the stomach lining and can stay there for years, maintaining the chronic inflammation. Our modern food and water provide large amounts of toxins to damage our stomachs: agricultural chemicals, GMOs, flavourings, preservatives and other food additives. Modern dental care is a considerable source of toxic chemicals, which are swallowed and can damage the stomach lining: mercury from amalgam fillings, toothpaste and mouthwashes (particularly with fluoride), chemicals in your fillings, crowns and anything else put in your mouth by the dentist.[70] Smoking and drinking to excess are also known to cause chronic gastritis. Chronic stress and negative mental attitudes can also contribute to this problem.[69]

When the stomach lining gets inflamed and sore, the body downregulates stomach acid production, so the stomach lining doesn't get further damaged and ulcers do not form; this condition is called *hypochlorhydria* or low stomach acid.[71] This presents its own problem: the stomach acid is the natural barrier for pathogenic microbes and parasites. When the stomach is not producing enough acid, these pathogens overgrow in the whole of your digestive system, including the stomach itself. Normally the stomach is the least-populated area of the digestive system due to its extremely acid environment. It has a natural resident flora, which normally lives on the stomach mucosa, maintaining its health and function (largely yeast, lactobacilli and *Helicobacter pylori*).[72] However, in a person with hypochlorhydria resident microbes get out of control and all sorts of pathogenic and opportunistic bacteria and fungi grow in the stomach. The most research in this area has been done in stomach cancer patients, the majority of whom show low levels of stomach acid production.[73]

The microbes, which populate a low-acid stomach, play a very important role in causing stomach cancer, ulcers and gastritis.[72,73] Many of these microbes love to eat carbohydrates, particularly the processed kind. In the stomach with low acidity, overgrowing microbes start fermenting dietary carbohydrates with the production of various toxins and gases (including carbon dioxide and methane). Accumulating gases cause excessive belching and burping, while toxins make the inflammation in the stomach even worse, increasing the severity of gastritis. Some of these microbial toxins cause a partial paralysis of the stomach muscle, called gastroparesis, which slows down stomach activity.[74] People with this condition complain that food stays in their stomach for long periods of time, not digesting and not moving. When pathogens grow around the sphincter muscle at the top of the stomach (this round muscle normally separates the stomach from the oesophagus and does not allow food to go back up), they partially paralyse this sphincter. This causes reflux: regurgitation of food back up into the oesophagus. Even with low stomach acid production there is some acid in the regurgitated food, which burns the walls of the oesophagus, giving the person typical symptoms of 'acid indigestion' or heartburn, leading to a common condition called GORD or GERD (gastroesophageal reflux disease). Antacids are usually prescribed for acid indigestion and reflux, which may alleviate the immediate symptoms but, in the long run, make the whole situation worse, as they reduce stomach acid production even further.

To protect the inflamed stomach lining from damage, the liver and pancreas come to help by pumping their juices up into the stomach (yes, things don't just travel 'down' in the gut, but can travel up as well).[76] The pancreas produces an alkaline solution, similar to bicarbonate of soda, which on contact with the stomach acid produces gas, sometimes a lot of gas. As a result, one of the most common symptoms of gastritis is voluminous burping, which can happen after food, between food and on an empty stomach.[75] This process can be particularly active in the middle of the night, waking the person up several times so the gas can be belched out, which disrupts sleep. Some gases can be flammable and can cause a hot flush when being released: these hot flushes can happen at any age (not only in menopause, but in young adults and even children).

Many people with low stomach acid production and an overgrowth of microbes in the stomach suffer from belching and bloating, because yeasts, archaea and other microbes in their stomachs produce too much gas. Your stomach is positioned underneath your heart (separated by the diaphragm). When the stomach fills with gas, it can push the heart up into an unnatural position, which can cause a heart problem: heart racing, abnormal rhythm and palpitations. This usually happens when the person is driving or sitting in a way that doesn't give their abdomen much room to expand. Releasing the gas though belching can stop the heart symptoms. If belching does not happen naturally, stimulating a vomiting reflex by tickling the back of your throat with your fingers can help to release the gas. Sometimes, it is better to do that than suffer from heart problems.

Another common symptom of chronic gastritis is *Recurrent Vomiting Syndrome*.[77] The stomach lining is inflamed and sore; when another irritant comes in with food or drink (a pesticide-laden piece of fruit or vegetable, water full of chlorine or fluoride, junk food full of chemicals, etc.), the body triggers the vomiting reflex and the person vomits again and again until the stomach is more or less empty. Sometimes the vomiting is accompanied by diarrhoea and a headache – the body is unloading toxins. These vomiting episodes can happen every few weeks to every few months; in some people they happen more often. Activity of worms, flukes and other residents of the digestive system can play an important role in this condition. The vomiting often coincides with a particular stage in these creatures' life cycle (when they lay eggs, hatch into larvae, etc). Their life cycle is connected to the moon cycle, so many people notice that they feel worse on the full moon or coming up to it.

In a person with chronic gastritis there is a distant burning sensation in the stomach, which can feel as if you are hungry. Many people, particularly in the initial stages, do think that they are hungry and eat as often as they can. The immediate relief of this 'hunger' is often achieved by eating bread and other starchy foods. But, in the long run, that makes the situation worse, as these foods feed the pathogens in the stomach; these pathogens produce more toxins leading to more inflammation. So, having consumed almost a loaf of bread, you are invariably 'hungry' again fairly soon.

A person with chronic gastritis cannot tolerate many foods. Coffee, chocolate, milk, raw fruit and vegetables, nuts and seeds, anything made with flour and sugar and spices aggravate the inflammation in the stomach and make the gastritis worse. In order to heal the stomach, many foods have to be avoided for as long as it takes to accomplish the healing. A simple test for your stomach acid production is to eat some freshly cooked beetroot. If, for the following 1-3 days, your urine and/or your stool become red, then it is likely that your stomach acid production is low. Your body cannot digest the red pigment from the beetroot and it finishes up in your urine and stool.

In my experience it is essential to follow the *GAPS Introduction Diet* to the letter to heal the stomach lining and get rid of gastritis permanently. Meat stocks are essential (lamb, beef, poultry and game). Many people find chicken stock, made with chicken giblets, feet and carcasses, particularly soothing. Soups made with meat stock and a few low-fibre vegetables (carrot, onion and pumpkin or courgettes/zucchini) will nourish and heal. Homemade whey and kefir are essential for the majority of people, so add some into every cup of the meat stock you drink. Many adults find it very helpful to take a good quality probiotic from the start. Drinking a soothing tea (ginger, mint, calendula) between meals is helpful. When the burning sensation in the stomach subsides, it is a good idea to introduce daily GAPS shakes. They will help to remove toxins stored in your stomach lining, because these toxins will not allow your stomach to heal. They will also help your liver to unload gall stones and improve its functions. One of these functions is bile production and digestion of fats, which many people with gastritis find difficult. It is important to introduce fats gradually following your tolerance level. Consuming animal fats is essential for the healing process, but you need to be able to digest them.

In order to heal your stomach, you have to look at what kind of toxins are coming into it. Do you have dental materials in your mouth which may be leaching toxins (amalgam fillings in particular)? Are you using conventional toothpaste or mouthwash, full of fluoride and other toxins? Are you drinking conventional tap water without filtering it (containing chlorine, agricultural chemicals, pharmaceuticals and other poisons)? Are you taking pharmaceutical drugs? As long as these toxins keep coming into your stomach, there can be no healing. You have to take steps to remove them from your life.

It can take from a couple of weeks to a few years to heal chronic gastritis, but it is essential to do it. So many people in our modern world live with chronic gastritis and think it is 'normal', taking antacids and other medications for 'indigestion'. Long term this situation can lead to development of stomach ulcers and stomach cancers, and problems in the rest of the digestive system.

As the whole digestive process really begins in the stomach, chronic gastritis will not allow you to digest your food properly. As a result, people suffer from food intolerances and allergies: the food does not digest properly and absorbs in a partially digested state, triggering food allergy and intolerances. As the inflamed stomach is unable to provide the natural acid barrier, pathogens overgrow in the whole of the digestive system bringing many symptoms of GAPS. When they overgrow in the intestines, the person may be diagnosed with SIBO (Small Intestinal Bacterial Overgrowth).

It is helpful for people with low stomach acidity to take stomach acid supplements at the beginning of their meals: Betaine HCl with pepsin or HCl with pepsin. For the majority of people, particularly for children, I recommend using fermented vegetables (particularly fermented cabbage) for this purpose: eating a small helping with every meal or at the beginning of the meal will help to stimulate natural stomach acid production. A small fresh cabbage salad at the beginning of the meal can also be helpful. To understand this subject in more detail, please read the chapter *Digestive Enzymes*.

Stuttering

In my opinion, stuttering (or stammering) is a GAPS condition in the majority of people with this affliction. Toxicity in the brain does not allow the brain to produce and regulate normal speech. Following the GAPS Diet is the first and the most important intervention I would recommend, because it will remove the physiological reason for stuttering. Once that is taken care off, speech therapy, cranial osteopathy and other interventions can be much more fruitful and helpful. Many people will recover from this problem just with the GAPS Diet.

Sugar cravings, chocolate cravings

Cravings for sweet things and chocolate are due to unstable blood sugar level. In order to remove your sugar cravings, you need to keep your blood sugar at a steady level. To do that, I recommend making a *butter/honey mixture*. Put this mixture in a glass jar and carry that jar with you everywhere. Eat 2–3 tablespoons of this mixture every 15–25 minutes all day long. Do this for a month or longer, depending on the severity of your sugar cravings. In the meantime, focus on implementing the GAPS Diet, which will normalise your blood sugar permanently. Once your blood sugar is normal, your cravings will be gone, and at that stage you can stop carrying a jar of butter/honey mixture with you.

The butter/honey mixture To make butter/honey mixture soften 200–400 g (7–14 oz) of raw organic unsalted butter at room temperature or in the sun, add raw honey to taste (about 1–4 tablespoons) and mix well. Your taste buds will tell you how much honey to add to the butter: the mixture should taste pleasant for you. It is possible that at the beginning you would want to add more honey. Later on, as your sugar cravings reduce, less honey in the mixture will taste nicer for you. Listen to your taste buds; they will guide you well! If, for some reason, you cannot have butter, use coconut oil, sour cream, tallow, lard or any other animal fat.

In most cases, craving for sweet things is due to deficiency of fats in the body. Make sure that every meal you eat is rich in animal fats. If the meal doesn't have enough, add more fat to it (bacon fat, pork, beef, lamb, goose, duck fat, butter and ghee). An excellent food for people with this problem is home-cured pork fat, called lardo in Italy and salo in Russia and Ukraine. Please look in the chapter *What we shall eat and why, with some recipes* for how to make it.

Vitiligo

The pigment in our skin is produced by cells called melanocytes. These cells have the same origin as the cells of our nervous system in the glia and myelin – they all come from the same place during our foetal development (the neural crest).[78] All of these cells are very vulnerable to accumulation of toxic metals and other environmental toxins. These toxins attach themselves to proteins in the cellular structure, triggering inflammation and autoimmune attack on the cell. This attack destroys the ability of melanocytes to produce melanin – the pigment which gives colour to our skin and hair, and it can destroy the cells themselves.[79] There are many different diagnoses people can receive, but vitiligo is the most common. In a person with vitiligo the skin develops white patches with sharp margins. Vitiligo and other depigmentation disorders often coincide with other autoimmune and inflammatory diseases, such as scleroderma, type one diabetes, psoriasis, alopecia areata, lupus erythematosus, Hashimoto's thyroiditis and rheumatoid arthritis. [79] People with pernicious anaemia also can have vitiligo.[80] Pernicious anaemia happens in people with vitamin B12 deficiency, and the state of the gut flora plays an important role in this disease, because it is the major source of B12 in the body.

I have no doubt that all autoimmunity is born in the gut. The GAPS Nutritional Protocol will rebalance your immunity. In the meantime, it is important to work on removing toxins from your skin. First remove all man-made chemicals: soaps, shampoo, skin creams, make-up and all other personal care products, laundry detergent, dishwashing liquid and any other man-made chemicals you can think of. Replace them with natural alternatives (please, see the chapter *Detoxification*). Take a course of beta-carotene supplements (and/or drink freshly pressed carrot juice, watermelon juice and juices from greens, which are rich in beta-carotene). Beta-carotene is a powerful antioxidant which targets the skin and helps to remove many toxins. Regular baths with Epsom salt, sea salt, bicarbonate of soda and seaweed powder, as well as clay and honey applications, will help to remove toxicity from your skin. Regular use of traditional saunas helps to remove toxins through sweat. Traditional mud treatments help many people as they also detoxify the skin. It is best to do mud baths and applications at an established natural mud spa.

The good news is that human skin has a very rapid cell turnover (cell regeneration process). Skin cells, including melanocytes, are born in the deep layers of the skin. As the outer layer of the skin sheds cells all the time, the deeper layers mature and become the outer layers, until they also get shed.[78] A good example of how fast your skin renews itself is tanning. When we sunbathe, melanocytes in the deep skin layers produce a pigment called melanin. This pigment is released and absorbed by surrounding skin cells, turning your skin brown. As these cells slowly move to the surface of the skin and are shed, the tan gets 'washed off' as well, demonstrating how quickly your skin renews itself. As your gut heals and autoimmunity stops, your skin will have a chance to give birth to new healthy melanocytes able to produce normal amounts of pigment in your skin. And the old damaged skin cells will just be shed.

Wet nursing

No matter how well you try to organise your pregnancy and plan your breastfeeding, you may find that you cannot produce enough milk for your baby or cannot produce milk at all. There may be many different reasons for that. When this happens, in our modern world the child is fed formula; there are many brands on the market and every company advertises its formula as the best. However, no matter how much effort has been put into creating those formulas, none of them will ever come close to the quality of human breast milk flowing straight from the mother to the baby! Why? Because the milk of any animal (including human) is alive; it is, in effect, the female's white blood. It has alive and active immune cells, immune complexes, hormones, enzymes, neurotransmitters, proteins, fats, carbohydrates, vitamins, minerals and many other substances. All of these molecules and substances in mother's milk are in the right bio-chemical and bio-physical form for the baby, and in the right balance with each other. On top of that, breast milk is a probiotic food; it has probiotic microbes in it, necessary for the baby to develop normal gut flora.[81] When we process milk, we damage it: all the living active immune cells in the milk get killed, the structure of hormones, enzymes, neurotransmitters and other complex molecules gets altered and denatured, and many molecules get destroyed. Processed milk loses its many beneficial properties and can even become harmful. Baby formulas are highly processed substances; they can never come close to the living milk coming directly from the mother to the baby. So, it is not in your baby's best interest to be fed formula milk! We now have plenty of evidence showing that formula-fed babies are prone to all sorts of illnesses, and generally have a poorer constitution than breastfed babies.[82]

But what do we do if the mother cannot feed her baby? Well, let us think, what have women done for all of our existence on this planet? For millennia humanity did not have formula milk! If a woman was ill or, worse than that, died in labour, what did her family do to feed the baby? People used to live in close communities where a number of women would have babies at the same time. So, if any of those women could not feed her baby, other women in the community would do that for her. This practice was called wet nursing and we must bring it back to life!

So, here is what I recommend to all pregnant women: go to antenatal classes or any other place where you can meet pregnant women in your local area. Talk to those women and form a *Wet-Nursing Group*. When any of you give birth to your baby, you can support those who cannot breastfeed for whatever reason. Many breastfeeding women produce a lot of milk, enough to feed more than one baby, and they may be happy to share their milk. Even one breastfeeding session per day will do wonders for a bottle-fed baby's health! It is best if the baby can be put directly to the breast of the woman. Pumping breast milk out, putting it in a bottle, keeping it in the refrigerator and then rewarming it will damage the milk to a certain degree and make it less beneficial for the baby. Still, it is infinitely better than any formula! Never use microwave ovens to warm the milk; use traditional sources of heat (microwaves destroy food and turn it carcinogenic).

Many women will be wondering if it is safe to have milk from another person. Healthy milk is produced by healthy women! Make sure that the woman you have chosen to wet-nurse your baby, is healthy. The best indicator of that is the health of her own baby: if her baby is healthy and thriving, then the milk of this woman is likely to be healthy and will do your baby a lot of good. There is no need to worry about microbes: the living milk of any animal is full of probiotic microbes and active immune cells; it destroys any pathogenic microbes which get in it. However, dead milk from formula is a perfect medium for any pathogens to grow and thrive if they get in it.

It is essential for all of our babies to get colostrum in the first few days of their life. Colostrum is the very rich milk produced by a woman in the first two weeks after delivering a baby. If your baby did not get it, do your best to find women who have just given birth and are producing colostrum. Newborn babies take very little from the mother's breast; a lot of colostrum is left and can be shared with other babies. If your baby is suffering from eczema, colic, asthma, allergies or any other illness, feeding it fresh colostrum as often as possible can just be enough to remove any of those problems.

In our modern world increasing numbers of babies suffer from poor health. We have already mentioned allergies, eczema, colic and asthma. But other, more severe health problems are also on the increase: type one diabetes, FPIES (Food Protein Induced Enterocolitis Syndrome), failure to thrive, learning disabilities and epilepsy. Many of these babies are exclusively breastfed! What does this mean? It means that the mother is not healthy and is producing unhealthy milk. I have seen some of these babies improve and recover, when the mother stopped breastfeeding and found a healthy wet nurse. Colostrum is particularly important for these babies. If the baby is old enough to start having solids, it is important to follow the GAPS Diet for babies (described in detail in my first GAPS book

Gut and Psychology Syndrome, chapter New Baby). Working on this diet will allow the mother, who is producing unhealthy milk, to stop breastfeeding sooner. Supplementing the baby's diet with some wet nursing will ensure the best chance for the baby to recover.

Breastfeeding is one of the joys of having children! It is a wonderful experience, but if you are unable to do it for some reason there is no need to despair. Focus on finding a good wet nurse for your baby. This way you will know that you have done the best for your baby's health! Many women in the Western world find it easier to look for a healthy wet nurse from immigrant communities, particularly among women who have immigrated recently. Western industrialised countries have created an environment which damages people's health. Nations which follow a more traditional way of life have better health overall; their women are stronger and, on average, have healthier pregnancies and produce healthier babies. If you have such a traditional immigrant community in your local area, you may want to try to look for a wet nurse there. Wet nursing used to be a profession in traditional societies; these women looked after their diet and their health to make sure that they produced good quality milk. We need to bring this profession back! This will provide babies, whose mothers cannot breastfeed them, with a much better solution than commercial formula milk will ever be able to do.

Recommended Reading

This is a short alphabetic list of books, which will help to expand your understanding, dear reader. This list is not exhaustive by any means, but is a good start.

Douglass J. *Living soul*. 2008. SPS publications.

Enig MG. *Know Your Fats: The Complete Primer for Understanding the Nutrition of Fats, Oils, and Cholesterol*. Bethesda Press, Silver Spring, MD, 2000.

Fallon S, Enig MG. *Nourishing Traditions. The cookbook that challenges politically correct nutrition and the diet dictocrats*. 1999. New Trends Publishing, Washington DC 20007.

Gerber R. *Vibrational medicine*. 2001. Bear & company.

Graveline D. *The statin damage crisis*. 2014. Infinity Publishing.

Harvey G. *The carbon fields. How our countryside can save Britain*. 2008. GrassRoots.

Harvey G. *The forgiveness of nature. The story of grass*. 2001. Published by Jonathan Cape.

Harvey G. *We want real food*. 2006. Constable. London.

Hawkins DR. *Power versus force. The hidden determinants of human behaviour*. 2002. Hay house Inc.

Hay L. *Heal your body*. 1988. Hay house Inc.

Huggins HA and Levy TE. *Uninformed consent. Hidden dangers in dental care*. 1999. Hampton Roads Pub Co.

Keith L. *The vegetarian myth. Food, justice and sustainability*. 2009. Flashpoint Press, California.

Lipton BH. *The biology of belief. Unleashing the power of consciousness, matter and miracles*. 2008. Hay house Inc.

McTaggart L. *The field*. 2003. HarperCollins publishing Ltd.

Price WA. *Nutrition and physical degeneration. A comparison of primitive and modern diets and their effects*. 1938. Price.

Ravnskov U. *The Cholesterol Myths. Exposing the fallacy that saturated fat and cholesterol cause heart disease*. 2000. NewTrends Publishing.

Salatin J. *Pastured poultry profits*. 1996. Polyface, Inc.

Salatin J. *You Can Farm: The Entrepreneur's Guide to Start & Succeed in a Farming Enterprise*. 2006. Polyface, Inc.

Savory A. *Holistic Management. A new framework for decision making*. 1999. Island Press.

Schmid R. *The untold story of milk. The history, politics and science of nature's perfect food: raw milk from pastured cows*. New trends publishing. 2009.

Sheldrake R. *The science delusion*. 2013. Coronet.

Silva J, Stone RB. You the healer. 1989. HJ Kramer Inc.

Tsabary S. *The awakened family*. 2018. Yellow kite publishing.

Campbell-McBride N. *GAPS Stories. Personal Accounts of improvement and recovery through the GAPS Nutritional protocol*. 2012. Medinform Publishing.

Campbell-McBride N. *Gut and psychology syndrome. Natural treatment for autism, dyspraxia, dyslexia, ADD/ADHD, depression and schizophrenia*. 2010. Medinform Publishing.

Campbell-McBride N. *Put your heart in your mouth. What really is heart disease and what can we do to prevent and even reverse it*. 2007. Medinform Publishing.

Campbell-McBride N. *Vegetarianism explained*. 2017. Medinform Publishing.

References

Good health begins in the soil inside us!

1. Joel Faintuch, Salomao Faintuch. *Microbiome and Metabolome in Diagnosis, Therapy, and other Strategic Applications*. 2019, Elsevier Inc.
2. Sender R, Fuchs S, Milo R. Revised Estimates for the Number of Human and Bacteria Cells in the Body. *PLoS Biol*. 2016; 14(8):e1002533.
3. *Study Shows Gut Bacteria Can Spread to Other Organs and Trigger Disease* [Internet]. [cited 2020 Feb 14]. Available from: https://www.sciencealert.com/gut-bacteria-can-spread-to-organs-and-trigger-disease
4. Tytgat HLP, Nobrega FL, Oost J van der, Vos WM de. Bowel Biofilms: Tipping Points between a Healthy and Compromised Gut? *Trends in Microbiology*. 2019 Jan 1;27(1):17–25.
5. Brunetti Jerry. *The Farm as Ecosystem: Tapping Nature's Reservoir – Geology, Biology, Diversity*. 2014. Acres USA
6. Sugar Transport in Plants: Phloem [Internet]. *Biology* 1520. 2016 [cited 2020 Feb 14]. Available from: http://bio1520.biology.gatech. edu/nutrition-transport-and-homeostasis/plant-transport-processes-ii/
7. Michael Phillips. *Mycorrhizal Planet. How Symbiotic Fungi Work with Roots to Support Plant Health and Build Soil Fertility*. 2017. Chelsea Green Publishing
8. Berruti A, Lumini E, Balestrini R, Bianciotto V. Arbuscular Mycorrhizal Fungi as Natural Biofertilizers: Let's Benefit from Past Successes. *Front Microbiol* [Internet]. 2016 Jan 19 [cited 2020 Feb 14];6. Available from: https://www.ncbi.nlm.nih.gov/pmc/articles/PMC4717633/
9. Chen M, Arato M, Borghi L, Nouri E, Reinhardt D. Beneficial Services of Arbuscular Mycorrhizal Fungi – From Ecology to Application. *Front Plant Sci* [Internet]. 2018 Sep 4 [cited 2020 Feb 14];9. Available from: https://www.ncbi.nlm.nih.gov/pmc/articles/PMC6132195/
10. Hallen-Adams HE, Suhr MJ. Fungi in the healthy human gastrointestinal tract. *Virulence*. 2016 Oct 13;8(3):352–8.
11. Charles A Janeway J, Travers P, Walport M, Shlomchik MJ. The mucosal immune system. *Immunobiology: The Immune System in Health and Disease*, 5th edition [Internet]. 2001 [cited 2020 Feb 14]; Available from: https://www.ncbi.nlm.nih.gov/books/NBK27169/
12. Huffnagle GB, Noverr MC. The emerging world of the fungal microbiome. *Trends in Microbiology*. 2013 Jul 1;21(7):334–41.
13. Rodríguez IA, Cárdenas-González JF, Juárez VMM, Pérez AR, Zarate M de GM, Castillo NCP. Biosorption of Heavy Metals by Candida albicans. *Advances in Bioremediation and Phytoremediation* [Internet]. 2017 Dec 20 [cited 2020 Feb 14]; Available from: https://www.intechopen. com/books/advances-in-bioremediation-and-phytoremediation/ biosorption-of-heavy-metals-by-candida-albicans
14. Mutter J. Is dental amalgam safe for humans? The opinion of the scientific committee of the European Commission. *J Occup Med Toxicol*. 2011 Jan 13;6:2.
15. Rybalchenko OV, Bondarenko VM, Orlova OG, Markov AG, Amasheh S. Inhibitory effects of Lactobacillus fermentum on microbial growth and biofilm formation. *Arch Microbiol*. 2015 Oct 1;197(8):1027–32.

16. Matsubara VH, Bandara HMHN, Mayer MPA, Samaranayake LP. Probiotics as Antifungals in Mucosal Candidiasis. *Clin Infect Dis*. 2016 May 1;62(9): 1143–53.
17. Yoon MY, Yoon SS. Disruption of the Gut Ecosystem by Antibiotics. *Yonsei Med J*. 2018 Jan 1;59(1):4–12.
18. Chang Q, Wang W, Regev-Yochay G, Lipsitch M, Hanage WP. Antibiotics in agriculture and the risk to human health: how worried should we be? *Evol Appl*. 2015 Mar;8(3):240–7.
19. Landers TF, Cohen B, Wittum TE, Larson EL. *A Review of Antibiotic Use in Food Animals: Perspective, Policy, and Potential. Public Health Rep*. 2012;127(1):4–22.
20. Kurenbach B, Hill AM, Godsoe W, van Hamelsveld S, Heinemann JA. Agrichemicals and antibiotics in combination increase antibiotic resistance evolution. *Peer J* [Internet]. 2018 Oct 12 [cited 2020 Feb 14];6. Available from: https://www.ncbi.nlm.nih.gov/pmc/articles/ PMC6188010/
21. Cimitile M. Worried about Antibiotics in Your Beef? Vegetables May Be No Better [Internet]. *Scientific American*. [cited 2020 Feb 14]. Available from: https://www.scientificamerican.com/article/vegetables-contain-antibiotics/
22. Driver JD, Holben WE, Rillig MC (2005) Characterization of glomalin as a hyphal wall component of arbuscular mycorrhizal fungi. *Soil Biol Biochem* 37:101–106 Feeney DS, Daniell T, Hallett P
23. Mendes Giannini MJS, Bernardi T, Scorzoni L, Fusco-Almeida AM, Sardi JCO. Candida species: current epidemiology, pathogenicity, biofilm formation, natural antifungal products and new therapeutic options. *Journal of Medical Microbiology*. 2013 Jan 1;62(1):10–24.
24. Stephen AM, Cummings JH. The microbial contribution to human faecal mass. *J Med Microbiol*. 1980 Feb;13(1):45–56.
25. Momozawa Y, Deffontaine V, Louis E, Medrano JF. Characterization of Bacteria in Biopsies of Colon and Stools by High Throughput Sequencing of the V2 Region of Bacterial 16S rRNA Gene in Human. *PLoS One* [Internet]. 2011 Feb 10 [cited 2020 Feb 14];6(2). Available from: https://www.ncbi.nlm.nih.gov/pmc/articles/PMC3037395/
26. Senghor B, Sokhna C, Ruimy R, Lagier J-C. Gut microbiota diversity according to dietary habits and geographical provenance. *Human Microbiome Journal*. 2018 Apr 1;7–8:1–9.
27. Tomova A, Bukovsky I, Rembert E, Yonas W, Alwarith J, Barnard ND, *et al*.The Effects of Vegetarian and Vegan Diets on Gut Microbiota. *Front Nutr* [Internet]. 2019 Apr 17 [cited 2020 Feb 14];6. Available from: https://www.ncbi.nlm.nih.gov/pmc/articles/PMC6478664/
28. Ling J, O'Donoghue P, Söll D. Genetic code flexibility in microorganisms: novel mechanisms and impact on physiology. *Nat Rev Microbiol*. 2015 Nov;13(11):707–21.
29. Majewski J, Zawadzki P, Pickerill P, Cohan FM, Dowson CG. Barriers to Genetic Exchange between Bacterial Species: Streptococcus pneumoniae Transformation. *J Bacteriol*. 2000 Feb;182(4):1016–23.
30. Hyeonsoo Jeong, Bushra Arif, Gustavo Caetano-Anollés, Kyung Mo Kim, Arshan Nasir. Horizontal gene transfer in human-associated microorganisms inferred by phylogenetic reconstruction and reconciliation. *Scientific Reports*, 2019; 9 (1).

31. Palmer RJ. Composition and development of oral bacterial communities. *Periodontol 2000* [Internet]. 2014 Feb [cited 2020 Feb 14];64(1). Available from: https://www.ncbi.nlm.nih.gov/pmc/articles/PMC3876289/
32. Thursby E, Juge N. Introduction to the human gut microbiota. *Biochem J.* 2017 Jun 1;474(11):1823–36.
33. O'May GA, Reynolds N, Macfarlane GT. Effect of pH on an In Vitro Model of Gastric Microbiota in Enteral Nutrition Patients. *Appl Environ Microbiol.* 2005 Aug;71(8):4777–83.
34. Smith JL. The role of gastric acid in preventing foodborne disease and how bacteria overcome acid conditions. *J Food Prot.* 2003 Jul;66(7):1292–303.
35. Anti-inflammatory drug and gut bacteria have a dynamic interplay [Internet]. *ScienceDaily*. [cited 2020 Feb 14]. Available from: https://www.sciencedaily.com/releases/2016/01/160104132151.htm
36. Zhang Y-J, Li S, Gan R-Y, Zhou T, Xu D-P, Li H-B. Impacts of Gut Bacteria on Human Health and Diseases. *Int J Mol Sci.* 2015 Apr 2;16(4):7493–519.
37. Cheung KS, Leung WK. Long-term use of proton-pump inhibitors and risk of gastric cancer: a review of the current evidence. *Therap Adv Gastroenterol* [Internet]. 2019 Mar 11 [cited 2020 Feb 14];12. Available from: https://www.ncbi.nlm.nih.gov/pmc/articles/PMC6415482/
38. Lender N, Talley NJ, Enck P, Haag S, Zipfel S, Morrison M, *et al.*Review article: associations between Helicobacter pylori and obesity – an ecological study. *Alimentary Pharmacology & Therapeutics*. 2014;40(1):24–31.
39. Jeffery PL, McGuckin MA, Linden SK. Endocrine impact of Helicobacter pylori: Focus on ghrelin and ghrelin o-acyltransferase. *World J Gastroenterol.* 2011 Mar 14;17(10):1249–60.
40. Hao WL, Lee YK. Microflora of the gastrointestinal tract: a review. *Methods Mol Biol.* 2004;268:491–502.
41. Quigley EMM. Gut Bacteria in Health and Disease. *Gastroenterol Hepatol (NY).* 2013 Sep;9(9):560–9.
42. Jandhyala SM, Talukdar R, Subramanyam C, Vuyyuru H, Sasikala M, Reddy DN. Role of the normal gut microbiota. *World J Gastroenterol.* 2015 Aug 7;21(29):8787–803.
43. Rinninella E, Raoul P, Cintoni M, Franceschi F, Miggiano GAD, Gasbarrini A, *et al.* What is the Healthy Gut Microbiota Composition? A Changing Ecosystem across Age, Environment, Diet, and Diseases. *Microorganisms* [Internet]. 2019 Jan 10 [cited 2020 Feb 15];7(1). Available from: https://www.ncbi.nlm.nih.gov/pmc/articles/PMC6351938/
44. Hungate, R.E. 1966. *The rumen and its microbes*. Academic Press, NY.
45. den Besten G, van Eunen K, Groen AK, Venema K, Reijngoud D-J, Bakker BM. The role of short-chain fatty acids in the interplay between diet, gut microbiota, and host energy metabolism. *J Lipid Res.* 2013 Sep;54(9):2325–40.
46. Vyas U, Ranganathan N. Probiotics, Prebiotics, and Synbiotics: Gut and Beyond. *Gastroenterol Res Pract* [Internet]. 2012 [cited 2020 Feb 15];2012. Available from: https://www.ncbi.nlm.nih.gov/pmc/articles/PMC3459241/
47. Methanobrevibacter Smithii – an overview | *ScienceDirect Topics* [Internet]. [cited 2020 Feb 15]. Available from: https://www.sciencedirect.com/topics/immunology-and-microbiology/methanobrevibacter-smithii
48. Gaci N, Borrel G, Tottey W, O'Toole PW, Brugère J-F. Archaea and the human gut: New beginning of an old story. *World J Gastroenterol.* 2014 Nov 21;20(43):16062–78.

49. Lurie-Weinberger MN, Gophna U (2015) Archaea in and on the Human Body: Health Implications and Future Directions. *PLoS Pathog* 11(6): e1004833. https://doi.org/10.1371/journal.ppat.1004833
50. Moye ZD, Woolston J, Sulakvelidze A. Bacteriophage Applications for Food Production and Processing. *Viruses* [Internet]. 2018 Apr 19 [cited 2020 Feb 15];10(4). Available from: https://www.ncbi.nlm.nih.gov/pmc/articles/PMC5923499/
51. Curtin JJ, Donlan RM. Using Bacteriophages To Reduce Formation of Catheter-Associated Biofilms by Staphylococcus epidermidis. *Antimicrob Agents Chemother*. 2006 Apr;50(4):1268–75.
52. Myelnikov D. An Alternative Cure: The Adoption and Survival of Bacteriophage Therapy in the USSR, 1922–1955. *J Hist Med Allied Sci*. 2018 Oct;73(4):385–411.
53. Sutton TDS, Hill C. Gut Bacteriophage: Current Understanding and Challenges. *Front Endocrinol* [Internet]. 2019 [cited 2020 Feb 15];10. Available from: https://www.frontiersin.org/articles/10.3389/fendo.2019.00784/full
54. Whitley RJ. Herpesviruses. In: Baron S, editor. *Medical Microbiology* [Internet]. 4th ed. Galveston (TX): University of Texas Medical Branch at Galveston; 1996 [cited 2020 Feb 15]. Available from: http://www.ncbi.nlm.nih.gov/books/NBK8157/
55. Shen Y, Nemunaitis J. Herpes simplex virus 1 (HSV-1) for cancer treatment. *Cancer Gene Therapy*. 2006 Nov;13(11):975–92.
56. Antonsson A, Forslund O, Ekberg H, Sterner G, Hansson BG (December 2000). "The ubiquity and impressive genomic diversity of human skin papillomaviruses suggest a commensalic nature of these viruses". *Journal of Virology*. 74 (24): 11636–41.
57. Belkaid Y, Hand T. Role of the Microbiota in Immunity and inflammation. *Cell*. 2014 Mar 27;157(1):121–41.
58. PennisiNov. 19 E, 2014, Pm 1:00. Viruses help keep the gut healthy [Internet]. *Science* | AAAS. 2014 [cited 2020 Feb 16]. Available from: https://www.sciencemag.org/news/2014/11/viruses-help-keep-gut-healthy
59. Bhatia LA. *Textbook of environmental biology*. 2010. International Publishing House.
60. *Soil Microorganisms* [Internet]. [cited 2020 Feb 16]. Available from: https://www.sare.org/Learning-Center/Books/Building-Soils-for-Better-Crops-3rd-Edition/Text-Version/The-Living-Soil/Soil-Microorganisms
61. Helmby H. Human helminth therapy to treat inflammatory disorders- where do we stand? *BMC Immunol* [Internet]. 2015 Mar 26 [cited 2020 Feb 16];16. Available from: https://www.ncbi.nlm.nih.gov/pmc/articles/PMC4374592/
62. Moreels TG, Pelckmans PA. Gastrointestinal parasites: potential therapy for refractory inflammatory bowel diseases. *Inflamm Bowel Dis*. 2005 Feb;11(2): 178–84.
63. Baggaley K. Scientists are trying to treat autoimmune disease with intestinal worms [Internet]. *Popular Science*. 2017 [cited 2020 Feb 16]. Available from: https://www.popsci.com/can-intestinal-worms-treat-autoimmune-disease/
64. Berrilli F, Di Cave D, Cavallero S, D'Amelio S. Interactions between parasites and microbial communities in the human gut. *Front Cell Infect Microbiol* [Internet]. 2012 Nov 16 [cited 2020 Feb 16];2. Available from: https://www.ncbi.nlm.nih.gov/pmc/articles/PMC3499702/
65. Domingue GJ. Demystifying Pleomorphic Forms in Persistence and

Expression of Disease: Are They Bacteria, and Is Peptidoglycan the Solution? *Discovery Medicine* [Internet]. 2010 Sep 23 [cited 2020 Jan 31]; Available from: http://www.discoverymedicine.com/Gerald-J-Domingue/2010/09/23/demystifying-pleomorphic-forms-in-persistence-and-expression-of-disease-are-they-bacteria-and-is-peptidoglycan-the-solution/

66. Allan EJ, Hoishen C, Gumpert J. Bacterial L-forms. *Adv Appl Microbiol* 68:1-39, 2009.
67. Markova N. L-form Bacteria Cohabitants in Human Blood: Significance for Health and Diseases. *Discovery Medicine*. 2017 May 28;23(128):305–13.
68. Markova N. L-form Bacteria Cohabitants in Human Blood: Significance for Health and Diseases. *Discovery Medicine*. 2017 May 28;23(128):305–13.
69. Macomber PB. Cancer and cell wall deficient bacteria. *Med Hypotheses*. 1990 May;32(1):1–9.
70. Markova N. Dysbiotic microbiota in autistic children and their mothers: persistence of fungal and bacterial wall-deficient L-form variants in blood. *Scientific Reports*. 2019 Sep 16;9(1):13401.
71. Errington J. Cell wall-deficient, L-form bacteria in the 21st century: a personal perspective. *Biochem Soc Trans*. 2017 Apr 15;45(2):287–95.
72. Errington J, Mickiewicz K, Kawai Y, Wu LJ. L-form bacteria, chronic diseases and the origins of life. *Philos Trans R Soc Lond B Biol Sci* [Internet]. 2016 Nov 5 [cited 2020 Feb 16];371(1707). Available from: https://www.ncbi.nlm.nih.gov/pmc/articles/PMC5052740/
73. Orefici G, Cardona F, Cox CJ, Cunningham MW. Pediatric Autoimmune Neuropsychiatric Disorders Associated with Streptococcal Infections (PANDAS). In: Ferretti JJ, Stevens DL, Fischetti VA, editors. *Streptococcus pyogenes: Basic Biology to Clinical Manifestations* [Internet]. Oklahoma City (OK): University of Oklahoma Health Sciences Center; 2016 [cited 2020 Feb 17]. Available from: http://www.ncbi.nlm.nih.gov/books/NBK333433/
74. Mattman LH. *Cell Wall Deficient Forms. Stealth Pathogens*. CRC Press Inc., Boca Raton, FL, 2001.
75. McLaughlin RW, Vali H, Lau PC, Palfree RG, De Ciccio A, Sirois M, Ahmad D, Villemur R, Desrosiers M, Chan EC. Are there naturally occurring pleomorphic bacteria in the blood of healthy humans? *J Clin Microbiol* 40:4771–4775, 2002.
76. Prozorovski SV, Kaz LN, Kagan GJ. *Bacterial L-forms: Mechanisms of Formation, Structure, Role in Pathology*. Medicine Publishing, Moscow, Russia, 1981.
77. Pease PE, Tallack JE. A permanent endoparasite of man. The silent zoogleal/symplasm/L-form phase. *Microbios* 64:173–80, 1990.
78. Khandel P, Yadaw RK, Soni DK, Kanwar L, Shahi SK. Biogenesis of metal nanoparticles and their pharmacological applications: present status and application prospects. *J Nanostruct Chem*. 2018 Sep 1;8(3):217–54.
79. Meiring P. Researchers have directly proven that bacteria can change shape inside humans to avoid antibiotics [Internet]. *Cape Business News*. 2019 [cited 2020 Feb 15]. Available from: https://www.cbn.co.za/featured/researchers-have-directly-proven-that-bacteria-can-change-shape-inside-humans-to-avoid-antibiotics/
80. Markova N, Michailova L, Jourdanova M, Kussovski V, Valcheva V, Mokrousov I, Radoucheva T. Exhibition of persistent and drug-tolerant L-form habit of Mycobacterium tuberculosis during infection in rats. *Cent Eur J Biol* 23:407–416, 2008b.

81. Markova N, Slavchev G, Michailova L, Jourdanova M. Survival of Escherichia coli under lethal heat stress by L-form conversion. *Int J Biol Sci* 6:303–315, 2010.
82. Rodríguez EA, Cárdenas-González JF, Martínez Juárez VM, *et al.* (December 20th 2017). Biosorption of Heavy Metals by Candida albicans, *Advances in Bioremediation and Phytoremediation*, Naofumi Shiomi, IntechOpen, DOI: 10.5772/intechopen.72454. Available from: https://www.intechopen.com/books/advances-in-bioremediation-and-phytoremediation/biosorption-of-heavy-metals-by-candida-albicans
83. Antoine Bechamp. *The Blood And Its Third Anatomical Element*. Trans. Montague R Leverson (London: John Ouseley Ltd, 1912; reprinted Pomeroy, Washington: Health Research).
84. RB Pearson. *Plagiarist Impostor! The Germ Theory Exploded!* (United states: RB Pearson, 1942; reprinted, Pomeroy, Washington: Health Research, 1964).
85. E Enby *et al.* Hidden Killers: The Revolutionary Medical Discoveries of Professor Guenther Enderlein (California: Sheehan Communications, 1990), 31.
86. Günther Enderlein. *Bacterial Cyclogeny: Prolegomena To Study of the Structure, Sexual and Asexual Reproduction and Development of Bacteria.*1999, English translation. (Originally published in 1925 in German).
87. Wilhelm Reich. *The Bion Experiment: On the Origin of Life*. (New York: Farrar Straus Giroux, 1979).
88. Rosenberg E, Zilber-Rosenberg I. The hologenome concept of evolution after 10 years. *Microbiome*. 2018 Apr 25;6(1):78.
89. Nenah Sylver. *The Rife Handbook of Frequency Therapy and Holistic Health*. 2018, 5th edition. Desert Gate Productions LLC, Surprise, Arizona. 189–241.
90. Grice EA, Segre JA. The Human Microbiome: Our Second Genome. *Annu Rev Genomics Hum Genet*. 2012;13:151–70.
91. Kramer P, Bressan P. Humans as superorganisms: How microbes, viruses, imprinted genes, and other selfish entities shape our behavior. *Perspectives on Psychological Science*. 2015. 10 (4): 464–481.
92. The Influence of Cooperative Bacteria on Animal Host Biology, In: *Advances in Molecular and Cellular Microbiology*. 2005, University College London, editors: MJ McFall Ngai, B Henderson, EG Ruby.
93. Irving M. New study suggests antibiotics can weaken the immune system [Internet]. *New Atlas*. 2017 [cited 2020 Feb 17]. Available from: https://newatlas.com/antibiotics-counteract-immune-system/52457/
94. Savory A. *Holistic Management. A new framework for decision making*. 1999. Island Press.

What does gut flora do for us?

1. Macfarlane S, Bahrami B, Macfarlane GT. Mucosal biofilm communities in the human intestinal tract. *Adv Appl Microbiol*. 2011;75:111–43.
2. De Weirdt R, Van de Wiele T. Micromanagement in the gut: microenvironmental factors govern colon mucosal biofilm structure and functionality. *Biofilms and Microbiomes*. 2015 Dec 16;1(1):1–6.
3. Perez-Vilar J, Hill RL (2004). "Mucin Family of Glycoproteins". *Encyclopedia of Biological Chemistry* (Lennarz & Lane, EDs.). Oxford: Academic Press/Elsevier. 2: 758–764.
4. Garcia-Gutierrez E, Mayer MJ, Cotter PD, Narbad A. Gut microbiota as a source of novel antimicrobials. *Gut Microbes*. 2018 May 22;10(1):1–21.

5. Conlon MA, Bird AR. The Impact of Diet and Lifestyle on Gut Microbiota and Human Health. *Nutrients*. 2014 Dec 24;7(1):17–44.
6. Joutey NT, Bahafid W, Sayel H, ElGhachtouli N. Biodegradation: Involved Microorganisms and Genetically Engineered Microorganisms. *Biodegradation – Life of Science* [Internet]. 2013 Jun 14 [cited 2020 Feb 19]; Available from: https://www.intechopen.com/books/biodegradation-life-of-science/biodegradation-involved-microorganisms-and-genetically-engineered-microorganisms
7. Isotrope. Detox: Gut Bacteria & Heavy Metal Chelation [Internet]. *Isotrope*. 2019 [cited 2020 Feb 19]. Available from: https://www.isotrope.com/gut-bacteria-heavy-metal-chelation/
8. Cutler AH. *Amalgam Illness, Diagnosis and Treatment*. 2017. Andy Cutler Publishing.
9. George GN, Singh SP, Hoover J, Pickering IJ. The Chemical Forms of Mercury in Aged and Fresh Dental Amalgam Surfaces. *Chem Res Toxicol*. 2009 Nov;22(11):1761–4.
10. Rice KM, Walker EM, Wu M, Gillette C, Blough ER. Environmental Mercury and Its Toxic Effects. *J Prev Med Public Health*. 2014 Mar;47(2):74–83.
11. Li H, He J, Jia W. The influence of gut microbiota on drug metabolism and toxicity. *Expert Opin Drug Metab Toxicol*. 2016;12(1):31–40.
12. Anthony Atala; Darrell J. Irvine; Marsha Moses; Sunil Shaunak (1 August 2010). "Wound Healing Versus Regeneration: Role of the Tissue Environment in Regenerative Medicine". *MRS Bull*. 35 (8): 597–606.
13. Michalopoulos GK, DeFrances MC (April 1997). "Liver regeneration". *Science*. 276 (5309): 60–6.
14. Salem I, Ramser A, Isham N, Ghannoum MA. The Gut Microbiome as a Major Regulator of the Gut-Skin Axis. *Front Microbiol* [Internet]. 2018 Jul 10 [cited 2020 Feb 19];9. Available from: https://www.ncbi.nlm.nih.gov/pmc/articles/PMC6048199/
15. Cénit MC, Matzaraki V, Tigchelaar EF, Zhernakova A. Rapidly expanding knowledge on the role of the gut microbiome in health and disease. *Biochim Biophys Acta*. 2014 Oct;1842(10):1981–1992. doi: 10.1016/j.bbadis. 2014.05. 023. Review.
16. Yoshii K, Hosomi K, Sawane K, Kunisawa J. Metabolism of Dietary and Microbial Vitamin B Family in the Regulation of Host Immunity. *Front Nutr* [Internet]. 2019 [cited 2020 Feb 19];6. Available from: https://www.frontiersin.org/articles/10.3389/fnut.2019.00048/full
17. Bio-K+. The Link between iron absorption and the microbiome | *Bio-K+* [Internet]. Bio-K+ Community. [cited 2020 Feb 19]. Available from: https://www.biokplus.com/blog/en_CA/gut-health/iron-deficiency-anemia-how-our-microbiome-impacts-iron-absorption/
18. *Human Intestinal microflora in health and disease*. Edited by David J Hentges. Academic Press, London. 1983.
19. Masterjohn C. On the trail of the elusive x factor: a sixty-two-year-old mystery finally solved. *Wise Traditions*. 2007;8(1).
20. vom Steeg LG, Klein SL. Sex Steroids Mediate Bidirectional Interactions Between Hosts and Microbes. *Horm Behav*. 2017 Feb;88:45–51.
21. Clarke G, Stilling RM, Kennedy PJ, Stanton C, Cryan JF, Dinan TG. Minireview: Gut Microbiota: The Neglected Endocrine Organ. *Mol Endocrinol*. 2014 Aug;28(8):1221–38.
22. Kwa M, Plottel CS, Blaser MJ, Adams S. The Intestinal Microbiome and Estrogen Receptor–Positive Female Breast Cancer. *J Natl Cancer Inst* [Internet].

2016 Apr 22 [cited 2020 Feb 24];108(8). Available from: https://www.ncbi.nlm.nih.gov/pmc/articles/PMC5017946/

23. Baker JM, Al-Nakkash L, Herbst-Kralovetz MM. Estrogen-gut microbiome axis: Physiological and clinical implications. *Maturitas*. 2017 Sep;103:45–53.
24. Strandwitz P. Neurotransmitter modulation by the gut microbiota. *Brain Res*. 2018 15;1693(Pt B):128–33.
25. Naseribafrouei A, Hestad K, Avershina E, Sekelja M, Linlokken A, Wilson R, *et al*.Correlation between the human fecal microbiota and depression. *Neurogastroenterology & Motility*. 2014 May 1;26.
26. Strandwitz P, Kim KH *et al*.GABA-modulating bacteria of the human gut microbiota. *Nat Microbiol*. 2019 Mar;4(3):396-403. doi: 10.1038/s41564-018-0307-3. Epub 2018 Dec 10.
27. Alcock J, Maley CC, Aktipis CA. Is eating behavior manipulated by the gastrointestinal microbiota? Evolutionary pressures and potential mechanisms. *Bioessays*. 2014 Oct;36(10):940–9.
28. Parkar SG, Kalsbeek A, Cheeseman JF. Potential Role for the Gut Microbiota in Modulating Host Circadian Rhythms and Metabolic Health. *Microorganisms* [Internet]. 2019 Jan 31 [cited 2020 Feb 24];7(2). Available from: https://www.ncbi.nlm.nih.gov/pmc/articles/PMC6406615/
29. Carvalho Cabral P, Olivier M, Cermakian N. The Complex Interplay of Parasites, Their Hosts, and Circadian Clocks. *Front Cell Infect Microbiol* [Internet]. 2019 [cited 2020 Feb 20];9. Available from: https://www.frontiersin.org/articles/10.3389/fcimb.2019.00425/full
30. Yuanyuan Li, Yanli Hao *et al*.The Role of Microbiome in Insomnia, Circadian Disturbance and Depression. *Front Psychiatry*. 2018; 9: 669. Published online 2018 Dec 5.
31. Stinson LF, Boyce MC, Payne MS, Keelan JA. The Not-so-Sterile Womb: Evidence That the Human Fetus Is Exposed to Bacteria Prior to Birth. *Front Microbiol* [Internet]. 2019 Jun 4 [cited 2020 Feb 20];10. Available from: https://www.ncbi.nlm.nih.gov/pmc/articles/PMC6558212/
32. Amabebe E, Anumba DOC. The Vaginal Microenvironment: The Physiologic Role of Lactobacilli. *Front Med* [Internet]. 2018 [cited 2020 Feb 20];5. Available from: https://www.frontiersin.org/articles/10.3389/fmed.2018.00181/full
33. Milani C, Duranti S, Bottacini F, Casey E, Turroni F, Mahony J, *et al*.The First Microbial Colonizers of the Human Gut: Composition, Activities, and Health Implications of the Infant Gut Microbiota. *Microbiol Mol Biol Rev* [Internet]. 2017 Nov 8 [cited 2020 Feb 10];81(4). Available from: https://www.ncbi.nlm.nih.gov/pmc/articles/PMC5706746/
34. Neu J, Rushing J. Cesarean versus Vaginal Delivery: Long term infant outcomes and the Hygiene Hypothesis. *Clin Perinatol*. 2011 Jun;38(2):321–31.
35. Environmental Working Group. Body Burden: The Pollution in Newborns [Internet]. EWG. 5AD [cited 2020 Feb 20]. Available from: https://www.ewg.org/research/body-burden-pollution-newborns
36. Walker M. *Breastfeeding Management for the Clinician*. Jones & Bartlett Publishers; 2013. 636 p.
37. O'Sullivan A, Farver M, Smilowitz JT. The Influence of Early Infant-Feeding Practices on the Intestinal Microbiome and Body Composition in Infants. *Nutr Metab Insights*. 2015 Dec 16;8(Suppl 1):1–9.
38. Maier L, Pruteanu M, Kuhn M, Zeller G, Telzerow A, Anderson EE, *et al*.Extensive impact of non-antibiotic drugs on human gut bacteria. *Nature*. 2018 Mar 29;555(7698):623–8.

39. Ding HT, Taur Y, Walkup JT. Gut Microbiota and Autism: Key Concepts and Findings. *J Autism Dev Disord*. 2017 Feb 1;47(2):480–9.
40. Yue H, Bing J, Zheng Q, Zhang Y, Hu T, Du H, *et al.*Filamentation in Candida auris, an emerging fungal pathogen of humans: passage through the mammalian body induces a heritable phenotypic switch. *Emerg Microbes Infect* [Internet]. 2018 Nov 28 [cited 2020 Feb 20];7. Available from: https://www.ncbi.nlm.nih.gov/pmc/articles/PMC6258701/
41. Albacker, L., Chaudhary, V., Chang, Y. *et al.*Invariant natural killer T cells recognize a fungal glycosphingolipid that can induce airway hyperreactivity. *Nat Med* 19, 1297–1304 (2013). https://doi.org/10.1038/nm.3321
42. Wu J, Yan L-J. Streptozotocin-induced type 1 diabetes in rodents as a model for studying mitochondrial mechanisms of diabetic cell glucotoxicity. *Diabetes Metab Syndr Obes*. 2015 Apr 2;8:181–8.
43. Rashid T, Ebringer A. Autoimmunity in Rheumatic Diseases Is Induced by Microbial Infections via Crossreactivity or Molecular Mimicry [Internet]. *Autoimmune Diseases*. 2012 [cited 2020 Feb 20]. Available from: https://www.hindawi.com/journals/ad/2012/539282/
44. Scher JU, Sczesnak A, Longman RS, Segata N, Ubeda C, Bielski C, *et al.* Expansion of intestinal Prevotella copri correlates with enhanced susceptibility to arthritis. *eLife* [Internet]. 2013 Nov 5 [cited 2020 Feb 20];2. Available from: https://www.ncbi.nlm.nih.gov/pmc/articles/PMC3816614/
45. Krakauer T, Pradhan K, Stiles BG. Staphylococcal Superantigens Spark Host-Mediated Danger Signals. *Front Immunol* [Internet]. 2016 Feb 2 [cited 2020 Feb 20];7. Available from: https://www.ncbi.nlm.nih.gov/pmc/articles/ PMC4735405/

Immune system

1. Guyton and Hall (2011). *Textbook of Medical Physiology*. U.S.: Saunders Elsevier.
2. Sender R, Fuchs S, Milo R. Revised Estimates for the Number of Human and Bacteria Cells in the Body. *PLoS Biol*. 2016;14(8):e1002533.
3. Wu H-J, Wu E. The role of gut microbiota in immune homeostasis and autoimmunity. *Gut Microbes*. 2012 Jan 1;3(1):4–14.
4. Belkaid Y, Hand T. Role of the Microbiota in Immunity and inflammation. *Cell*. 2014 Mar 27;157(1):121–41.
5. Yin C, Mohanta S, Maffia P, Habenicht AJ (6 March 2017). "Editorial: Tertiary Lymphoid Organs (TLOs): Powerhouses of Disease Immunity". *Frontiers in Immunology*. 8: 228.
6. Forchielli ML, Walker WA. The role of gut-associated lymphoid tissues and mucosal defence. *Br J Nutr*. 2005 Apr;93 Suppl 1:S41–48.
7. Malabsorption Syndrome: Causes, Symptoms, and Risk Factors [Internet]. *Healthline*. [cited 2020 Mar 2]. Available from: https://www.healthline.com/health/malabsorption
8. Carla Lintas, Altieri Lura *et al.*Association of autism with polyomavirus infection in post-mortem brains. *J Neurovirol*. 2010 Mar;16(2):141–9.
9. Quigley EMM. Gut Bacteria in Health and Disease. *Gastroenterol Hepatol* (N Y). 2013 Sep;9(9):560–9.
10. Graham NM, Burrell CJ, Douglas RM, Debelle P, Davies L. Adverse effects of aspirin, acetaminophen, and ibuprofen on immune function, viral shedding, and clinical status in rhinovirus-infected volunteers. *J Infect Dis*. 1990 Dec;162(6):1277–82.

11. Rosenblum MD, Gratz IK, Paw JS, Abbas AK. Treating Human Autoimmunity: Current Practice and Future Prospects. *Sci Transl Med.* 2012 Mar 14;4(125): 125sr1.
12. Lerner, A., Aminov, R., and Matthias, T. (2016). Dysbiosis may trigger autoimmune diseases via inappropriate posttranslational modification of host proteins. *Front. Microbiol.* 7:84. doi: 10.3389/fmicb.2016.00084
13. Rashid T, Ebringer A. Autoimmunity in Rheumatic Diseases Is Induced by Microbial Infections via Crossreactivity or Molecular Mimicry [Internet]. *Autoimmune Diseases.* 2012 [cited 2020 Feb 20]. Available from: https://www.hindawi.com/journals/ad/2012/539282/
14. Malandain H. Transglutaminases: a meeting point for wheat allergy, celiac disease, and food safety. *Eur Ann Allergy Clin Immunol.* 2005 Dec;37(10): 397–403.
15. Matthias T, Jeremias P, Neidhöfer S, Lerner A. The industrial food additive, microbial transglutaminase, mimics tissue transglutaminase and is immunogenic in celiac disease patients. *Autoimmun Rev.* 2016 Dec;15(12):1111–9.
16. Lerner A, Aminov R, Matthias T. Transglutaminases in Dysbiosis As Potential Environmental Drivers of Autoimmunity. *Front Microbiol* [Internet]. 2017 Jan 24 [cited 2020 Feb 28];8. Available from: https://www.ncbi.nlm.nih.gov/pmc/articles/PMC5258703/
17. Lerner A, Matthias T. Possible association between celiac disease and bacterial transglutaminase in food processing: a hypothesis. *Nutr Rev.* 2015 Aug;73(8): 544–52.
18. Vieira SM, Hiltensperger M, Kumar V, Zegarra-Ruiz D, Dehner C, Khan N, *et al.*Translocation of a gut pathobiont drives autoimmunity in mice and humans. *Science.* 2018 Mar 9;359(6380):1156–61.
19. *Mosaic of Autoimmunity. The Novel Factors of Autoimmune Diseases.* 1st Edition. Editors: Carlo Perricone, Yehuda Shoenfeld. 2019. Academic Press.
20. Hall, D. A. (ed) (1964) *International Review of Connective Tissue Research*, Vol. 2, F. Verzár, Aging of the Collagen Fiber, Academic Press, New York, p. 244 top paragraph
21. Di Lullo, Gloria A.; Sweeney, Shawn M.; Körkkö, Jarmo; Ala-Kokko, Leena & San Antonio, James D. (2002). "Mapping the Ligand-binding Sites and Disease-associated Mutations on the Most Abundant Protein in the Human, Type I Collagen". *J. Biol. Chem.* 277 (6): 4223–4231.
22. Ben-Amram H, Bashi T, Werbner N, Neuman H, Fridkin M, Blank M, *et al.*Tuftsin-Phosphorylcholine Maintains Normal Gut Microbiota in Collagen Induced Arthritic Mice. *Front Microbiol* [Internet]. 2017 Jul 10 [cited 2020 Feb 28];8. Available from: https://www.ncbi.nlm.nih.gov/pmc/articles/PMC5502260/
23. Samsel A, Seneff S. Glyphosate pathways to modern diseases VI: Prions, amyloidoses and autoimmune neurological diseases. *JBPC.* 2017 Mar 30;17(1):8–32.
24. Beecham J, Seneff S. The possible link between autism and glyphosate acting as glycine mimetic – a review of evidence from the literature with analysis. *J Mol Genet Med* 2015; 9:4.
25. *Glyphosate in Collagen.* February 1, 2017 By Stephanie Seneff, PhD https://www.westonaprice.org/health-topics/environmental-toxins/ glyphosate-in-collagen/
26. Solhjoo M, Bansal P, Goyal A, Chauhan K. Drug-Induced Lupus Erythematosus. In: *StatPearls* [Internet]. *Treasure Island* (FL): StatPearls Publishing; 2020 [cited 2020 Mar 3]. Available from: http://www.ncbi.nlm.nih.gov/books/NBK441889/

27. Hart FD. Drug-induced arthritis and arthralgia. *Drugs*. 1984 Oct;28(4):347–54.
28. T Cutler AH. *Amalgam Illness, Diagnosis and Treatment*. 2017. Andy Cutler Publishing.
29. Wiemels J. Perspectives on the Causes of Childhood Leukaemia. *Chem Biol Interact* [Internet]. 2012 Apr 5 [cited 2020 Mar 3];196(3). Available from: https://www.ncbi.nlm.nih.gov/pmc/articles/PMC3839796/
30. Carpenter DO, Bushkin-Bedient S. Exposure to Chemicals and Radiation During Childhood and Risk for Cancer Later in Life. *Journal of Adolescent Health*. 2013 May 1;52(5, Supplement):S21–9.
31. Alessio Fasano. Leaky Gut and Autoimmune Diseases. *Clin Rev Allergy Immunol*, 2012 Feb;42(1):71-8.
32. Khazan O. *The Reason Anxious People Often Have Allergies* [Internet]. The Atlantic. 2019 [cited 2020 Mar 3]. Available from: https://www.theatlantic.com/health/archive/2019/07/allergies-anxiety/593572/
33. Lee N, Kim W-U. Microbiota in T-cell homeostasis and inflammatory diseases. *Exp Mol Med*. 2017 May;49(5):e340.
34. Devereux, Graham; Seaton, A. (December 2004). "Diet as a risk factor for atopy and asthma". *J Allergy Clin Immunol*. 115 (6): 1109–1117.
35. da Silva EZ, Jamur MC, Oliver C (2014). "Mast cell function: a new vision of an old cell". *J. Histochem. Cytochem*. 62 (10): 698–738.
36. Cookson H, Grattan C. An update on mast cell disorders. *Clin Med* (Lond). 2016 Dec;16(6):580–3.
37. Frontiers | Biogenic Amines: Signals Between Commensal Microbiota and Gut Physiology | *Endocrinology* [Internet]. [cited 2020 Mar 3]. Available from: https://www.frontiersin.org/articles/10.3389/fendo.2019.00504/full
38. Lombardi VC, De Meirleir KL, Subramanian K, Nourani SM, Dagda RK, Delaney SL, *et al*. Nutritional modulation of the intestinal microbiota; future opportunities for the prevention and treatment of neuroimmune and neuroinflammatory disease. *The Journal of Nutritional Biochemistry*. 2018 Nov 1;61:1–16.
39. Li L, Ruan L, Ji A, Wen Z, Chen S, Wang L, *et al*.Biogenic amines analysis and microbial contribution in traditional fermented food of Douchi. *Scientific Reports*. 2018 Aug 22;8(1):1–10.
40. Chilton SN, Burton JP, Reid G. Inclusion of Fermented Foods in Food Guides around the World. *Nutrients*. 2015 Jan 8;7(1):390–404.
41. Priyadarshani WMD, Rakshit SK. Screening selected strains of probiotic lactic acid bacteria for their ability to produce biogenic amines (histamine and tyramine). *International Journal of Food Science & Technology*. 2011;46(10):2062–9.
42. Evans SS, Repasky EA, Fisher DT. Fever and the thermal regulation of immunity: the immune system feels the heat. *Nature Reviews Immunology*. 2015 Jun;15(6):335–49.
43. Hussain J, Cohen M. Clinical Effects of Regular Dry Sauna Bathing: A Systematic Review. *Evid Based Complement Alternat Med* [Internet]. 2018 Apr 24 [cited 2020 Mar 3];2018. Available from: https://www.ncbi.nlm.nih.gov/pmc/articles/PMC5941775/
44. Yu JC, Khodadadi H, Malik A, Davidson B, Salles É da SL, Bhatia J, *et al*. Innate Immunity of Neonates and Infants. *Front Immunol* [Internet]. 2018 Jul 30 [cited 2020 Mar 3];9. Available from: https://www.ncbi.nlm.nih.gov/pmc/articles/PMC6077196/
45. PennisiNov. 19 E, 2014, Pm 1:00. Viruses help keep the gut healthy [Internet]. *Science* | AAAS. 2014 [cited 2020 Feb 16]. Available from: https://www.sciencemag.org/news/2014/11/viruses-help-keep-gut-healthy

46. Bradford AB. *What Is the Hygiene Hypothesis?* [Internet]. livescience.com. 2016 [cited 2020 Mar 3]. Available from: https://www.livescience.com/54078-hygiene-hypothesis.html
47. Katona P, Katona-Apte J. The Interaction between Nutrition and Infection. *Clin Infect Dis*. 2008 May 15;46(10):1582–8.
48. Grammatikos AP, Tsokos GC. Immunodeficiency and autoimmunity: lessons from systemic lupus erythematosus. *Trends Mol Med*. 2012 Feb;18(2):101–8.
49. Tsoupras A, Lordan R, Zabetakis I. Inflammation, not Cholesterol, Is a Cause of Chronic Disease. *Nutrients* [Internet]. 2018 May 12 [cited 2020 Mar 3];10(5). Available from: https://www.ncbi.nlm.nih.gov/pmc/articles/PMC5986484/
50. Bhakdi S, Tranum-Jensen J, Utermann G, Füssle R. Binding and partial inactivation of Staphylococcus aureus alpha-toxin by human plasma low density lipoprotein. *J Biol Chem*. 1983 May 10;258(9):5899–904.
51. Ravnskov U. High cholesterol may protect against infections and atherosclerosis. *QJM*. 2003 Dec 1;96(12):927–34.
52. Elmehdawi R. Hypolipidemia: A Word of Caution. *Libyan J Med*. 2008 Jun 1;3(2):84–90.
53. Andersen CJ. Bioactive Egg Components and Inflammation. *Nutrients*. 2015 Sep 16;7(9):7889–913.
54. Daisy Coyle. Food Fermentation: Benefits, Safety, Food List, and More [Internet]. Healthline. 2019 [cited 2020 Mar 2]. Available from: https://www.healthline.com/nutrition/fermentation
55. Singh RK, Chang H-W, Yan D, Lee KM, Ucmak D, Wong K, *et al*. Influence of diet on the gut microbiome and implications for human health. *J Transl Med* [Internet]. 2017 Apr 8 [cited 2020 Mar 3];15. Available from: https://www.ncbi.nlm.nih.gov/pmc/articles/PMC5385025/
56. Medawar E, Huhn S, Villringer A, Veronica Witte A. The effects of plant-based diets on the body and the brain: a systematic review. *Translational Psychiatry*. 2019 Sep 12;9(1):1–17.
57. Guggenheim AG, Wright KM, Zwickey HL. Immune Modulation from Five Major Mushrooms: Application to Integrative Oncology. *Integr Med (Encinitas)*. 2014 Feb;13(1):32–44.
58. Bloomfield S, Stanwell-Smith R, Crevel R, Pickup J. Too clean, or not too clean: the Hygiene Hypothesis and home hygiene. *Clin Exp Allergy*. 2006 Apr;36(4):402–25.
59. Aminov RI. 2010. A brief history of the antibiotic era: lessons learned and challenges for the future. *Front Microbiol* 1:134.

Hormones

1. Mittal R, Debs LH, Patel AP, Nguyen D, Patel K, O'Connor G, *et al*. Neurotransmitters: The critical modulators regulating gut-brain axis. *J Cell Physiol*. 2017 Sep;232(9):2359–72.
2. Claus SP, Guillou H, Ellero-Simatos S. The gut microbiota: a major player in the toxicity of environmental pollutants? *NPJ Biofilms Microbiomes*. 2016 May 4;2:16003.
3. *Endocrine Disruptors* [Internet]. National Institute of Environmental Health Sciences. [cited 2020 Mar 9]. Available from: https://www.niehs.nih.gov/health/topics/agents/endocrine/index.cfm
4. Lauretta R, Sansone A, Sansone M, Romanelli F, Appetecchia M. Endocrine

Disrupting Chemicals: Effects on Endocrine Glands. *Front Endocrinol* (Lausanne) [Internet]. 2019 Mar 21 [cited 2020 Mar 9];10. Available from: https://www.ncbi.nlm.nih.gov/pmc/articles/PMC6448049/

5. Street ME, Angelini S, Bernasconi S, Burgio E, Cassio A, Catellani C, *et al.* Current Knowledge on Endocrine Disrupting Chemicals (EDCs) from Animal Biology to Humans, from Pregnancy to Adulthood: Highlights from a National Italian Meeting. *Int J Mol Sci* [Internet]. 2018 Jun 2 [cited 2020 Mar 9];19(6). Available from: https://www.ncbi.nlm.nih.gov/pmc/articles/PMC6032228/
6. Vilahur N, Fernández MF, Bustamante M, Ramos R, Forns J, Ballester F, *et al.* In utero exposure to mixtures of xenoestrogens and child neuropsychological development. *Environ Res.* 2014 Oct;134:98–104.
7. Schug TT, Janesick A, Blumberg B, Heindel JJ. Endocrine Disrupting Chemicals and Disease Susceptibility. *J Steroid Biochem Mol Biol.* 2011 Nov;127(3–5):204–15.
8. Patisaul HB. Endocrine disruption by dietary phyto-oestrogens: impact on dimorphic sexual systems and behaviours. *Proc Nutr Soc.* 2017 May;76(2):130–44.
9. Nkhata SG, Ayua E, Kamau EH, Shingiro J. Fermentation and germination improve nutritional value of cereals and legumes through activation of endogenous enzymes. *Food Sci Nutr.* 2018 Oct 16;6(8):2446–58.
10. Rizzo G, Baroni L. Soy, Soy Foods and Their Role in Vegetarian Diets. *Nutrients* [Internet]. 2018 Jan 5 [cited 2020 Mar 9];10(1). Available from: https://www.ncbi.nlm.nih.gov/pmc/articles/PMC5793271/
11. Datis Kharrazian. Good thyroid health depends on good gut health [Internet]. *Dr. K. News.* 2010 [cited 2020 Mar 9]. Available from: https://drknews.com/good-thyroid-health-depends-on-good-gut-health/
12. Nussey S, Whitehead S. *The thyroid gland* [Internet]. BIOS Scientific Publishers; 2001 [cited 2020 Mar 9]. Available from: https://www.ncbi.nlm.nih.gov/books/NBK28/
13. Lerner A, Jeremias P, Matthias T. *Gut-thyroid axis and celiac disease.* 2017 Apr 5;6(4):R52–8.
14. Kheradpisheh Z, Mirzaei M, Mahvi AH, Mokhtari M, Azizi R, Fallahzadeh H, *et al.* Impact of Drinking Water Fluoride on Human Thyroid Hormones: A Case-Control Study. *Sci Rep* [Internet]. 2018 Feb 8 [cited 2020 Mar 9];8. Available from: https://www.ncbi.nlm.nih.gov/pmc/articles/PMC5805681/
15. Yang RS, Witt KL, Alden CJ, Cockerham LG. Toxicology of methyl bromide. *Rev Environ Contam Toxicol.* 1995;142:65–85.
16. Boston 677 Huntington Avenue, Ma 02115 +1495 1000. Is Fluoridated Drinking Water Safe? [Internet]. *Harvard Public Health Magazine.* 2016 [cited 2020 Mar 9]. Available from: https://www.hsph.harvard.edu/magazine/magazine_article/fluoridated-drinking-water/
17. Stadel BV. Dietary iodine and risk of breast, endometrial, and ovarian cancer. *Lancet.* 1976 Apr 24;1(7965):890–1.
18. Patricia Wu. Thyroid Disease and Diabetes. *Clinical Diabetes* [Internet]. 2000 [cited 2020 Mar 9];VOL. 18 NO. 1(Winter). Available from: http://journal.diabetes.org/clinicaldiabetes/v18n12000/pg38.htm
19. Klein JR. The immune system as a regulator of thyroid hormone activity. *Exp Biol Med* (Maywood). 2006 Mar;231(3):229–36.
20. Cutler AH. *Amalgam Illness, Diagnosis and Treatment.* 2017. Andy Cutler Publishing.

21. Farzi A, Fröhlich EE, Holzer P. Gut Microbiota and the Neuroendocrine System. *Neurotherapeutics*. 2018 Jan;15(1):5–22.
22. Terry Wahls. *7 Foods To Eat To Heal Adrenal Fatigue* [Internet]. mindbodygreen. 2016 [cited 2020 Mar 9]. Available from: https://www.mindbodygreen.com/0-25960/7-foods-to-eat-to-heal-adrenal-fatigue.html
23. Cham S, Koslik HJ, Golomb BA. Mood, Personality, and Behaviour Changes During Treatment with Statins: A Case Series. *Drug Saf Case Rep* [Internet]. 2015 Dec 29 [cited 2020 Mar 9];3. Available from: https://www.ncbi.nlm.nih.gov/pmc/articles/PMC5005588/
24. Neuman H, Debelius JW, Knight R, Koren O. Microbial endocrinology: the interplay between the microbiota and the endocrine system. *FEMS Microbiol Rev*. 2015 Jul 1;39(4):509–21.
25. Clarke G, Stilling RM, Kennedy PJ, Stanton C, Cryan JF, Dinan TG. Minireview: Gut Microbiota: The Neglected Endocrine Organ. *Mol Endocrinol*. 2014 Aug;28(8):1221–38.
26. *Menopausal Hormone Therapy and Cancer* [Internet]. National Cancer Institute. 2011 [cited 2020 Mar 9]. Available from: https://www.cancer.gov/about-cancer/causes-prevention/risk/hormones/mht-fact-sheet
27. Chaban B, Jayaprakash T, Wagner E, Bourque D, Lohn Z, Albert A, *et al*. Characterization of the vaginal microbiota of healthy Canadian women through the menstrual cycle. *Microbiome*. 2014 Jul 4;2:23.
28. Baker JM, Al-Nakkash L, Herbst-Kralovetz MM. Oestrogen-gut microbiome axis: Physiological and clinical implications. *Maturitas*. 2017 Sep;103:45–53.
29. Bourrie BCT, Willing BP, Cotter PD. The Microbiota and Health Promoting Characteristics of the Fermented Beverage Kefir. *Front Microbiol* [Internet]. 2016 May 4 [cited 2020 Mar 9];7. Available from: https://www.ncbi.nlm.nih.gov/pmc/articles/PMC4854945/

The liver and the lungs

1. Canadian Liver Foundation. Your liver is essential to your life. *The Canadian Liver Foundation* [Internet]. Canadian Liver Foundation. 2017 [cited 2020 Mar 31]. Available from: https://www.liver.ca/your-liver/
2. Chris Kresser. *Liver: Nature's Most Potent Superfood* [Internet]. Chris Kresser. 2008 [cited 2020 Mar 31]. Available from: https://chriskresser.com/natures-most-potent-superfood/
3. Garrow JS, James WPT, Ralph A. *Human nutrition and dietetics*. 2000. 10th edition. Churchill Livingstone.
4. Stokes, Caroline S.; Gluud, Lise Lotte; Casper, Markus; Lammert, Frank (2014-07-01). "Ursodeoxycholic Acid and Diets Higher in Fat Prevent Gallbladder Stones During Weight Loss: A Meta-analysis of Randomized Controlled Trials". *Clinical Gastroenterology and Hepatology*. 12 (7): 1090–1100.e2.
5. Njeze GE. Gallstones. *Niger J Surg*. 2013;19(2):49–55.
6. Abdallah AA, Krige JEJ, Bornman PC. Biliary tract obstruction in chronic pancreatitis. *HPB* (Oxford). 2007;9(6):421–8.
7. DeLoid GM, Sohal IS, Lorente LR, Molina RM, Pyrgiotakis G, Stevanovic A, *et al*. Reducing Intestinal Digestion and Absorption of Fat Using a Nature-Derived Biopolymer: Interference of Triglyceride Hydrolysis by Nanocellulose. *ACS Nano*. 2018 Jul 24;12(7):6469–79.

8. Johns Hopkins Medicine. *Gallbladder Removal Is Common. But Is It Necessary?* – 04/03/2017 [Internet]. 2017 [cited 2020 Mar 31]. Available from: https://www.hopkinsmedicine.org/news/media/releases/gallbladder_removal_is_common_but_is_it_necessary
9. Pannu HK, Fishman EK. Complications of Endoscopic Retrograde Cholangiopancreatography: Spectrum of Abnormalities Demonstrated with CT. *RadioGraphics*. 2001 Nov 1;21(6):1441–53.
10. Jagmohan B. Remove Gall Stones Without Surgery [Internet]. *Health is About You*. 2018 [cited 2020 Mar 31]. Available from: https://www.healthisaboutyou.com/home-remedies/remove-gallstones-without-surgery/
11. Association for the Advancement of Restorative Medicine. Peppermint oil [Internet]. *Restorative Medicine*. [cited 2020 Mar 31]. Available from: https://restorativemedicine.org/library/monographs/peppermint-oil/
12. Kim ES, Chun HJ, Keum B, Seo YS, Jeen YT, Lee HS, *et al*. Coffee Enema for Preparation for Small Bowel Video Capsule Endoscopy: A Pilot Study. *Clin Nutr Res*. 2014;3(2):134.
13. Griffiths DJ. Endogenous retroviruses in the human genome sequence. *Genome Biol*. 2001;2(6): reviews 1017.1–reviews1017.5.
14. Popkin BM, D'Anci KE, Rosenberg IH. Water, Hydration and Health. *Nutr Rev*. 2010 Aug;68(8):439–58.
15. Hobbs C. Natural Therapy for Your Liver: Herbs and Other Natural Remedies for a Healthy Liver. *Penguin*; 2002. 148 p.
16. Suzuki T, Chow C-W, Downey GP. Role of innate immune cells and their products in lung immunopathology. *The International Journal of Biochemistry & Cell Biology*. 2008 Jun 1;40(6):1348–61.
17. Malaguarnera G, Cataudella E, Giordano M, Nunnari G, Chisari G, Malaguarnera M. Toxic hepatitis in occupational exposure to solvents. *World J Gastroenterol*. 2012 Jun 14;18(22):2756–66.
18. MARY ENIG, PHD. *Saturated Fats and the Lungs* [Internet]. The Weston A. Price Foundation. [cited 2020 Mar 11]. Available from: https://www.westonaprice.org/health-topics/know-your-fats/saturated-fats-and-the-lungs/
19. Glasser JR, Mallampalli RK. Surfactant and its role in the pathobiology of pulmonary infection. *Microbes Infect*. 2012 Jan;14(1):17–25.
20. Chakraborty M, Kotecha S. Pulmonary surfactant in new-born infants and children. *Breathe*. 2013 Dec 1;9(6):476–88.
21. He Y, Wen Q, Yao F, Xu D, Huang Y, Wang J. Gut–lung axis: The microbial contributions and clinical implications. *Critical Reviews in Microbiology*. 2017 Jan 2;43(1):81–95.
22. Moffatt MF, Cookson WO. The lung microbiome in health and disease. *Clin Med (Lond)*. 2017 Dec;17(6):525–9.
23. Cushion MT. Are Members of the Fungal Genus Pneumocystis (a) Commensals; (b) Opportunists; (c) Pathogens; or (d) All of the Above? *PLoS Pathog* [Internet]. 2010 Sep 23 [cited 2020 Apr 1];6(9). Available from: https://www.ncbi.nlm.nih.gov/pmc/articles/PMC2944789/
24. Frati F, Salvatori C, Incorvaia C, Bellucci A, Di Cara G, Marcucci F, *et al*. The Role of the Microbiome in Asthma: The Gut–Lung Axis. *Int J Mol Sci* [Internet]. 2018 Dec 30 [cited 2020 Apr 1];20(1). Available from: https://www.ncbi.nlm.nih.gov/pmc/articles/PMC6337651/
25. Service HEA. *Food intolerance* [Internet]. 2014 [cited 2020 Apr 1]. Available from: https://heas.health.vic.gov.au/early-childhood-services/allergy-and-intolerance/food-intolerance

26. Kudo M, Ishigatsubo Y, Aoki I. Pathology of asthma. *Front Microbiol* [Internet]. 2013 [cited 2020 Apr 1];4. Available from: https://www.frontiersin.org/articles/10.3389/fmicb.2013.00263/full
27. Doeing DC, Solway J. Airway smooth muscle in the pathophysiology and treatment of asthma. *J Appl Physiol* (1985). 2013 Apr 1;114(7):834–43.
28. D Freed, J Mansfield. Asthma: What we do and why we do it. *JNutr&EnvirMed*, June 2008,17(2):97–110
29. Dharmage SC, Perret JL, Custovic A. Epidemiology of Asthma in Children and Adults. *Front Pediatr* [Internet]. 2019 Jun 18 [cited 2020 Apr 1];7. Available from: https://www.ncbi.nlm.nih.gov/pmc/articles/PMC6591438/

Toxins and parasites

1. Roundtable on Environmental Health Sciences R, Practice B on PH and PH, Medicine I of. The Challenge: Chemicals in Today's Society [Internet]. Identifying and Reducing Environmental Health Risks of Chemicals in Our Society: Workshop Summary. National Academies Press (US); 2014 [cited 2020 Apr 8]. Available from: https://www.ncbi.nlm.nih.gov/books/NBK268889/
2. Environmental Working Group. *Body Burden: The Pollution in Newborns* [Internet]. EWG. 5AD [cited 2020 Feb 20]. Available from: https://www.ewg.org/research/body-burden-pollution-newborns
3. Chance GW. Environmental contaminants and children's health: Cause for concern, time for action. *Paediatr Child Health*. 2001 Dec; 6(10):731–43.
4. Prasad R. *Mycoremediation and Environmental Sustainability*: Volume 1. pg. 5: Springer; 2018. 243 p.
5. Jillian Levy, CHHC. *What Is Candida Die Off? 6 Ways to Manage Symptoms* [Internet]. Dr. Axe. 2019 [cited 2020 Apr 9]. Available from: https://draxe.com/health/candida-die-off/
6. Vaccaro DE. Symbiosis Therapy: The Potential of Using Human Protozoa for Molecular Therapy. *Molecular Therapy*. 2000 Dec 1;2(6):535–8.
7. Helmby H. Human helminth therapy to treat inflammatory disorders – where do we stand? *BMC Immunol* [Internet]. 2015 Mar 26 [cited 2020 Feb 16];16. Available from: https://www.ncbi.nlm.nih.gov/pmc/articles/PMC4374592/
8. Rushton S, Spake A, Chariton L. *The Unintended Consequences of Using Glyphosate*. 2016 Jan;27.
9. Benbrook CM. Trends in glyphosate herbicide use in the United States and globally. *Environ Sci Eur* [Internet]. 2016 [cited 2020 Apr 8];28(1). Available from: https://www.ncbi.nlm.nih.gov/pmc/articles/PMC5044953/
10. NIH: National Institute of Allergy and Infectious Diseases. *Lyme Disease Co-Infection* | NIH: National Institute of Allergy and Infectious Diseases [Internet]. 2018 [cited 2020 Apr 9]. Available from: https://www.niaid.nih.gov/diseases-conditions/lyme-disease-co-infection
11. Citera M, Freeman PR, Horowitz RI. Empirical validation of the Horowitz Multiple Systemic Infectious Disease Syndrome Questionnaire for suspected Lyme disease. *Int J Gen Med*. 2017 Sep 4;10:249–73.
12. Cummins J, Tangney M. Bacteria and tumours: causative agents or opportunistic inhabitants? *Infect Agent Cancer*. 2013 Mar 28;8:11.
13. The American Cancer Society medical and editorial content team. *Parasites that can lead to cancer* | American Cancer Society [Internet]. 2016 [cited 2020 Apr 9]. Available from: https://www.cancer.org/cancer/cancer-causes/infectious-agents/infections-that-can-lead-to-cancer/parasites.html

14. Muehlenbachs A, Bhatnagar J, Agudelo CA, Hidron A, Eberhard ML, Mathison BA, *et al.* Malignant Transformation of Hymenolepis nana in a Human Host. *New England Journal of Medicine.* 2015 Nov 5;373(19):1845–52.
15. Iranzo J, Puigbò P, Lobkovsky AE, Wolf YI, Koonin EV. Inevitability of Genetic Parasites. *Genome Biol Evol.* 2016 Aug 8;8(9):2856–69.
16. Liberti MV, Locasale JW. The Warburg Effect: How Does it Benefit Cancer Cells? *Trends Biochem Sci.* 2016 Mar;41(3):211–8.
17. Kittle AM, Bukombe JK, Sinclair ARE, Mduma SAR, Fryxell JM. Landscape-level movement patterns by lions in western Serengeti: comparing the influence of inter-specific competitors, habitat attributes and prey availability. *Mov Ecol* [Internet]. 2016 Jul 1 [cited 2020 Apr 9];4. Available from: https://www.ncbi.nlm.nih.gov/pmc/articles/PMC4929767/

Bones and teeth

1. Hal Huggins and Thomas E Levy. *Uninformed Consent: The Hidden Dangers In Dental Care.* Hampton Roads Publishing; 1 edition (January 1, 1999).
2. Raggatt, L. J. *et al.* (May 25, 2010). "Cellular and Molecular Mechanisms of Bone Remodelling". *The Journal of Biological Chemistry.* 285 (33): 25103–25108.
3. Steven Lin. *The Dental Diet: The Surprising Link Between Your Teeth, Real Food And Life-Changing Natural Health.* London: Hay House, 2018.
4. Health NRC (US) *C on D and. Fat-Soluble Vitamins* [Internet]. Diet and Health: Implications for Reducing Chronic Disease Risk. National Academies Press (US); 1989 [cited 2020 Apr 17]. Available from: https://www.ncbi.nlm.nih.gov/books/NBK218749/
5. Kreider RB, Campbell B. Protein for exercise and recovery. *Phys Sportsmed.* 2009 Jun;37(2):13–21.
6. Abou Neel EA, Aljabo A, Strange A, Ibrahim S, Coathup M, Young AM, *et al.* Demineralization–remineralization dynamics in teeth and bone. *Int J Nanomedicine.* 2016 Sep 19;11:4743–63.
7. Dominik Nischwitz. *It's All In Your Mouth. Biological Dentistry And The Surprising Impact Of Oral Health On The Whole Body Wellness.* Chelsea Green.2020.
8. Masterjohn C. On the trail of the elusive x factor: a sixty-two-year-old mystery finally solved. *Wise Traditions.* 2007;8(1).
9. Song I-S, Han K, Ko Y, Park Y-G, Ryu J-J, Park J-B. Associations between the consumption of carbonated beverages and periodontal disease: The 2008–2010 Korea national health and nutrition examination survey. *Medicine* [Internet]. 2016 Jul [cited 2020 Apr 20];95(28). Available from: insights.ovid.com
10. Laine CM, Laine T. Diagnosis of Osteoporosis in Children and Adolescents. *Eur Endocrinol.* 2013 Aug;9(2):141–4.
11. Originally written in August 2012 by:Giana Angelo, Ph.D. *Bone Health In Depth* [Internet]. Linus Pauling Institute. 2016 [cited 2020 Apr 20]. Available from: https://lpi.oregonstate.edu/mic/health-disease/bone-health
12. Dominik Nischwitz. *It's All In Your Mouth. Biological Dentistry And The Surprising Impact Of Oral Health On The Whole Body Wellness.* Chelsea Green.2020.
13. Sahay M, Sahay R. Rickets–vitamin D deficiency and dependency. *Indian J Endocrinol Metab.* 2012;16(2):164–76.

14. Masterjohn C. On the trail of the elusive x factor: a sixty-two-year-old mystery finally solved. *Wise Traditions*. 2007;8(1).
15. Price WA. *Nutrition and physical degeneration. A comparison of primitive and modern diets and their effects*. 1938. Price.
16. Price WA, Studies of Relationships Between Nutritional Deficiencies and (a) Facial and Dental Arch Deformities and (b) Loss of Immunity to Dental Caries Among South Sea Islanders and Florida Indians. *Dental Cosmos*. 1935;77(11):1033-45.
17. https://www.westonaprice.org/health-topics/childrens-health/vitamin-a-for-fetal-development/
18. https://www.westonaprice.org/health-topics/childrens-health/sacred-foods-for-exceptionally-healthy-babies-and-parents-too/
19. Pillai SM, Sereda NH, Hoffman ML, Valley EV, Crenshaw TD, Park Y-K, *et al.* Effects of Poor Maternal Nutrition during Gestation on Bone Development and Mesenchymal Stem Cell Activity in Offspring. *PLoS One* [Internet]. 2016 Dec 12 [cited 2020 May 5];11(12). Available from: https://www.ncbi.nlm.nih.gov/pmc/articles/PMC5152907/
20. D Kersten, G Graham, L Scherwitz. *Pottenger's Prophecy: How Food Resets Genes For Wellness Or Illness*. Destiny Health Publishing (June 6, 2011).
21. Dr Eric Davis. *Symptoms Of Toxicity* [Internet]. Eric Davis Dental. [cited 2020 May 5]. Available from: https://www.ericdavisdental.com/biological-dentistry/symptoms-of-toxicity/
22. Deo PN, Deshmukh R. Oral microbiome: Unveiling the fundamentals. *J Oral Maxillofac Pathol*. 2019;23(1):122–8.
23. Turner MD, Ship JA. Dry Mouth and Its Effects on the Oral Health of Elderly People. *The Journal of the American Dental Association*. 2007 Sep;138:S15–20.
24. Dominik Nischwitz. *It's All In Your Mouth. Biological Dentistry And The Surprising Impact Of Oral Health On The Whole Body Wellness*. Chelsea Green.2020.
25. Naumova EA, Sandulescu T, Bochnig C, Khatib PA, Lee W-K, Zimmer S, *et al.* Dynamic changes in saliva after acute mental stress. *Scientific Reports*. 2014 May 8;4(1):1–9.
26. Baek JH, Krasieva T, Tang S, Ahn Y, Kim CS, Vu D, *et al.* Optical approach to the salivary pellicle. *J Biomed Opt*. 2009;14(4):044001.
27. An TD, Pothiraj C, Gopinath RM, Kayalvizhi B. *Effect of oil-pulling on dental caries causing bacteria*. Vol. 2. pg 63-66; 2008.
28. Price WA. *Nutrition and physical degeneration. A comparison of primitive and modern diets and their effects*. 1938. Price.
29. Masterjohn C. On the trail of the elusive x factor: a sixty-two-year-old mystery finally solved. *Wise Traditions*. 2007;8(1).
30. Sheetal A, Hiremath VK, Patil AG, Sajjansetty S, Kumar SR. Malnutrition and its Oral Outcome – A Review. *J Clin Diagn Res*. 2013 Jan;7(1):178–80.
31. Joshipura KJ, Muñoz-Torres FJ, Morou-Bermudez E, Patel RP. Over-the-counter mouthwash use and risk of pre-diabetes/diabetes. *Nitric Oxide*. 2017 Dec 1;71:14–20.
32. Wong MC, Glenny AM, Tsang BW, Lo EC, Worthington HV, Marinho VC (January 2010). "Topical fluoride as a cause of dental fluorosis in children". *The Cochrane Database of Systematic Reviews* (1): CD007693.
33. Peckham S, Awofeso N. Water Fluoridation: A Critical Review of the Physiological Effects of Ingested Fluoride as a Public Health Intervention. *Scientific World Journal* [Internet]. 2014 Feb 26 [cited 2020 May 6];2014. Available from: https://www.ncbi.nlm.nih.gov/pmc/articles/PMC3956646/

34. Woods JO. Dr Hal Alan Huggins, Noted Dental Pioneer, Passes Away. *Integr Med (Encinitas)*. 2015 Feb;14(1):14–5.
35. Bates MN, Fawcett J, Garrett N, Cutress T, Kjellstrom T. Health effects of dental amalgam exposure: a retrospective cohort study. *Int J Epidemiol*. 2004 Aug 1;33(4):894–902.
36. Blanche D Grube, DMD, IMD. 2018 Integrative SIBO Conference Highlights. *Natural Medicine Journal* [Internet]. 2018 Jun [cited 2020 May 6];Vol. 10(6). Available from: https://www.naturalmedicinejournal.com/journal/2018-06/2018-integrative-sibo-conference-highlights
37. Sandborgh-Englund G, Einarsson C, Sandström M, Ekstrand J. Gastrointestinal absorption of metallic mercury. *Arch Environ Health*. 2004 Sep;59(9):449–54.
38. Chris Kresser, M.S. *How Dental Health Affects Your Whole Body*. With Steven Lin | RHR [Internet]. Chris Kresser. 2018 [cited 2020 May 6]. Available from: https://chriskresser.com/how-dental-health-affects-your-whole-body-with-steven-lin/
39. https://www.westonaprice.org/health-topics/dentistry/root-canal-dangers/
40. Hal Huggins and Thomas E Levy. *Uninformed Consent: The Hidden Dangers In Dental Care*. Hampton Roads Publishing; 1 edition (January 1, 1999).
41. Dominik Nischwitz. *It's All In Your Mouth. Biological Dentistry And The Surprising Impact Of Oral Health On The Whole Body Wellness*. Chelsea Green.2020.
42. Dr William P Glaros DDS. Oral-Electro Galvanism: Super-Charged Fillings [Internet]. *Biological Dentist*, Houston Texas. 2011 [cited 2020 May 6]. Available from: https://www.biologicaldentist.com/770/oral-electro-galvanism-super-charged-fillings/
43. Coventry BJ, Ashdown ML, Quinn MA, Markovic SN, Yatomi-Clarke SL, Robinson AP. CRP identifies homeostatic immune oscillations in cancer patients: a potential treatment targeting tool? *J Transl Med*. 2009 Nov 30;7:102.

Problems down below

1. *Organic Acids Test Book*. The great plains laboratory Inc. Published on Oct 7, 2015.
2. Grover S, Srivastava A, Lee R, Tewari AK, Te AE. Role of inflammation in bladder function and interstitial cystitis. *Ther Adv Urol*. 2011 Feb;3(1): 19–33.
3. Skypala IJ, Williams M, Reeves L, Meyer R, Venter C. Sensitivity to food additives, vaso-active amines and salicylates: a review of the evidence. *Clin Transl Allergy* [Internet]. 2015 Oct 13 [cited 2020 May 11];5. Available from: https://www.ncbi.nlm.nih.gov/pmc/articles/PMC4604636/
4. Schwiertz, Andreas (2016). *Microbiota of the human body : implications in health and disease*. Switzerland: Springer. p. 1. ISBN 978-3-319-31248-4.
5. Nienhouse V, Gao X, Dong Q, *et al*. Interplay between bladder microbiota and urinary antimicrobial peptides: mechanisms for human urinary tract infection risk and symptom severity. *PLoS One*. 2014;9(12):e114185. Published 2014 Dec 8. doi:10.1371/journal.pone.0114185
6. Porter, C.M., Shrestha, E., Peiffer, L.B. *et al*. The microbiome in prostate inflammation and prostate cancer. *Prostate Cancer Prostatic Dis* 21, 345–354 (2018). https://doi.org/10.1038/s41391-018-0041-1

7. Norman W Walker. *Colon Health: The Key To A Vibrant Life*. 1979. Norwalk Press US.
8. Franasiak, Jason M.; Scott, Richard T. (2015). "Reproductive tract microbiome in assisted reproductive technologies". *Fertility and Sterility*. 104 (6): 1364–1371.
9. Amabebe E, Anumba DOC. The Vaginal Microenvironment: The Physiologic Role of Lactobacilli. *Front Med* [Internet]. 2018 [cited 2020 Feb 20];5. Available from: https://www.frontiersin.org/articles/10.3389/fmed.2018.00181/full
10. Fox C, Eichelberger K. Maternal microbiome and pregnancy outcomes. *Fertility and Sterility*. 2015 Dec 1;104(6):1358–63.
11. Stout MJ, Conlon B, Landeau M, Lee I, Bower C, Zhao Q, *et al*. Identification of intracellular bacteria in the basal plate of the human placenta in term and preterm gestations. *American Journal of Obstetrics & Gynecology*. 2013 Mar 1;208(3):226.e1-226.e7.
12. Baker JM, Chase DM, Herbst-Kralovetz MM. Uterine Microbiota: Residents, Tourists, or Invaders? *Front Immunol* [Internet]. 2018 Mar 2 [cited 2020 May 11];9. Available from: https://www.ncbi.nlm.nih.gov/pmc/articles/PMC5840171/
13. Zheng J, Xiao X, Zhang Q, Mao L, Yu M, Xu J. The Placental Microbiome Varies in Association with Low Birth Weight in Full-Term Neonates. *Nutrients*. 2015 Aug;7(8):6924–37.
14. Mueller NT, Bakacs E, Combellick J, Grigoryan Z, Dominguez-Bello MG. The infant microbiome development: mom matters. *Trends Mol Med*. 2015 Feb;21(2):109–17.
15. Bretveld RW, Thomas CM, Scheepers PT, Zielhuis GA, Roeleveld N. Pesticide exposure: the hormonal function of the female reproductive system disrupted? *Reprod Biol Endocrinol*. 2006 May 31;4:30.
16. Guyton and Hall (2011). *Textbook of Medical Physiology*. U.S.: Saunders Elsevier.
17. Huggins C. Endocrine Control of Prostatic Cancer. *Science*. 1943 Jun 18;97(2529):541–4.
18. Wang P-H, Chen Y-L, Wei ST-S, Wu K, Lee T-H, Wu T-Y, *et al*. Retroconversion of oestrogens into androgens by bacteria via a cobalamin-mediated methylation. *Proc Natl Acad Sci USA*. 2020 21;117(3):1395–403.
19. Bosland MC. The Role of Oestrogens in Prostate Carcinogenesis: A Rationale for Chemoprevention. *Rev Urol*. 2005;7(Suppl 3):S4–10.
20. Huggins Charles, Hodges Clarence V. Studies on Prostatic Cancer: I. The Effect of Castration, of Oestrogen and of Androgen Injection on Serum Phosphatases in Metastatic Carcinoma of the Prostate*. *Journal of Urology*. 2002 Jul 1;168(1):9–12.
21. De Marzo AM, Platz EA, Sutcliffe S, Xu J, Grönberg H, Drake CG, *et al*. Inflammation in prostate carcinogenesis. *Nat Rev Cancer*. 2007 Apr;7(4):256–69.
22. Massari F, Mollica V, Di Nunno V, Gatto L, Santoni M, Scarpelli M, *et al*. The Human Microbiota and Prostate Cancer: Friend or Foe? *Cancers* (Basel) [Internet]. 2019 Mar 31 [cited 2020 May 11];11(4). Available from: https://www.ncbi.nlm.nih.gov/pmc/articles/PMC6521295/
23. Tang J. Microbiome in the urinary system—a review. *AIMS Microbiol*. 2017 Mar 20;3(2):143–54.
24. *Organic Acids Test Book*. The great plains laboratory Inc. Published on Oct 7, 2015.

25. Nienhouse V, Gao X, Dong Q, *et al*. Interplay between bladder microbiota and urinary antimicrobial peptides: mechanisms for human urinary tract infection risk and symptom severity. *PLoS One*. 2014;9(12):e114185. Published 2014 Dec 8. doi:10.1371/journal.pone.0114185.

GAPS behaviour

1. Jeffrey Norris. *Do Gut Bacteria Rule Our Minds?* [Internet]. Do Gut Bacteria Rule Our Minds? | UC San Francisco. 2014 [cited 2020 Mar 4]. Available from: https://www.ucsf.edu/news/2014/08/116526/do-gut-bacteria-rule-our-minds
2. Galland L. The gut microbiome and the brain. *J Med Food*. 2014;17(12): 1261 1272. doi:10.1089/jmf.2014.7000
3. Schwiertz, Andreas (2016). *Microbiota of the human body: implications in health and disease*. Switzerland: Springer. p. 1. ISBN 978-3-319-31248-4.
4. Christian LM, Galley JD *et al*.Gut microbiome composition is associated with temperament during early childhood. *Brain, Behaviour, and Immunity*, Volume 45, March 2015, Pages 118-127.
5. O'Mahony, S. M., Clarke, G., Borre, Y. E., Dinan, T. G., & Cryan, J. F. (2015). Serotonin, tryptophan metabolism and the brain-gut-microbiome axis. *Behavioural brain research*, 277, 32-48.
6. de Weerth C. Do bacteria shape our development? Crosstalk between intestinal microbiota and HPA axis. *Neurosci Biobehav Rev*. 2017;83:458 471. doi:10.1016/j.neubiorev.2017.09.016
7. Cannabis-Induced Psychosis in Teenagers and Young Adults: Risk Factors, Detection, Management [Internet]. *Psychiatry Advisor*. 2019 [cited 2020 Mar 4]. Available from: https://www.psychiatryadvisor.com/home/topics/addiction/cannabis-use-disorder/cannabis-induced-psychosis-in-teenagers-and-young-adults-risk-factors-detection-management/
8. Lu DL, Lin XL. Development of psychotic symptoms following ingestion of small quantities of alcohol. *Neuropsychiatr Dis Treat*. 2016;12:2449 2454. Published 2016 Sep 22. doi:10.2147/NDT.S112825

Food addictions

1. Alcock J, Maley CC, Aktipis CA. Is eating behaviour manipulated by the gastrointestinal microbiota? Evolutionary pressures and potential mechanisms. *Bioessays*. 2014 Oct;36(10):940–9.
2. Flint HJ, Scott KP, Duncan SH, Louis P, Forano E. Microbial degradation of complex carbohydrates in the gut. *Gut Microbes*. 2012 Jul 1;3(4):289–306.
3. Galland L. The Gut Microbiome and the Brain. *J Med Food*. 2014 Dec 1;17(12):1261–72.
4. Painter K, Cordell BJ, Sticco KL. Auto-brewery Syndrome (Gut Fermentation). In: *StatPearls* [Internet]. Treasure Island (FL): StatPearls Publishing; 2020 [cited 2020 Mar 10]. Available from: http://www.ncbi.nlm.nih.gov/books/ NBK513346/
5. Ahmed SH, Guillem K, Vandaele Y. Sugar addiction: pushing the drug-sugar analogy to the limit. *Curr Opin Clin Nutr Metab Care*. 2013 Jul;16(4):434–9.
6. Melissa Kravitz Hoeffner. Food companies intentionally make their products addictive, and it's making us sick [Internet]. *Salon*. 2019 [cited 2020 Mar 10]. Available from: https://www.salon.com/2019/03/28/food-companies-intentionally-make-their-products-addictive-and-its-making-us-sick_partner/

7. Zhang Y-J, Li S, Gan R-Y, Zhou T, Xu D-P, Li H-B. Impacts of Gut Bacteria on Human Health and Diseases. *Int J Mol Sci*. 2015 Apr 2;16(4):7493–519.
8. Liester MB, Moore-Liester JD. Is Sugar a Gateway Drug? *Journal of Drug Abuse* [Internet]. 2015 Dec 16 [cited 2020 Mar 10];1(1). Available from: https://drugabuse.imedpub.com/abstract/is-sugar-a-gateway-drug-7783.html
9. Rogers GB, Keating DJ, Young RL, Wong M-L, Licinio J, Wesselingh S. From gut dysbiosis to altered brain function and mental illness: mechanisms and pathways. *Molecular Psychiatry*. 2016 Jun;21(6):738–48.

Food

What GAPS people should eat and what should be avoided

1. Campbell-McBride N. *Gut and psychology syndrome. Natural treatment for autism, dyspraxia, dyslexia, ADD/ADHD, depression and schizophrenia*. 2010. Medinform Publishing.
2. Grundmann O. The gut microbiome and pre-systemic metabolism: current state and evolving research. *J. Drug Metab. Toxicol*, 2010. pdfs.semanticscholar.org
3. Turroni S, Rampelli S *et al*. Enterocyte-Associated Microbiome of the Hadza Hunter-Gatherers. *Front. Microbiol*, 06 June 2016. https://doi.org/10.3389/fmicb.2016.00865
4. Garrow JS, James WPT, Ralph A. *Human nutrition and dietetics*. 2000. 10th edition. Churchill Livingstone.
5. Eaton KK. Sugars in food intolerance and abnormal gut fermentation. *J Nutr Med* 1992;3:295-301.
6. Poley, J. R.; Bhatia, M.; Welsh, J. D. (1978). "Disaccharidase deficiency in infants with cow's milk protein intolerance. Response to treatment". *Digestion*. 17 (2): 97–107.
7. Millward, C; Ferriter, M; Calver, S; Connell-Jones, G (2008). "Gluten- and casein-free diets for autistic spectrum disorder". *Cochrane Database of Systematic Reviews* (2): CD003498. doi:10.1002/14651858
8. Sanz Y. Microbiome and Gluten. *Ann Nutr Metab*. 2015;67 Suppl 2:28 41. doi:10.1159/000440991
9. William Davis. *Wheat Belly (Revised and Expanded Edition): Lose the Wheat, Lose the Weight, and Find Your Path Back to Health*. Penguin Random House USA; Revised, Expanded edition (28 Jan. 2020).
10. Hoffman JR *et al*. Protein – which is best? *J Sports Sci Med*. 2004 Sep;3(3). Published online 2004 Sep1.
11. Fallon S, Enig M. *Nourishing Traditions. The cookbook that challenges politically correct nutrition and the diet dictocrats*. 1999. New Trends Publishing, Washington DC 2007.
12. Sandstead HH. Fibre, phytates, and mineral nutrition. *Nutr Rev* 1992; 50:30–1.
13. Freed DL. Lectins in food: their importance in health and disease. *J Nutr Med* 1991; 2: 45-64.
14. Freed DL. Do dietary lectins cause disease? *Br Med J* 1999; 318(71090):1023–4.
15. Pusztai A, Ewen SW, Grant G. *et al*. Antinutritive effects of wheat-germ agglutinin and other N-acetylglucosamine-specific lectins. *Br J Nutr* 1993; 70: 313–21.
16. Cordain L. Cereal grains: humanity's double-edged sword. *World Rev Nutr Diet* 1999; 84:19–73.

17. Els JM, Van Damme *et al.* (1998). *Handbook of Plant Lectins: Properties and Biomedical Applications*. John Wiley & Sons.
18. Malik, TF; Panuganti, KK (January 2020). "*Lactose Intolerance*". PMID 30335318.
19. *Common Methods of Processing and Preserving Food*. Streetdirectory.com. April 7, 2015.
20. *Food Processing Lesson Plan*. Johns Hopkins Bloomberg School of Public Health. April 7, 2015.
21. Levenstein H.: '*Paradox of Plenty*', p.106–107. University of California Press, 2003.
22. *Most packaged supermarket food is unhealthy* – study. http://www.radionz.co.nz/news/national/280056/%27supermarket-food-largely-unhealthy%27.
23. *Ultra processed foods prevalent and unhealthy research*. http://www.sciencemediacentre.co.nz/2015/07/30/ultra-processed-foods-prevalent-unhealthy-research/.
24. Gracy-Whitman L, Ell S. Artificial colourings and adverse reactions. *BMJ* 1995; 310:1204.
25. Rogers S. *Tired or toxic? A blueprint for health*. 1990. Prestige Publishers.
26. Rowe KS, Rose KJ. Synthetic food colouring and behaviour: A dose response effect in a double-blind, placebo-controlled, repeated-measures study. *Journal of Paediatrics* 12: 691-698, 1994.
27. Rowe KS. Synthetic food colouring and hyperactivity: a double-blind crossover study. *Aust Paediatr J*, 24: 143-47, 1988.
28. Boris M, Mandel F. Food and additives are common causes of the attention deficit hyperactive disorder in children. *Annals of Allergy* 72: 462-68, 1994.
29. Rea WJ. *Chemical Sensitivity*. Vols. 1,2,3,4. Lewis, Boca Raton, 1994-1998.
30. Pizzorno JE, Murray MT. *Textbook of natural medicine*. 4th edition, 2012.
31. Mirkkunen M. (1982). Reactive hypoglycaemia tendency among habitually violent offenders. *Neuropsychopharmacol* 8:35-40.
32. Geary A. *The food and mood handbook*. 2001. Thorsons.
33. Eaton KK. Sugars in food intolerance and abnormal gut fermentation. *J Nutr Med* 1992;3:295-301.
34. Fayemiwo SA *et al.*Gut fermentation syndrome. *African J Cl Exp Microbiol*, Vol 15, No 1 (2014).
35. Bivin WS *et al.* Production of ethanol from infant food formulas by common yeasts. *J Appl Bacteriol*, Vol 58, 4, pp 355–357, April 1985.
36. Round JL, Mazmanian SK. (2009). "The gut microbiota shapes intestinal immune responses during health and disease". *Nature Reviews: Immunology*, 9 (5): 313–323.
37. Yudkin J. *Pure, white and deadly. How sugar is killing us and what we can do to stop it*. 2012.
38. Hurst AF, Knott FA. Intestinal carbohydrate dyspepsia. *Quart J Med* 1930-31;24:171-80.
39. Kaur J (2014). "A comprehensive review on metabolic syndrome". *Cardiology Research and Practice*. 2014: 1–21.
40. Campbell-McBride N. *Put your heart in your mouth. What really is heart disease and what can we do to prevent and even reverse it*. 2007. Medinform Publishing.
41, Hurst AF, Knott FA. Intestinal carbohydrate dyspepsia. *Quart J Med* 1930-31;24:171-80.
42. Fallon S, Enig M. *Nourishing Traditions. The cookbook that challenges politically correct nutrition and the diet dictocrats*. 1999. New Trends Publishing, Washington DC 20007.

43. Sandstead HH. Fibre, phytates, and mineral nutrition. *Nutr Rev* 1992; 50:30-1.
44. Cordain L. Cereal grains: humanity's double-edged sword. *World Rev Nutr Diet* 1999; 84:19-73.
45. Enig MG. *Know Your Fats: The Complete Primer for Understanding the Nutrition of Fats, oils, and Cholesterol*. Bethesda Press, Silver Spring, MD, 2000.
46. Centers for Disease Control and Prevention (1994). "Documentation for Immediately Dangerous To Life or Health Concentrations (IDLHs) – Acrylamide". http://www.cdc.gov/niosh/idlh/79061.html
47. Xu Y *et al.* (Apr 5, 2014). "Risk assessment, formation, and mitigation of dietary acrylamide: Current status and future prospects.". *Food and chemical toxicology: an international journal published for the British Industrial Biological Research Association* 69C: 1–12.
48. Tareke E, Rydberg P *et al.*(2002). "Analysis of acrylamide, a carcinogen formed in heated foodstuffs". *J. Agric. Food. Chem.* 50 (17): 4998–5006.
49. Fallon S, Enig M. *Nourishing Traditions. The cookbook that challenges politically correct nutrition and the diet dictocrats.* 1999. New Trends Publishing, Washington DC 2007.
50. COMA Report. Dietary sugars and human disease: conclusions and recommendations. *Br Dent J.* 1990; 165:46.
51. http://www.statista.com/statistics/249681/total-consumption-of-sugar-worldwide/
52. Berg JM, Tymoczko JL and Stryer L. *Biochemistry*, 2006.
53. Tran G, 2015. *Sugarcane press mud. Feedipedia, a programme by INRA, CIRAD, AFZ and FAO.* http://www.feedipedia.org/node/563 Last updated on May 27, 2015, 18:02.
54. Dowling RN. (1928). *Sugar Beet and Beet Sugar*. London: Ernest Benn Limited.
55. Altura BM, Zhang A, Altura BT. Magnesium, hypertensive vascular diseases, atherogenesis, subcellular compartmentation of Ca2+ and Mg2+ and vascular contractility. *Miner Electrolyte Metab.* 1993;19:323–336.
56. Altura BM, Altura BT. Magnesium and cardiovascular biology: an important link between cardiovascular risk factors and atherogenesis. *Cell Mol Biol Res.* 1995;41:347–359.
57. Yudkin J. *Pure, white and deadly. How sugar is killing us and what we can do to stop it.* 2012.
58. Staff writers (March 2010). "The lowdown on high-fructose corn syrup". *Consumer Reports.*
59. Engber D. (28 April 2009). "The decline and fall of high-fructose corn syrup". *Slate Magazine*. Slate.com.
60. Lim U, Subar AF, Mouw T. *et al.* Consumption of aspartame-containing beverages and incidence of hematopoietic and brain malignancies. *Cancer Epidemiology, Biomarkers and Prevention* 2006; 15(9):1654–1659.
61. Roberts HJ. (2004). "Aspartame disease: a possible cause for concomitant Graves' disease and pulmonary hypertension". *Texas Heart Institute Journal* 31 (1): 105; author reply 105–6. PMC 387446. PMID 15061638.
62. Humphries P, Pretorius E, Naudé H. (2008). "Direct and indirect cellular effects of aspartame on the brain". *Eur J Clin Nutrition* 62 (4): 451–462. doi:10.1038/sj.ejcn.1602866. PMID 17684524.
63. Trocho C, Pardo R, Rafecas I. *et al.* (1998). "Formaldehyde derived from dietary aspartame binds to tissue components in vivo". *Life Sciences* 63 (5): 337–49.
64. Daniel KT. *The Whole Soy Story*. 2006. New Trends Publishing.
65. "History of Soy Sauce, Shoyu, and Tamari – Page 1". soyinfocenter.com.

66. Endres Joseph G. (2001). *Soy Protein Products*. Champaign-Urbana, IL: AOCS Publishing. pp. 43–44.
67. http://www.alkalizeforhealth.net/Lsoy.htm Soy, aluminium and Alzheimer's disease.
68. Shcherbatykh I, Carpenter DO. The Role of Metals in the Etiology of Alzheimer's Disease. *Journal of Alzheimer's Disease*. 2007;11(2):191–205.
69. Henkel J. (May–June 2000). "Soy: Health Claims for Soy Protein, Question About Other Components". *FDA Consumer* (Food and Drug Administration) 34 (3): 18–20.
70. Messina M, McCaskill-Stevens W, Lampe JW. (September 2006). "Addressing the Soy and Breast Cancer Relationship: Review, Commentary, and Workshop Proceedings". *JNCI Journal of the National Cancer Institute* (National Cancer Institute) 98 (18): 1275–1284.
71. Doerge DR, Sheehan DM. Goitrogenic and estrogenic activity of soy isoflavones. *Environ Health Perspect*. 2002 Jun;110 Suppl 3:349-53.
72. Song TT, Hendrich S, Murphy PA. (1999). "Estrogenic activity of glycitein, a soy isoflavone". *Journal of Agricultural and Food Chemistry* 47 (4): 1607–1610.
73. Dendougui Ferial, Schwedt Georg (2004). "In vitro analysis of binding capacities of calcium to phytic acid in different food samples". *European Food Research and Technology* 219 (4).
74. Committee on Food Protection, Food and Nutrition Board, National Research Council (1973). "Phytates". Toxicants Occurring Naturally in Foods. National Academy of Sciences. pp. 363–371.
75. Miniello VL *et al.* (2003). "Soy-based formulas and phyto-oestrogens: A safety profile". *Acta Paediatrica* (Wiley-Blackwell) 91 (441): 93–100.
76. Strom BL *et al.* (2001). "Exposure to soy-based formula in infancy and endocrinological and reproductive outcomes in young adulthood". *JAMA: the Journal of the American Medical Association* (American Medical Association) 286 (7): 807–814.
77. Garrow JS, James WPT, Ralph A. *Human nutrition and dietetics*. 2000. 10th edition. Churchill Livingstone.
78. Ensimger AH *et al. The Concise Encyclopedia of Food and Nutrition*. CRC Press, 1995.
79. Pizzorno JE, Murray MT. T*extbook of natural medicine*. 4th edition, 2012.
80. Stipanuk MH. (2006). *Biochemical, Physiological and Molecular Aspects of Human Nutrition* (2nd ed.). Philadelphia: Saunders.
81. Shoenfeld P. Vitamin A-mazing. *Wise Traditions*, Spring 2020, p.13–26.
82. Seneff S. Sunlight and Vitamin D: They're Not The Same Thing! *Wise Traditions*, Spring 2020, p.27–35.
83. Bailey LB, Caudill MA (2012). "Folate". In Eardman JW Jr, MacDonald IA, Zeisel SH (eds.). *Present Knowledge in Nutrition*, Tenth Edition. Ames, IA: ILSI Press/Wiley-Blackwell. pp. 321–342.
84. Masterjohn C. On the trail of the elusive x factor: a sixty-two-year-old mystery finally solved. *Wise Traditions*. 2007;8(1).
85. Stipanuk MH. (2006). *Biochemical, Physiological and Molecular Aspects of Human Nutrition* (2nd ed.). Philadelphia: Saunders.
86. Garrow JS, James WPT, Ralph A. *Human nutrition and dietetics*. 2000. 10th edition. Churchill Livingstone.
87. Fallon S, Enig M. *Nourishing Traditions. The cookbook that challenges politically correct nutrition and the diet dictocrats*. 1999. New Trends Publishing, Washington DC 2007.

88. Pizzorno JE, Murray MT. *Textbook of natural medicine*. 4th edition, 2012.
89. Gray N. "No link between eggs and heart disease or stroke, says BMJ meta-analysis." January 25, 2013. foodnavigator.com/Science/No-link-between-eggs-and-heart-disease-or-stroke-says-BMJ-meta-analysis
90. nhs.uk/conditions/Lactose-intolerance/Pages/Introduction.aspx
91. Review of the potential health impact of -casomorphins and related peptides. *European Food Safety Authority*, doi: 10.2903/j.efsa.2009.231r
92. Cade, R.; Privette, R.; Fregly, M.; Rowland, N.; Sun, Z.; Zele, V. Autism and schizophrenia: Intestinal disorders. *Nutritional Neuroscience* 2000, 3, 57–72.
93. Sador Ellix Katz. *The Art of Fermentation: An In-depth Exploration of Essential Concepts and Processes from Around the World*. Chelsea Green Publishing Co; First Edition (7 Jun. 2012).
94. A campaign for real milk. Weston A. Price Foundation. http://www.food.gov.uk/sites/default/files/multimedia/pdfs/publication/raw-milk-weston-foundation-presentation.pdf
95. Schmid R. *The untold story of milk. The history, politics and science of nature's perfect food: raw milk from pastured cows*. New trends publishing. 2009.
96. Raw Milk: *What the Scientific Literature Really Says. A Response to Bill Marler, JD*. Prepared by the Weston A. Price Foundation. http://www.realmilk.com/wp-content/uploads/2012/11/ResponsetoMarler ListofStudies.pdf
97. Dreher ML, Maher CV, Kearney P. The traditional and emerging role of nuts in healthful diets. *Nutr Rev* 1996; 54:241–5.
98. Honey: health benefits and uses in medicine. http://www.medicalnewstoday.com/articles/264667.php
99. Honey kills antibiotic-resistant bugs. Published online 19 November 2002 | Nature. doi:10.1038/news021118-1.
100. Herman AC *et al*. Effect of honey on nocturnal cough and sleep quality: a double-blind, randomized, placebo-controlled study. *Paediatrics* Volume 130, Number 3, September 2012.
101. *Honey holds some promise for treating burns*. Published: 9 October 2008, http://www.hbns.org
102. Haffejee IE, Moosa A. Honey in the treatment of infantile gastroenteritis. *Br Med J (Clin Res Ed)* 1985;290:1866.
103. Oesophagus: heartburn and honey. Clinical review. *BMJ* 2001;323:736.
104. Oduwole O, Meremikwu MM, Oyo-Ita A, Udoh EE. (2014). "Honey for acute cough in children". *Cochrane Database Syst Rev* (Systematic review) 3 (12): CD007094.
105. Majtan J. (2014). "Honey: an immunomodulator in wound healing". *Wound Repair Regen*. 22 (2 Mar–Apr): 187–192.
106. Enig M. Know *Your Fats: The Complete Primer for Understanding the Nutrition of Fats, Oils and Cholesterol*. Silver Spring: Bethseda Press, 2000.
107. About salt: production. The Salt Manufacturers Association. http://web.archive.org/web/20090409144219/http://www.saltsense.co.uk/aboutsalt-prod02.htm
108. "A brief history of salt". *Time Magazine*. 15 March 1982. Retrieved 11 October 2013.
109. Fallon S, Enig M. *Nourishing Traditions. The cookbook that challenges politically correct nutrition and the diet dictocrats*. 1999. New Trends Publishing, Washington DC 2007.
110. Lopez BA. "Hallstatt's White Gold: Salt". *Virtual Vienna Net*. Retrieved 3 March 2013.

111. Strazzullo *et al.* (2009). "Salt intake, stroke, and cardiovascular disease: meta-analysis of prospective studies". *British Medical Journal* 339 (b4567).
112, "References on food salt & health issues". *Salt Institute*. 2009. Retrieved 5 December 2010.
113. The national organic programme and its discontents. *The Natural Farmer*. Winter 2018-19; B1-3. Published by NOFA (Northeast Organic Farming Association).
114. https://www.dutchnews.nl/news/2019/08/food-companies-caught-selling-fake-organic-products-escape-prosecution/
115. https://www.grubstreet.com/2017/09/millions-of-pounds-of-fake-organic-food-entering-america.html
116. https://www.marketwatch.com/story/how-to-avoid-wasting-money-on-fake-organic-food-2017-12-27
117. Fake Italian organic food sold around Europe, https://www.eubusiness.com/news-eu/italy-environment.dwq

Treatment

1. Dr Sidney V. Haas and Merrill P. Haas. *The Management of Celiac Disease*, originally published in 1951. Muriwai Books, 2017.
2. Gottschall E. *Breaking the vicious cycle. Intestinal health through diet*. 1996. The Kirkton Press.
3. https://microbiomepost.com/some-commensal-bacteria-support-gut-epithelial-regeneration/
4. Campbell-McBride N. *Gut and psychology syndrome. Natural treatment for autism, dyspraxia, dyslexia, ADD/ADHD, depression and schizophrenia*. 2010. Medinform Publishing.
5. Russian: (Electro-magnetic field and human health). 2002, 177.
6. Russian: (Radiation biophysics: radio-frequencies and microwave electro-magnetic radiation.) (Textbook for university physics). 2008. 184.
7. Debunking the myth that microwave ovens are harmless. https://www.westonaprice.org/?s=microwave+oven
8. Garrow JS, James WPT, Ralph A. *Human nutrition and dietetics*. 2000. 10th edition. Churchill Livingstone.
9. FG Young. Claude Bernard and the Discovery of Glycogen. *Br Med J* 1957;1:1431.
10. Stipanuk MH. (2006). *Biochemical, Physiological and Molecular Aspects of Human Nutrition* (2nd ed.). Philadelphia: Saunders.
11. Sador Ellix Katz. *The Art of Fermentation: An In-depth Exploration of Essential Concepts and Processes from Around the World*. Chelsea Green Publishing Co; First Edition (7 Jun. 2012).
12. Holmes AJ *et al.* Diet-Microbiome Interactions in Health Are Controlled by Intestinal Nitrogen Source Constraints. *Cell Metabolism*, Volume 25, Issue 1;2017, 140-151.
13. Freeman JM, Kossoff EH, Hartman AL. The ketogenic diet: one decade later. *Pediatrics*. 2007 Mar;119(3):535–43.
14. Weber DD, Aminazdeh-Gohari S, Kofler B. Ketogenic diet in cancer therapy. *Aging* (Albany NY). 2018 Feb 11;10(2):164–165.
15. FilipeDeVadde *et al.* Microbiota-Produced Succinate Improves Glucose Homeostasis via Intestinal Gluconeogenesis. *Cell Metabolism*. Volume 24, Issue 1, 12 July 2016, Pages 151–157.

16. Dr Nasha Winters and Jess Higgins Kelley. *The Metabolic Approach To Cancer*. 2017. Chelsea Green Publishing.

What we shall eat and why, with some recipes

1. Mathews, M.B. (1975). *Connective Tissue, Macromolecular Structure Evolution*. Springer-Verlag, Berlin and New York.
2. Garrow JS, James WPT, Ralph A. *Human nutrition and dietetics*. 2000. 10th edition. Churchill Livingstone.
3. Sador Ellix Katz. *The Art of Fermentation: An In-depth Exploration of Essential Concepts and Processes from Around the World*. Chelsea Green Publishing Co; First Edition (7 Jun. 2012).
4. Sally Fallon Morell. *Nourishing Diets. How Paleo, Ancestral And Traditional Peoples Really Ate*. 2018. Grand central L&S.
5. Fallon S, Enig M. *Nourishing Traditions. The cookbook that challenges politically correct nutrition and the diet dictocrats*. 1999. New Trends Publishing, Washington DC, 20007.
6. Kirstain K. Shockey & Christoopher Shockey. *Miso, Tempeh. Natto and other tasty ferments*. 2019. Storey Publishing.
7. Bevely Rubik. *How Does Pork Prepared in Various Ways Affect the Blood. Wise Traditions in Food, Farming and the Healing Arts*, the quarterly journal of the Weston A. Price Foundation, Fall 2011. https://www.westonaprice.org/health-topics/food-features/how-does-pork-prepared-in-various-ways-affect-the-blood/

Vegetarianism

1. N Campbell-McBride. *Vegetarianism Explained. Making an Informed Decision*. 2017. Medinform Publishing.
2. Bhatia LA. *Textbook of environmental biology*. 2010. International Publishing House.
3. Sejrsen K., Torben Hvelplund, Mette Olaf Nielsen. *Ruminant Physiology: Digestion, metabolism and impact of nutrition on gene expression, immunology and stress*. 2006. Wageningen Academic Publisher.
4. Hungate RE. *The rumen and its microbes*. 1966. Academic Press. New York and London.
5. Comparative digestion. *Veterinary Science*. http://vetsci.co.uk/2010/05/14/comparative-digestion/
6. Garrow JS, James WPT, Ralph A. *Human nutrition and dietetics*. 2000. 10th edition. Churchill Livingstone.
7. Guyton and Hall (2011). *Textbook of Medical Physiology*. U.S.: Saunders Elsevier.
8. Price WA, Studies of Relationships Between Nutritional Deficiencies and (a) Facial and Dental Arch Deformities and (b) Loss of Immunity to Dental Caries Among South Sea Islanders and Florida Indians. *Dental Cosmos*. 1935;77(11):1033–45.
9. Sally Fallon Morell. *Nourishing Diets. How Paleo, Ancestral And Traditional Peoples Really Ate*. 2018. Grand central L&S.
10. *Plant Foods for Human Nutrition*. International Journal presenting research on nutritional quality of plant foods. ISSN: 0921–9668

11. Hoffman JR *et al*. Protein – which is best? *J Sports Sci Med*. 2004 Sep;3(3). Published online 2004 Sep1.
12. Enig MG. *Know Your Fats: The Complete Primer for Understanding the Nutrition of Fats, Oils, and Cholesterol*. Bethesda Press, Silver Spring, MD, 2000.
13. Pizzorno JE, Murray MT. *Textbook of natural medicine*. 4th edition, 2012.
14. Erasmus U. *Fats that heal, fats that kill*. 1993. Alive books.
15. Oregon State University. 'Eat Your Broccoli: Study Finds Strong Anti-Cancer Properties In Cruciferous Veggies'. *Science Daily*. 18 May 2007.
16. Ambrosone CB, Tang L. Cruciferous vegetable intake and cancer prevention: role of nutrigenetics. *Cancer Prev Res* (Phila Pa). 2009 Apr;2(4):298–300. 2009.
17. Cheney G. Vitamin U therapy of peptic ulcer. *Calif Med*. 1952 Oct;77(4):248–52.
18. Blomhoff R, Carlsen MH, Andersen LF, Jacobs DR. Health benefits of nuts: potential role of antioxidants. *Br J Nutr*. 2006 Nov;96 Suppl 2:S52–60. 2006. PMID:17125534.
19. Gerson C and Walker M. *The Gerson Therapy. The amazing nutritional programme for cancer and other illnesses*. 2001. Twin Streams Kensington Publishing.
20. Slavin J. Fiber and prebiotics: mechanisms and health benefits. *Nutrients*. 2013 Apr; 5(4): 1417–1435.
21. Harcombe Z. *The obesity epidemic*. 2010. Columbus Publishing.
22. Ephrata *Cloister in 1732 promoted celibacy and veganism*. https://en.wikipedia.org/wiki/Ephrata_Cloister
23. Enig MG. *Know Your Fats: The Complete Primer for Understanding the Nutrition of Fats, Oils, and Cholesterol*. Bethesda Press, Silver Spring, MD, 2000.
24. Garrow JS, James WPT, Ralph A. *Human nutrition and dietetics*. 2000. 10th edition. Churchill Livingstone.
25. https://theconversation.com/the-myth-of-a-vegetarian-india-102768
26. The myth of the Indian vegetarian nation. https://www.bbc.com/news/world-asia-india-43581122
27. Most packaged supermarket food is unhealthy – study. http://www.radionz.co.nz/news/national/280056/%27supermarket-food-largely-unhealthy%27.
28. Geary A. *The food and mood handbook*. 2001. Thorsons.
29. Ravnskov U. *The Cholesterol Myths. Exposing the fallacy that saturated fat and cholesterol cause heart disease*. 2000. NewTrends Publishing.
30. Fallon S. Twenty-two reasons not to go vegetarian. *Wise traditions in food, farming and healing arts*. Spring 2008; vol 9; 1:37–48.
31. Price WA. *Nutrition and physical degeneration. A comparison of primitive and modern diets and their effects*. 1938. Price.

One man's meat is another man's poison!

1. Price WA. *Nutrition and physical degeneration. A comparison of primitive and modern diets and their effects*. 1938. Price.
2. Deepak Chopra. *Perfect health. The complete mind body guide*.1990. Bantam books.
3. Sally Fallon Morell. *Nourishing Diets. How Paleo, Ancestral And Traditional Peoples Really Ate*. 2018. Grand central L&S.
4. Roger Williams. *Biochemical Individuality*. University of Texas Press (1956).
5. Gonzalez NJ. *One man alone. An investigation of nutrition, cancer and William Donald Kelley*. 2010. New Spring Press.

6. William Walcott and Trish Fahey. *The Metabolic Typing Diet.* 2000, Broadway Books New York.
7. Purves W, Sadava D, Orians G and Heller C. 2004. Life: *The Science of Biology*, 7th edition. Sunderland, MA: Sinauer.
8. Garrow JS, James WPT, Ralph A. *Human nutrition and dietetics*. 2000. 10th edition. Churchill Livingstone. Alberts *et al. Molecular Biology of the Cell*: 4th edition, NY: Garland Science, 2002.
9. Robertson D. *Primer on the autonomic nervous system*. 3rd edition. 2011. Academic Press.
10. Gonzalez NJ. *One man alone. An investigation of nutrition, cancer and William Donald Kelley*. 2010. New Spring Press.
11. Vasey C. *The Acid-Alkaline Diet for Optimum Health.*1999. Healing Arts Press.
12. Pizzorno JE, Murray MT. *Textbook of natural medicine*. 4th edition, 2012.
13. Nelson DL and Cox MM. *Lehninger Principles of Biochemistry*, 4th edition, 2004.
14. "A brief history of salt". *Time Magazine*. 15 March 1982. Retrieved 11 October 2013.
15. Hansen, Julieann. "The Science of Sweat". American College of Sports Medicine. Archived from the original on 2013-09-21. Retrieved 19 September 2013.
16. Sally Fallon Morell. *Nourishing Diets. How Paleo, Ancestral And Traditional Peoples Really Ate.* 2018. Grand central L&S.
17. https://www.manataka.org/page1476.html Health Alert.
18. http://articles.mercola.com/sites/articles/archive/2013/12/30/worst-food-ingredients.aspx 7 worst ingredients in food.
19. https://airfreshenerlawsuit.com/use-of-perfumes/Air fresheners class action. University of Toronto.
20. https://en.wikipedia.org/wiki/Olfactory_fatigue Olfactory fatigue.
21. Gravitz L. Food science: taste bud hackers. *Nature* 486, S14-S15, 21 June 2012. doi:10.1038/486S14a
22. BSAEM/BSNM. *Effective Nutritional Medicine: the application of nutrition to major health problems*. 1995. From the British Society for Allergy Environmental and Nutritional Medicine, PO Box 7 Knighton, LD7 1WT.
23. Pizzorno JE, Murray MT. *Textbook of natural medicine*. 4th edition, 2012.
24. Sansouce J. Can oil pulling help you detox? http://www.drfranklipman.com/can-oil-pulling-help-you-detox/
25. Huggins HA and Levy TE. *Uninformed consent. Hidden dangers in dental care.* 1999. Hampton Roads Pub Co.
26. Garrow JS, James WPT, Ralph A. *Human nutrition and dietetics*. 2000. 10th edition. Churchill Livingstone. Alberts *et al. Molecular Biology of the Cell*: 4th edition, NY: Garland Science, 2002.
27. Richardson A. *They are what you feed them. How food can improve your child's behaviour, mood and learning*. 2006. Harper Thornsons.
28. Rapley G and Murkett T. *Baby-led weaning: helping your baby to love good food.* 2008. Random House.
29. Clark S. *What really works for kids*. 2002. Transworld Publishers.

Nutritional supplements for GAPS people

1. Probiotics

1. Salminen, Seppo, Sonja Nybom, Jussi Meriluoto, Maria Carmen Collado, Satu

Vesterlund, and Hani El-Nezami. "Interaction of Probiotics and Pathogens—Benefits to Human Health?" *Current Opinion in Biotechnology* 21, no. 2 (April 2010): 157–67. https://doi.org/10.1016/j.copbio.2010.03.016.

2. Stanton, Catherine, R. Paul Ross, Gerald F. Fitzgerald, and Douwe Van Sinderen. "Fermented Functional Foods Based on Probiotics and Their Biogenic Metabolites." *Current Opinion in Biotechnology* 16, no. 2 (April 2005): 198–203. https://doi.org/10.1016/j.copbio.2005.02.008.
3. Sandor KE. *The Art of Fermentation: An In-Depth Exploration of Essential Concepts and Processes from Around the World*. 2012. Chelsea Green Publishing.
4. Vikhanski, Luba (2016). *Immunity: How Elie Metchnikoff Changed the Course of Modern Medicine*. Chicago Review Press. p. 278.
5. Liu Y, Tran DQ, Rhoads JM. Probiotics in Disease Prevention and Treatment. *J Clin Pharmacol*. 2018;58 Suppl 10(Suppl 10):S164 S179. doi:10.1002/jcph.1121
6. Reid G Probiotics: definition, scope and mechanisms of action. *Best Pract Res Clin Gastroenterol* 2016;30:17–25.
7. Chang HY, Chen JH, Chang JH, Lin HC, Lin CY, Peng CC. Multiple strains probiotics appear to be the most effective probiotics in the prevention of necrotizing enterocolitis and mortality: an updated meta-analysis. *PLoS ONE*. 2017;12:e0171579.
8. Szajewska H, Skorka A, Ruszczynski M, Gieruszczak-Bialek D. Meta-analysis: Lactobacillus GG for treating acute gastroenteritis in children—updated analysis of randomised controlled trials. *Aliment Pharmacol Ther*. 2013;38:467–476.
9. Tuomola EM, Ouwehand AC, Salminen SJ. The effect of probiotic bacteria on the adhesion of pathogens to human intestinal mucus. *FEMS Immunol Med Microbiol*. 1999;26:137–142. [PubMed] [Google Scholar]
10. Bermudez-Brito M, Plaza-Diaz J, Munoz-Quezada S, Gomez-Llorente C, Gil A. Probiotic mechanisms of action. *Ann Nutr Metab*. 2012;61:160–174.
11. Ukena SN, Singh A, Dringenberg U, *et al.*Probiotic Escherichia coli Nissle 1917 inhibits leaky gut by enhancing mucosal integrity. *PLoS ONE*. 2007;2:e1308.
12. Fiocchi C Probiotics in inflammatory bowel disease: yet another mechanism of action? *Gastroenterology*. 2006;131:2009–2012.
13. Mantegazza C, Molinari P, D'Auria E, Sonnino M, Morelli L, Zuccotti GV. Probiotics and antibiotic-associated diarrhea in children: a review and new evidence on Lactobacillus rhamnosus GG during and after antibiotic treatment. *Pharmacol Res*. 2017;128:63–72.
14. Sandhu BK, Paul SP. Irritable bowel syndrome in children: pathogenesis, diagnosis and evidence-based treatment. *World J Gastroenterol*. 2014;20:6013–6023.
15. Ford AC, Quigley EM, Lacy BE, *et al.* Efficacy of prebiotics, probiotics, and synbiotics in irritable bowel syndrome and chronic idiopathic constipation: systematic review and meta-analysis. *Am J Gastroenterol*. 2014;109:1547–1561.
16. Schmid R. *The untold story of milk. The history, politics and science of nature's perfect food: raw milk from pastured cows*. New trends publishing. 2009.
17. Lomax, A. R., and P. C. Calder. "Probiotics, Immune Function, Infection and Inflammation: A Review of the Evidence from Studies Conducted in Humans." *Current Pharmaceutical Design* 15, no. 13 (2009): 1428–1518.
18. Savino F, Cresi F, Pautasso S, *et al.* Intestinal microflora in breastfed colicky and non-colicky infants. *Acta Paediatr*. 2004;93:825–829.
19. Xu M, Wang J, Wang N, Sun F, Wang L, Liu XH. The efficacy and safety of the

probiotic bacterium Lactobacillus reuteri DSM 17938 for infantile colic: a meta-analysis of randomized controlled trials. *PLoS ONE*. 2015;10: e0141445.
20. Osborn DA, Sinn JK. Probiotics in infants for prevention of allergic disease and food hypersensitivity. *Cochrane Database Syst Rev*. 2007;CD006475.
21. West CE, Jenmalm MC, Kozyrskyj AL, Prescott SL. Probiotics for treatment and primary prevention of allergic diseases and asthma: looking back and moving forward. *Expert Rev Clin Immunol*. 2016;12:625–639. [PubMed] [Google Scholar]
22. Cuello-Garcia CA, Brozek JL, Fiocchi A, *et al*. Probiotics for the prevention of allergy: a systematic review and meta-analysis of randomized controlled trials. *J Allergy Clin Immunol*. 2015;136:952–961. [PubMed] [Google Scholar]
23. Dang D, Zhou W, Lun ZJ, Mu X, Wang DX, Wu H. Meta-analysis of probiotics and/or prebiotics for the prevention of eczema. *J Int Med Res*. 2013;41: 1426–1436. [PubMed] [Google Scholar]
24. Zhang GQ, Hu HJ, Liu CY, Zhang Q, Shakya S, Li ZY. Probiotics for prevention of atopy and food hypersensitivity in early childhood: a PRISMA-compliant systematic review and meta-analysis of randomized controlled trials. *Medicine* (Baltimore). 2016;95:e2562. [PMC free article] [PubMed] [Google Scholar]
25. Zuccotti G, Meneghin F, Aceti A, *et al*.Probiotics for prevention of atopic diseases in infants: systematic review and meta-analysis. *Allergy*. 2015;70: 1356–1371.
26. Tang ML, Ponsonby AL, Orsini F, *et al*.Administration of a probiotic with peanut oral immunotherapy: a randomized trial. *J Allergy Clin Immunol*. 2015;135:737–744. [PubMed] [Google Scholar]
27. Vliagoftis H, Kouranos VD, Betsi GI, Falagas ME. Probiotics for the treatment of allergic rhinitis and asthma: systematic review of randomized controlled trials. *Ann Allergy Asthma Immunol*. 2008;101:570–579.
28. Kang, Dae-Wook, James B. Adams, Ann C. Gregory, Thomas Borody, Lauren Chittick, Alessio Fasano, Alexander Khoruts, *et al*."Microbiota Transfer Therapy Alters Gut Ecosystem and Improves Gastrointestinal and Autism Symptoms: An Open-Label Study." *Microbiome* 5, no. 1 (January 23, 2017): 10.
29. Rudzki, Leszek, and Agata Szulc. "'Immune Gate' of Psychopathology—The Role of Gut Derived Immune Activation in Major Psychiatric Disorders." *Frontiers in Psychiatry* 9 (May 29, 2018).
30. Corthesy B, Gaskins HR, Mercenier A. Cross-talk between probiotic bacteria and the host immune system. *J Nutr*. 2007;137:781S–790S.
31. Wang Y, Li X, Ge T, *et al*. Probiotics for prevention and treatment of respiratory tract infections in children: a systematic review and meta-analysis of randomized controlled trials. *Medicine* (Baltimore). 2016;95:e4509.
32. Gleeson M, Bishop NC, Oliveira M, Tauler P. Daily probiotic's (Lactobacillus casei Shirota) reduction of infection incidence in athletes. *Int J Sport Nutr Exerc Metab*. 2011;21:55–64.
33. Spinler JK, Auchtung J, Brown A, *et al*. Next-generation probiotics targeting Clostridium difficile through precursor-directed antimicrobial biosynthesis. *Infect Immun*. 2017;85.
34. Li, Zhiping, Shiqi Yang, Huizhi Lin, Jiawen Huang, Paul A. Watkins, Ann B. Moser, Claudio Desimone, Xiao-yu Song, and Anna Mae Diehl. "Probiotics and Antibodies to TNF Inhibit Inflammatory Activity and Improve Nonalcoholic Fatty Liver Disease." *Hepatology* (Baltimore, Md.) 37, no. 2 (February 2003): 343–50.
35. Liu Y, Tran DQ, Rhoads JM. Probiotics in Disease Prevention and Treatment.

J Clin Pharmacol. 2018;58 Suppl 10(Suppl 10):S164 S179. doi:10.1002/jcph.1121

36. Reid G Probiotics: definition, scope and mechanisms of action. *Best Pract Res Clin Gastroenterol* 2016;30:17–25.
37. Wang F, Feng J, Chen P, *et al.*Probiotics in Helicobacter pylori eradication therapy: Systematic review and network meta-analysis. *Clin Res Hepatol Gastroenterol*. 2017;41:466–475.
38. Hendijani F, Akbari V. Probiotic supplementation for management of cardiovascular risk factors in adults with type II diabetes: A systematic review and meta-analysis. *Clin Nutr*. 2018;37(2):532–541. [PubMed] [Google Scholar]
39. Wu Y, Zhang Q, Ren Y, Ruan Z. Effect of probiotic Lactobacillus on lipid profile: a systematic review and meta-analysis of randomized, controlled trials. *PLoS ONE*. 2017;12:e0178868.
40. Liu PC, Yan YK, Ma YJ, *et al.* Probiotics reduce postoperative infections in patients undergoing colorectal surgery: a systematic review and meta-analysis. *Gastroenterol Res Pract*. 2017;2017:6029075.
41. Lee JY, Chu SH, Jeon JY, *et al.* Effects of 12 weeks of probiotic supplementation on quality of life in colorectal cancer survivors: a double-blind, randomized, placebo-controlled trial. *Dig Liver Dis*. 2014;46(12):1126 1132. doi:10.1016/j.dld.2014.09.004
42. Górska A, Przystupski D, Niemczura MJ, Kulbacka J. Probiotic Bacteria: A Promising Tool in Cancer Prevention and Therapy. *Curr Microbiol*. 2019;76(8):939 949. doi:10.1007/s00284-019-01679-8
43. Mohammed AT, Khattab M *et al.* The Therapeutic Effect of Probiotics on Rheumatoid Arthritis: A Systematic Review and Meta-Analysis of Randomized Control Trials. *Clin. Rheumatol*. 2017 Sep 15.
44. Kobyliak N, Conte C, Cammarota G, *et al.*Probiotics in prevention and treatment of obesity: a critical view. *Nutr Metab* (Lond). 2016;13:14. Published 2016 Feb 20. doi:10.1186/s12986-016-0067-0
45. Brink, B. ten; Minekus, M.; van der Vossen, J.M.B.M.; Leer, R.J.; Huis in't Veld, J.H.J. (August 1994). "Antimicrobial activity of lactobacilli: preliminary characterization and optimization of production of acidocin B, a novel bacteriocin produced by Lactobacillus acidophilus M46". *Journal of Applied Microbiology*. 77 (2): 140–148.
46. Inglin RC, Stevens MJ, Meile L, Lacroix C, Meile L (July 2015). "High-throughput screening assays for antibacterial and antifungal activities of Lactobacillus species". *Journal of Microbiological Methods*. 114 (July 2015): 26–9.
47. Fettweis JM, Brooks JP, Serrano MG, Sheth NU, Girerd PH, Edwards DJ, Strauss JF, Jefferson KK, Buck GA (October 2014). "Differences in vaginal microbiome in African American women versus women of European ancestry". *Microbiology*. 160 (Pt 10): 2272–2282.
48. Soto A, Martín V, Jiménez E, Mader I, Rodríguez JM, Fernández L. Lactobacilli and bifidobacteria in human breast milk: influence of antibiotherapy and other host and clinical factors. *J Pediatr Gastroenterol Nutr*. 2014;59(1):78 88.
49. Schell MA, Karmirantzou M, Snel B, Vilanova D, Berger B, Pessi G, Zwahlen MC, Desiere F, Bork P, Delley M, Pridmore RD, Arigoni F (October 2002). "The genome sequence of Bifidobacterium longum reflects its adaptation to the human gastrointestinal tract". *Proceedings of the National Academy of Sciences of the United States of America*. 99 (22): 14422–7.
50. Turroni, Francesca, Julian R. Marchesi, Elena Foroni, Miguel Gueimonde, Fergus Shanahan, Abelardo Margolles, Douwe van Sinderen, and Marco

Ventura. "Microbiomic Analysis of the Bifidobacterial Population in the Human Distal Gut." *The ISME Journal* 3, no. 6 (June 2009): 745–51. https://doi.org/10.1038/ismej.2009.19.

51. Turroni, Francesca, Clelia Peano, Daniel A. Pass, Elena Foroni, Marco Severgnini, Marcus J. Claesson, Colm Kerr, *et al.* "Diversity of Bifidobacteria within the Infant Gut Microbiota." *PloS One* 7, no. 5 (2012): e36957. https://doi.org/10.1371/journal.pone.0036957.
52. Turroni, Francesca, Douwe van Sinderen, and Marco Ventura. "Genomics and Ecological Overview of the Genus Bifidobacterium." *International Journal of Food Microbiology* 149, no. 1 (September 1, 2011): 37–44. https://doi.org/10.1016/j.ijfoodmicro.2010.12.010.
53. Vogt RL, Dippold L (2005). "Escherichia coli O157:H7 outbreak associated with consumption of ground beef, June–July 2002". *Public Health Reports*. 120 (2): 174–8.
54. Tenaillon O, Skurnik D, Picard B, Denamur E (March 2010). "The population genetics of commensal Escherichia coli". *Nature Reviews. Microbiology*. 8 (3): 207–17.
55. Lodinová-Zádníková R, Cukrowska B, Tlaskalova-Hogenova H (July 2003). "Oral administration of probiotic Escherichia coli after birth reduces frequency of allergies and repeated infections later in life (after 10 and 20 years)". *International Archives of Allergy and Immunology*. 131 (3): 209–11.
56. Grozdanov L, Raasch C, Schulze J, Sonnenborn U, Gottschalk G, Hacker J, Dobrindt U (August 2004). "Analysis of the genome structure of the nonpathogenic probiotic Escherichia coli strain Nissle 1917". *Journal of Bacteriology*. 186 (16): 5432–41.
57. https://www.mutaflor.com/index.html
58. "The Genus Enterococcus as Probiotic." *Brazilian Archives of Biology and Technology* 56.3 (2013): 457–466. Web. 10 Jan. 2017.
59. Hong, H. A. *et al.* (2009) Bacillus subtilis isolated from the human gastronintestinal tract. *Research in Microbiology*. 160 (2):134-143.
60. Eckburg PB, Bik EM, Bernstein CN *et al.* (2005). "Diversity of the human intestinal microbial flora". *Science* 308 (5728): 1635–8.
61. Shylakhovenko VA (June 2003). "Anticancer and Immunostimulatory effects of Nucleoprotein Fraction of 'Bacillus subtilis'". *Experimental Oncology*. 25: 119–23.
62. http://retronprobiotics.com/strain/bacillus-subtilis-natto/
63. Szajewska, H; Kołodziej, M (October 2015). "Systematic review with meta-analysis: Saccharomyces boulardii in the prevention of antibiotic-associated diarrhoea". *Alimentary Pharmacology & Therapeutics*. 42 (7): 793–801.
64. Tung, Jennifer M; Dolovich, Lisa R; Lee, Christine H (December 2009). "Prevention of Clostridium difficile infection with Saccharomyces boulardii: A systematic review". *Canadian Journal of Gastroenterology*. 23 (12): 817–21.
65. Huffnagle GB, Noverr MC. The emerging world of the fungal microbiome. *Trends Microbiol*. 2013;21(7):334 341. doi:10.1016/j.tim.2013.04.002
66. AlmadaCarine CN *et al.* Review. Paraprobiotics: Evidences on their ability to modify biological responses, inactivation methods and perspectives on their application in foods. T*rends in Food Science & Technology*, Volume 58, December 2016, Pages 96–114.

2. Fats: the Good and the Bad

1. Garrow JS, James WPT, Ralph A. *Human nutrition and dietetics*. 2000. 10th

edition. Churchill Livingstone. Alberts *et al. Molecular Biology of the Cell:* 4th edition, NY: Garland Science, 2002.
2. Enig M. *Know Your Fats: The Complete Primer for Understanding the Nutrition of Fats, Oils and Cholesterol.* Silver Spring: Bethseda Press, 2000.
3. Gupta MK. (2007). *Practical guide for vegetable oil processing.* AOCS Press, Urbana, Illinois.
4. Dam H, Sondergaard E. The encephalomalacia producing effect of arachidonic and linoleic acids. *Zeitschrift fur Ernahrungswissenschaft* 2, 217–222, 1962.
5. Pinckney ER. The potential toxicity of excessive polyunsaturates. Do not let the patient harm himself. *American Heart Journal* 85, 723–726, 1973.
6. West CE, Redgrave TG. Reservations on the use of polyunsaturated fats in human nutrition. *Search* 5, 90–96, 1974.
7. McHugh MI *et al.* Immunosuppression with polyunsaturated fatty acids in renal transplantation. *Transplantation* 24, 263–267, 1977.
8. Alexander JC, Valli VE, Chanin BE. Biological observations from feeding heated corn oil and heated peanut oil to rats. *Journal of Toxicology and Environmental Health* 21, 295–309, 1087.
9. Ravnskov U. *The Cholesterol Myths. Exposing the fallacy that saturated fat and cholesterol cause heart disease.* 2000. NewTrends Publishing.
10. Enig M. *Know Your Fats: The Complete Primer for Understanding the Nutrition of Fats, Oils and Cholesterol.* Silver Spring: Bethseda Press, 2000.
11. Pizzorno JE, Murray MT. *Textbook of natural medicine.* 4th edition, 2012.
12. Horrobin D. *The madness of Adam and Eve.* Bantam Press. ISBN 0 593 04649 8, 2001.
13. Garrow JS, James WPT, Ralph A. *Human nutrition and dietetics.* 2000. 10th edition. Churchill Livingstone. Alberts *et al. Molecular Biology of the Cell*: 4th edition, NY: Garland Science, 2002.
14. Campbell-McBride N. *Put your heart in your mouth. What really is heart disease and what can we do to prevent and even reverse it.* 2007. Medinform Publishing.
15. Mann GV. Coronary heart disease: "Doing the wrong things." *Nutrition Today* July/August, p.12–14, 1985.
16. Alberts *et al. Molecular Biology of the Cell*: 4th edition, NY: Garland Science, 2002.
17. Nelson DL and Cox MM. *Lehninger Principles of Biochemistry*, 4th edition, 2004.
18. Seeley RR, Stephens TD, Tate P. *Anatomy and physiology*, 2nd edition. Mosby Year Book, 1992.
19. Enig M. *Know Your Fats: The Complete Primer for Understanding the Nutrition of Fats, Oils and Cholesterol.* Silver Spring: Bethseda Press, 2000.
20. Strauss E. Developmental Biology: one-eyed animals implicate cholesterol in development. *Science* 280;1528–1529;1998.
21. Dietschy JM, Turley SD. Cholesterol metabolism in the brain. *Curr Opin Lipidol.* 2001, 12: 105–112.
22. Moore KL, Persaud TV. (2011). *The developing human—clinical oriented embryology.* 9th edition. USA: Saunders, an imprint of Elsevier Inc.
23. Purves W, Sadava D, Orians G and Heller C. 2004. *Life: The Science of Biology*, 7th edition. Sunderland, MA: Sinauer.
24. Huttenlocher PR, Dabholkar AS. (1997). "Regional differences in synaptogenesis in human cerebral cortex". *The Journal of Comparative Neurology* 387 (2).
25. Graveline D. *Lipitor – thief of memory, statin drugs and the misguided war on cholesterol.* 2006. Infinity Publishing, Haverford, Pennsylvania.

26. Ravnskov U. *The Cholesterol Myths. Exposing the fallacy that saturated fat and cholesterol cause heart disease.* 2000. NewTrends Publishing.
27. Enig M. *Know Your Fats: The Complete Primer for Understanding the Nutrition of Fats, Oils and Cholesterol.* Silver Spring: Bethseda Press, 2000.
28. Graveline D. The statin damage crisis. 2014. Infinity Publishing.
29. UCSF Medical Centre data: /ucsfhealth.org/education/cholesterol_content_of_foods
30. USDA food composition nutrient database online.
31. Fallon S, Enig M. Nourishing Traditions. *The cookbook that challenges politically correct nutrition and the diet dictocrats.* 1999. New Trends Publishing, Washington DC 20007.
32. Campbell-McBride N. *Gut and psychology syndrome. Natural treatment for autism, dyspraxia, dyslexia, ADD/ADHD, depression and schizophrenia.* 2010. Medinform Publishing.
33. Horrobin DF. Lowering cholesterol concentrations and mortality. *British Medical Journal* 301, 554, 1990.
34. Albert DJ *et al.* Aggression in humans: what is its biological foundation? *Neurosci Biobehav Rev.* 1993;17:405–425.
35. Golomb BA. Cholesterol and violence: is there a connection? *Annals of Internal Medicine* 128, 478–487, 1998.
36. Bahrke MS *et al.* Psychological and behavioural effects of endogenous testosterone levels and anabolic-androgenic steroids among males. *Review. Sports Med.* 1990; 10:303–337.
37. Bhasin S *et al.* Sexual dysfunction in men and women with endocrine disorders. *Lancet.* 2007 Feb 17;369(9561):597–-611. Review.
38. Jacobs D *et al.* Report of the conference on low blood cholesterol: Mortality associations. *Circulation* 86, 1046–1060, 1992.
39. Rosch PJ. Views on Cholesterol. Health and Stress. *The Newsletter of The American Institute of Stress,* volumes 1995: 1, 1998: 1, 1999: 8, 2001: 2,4,7.
40. Ravnskov U. High cholesterol may protect against infections and atherosclerosis. *Q J Med* 2003;96:927–34.
41. Harris HW *et al.* The lipemia of sepsis: triglyceride-rich lipoproteins as agents of innate immunity. *Journal of Endotoxin Research* 6, 421–430, 2001.
42. Iribarren C *et al.* Serum total cholesterol and risk of hospitalisation and death from respiratory disease. *Int J Epidemiol* 26, 1191–1202, 1997.
43. Iribarren C *et al.* Cohort study of serum total cholesterol and in-hospital incidence of infectious diseases. *Epidemiology and Infection* 121, 335–347, 1998.
44. Bhakdi S *et al.* Binding and partial inactivation of Staphylococcus aureus A-toxin by human plasma low density lipoprotein. *Journal of Biological Chemistry* 258, 5899–5904, 1983.
45. Claxton AJ *et al.* Association between serum total cholesterol and HIV infection in a high-risk cohort of young men. *Journal of acquired immune deficiency syndromes and human retrovirology* 17, 51–57, 1998.
46. Muldoon MF *et al.*Immune system differences in men with hypo- or hypercholesterolemia. *Clinical Immunology and Immunopathology* 84, 145–149, 1997.
47. Neaton JD, Wentworth DN. Low serum cholesterol and risk of death from AIDS. *AIDS* 11, 929–930, 1997.
48. Porter R (2006). *The Cambridge History of Medicine.* Cambridge University Press.
49. Enig MG. *Know Your Fats: The Complete Primer for Understanding the Nutrition of Fats, Oils, and Cholesterol.* Bethesda Press, Silver Spring, MD, 2000.

50. Garrow JS, James WPT, Ralph A. Human nutrition and dietetics. 2000. 10th edition. Churchill Livingstone. Alberts *et al. Molecular Biology of the Cell*: 4th edition, NY: Garland Science, 2002.
51. https://www.healthline.com/nutrition/17-health-benefits-of-omega-3#section5
52. Horrobin D. *The madness of Adam and Eve*. Bantam Press. ISBN 0 593 04649 8, 2001.
53. Nelson GJ *et al.* (1997). "The effect of dietary arachidonic acid on plasma lipoprotein distributions, apoproteins, blood lipid levels, and tissue fatty acid composition in humans". *Lipids* 32 (4): 427–33.
54. Kelley DS *et al.* (1998). "Arachidonic acid supplementation enhances synthesis of eicosanoids without suppressing immune functions in young healthy men". *Lipids* 33 (2): 125–30.
55. Udo Erasmus. *Fats that heal, fats that kill*. 1993. Alive books.
56. https://www.healthline.com/nutrition/11-proven-benefits-of-olive-oil#section3
57. Lieberman, S.; Enig, M. G.; Preuss, H. G. (2006). "A Review of Monolaurin and Lauric Acid: Natural Virucidal and Bactericidal Agents". *Alternative and Complementary Therapies*. 12 (6): 310–314.

3. Cod Liver Oil

1. Price WA. *Nutrition and physical degeneration. A comparison of primitive and modern diets and their effects*. 1938. Price.
2. Garrow JS, James WPT, Ralph A. *Human nutrition and dietetics*. 2000. 10th edition. Churchill Livingstone.
3. Gupta P, K Singhal, AK Jangra, V Nautiyal and A Pandey (2012) "Shark liver oil: A review" Archived 2013-01-23 at the Wayback Machine *Asian Journal of Pharmaceutical Education and Research*, 1 (2): 1–15.
4. Enig M. *Know Your Fats: The Complete Primer for Understanding the Nutrition of Fats, Oils and Cholesterol*. Silver Spring: Bethseda Press, 2000.
5. Anthony H, Birtwistle S, Eaton K, Maberly *J. Environmental Medicine in Clinical Practice*. BSAENM Publications 1997.
6. Tanumihardjo SA. Vitamin A: biomarkers of nutrition for development. *Am J Clin Nutr* 2011;94:658S–65S.
7. Sommer A. *Vitamin A deficiency and clinical disease: An historical overview*. J Nutr 2008;138:1835–9.
8. World Health Organization. *Global Prevalence of Vitamin A Deficiency in Populations at Risk 1995–2005: WHO Global Database on Vitamin A Deficiency*. Geneva: World Health Organization; 2009.
9. van den Broek N, Dou L, Othman M, Neilson JP, Gates S, Gulmezoglu AM. Vitamin A supplementation during pregnancy for maternal and newborn outcomes. *Cochrane Database Syst Rev* 2010:CD008666.
10. Mora JR, Iwata M, von Andrian UH (September 2008). "Vitamin effects on the immune system: vitamins A and D take centre stage". *Nature Reviews. Immunology*. 8 (9): 685–98.
11. Garrow JS, James WPT, Ralph A. *Human nutrition and dietetics*. 2000. 10th edition. Churchill Livingstone.
12. Richardson, D. P. (28 February 2007). "Food Fortification". *Proceedings of the Nutrition Society*. 49 (1): 39–50.
13. Khoury MJ and others. Vitamin A and birth defects [letter]. *Lancet* 1996;347:322.

14. Sally Fallon Morell. *Nourishing Diets. How Paleo, Ancestral And Traditional Peoples Really Ate.* 2018. Grand central L&S.
15. Price WA. *Nutrition and physical degeneration. A comparison of primitive and modern diets and their effects.* 1938. Price.
16. Enig M. *Know Your Fats: The Complete Primer for Understanding the Nutrition of Fats, Oils and Cholesterol.* Silver Spring: Bethseda Press, 2000.
17. Holick MF, Chen TC (April 2008). "Vitamin D deficiency: a worldwide problem with health consequences". *The American Journal of Clinical Nutrition.* 87 (4): 1080S–6S.
18. Seneff S. Sunlight and vitamin D: they're not the same thing. *Wise Traditions In Food, Farming And Healing Arts*, spring 2020.
19. An estimate of premature cancer mortality in the U.S. due to inadequate doses of solar ultraviolet-B radiation. *Cancer.* 2002 Mar 15; 94(6):1867–75.
20. Beneficial effects of sun exposure on cancer mortality. *Prev Med.* 1993 Jan; 22(1): 132–40. Review.
21. Does sunlight prevent cancer? A systematic review. *Eur J Cancer.* 2006 Sep; 42(14): 2222–32. Epub 2006 Aug 10. Review.
22. Does sunlight have a beneficial influence on certain cancers? *Prog Biophys Mol Biol.* 2006 Sep; 92(1): 132–9. Epub 2006 Feb 28. Review.
23. Ecologic studies of solar UVB radiation and cancer mortality rates. Recent Results. *Cancer Res.* 2003; 164: 371–7. Review.
24. Geographic patterns of prostate cancer mortality. Evidence for a protective effect of ultraviolet radiation. *Cancer.* 1992 Dec 15; 70(12):2861–9.
25. Multiple sclerosis and prostate cancer: what do their similar geographies suggest? *Neuroepidemiology.*1992; 11(4–6): 244–54.
26. Sunlight and vitamin D for bone health and prevention of autoimmune diseases, cancers, and cardiovascular disease. *Am J Clin Nutr.*2004 Dec; 80(6 Suppl): 1678S–88S. Review.
27. UV radiation and cancer prevention: what is the evidence? *Anticancer Res.* 2006 Jul–Aug; 26(4A) :2723–7. Review.
28. Plourde E. *Sunscreens—Biohazard: Treat as Hazardous Waste.* Irvine, CA: New Voice Publications; 2011.
29. Epstein SS. *Unreasonable risk. How to avoid cancer from cosmetics and personal care products.* 2001. Published by Environmental Toxicology, Chicago Illinois.
30. Vitamin D: its role in cancer prevention and treatment. *Prog Biophys Mol Biol.* 2006 Sep; 92(1): 49–59. Epub 2006 Mar 10. Review.
31. Vitamin D physiology. *Prog Biophys Mol Biol.* 2006 Sep; 92(1): 4–8. Epub 2006 Feb 28. Review.
32. Vitamin D and cancer. *Anticancer Res.* 2006 Jul–Aug; 26(4A): 2515–24. Review.
33. Heaney RP. The vitamin D requirement in health and disease. *Journal of Steroid Biochemistry & Molecular Biology*, 97 (2005), 13–19.
34. Garrow JS, James WPT, Ralph A. *Human nutrition and dietetics.* 2000. 10th edition. Churchill Livingstone.
35. https://www.westonaprice.org/health-topics/abcs-of-nutrition/vitamin-d-supplementation-panacea-potential-problem/
36. Infante M, Ricordi C, *et al.* Influence of Vitamin D on Islet Autoimmunity and Beta-Cell Function in Type 1 Diabetes. *Nutrients.* 2019 Sep 11;11(9):2185. doi: 10.3390/nu11092185.
37. Saponaro F, Marcocci C *et al.* Vitamin D status and cardiovascular outcome.

J Endocrinol Invest. 2019 Nov; 42(11):1285–1290. doi: 10.1007/s40618-019-01057-y. Epub 2019 Jun 6. PMID: 31172459.

38. Sogomonian R, Alkhawam H, *et al*. Serum vitamin D levels correlate to coronary artery disease severity: a retrospective chart analysis. *Expert Rev Cardiovasc Ther*. 2016 Aug;14(8):977–82.
39. Cuomo A, *et al*. Prevalence and Correlates of Vitamin D Deficiency in a Sample of 290 Inpatients With Mental Illness. *Front Psychiatry*. 2019. PMID: 31001150
40. Illescas-Montes R, Melguizo-Rodríguez L, Ruiz C, Costela-Ruiz VJ. Vitamin D and autoimmune diseases. *Life Sci*. 2019 Sep 15;233:116744. doi: 10.1016/j.lfs.2019.116744. Epub 2019 Aug 8. PMID: 31401314
41. Vrani L, Mikolaševi I, Mili S. Vitamin D Deficiency: Consequence or Cause of Obesity? *Medicina* (Kaunas). 2019 Aug 28;55(9):541. doi: 10.3390/medicina 55090541. PMID: 31466220
42. Vaishya R, Vijay V, Lama P, Agarwal A. Does vitamin D deficiency influence the incidence and progression of knee osteoarthritis? – A literature review. *J Clin Orthop Trauma*. 2019 Jan–Feb;10(1):9-15. doi: 10.1016/j.jcot.2018.05.012. Epub 2018 May 20.
43. Bouillon R, Marcocci C, *et al*. Skeletal and Extraskeletal Actions of Vitamin D: Current Evidence and Outstanding Questions. *J. Endocr Rev*. 2019 Aug 1;40(4):1109–1151.
44. Charoenngam N, Shirvani A, Holick MF. Vitamin D for skeletal and non-skeletal health: What we should know. *J Clin Orthop Trauma*. 2019 Nov–Dec;10(6): 1082–1093.
45. Marino R, Misra M. Extra-Skeletal Effects of Vitamin D. *Nutrients*. 2019 Jun 27;11(7):1460. doi: 10.3390/nu11071460. PMID: 31252594
46. Garland, Cedric F., Frank C. Garland, Edward D. Gorham, Martin Lipkin, Harold Newmark, Sharif B. Mohr, and Michael F. Holick. "The Role of Vitamin D in Cancer Prevention." *American Journal of Public Health* 96, no. 2 (February 2006): 252–61.
47. Machado MRM, de Sousa Almeida-Filho B, *et al*. Low pretreatment serum concentration of vitamin D at breast cancer diagnosis in postmenopausal women. *Menopause*. 2019 Mar;26(3):293–299. doi: 10.1097/GME.000000 0000001203. PMID: 30234730
48. Garland, C. F., and F. C. Garland. "Do Sunlight and Vitamin D Reduce the Likelihood of Colon Cancer?" *International Journal of Epidemiology* 9, no. 3 (September 1980): 227–31.
49. Cai C. Treating Vitamin D Deficiency and Insufficiency in Chronic Neck and Back Pain and Muscle Spasm: A Case Series. *Perm J*. 2019;23:18–241. doi: 10.7812/TPP/18.241.
50. Teymoori-Rad M, Shokri F, Salimi V, Marashi SM. The interplay between vitamin D and viral infections. *Rev Med Virol*. 2019 Mar;29(2):e2032.
51. Vélayoudom-Céphise FL, Wémeau JL. Primary hyperparathyroidism and vitamin D deficiency. *Ann Endocrinol* (Paris). 2015 May;76(2):153–62.
52. https://naturalsociety.com/why-synthetic-vitamins-should-be-avoided/
53. Garrow JS, James WPT, Ralph A. *Human nutrition and dietetics*. 2000. 10th edition. Churchill Livingstone.
54. Miller RK *et al*. Periconceptional Vitamin A use: how much is teratogenic? *Reprod Toxic*. 1998;12(1):75–88.
55. Cod liver oil manufacturing. https://www.westonaprice.org/health-topics/cod-liver-oil/cod-liver-oil-manufacturing/

4. Digestive Enzymes

1. Howden CW, Hunt RH. Spontaneous hypochlorhydria in man: possible causes and consequences. *Dig Dis*. 1986;4(1):26 32. doi:10.1159/000171134
2. Yago MR, Frymoyer AR, Smelick GS, *et al*. Gastric reacidification with betaine HCl in healthy volunteers with rabeprazole-induced hypochlorhydria. *Mol Pharm*. 2013;10(11):4032 4037.
3. Liu Z, Udenigwe CC. Role of food-derived opioid peptides in the central nervous and gastrointestinal systems. *J Food Biochem*. 2019;43(1):e12629.doi: 10.1111/jfbc.12629
4. Rayford PL, Miller TA, Thompson JC. Secretin, cholecystokinin and newer gastrointestinal hormones (first of two parts). *N Engl J Med*. 1976;294(20):1093 1101. doi:10.1056/NEJM197605132942006
5. Ovesen L, Bendtsen F, Tage-Jensen U, Pedersen NT, Gram BR, Rune SJ. Intraluminal pH in the stomach, duodenum, and proximal jejunum in normal subjects and patients with exocrine pancreatic insufficiency. *Gastroenterology*. 1986;90(4):958 962. doi:10.1016/0016-5085(86)90873-5
6. Campbell-McBride N. *Gut and psychology syndrome. Natural treatment for autism, dyspraxia, dyslexia, ADD/ADHD, depression and schizophrenia*. 2010. Medinform Publishing.
7. Khan MN, Raza SS, Hussain AK, Nadeem MD, Ullah F. *Pancreatic Duct Stones*. J Ayub Med Coll Abbottabad. 2017;29(1):154 156.
8. FRAZER JW Jr, ANLYAN WG, ISLEY JK. Studies in pancreatic exocrine insuffiency. *Surg Forum*. 1958;9:525 530.
9. Johnson CD, Besselink MG, Carter R. Acute pancreatitis. *BMJ*. 2014; 349:g4859. Published 2014 Aug 12. doi:10.1136/bmj.g4859
10. Noto JM, Peek RM Jr. The gastric microbiome, its interaction with Helicobacter pylori, and its potential role in the progression to stomach cancer. *PLoS Pathog*. 2017;13(10):e1006573. Published 2017 Oct 5. doi:10.1371/journal.ppat.1006573
11. Wroblewski LE, Peek RM Jr, Coburn LA. The Role of the Microbiome in Gastrointestinal Cancer. *Gastroenterol Clin North Am*. 2016;45(3):543 556. doi:10.1016/j.gtc.2016.04.010
12. Buddam A, Dacha S. Gastric Stasis. In: *StatPearls*. Treasure Island (FL): StatPearls Publishing; 2020.

5. Vitamin and Mineral Supplementation

1. Dietary supplements: what the industry does not want you to know. https://www.westonaprice.org/health-topics/health-issues/dietary-supplements-what-the-industry-does-not-want-you-to-know/
2. Bronner F. Calcium absorption—a paradigm for mineral absorption. *J Nutr*. 1998;128(5):917 920. doi:10.1093/jn/128.5.917
3. Ferraro PM, Curhan GC, Gambaro G, Taylor EN. Total, Dietary, and Supplemental Vitamin C Intake and Risk of Incident Kidney Stones. *Am J Kidney Dis*. 2016;67(3):400 407. doi:10.1053/j.ajkd.2015.09.005
4. Jäger R, Purpura M, Farmer S, Cash HA, Keller D. Probiotic Bacillus coagulans GBI-30, 6086 Improves Protein Absorption and Utilization. *Probiotics Antimicrob Proteins*. 2018;10(4):611 615. doi:10.1007/s12602-017-9354-y
5. LeBlanc JG, Milani C, de Giori GS, Sesma F, van Sinderen D, Ventura M. Bacteria as vitamin suppliers to their host: a gut microbiota perspective. *Curr Opin Biotechnol*. 2013;24(2):160 168. doi:10.1016/j.copbio.2012.08.005
6. Li L, Qi G, Wang B, Yue D, Wang Y, Sato T. Fulvic acid anchored layered

double hydroxides: A multifunctional composite adsorbent for the removal of anionic dye and toxic metal. *J Hazard Mater*. 2018;343:19 28. doi:10.1016/j.jhazmat.2017.09.006

Detoxification for People with Gut and Physiology Syndrome

1. Epstein SS. *Unreasonable risk. How to avoid cancer from cosmetics and personal care products*. 2001. Published by Environmental Toxicology, Chicago Illinois.
2. Anthony H, Birtwistle S, Eaton K, Maberly J. *Environmental Medicine in Clinical Practice*. BSAENM Publications 1997.
3. Physicians' Health Initiative for Radiation and Environment (PHIRE) 5th Nov 2018, London, UK. Press Conference on Health Effects of Non-Ionising Radiation (NIR) and the implementation of 5G.
4. British Society for Ecological Medicine (BSEM) 5G International Medical Conference, 27th Sept 2019 London, UK. 5G The Fact, Risks and Remedies.
5. Liska DJ. The detoxification enzyme systems. *Altern Med Rev*. 1998;3(3): 187 198.
6. Grant DM. Detoxification pathways in the liver. *J Inherit Metab Dis*. 1991; 14(4):421 430. doi:10.1007/BF01797915
7. Pogue JM, Tam VH. Toxicity in Patients. *Adv Exp Med Biol*. 2019;1145:289 304. doi:10.1007/978-3-030-16373-0_17
8. Joffin N, Noirez P, Antignac JP, *et al*. Release and toxicity of adipose tissue-stored TCDD: Direct evidence from a xenografted fat model. *Environ Int*. 2018;121(Pt 2):1113 1120. doi:10.1016/j.envint.2018.10.027
9. Stang S, Wang H, Gardner KH, Mo W. Influences of water quality and climate on the water-energy nexus: A spatial comparison of two water systems. J *Environ Manage*. 2018;218:613 621. doi:10.1016/j.jenvman.2018.04.095
10. Bauer T, Gath J, Hunkeler A, Ernst M, Böckmann A, Meier BH. Hexagonal ice in pure water and biological NMR samples. *J Biomol NMR*. 2017;67(1):15 22. doi:10.1007/s10858-016-0080-7
11. https://www.networx.com/article/8-unexpected-uses-for-mustard
12. Patel S. Fragrance compounds: The wolves in sheep's clothings. *Med Hypotheses*. 2017;102:106 111. doi:10.1016/j.mehy.2017.03.025
13. Epstein SS. *Unreasonable risk. How to avoid cancer from cosmetics and personal care products*. 2001. Published by Environmental Toxicology, Chicago Illinois.
14. Anthony H, Birtwistle S, Eaton K, Maberly J. *Environmental Medicine in Clinical Practice*. BSAENM Publications 1997.
15. Marwah H, Garg T, Goyal AK, Rath G. Permeation enhancer strategies in transdermal drug delivery. *Drug Deliv*. 2016;23(2):564 578. doi:10.3109/10717544.2014.935532
16. Darbre PD. Aluminium and the human breast. *Morphologie*. 2016;100(329): 65 74. doi:10.1016/j.morpho.2016.02.001
17. Darbre PD. Underarm antiperspirants/deodorants and breast cancer. *Breast Cancer Res*. 2009;11 Suppl 3(Suppl 3):S5. doi:10.1186/bcr2424
18. Aengenheister L, Dugershaw BB, Manser P, *et al*. Investigating the accumulation and translocation of titanium dioxide nanoparticles with different surface modifications in static and dynamic human placental transfer models. *Eur J Pharm Biopharm*. 2019;142:488 497. doi:10.1016/j.ejpb.2019.07.018
19. Panico A, Serio F, Bagordo F, *et al*.Skin safety and health prevention: an overview of chemicals in cosmetic products. *J Prev Med Hyg*. 2019;60(1): E50 E57. Published 2019 Mar 29. doi:10.15167/2421-4248/ jpmh2019.60.1. 1080

20. Epstein SS. *Unreasonable risk. How to avoid cancer from cosmetics and personal care products*. 2001. Published by Environmental Toxicology, Chicago Illinois.
21. Crinnion W. Components of practical clinical detox programs—sauna as a therapeutic tool. *Altern Ther Health Med*. 2007;13(2):S154 S156.
22. https://www.westonaprice.org/podcast/64-vaccine-industry-rights/
23. https://www.westonaprice.org/podcast/17-vaccines-whats-fuss-part-2/
24. https://www.westonaprice.org/health-topics/vaccinations/why-we-need-to-reexamine-the-riskbenefit-tradeoffs-of-vaccines/
25. https://www.westonaprice.org/are-vaccines-safe-by-mary-tocco/
26. https://www.westonaprice.org/nurses-against-mandatory-vaccines/
27. Hulsey E, Bland T. Immune overload: Parental attitudes toward combination and single antigen vaccines. *Vaccine*. 2015;33(22):2546 2550. doi:10.1016/j.vaccine.2015.04.020
28. Valeriani F, Margarucci LM, Romano Spica V. Recreational Use of Spa Thermal Waters: Criticisms and Perspectives for Innovative Treatments. *Int J Environ Res Public Health*. 2018;15(12):2675. Published 2018 Nov 28.
29. Font-Ribera L, Marco E, Grimalt JO, *et al*. Exposure to disinfection by-products in swimming pools and biomarkers of genotoxicity and respiratory damage - *The PISCINA2 Study*. *Environ Int*. 2019;131:104988. doi:10.1016/j.envint.2019.104988
30. Chevalier G, Sinatra ST, Oschman JL, Sokal K, Sokal P. Earthing: health implications of reconnecting the human body to the Earth's surface electrons. *J Environ Public Health*. 2012;2012:291541. doi:10.1155/2012/291541
31. Davidson, Robert M., and Stephanie Seneff. "The Initial Common Pathway of Inflammation, Disease, and Sudden Death." *Entropy*. 14.12 (2012): 1399–1442.
32. Seneff S. Sunlight and vitamin D: they're not the same thing. *Wise Traditions In Food, Farming And Healing Arts*, spring 2020.
33. An estimate of premature cancer mortality in the U.S. due to inadequate doses of solar ultraviolet-B radiation. *Cancer*. 2002 Mar 15; 94(6):1867–75.
34. Beneficial effects of sun exposure on cancer mortality. *Prev Med*. 1993 Jan; 22(1): 132–40. Review.
35. Does sunlight prevent cancer? A systematic review. *Eur J Cancer*. 2006 Sep; 42(14): 2222–32. Epub 2006 Aug 10. Review.
36. Does sunlight have a beneficial influence on certain cancers? *Prog Biophys Mol Biol*. 2006 Sep; 92(1): 132–9. Epub 2006 Feb 28. Review.
37. Ecologic studies of solar UVB radiation and cancer mortality rates. Recent Results. *Cancer Res*. 2003; 164: 371–7. Review.
38. Geographic patterns of prostate cancer mortality. Evidence for a protective effect of ultraviolet radiation. *Cancer*. 1992 Dec 15; 70(12):2861–9.
39. Multiple sclerosis and prostate cancer: what do their similar geographies suggest? *Neuroepidemiology*.1992; 11(4–6): 244–54.
40. Sunlight and vitamin D for bone health and prevention of autoimmune diseases, cancers, and cardiovascular disease. *Am J Clin Nutr*. 2004 Dec; 80(6 Suppl): 1678S–88S. Review.
41. UV radiation and cancer prevention: what is the evidence? *Anticancer Res*. 2006 Jul–Aug; 26(4A) :2723–7. Review.
42. Plourde E. *Sunscreens—Biohazard: Treat as Hazardous Waste*. Irvine, CA: New Voice Publications; 2011.
43. Epstein SS. *Unreasonable risk. How to avoid cancer from cosmetics and personal care products*. 2001. Published by Environmental Toxicology, Chicago Illinois.

44. Martin CA, Gowda U, Renzaho AM. The prevalence of vitamin D deficiency among dark-skinned populations according to their stage of migration and region of birth: A meta-analysis. *Nutrition*. 2016;32(1):21 32. doi:10.1016/j.nut.2015.07.007
45. Ibbotson S. Drug and chemical induced photosensitivity from a clinical perspective. *Photochem Photobiol Sci*. 2018;17(12):1885 1903. doi:10.1039/c8pp00011e
46. Mathews-Roth MM. Beta-carotene therapy for erythropoietic protoporphyria and other photosensitivity diseases. *Biochimie*. 1986;68(6):875 884. doi:10.1016/s0300-9084(86)80104-3
47. Ahmadi K, Hazrati M, Ahmadizadeh M, Noohi S. Effect of Radiance-Dimmer Devices Simulating Natural Sunlight Rhythm on the Plasma Melatonin Levels and Anxiety and Depression Scores of the Submarine Personnel. *Iran J Psychiatry*. 2019;14(2):147 153.
48. Cipolla-Neto J, Amaral FGD. Melatonin as a Hormone: New Physiological and Clinical Insights. *Endocr Rev*. 2018;39(6):990 1028. doi:10.1210/er.2018-00084
49. Owczarek G, Gralewicz G, Wolska A, Skuza N, Jurowski P. Potencjalny wpływ barwy filtrów w okularach chroni cych przed ol nieniem słonecznym na wydzielanie melatoniny [Potential impact of colors of filters used in sunglasses on the melatonin suppression process]. *Med Pr*. 2017;68(5):629 637. doi:10.13075/mp.5893.00550
50. van der Rhee HJ, de Vries E, Coebergh JW. Regular sun exposure benefits health. *Med Hypotheses*. 2016;97:34 37. doi:10.1016/j.mehy.2016.10.011
51. Gerson C with Bishop B. *Healing the Gerson way. Defeating cancer and other chronic diseases*. 2007. Totality Books.
52. Ter Horst KW, Serlie MJ. Fructose Consumption, Lipogenesis, and Non-Alcoholic Fatty Liver Disease. *Nutrients*. 2017;9(9):981. Published 2017 Sep 6. doi:10.3390/nu9090981
53. Porter RS, Bode RF. A Review of the Antiviral Properties of Black Elder (Sambucus nigra L.) Products. *Phytother Res*. 2017;31(4):533 554. doi:10.1002/ptr.5782
54. Elderberry. In: *Drugs and Lactation Database* (LactMed). Bethesda (MD): National Library of Medicine (US); 2006.
55. Rahman Z, Singh VP. The relative impact of toxic heavy metals (THMs) (arsenic (As), cadmium (Cd), chromium (Cr)(VI), mercury (Hg), and lead (Pb)) on the total environment: an overview. *Environ Monit Assess*. 2019;191(7):419. Published 2019 Jun 8.
56. Bjørklund G, Dadar M, Mutter J, Aaseth J. The toxicology of mercury: Current research and emerging trends. *Environ Res*. 2017;159:545 554. doi:10.1016/j.envres.2017.08.051
57. Zakaria A, Ho YB. Heavy metals contamination in lipsticks and their associated health risks to lipstick consumers. *Regul Toxicol Pharmacol*. 2015;73(1):191 195. doi:10.1016/j.yrtph.2015.07.005
58. Borowska S, Brzóska MM. Metals in cosmetics: implications for human health. *J Appl Toxicol*. 2015;35(6):551 572. doi:10.1002/jat.3129
59. Rehman K, Fatima F, Waheed I, Akash MSH. Prevalence of exposure of heavy metals and their impact on health consequences. *J Cell Biochem*. 2018;119(1):157 184. doi:10.1002/jcb.26234
60. Amadi CN, Offor SJ, Frazzoli C, Orisakwe OE. Natural antidotes and management of metal toxicity. *Environ Sci Pollut Res Int*. 2019;26(18):18032 18052. doi:10.1007/s11356-019-05104-2

61. Andrew Hall Cutler. *Amalgam illness. Diagnosis and treatment*. 2017. noamalgam.com
62. Kim JJ, Kim YS, Kumar V. Heavy metal toxicity: An update of chelating therapeutic strategies. *J Trace Elem Med Biol*. 2019;54:226 231. doi:10.1016/j.jtemb.2019.05.003
63. Mehta A, Flora SJ. Possible role of metal redistribution, hepatotoxicity and oxidative stress in chelating agents induced hepatic and renal metallothionein in rats. *Food Chem Toxicol*. 2001;39(10):1029 1038. doi:10.1016/s0278-6915(01)00046-1
64. Rebecca Rust Lee and Andrew Hall Cutler. *The mercury detoxification manual*. 2019. Andy Cutler Publishing.
65. Blaucok-Busch E, Amin OR, Dessoki HH, Rabah T. Efficacy of DMSA Therapy in a Sample of Arab Children with Autistic Spectrum Disorder. *Maedica* (Buchar). 2012;7(3):214 221.
66. Clarke D, Buchanan R, Gupta N, Haley B. Amelioration of Acute Mercury Toxicity by a Novel, Non-Toxic Lipid Soluble Chelator N,N'bis-(2-mercaptoethyl)isophthalamide: Effect on Animal Survival, Health, Mercury Excretion and Organ Accumulation. *Toxicol Environ Chem*. 2012;94(3):616 640. doi:10.1080/02772248.2012.657199
67. Alcántara C, Jadán-Piedra C, Vélez D, Devesa V, Zúñiga M, Monedero V. Characterization of the binding capacity of mercurial species in Lactobacillus strains. *J Sci Food Agric*. 2017;97(15):5107 5113. doi:10.1002/jsfa.8388
68. https://www.bioray.com/ndf-plus-organic.html
69. Tinkov AA, Gritsenko VA, Skalnaya MG, Cherkasov SV, Aaseth J, Skalny AV. Gut as a target for cadmium toxicity. *Environ Pollut*. 2018;235:429 434. doi:10.1016/j.envpol.2017.12.114
70. Hal A Huggins. *Solving the MS mystery: help, hope and recovery*. 2002. Dragon Slayer Publication.
71 Andrew Hall Cutler. *Hair test interpretation: finding hidden toxicities*. 2004. noamalgam.com
72. Valentine-Thon E, Schiwara HW. Validity of MELISA for metal sensitivity testing. *Neuro Endocrinol Lett*. 2003;24(1–2):57 64.
73. Puri BK, Segal DR, Monro JA. Diagnostic use of the lymphocyte transformation test-memory lymphocyte immunostimulation assay in confirming active Lyme borreliosis in clinically and serologically ambiguous cases. *Int J Clin Exp Med*.
74. Epstein SS. *Unreasonable risk. How to avoid cancer from cosmetics and personal care products*. 2001. Published by Environmental Toxicology, Chicago Illinois.
75. Clarkson TW, Magos L. The toxicology of mercury and its chemical compounds. *Crit Rev Toxicol*. 2006;36(8):609 662. doi:10.1080/10408440600845619
76. Kumarathilaka P, Seneweera S, Ok YS, Meharg A, Bundschuh J. Arsenic in cooked rice foods: Assessing health risks and mitigation options. *Environ Int*. 2019;127:584 591. doi:10.1016/j.envint.2019.04.004
77. Mima M, Greenwald D, Ohlander S. Environmental Toxins and Male Fertility. *Curr Urol Rep*. 2018;19(7):50. Published 2018 May 17. doi:10.1007/s11934-018-0804-1
78. Andrew Hall Cutler. *Amalgam illness. Diagnosis and treatment*. 2017. noamalgam.com

Bowel management

1. Iwamuro M, Kawai Y, Takata K, Miyabe Y, Okada H, Yamamoto K. Reactive lymphoid hyperplasia with a lipomatous component associated with fecal compaction in an appendiceal orifice. *Intern Med*. 2014;53(10):1049 1053.
2. Zhao W, Ke M. Report of an unusual case with severe fecal impaction responding to medication therapy. *J Neurogastroenterol Motil*. 2010;16(2):199 202. doi:10.5056/jnm.2010.16.2.199
3. Cheetham MJ, Malouf AJ, Kamm MA. Fecal incontinence. *Gastroenterol Clin North Am*. 2001;30(1):115 130. doi:10.1016/s0889–8553(05)70170-9
4. Prichard DO, Bharucha AE. Recent advances in understanding and managing chronic constipation. F1000Res. 2018;7:F1000 *Faculty Rev-1640*. Published 2018 Oct 15. doi:10.12688/f1000research.15900.1
5. Magner, Lois (1992). *A History of Medicine*. Boca Raton, Florida: CRC Press. p. 31. ISBN 978-0-8247-8673-1.
6. Gerson C and Walker M. *The Gerson Therapy*. 2001.Twin Streams, Kensington Publishing Corporation.
7. Gerson C & Bishop B. *Healing the Gerson way. Defeating cancer and other chronic diseases*. 2007. Totality books.
8. Lim S. Metabolic acidosis. *Acta Med Indones*. 2007;39(3):145–150.

Healing

1. Anthony H, Birtwistle S, Eaton K, Maberly J. *Environmental Medicine in Clinical Practice*. BSAENM Publications 1997.
2. Selye Hans. *Stress without Distress*. 1975, Penguin Books Ltd.
3. Garkavi LH, Kvakina EB, Kuzmenko TS. *Anti-Stress Reactions And Activation* Therapy.) 1998.
4. Straub RH, Cutolo M. Psychoneuroimmunology-developments in stress research. *Wien Med Wochenschr*. 2018;168(3–4):76 84. doi:10.1007/s10354-017-0574-2
5. Lee DY, Kim E, Choi MH. Technical and clinical aspects of cortisol as a biochemical marker of chronic stress. *BMB Rep*. 2015;48(4):209 216. doi:10.5483/bmbrep.2015.48.4.275
6. Zhai L, Zhang H, Zhang D. Sleep Duration and Depression Among Adults: A Meta-analysis of Prospective Studies. *Depress Anxiety*. 2015;32(9):664 670. doi:10.1002/da.22386
7. Tetel MJ, de Vries GJ, Melcangi RC, Panzica G, O'Mahony SM. Steroids, stress and the gut microbiome-brain axis. *J Neuroendocrinol*. 2018;30(2):10.1111/jne.12548. doi:10.1111/jne.12548
8. Panossian A. Understanding adaptogenic activity: specificity of the pharmacological action of adaptogens and other phytochemicals. *Ann N Y Acad Sci*. 2017;1401(1):49 64. doi:10.1111/nyas.13399
9. Tanaka A, Saeki J, Hayama SI, Kass PH. Effect of Pets on Human Behaviour and Stress in Disaster. *Front Vet Sci*. 2019;6:113. Published 2019 Apr 18. doi:10.3389/fvets.2019.00113
10. Winter J, Jurek B. The interplay between oxytocin and the CRF system: regulation of the stress response. *Cell Tissue Res*. 2019;375(1):85 91. doi:10.1007/s00441-018-2866-2

Mind over matter

1. Deter HC, Orth-Gomér K, Wasilewski B, Verissimo R. The European Network on Psychosomatic Medicine (ENPM) – history and future directions. *Biopsychosoc Med.* 2017;11:3. Published 2017 Jan 26. doi:10.1186/s13030-016-0086-0
2. Nisavic M, Shuster JL, Gitlin D, Worley L, Stern TA. Readings on psychosomatic medicine: survey of resources for trainees. *Psychosomatics.* 2015;56(4):319 328. doi:10.1016/j.psym.2014.12.006
3. Ulnik JC. Corrientes actuales del pensamiento psicosomático [Current trends in psychosomatic medicine]. *Vertex.* 2019;XXX(145):182 184.
4. Louise Hay. *You can heal your life.* 1988. Eden Grove Editions.
5. Dale Carnegie. *How to Stop Worrying and Start Living* 1948. New York, Simon and Schuster.
6. Tanaka A, Saeki J, Hayama SI, Kass PH. Effect of Pets on Human Behaviour and Stress in Disaster. *Front Vet Sci.* 2019;6:113. Published 2019 Apr 18. doi:10.3389/fvets.2019.00113
7. Bruce H Lipton. The biology of belief. 2008. Hay House.
8. https://health.usnews.com/health-news/patient-advice/articles/2016-09-27/the-danger-in-taking-prescribed-medications
9. Sailler L. Les diagnostiques difficiles en iatrogénie [Diagnosis of iatrogenic diseases]. *Rev Med Interne.* 2009;30 Suppl 4:S295 S298. doi:10.1016/j.revmed.2009.09.014
10. Taro Gold. Open Your Mind, Open Your Life: A Book of Eastern Wisdom. 2004. 2nd edition. Andrews McMeel Universal.

A few last notes

1. Dugdale, J. S. (1996). *Entropy and its Physical Meaning* (2nd ed.). Taylor and Francis (UK); CRC (US)
2. P. Davis. *The demon in the machine. How hidden webs of information are solving the mystery of life.* 2019. Penguin books.
3. https://www.unccd.int/Lists/SiteDocumentLibrary/Publications/V2_201309-UNCCD-BRO_WEB_final.pdf
4. Harvey G. *The carbon fields. How our countryside can save Britain.* 2008. GrassRoots.
5. Roberts P. *The end of food.* 2008. Houghton Mifflin Company.
6. India is overproducing and wasting grain now, which is damaging soil and will result in lower future food production. April 2014. Coverage of Disruptive Science and Technology. http://www.nextbigfuture.com/2013/04/india-is-overproducing-and-wasting.html
7. Savory A. *Holistic Management. A new framework for decision making.* 1999. Island Press.
8. https://savory.global/
9. https://www.expertsure.com/2009/11/14/turning-desert-into-a-garden/
10. https://www.ted.com/talks/allan_savory_how_to_fight_desertification_and_reverse_climate_change
11. https://metro.co.uk/2018/08/08/man-turned-desert-forest-planting-tree-every-day-40-years-7814241/
12. https://www.chinadaily.com.cn/kindle/2017-09/06/content_31635441.htm

13. Jean Giorno. *The man who planted trees*. 2005. Chelsea Green Publishing.
14. Sheldrake R. *The science delusion*. 2013. Coronet. pp.78-79.

A–Z: GAPS conditions in alphabetic order

1. Andrew Hall Cutler. *Hair test interpretation: finding hidden toxicities*. 2004. noamalgam.com
2. Trüeb RM, Dias MFRG. Alopecia Areata: a Comprehensive Review of Pathogenesis and Management. *Clin Rev Allergy Immunol*. 2018;54(1):68 87. doi:10.1007/s12016-017-8620-9
3. Andrew Hall Cutler. *Amalgam illness. Diagnosis and treatment*. 2017. noamalgam.com
4. Rossi A, Fortuna MC, Caro G, *et al*. Chemotherapy-induced alopecia management: Clinical experience and practical advice. *J Cosmet Dermatol*. 2017;16(4):537 541. doi:10.1111/jocd.12308
5. Francesco Ciccia, Giuliana Guggino, Aroldo Rizzo, Riccardo Alessandro, Michele Maria Luchetti, Simon Milling, Laura Saieva, Heleen Cypers, Tommaso Stampone, Paola Di Benedetto, Armando Gabrielli, Alessio Fasano, Dirk Elewaut, Giovanni Triolo. Dysbiosis and zonulin upregulation alter gut epithelial and vascular barriers in patients with ankylosing spondylitis. *Annals of the Rheumatic Diseases*, Jan 2017, annrheumdis-2016-210000; DOI: 10.1136/annrheumdis-2016-210000
6. Outi Maki-Ikola *et al*. Enhanced jejunal production of antibodies to Klebsiella and other Enterobacteria in patients with ankylosing spondylitis and rheumatoid arthritis. http://dx.doi.org/10.1136/ard.56.7.421
7. Taha Rashid, Clyde Wilson, and Alan Ebringer. The Link between Ankylosing Spondylitis, Crohn's Disease, Klebsiella, and Starch Consumption. *Clinical and Developmental Immunology*, Volume 2013 (2013), Article ID 872632, 9 pages. http://dx.doi.org/10.1155/2013/872632
8. Thage O. The myotomes L2—S2 in man. *Acta Neurol Scand Suppl*. 1965;13 Pt 1:241 243. doi:10.1111/j.1600-0404.1965.tb01878.x
9. Korpi A, Järnberg J, Pasanen AL. Microbial volatile organic compounds. *Crit Rev Toxicol*. 2009;39(2):139 193. doi:10.1080/10408440802291497
10. Bodeker GC. Ayurvedic medicine. *CMAJ*. 1991;145(1):9 12.
11. Lebwohl B, Sanders DS, Green PHR. Coeliac disease. *Lancet*. 2018;391(10115): 70 81. doi:10.1016/S0140-6736(17)31796-8
12. Huebener S *et al*. Specific non-gluten proteins of wheat are novel target antigens in celiac disease humoural response. *J proteome Res* 2014, epub Oct 20.
13. Campbell-McBride N. *GAPS Stories. Personal Accounts of improvement and recovery through the GAPS Nutritional protocol*. 2012. Medinform Publishing.
14. Campbell-McBride N. *Gut and psychology syndrome. Natural treatment for autism, dyspraxia, dyslexia, ADD/ADHD, depression and schizophrenia*. 2010. Medinform Publishing.
15. Su, R Dailey, *et al*. Determining Effects of Superfine Sheep wool in Infantile Eczema (DESSINE): a randomized paediatric cross over study *J.C.* 2017. https://www.mcri.edu.au/sites/default/files/media/sudessinewoolonlinebjdarticle.pdf
16. Nunnari J, Suomalainen A. Mitochondria: in sickness and in health. *Cell*. 2012;148(6):1145 1159. doi:10.1016/j.cell.2012.02.035
17. Finsterer J, Zarrouk-Mahjoub S. Anti-mitochondrial M2 Antibodies and Myopathy. *Intern Med*. 2018;57(8):1187. doi:10.2169/internalmedicine.9878–17

18. Caubet JC, Cianferoni A, Groetch M, Nowak-Wegrzyn A. Food protein-induced enterocolitis syndrome. *Clin Exp Allergy*. 2019;49(9):1178 1190. doi:10.1111/cea.13415
19. Du YJ, Nowak-W grzyn A, Vadas P. FPIES in adults. *Ann Allergy Asthma Immunol*. 2018;121(6):736 738. doi:10.1016/j.anai.2018.08.003
20. Shao T, Shao L, Li H, Xie Z, He Z, Wen C. Combined Signature of the Fecal Microbiome and Metabolome in Patients with Gout. *Front Microbiol*. 2017;8:268. Published 2017 Feb 21. doi:10.3389/fmicb.2017.00268
21. Tatu L, Moulin T, Vuillier F, Bogousslavsky J. Arterial territories of the human brain. *Front Neurol Neurosci*. 2012;30:99 110. doi:10.1159/000333602
22. Vander Borght M, Wyns C. Fertility and infertility: Definition and epidemiology. *Clin Biochem*. 2018;62:2 10. doi:10.1016/j.clinbiochem.2018.03.012
23. Lotti F, Maggi M. Sexual dysfunction and male infertility. *Nat Rev Urol*. 2018;15(5):287 307. doi:10.1038/nrurol.2018.20
24. Letavernier E, Daudon M. Vitamin D, Hypercalciuria and Kidney Stones. *Nutrients*. 2018;10(3):366. Published 2018 Mar 17. doi:10.3390/nu10030366
25. Masterjohn C. On the trail of the elusive x factor: a sixty-two-year-old mystery finally solved. *Wise Traditions*. 2007;8(1).
26. Ross Russell AL, Dryden MS, Pinto AA, Lovett JK. Lyme disease: diagnosis and management. *Pract Neurol*. 2018;18(6):455 464. doi:10.1136/practneurol-2018-001998
27. Horowitz RI, Freeman PR. *Precision Medicine: The Role of the MSIDS Model in Defining, Diagnosing, and Treating Chronic Lyme Disease/Post Treatment Lyme Disease Syndrome and Other Chronic Illness: Part 2*. Healthcare (Basel). 2018; 6(4):129. Published 2018 Nov 5. doi:10.3390/healthcare6040129
28. http://cowden-protocol.com/
29. Engin A. The Definition and Prevalence of Obesity and Metabolic Syndrome. *Adv Exp Med Biol*. 2017;960:1 17. doi:10.1007/978-3-319-48382-5_1
30. Grandl G, Wolfrum C. Hemostasis, endothelial stress, inflammation, and the metabolic syndrome. *Semin Immunopathol*. 2018;40(2):215 224. doi:10.1007/s00281-017-0666-5
31. Campbell-McBride N. *Put your heart in your mouth. What really is heart disease and what can we do to prevent and even reverse it*. 2007. Medinform Publishing.
32. Volpe SL. Magnesium in disease prevention and overall health. *Adv Nutr*. 2013;4(3):378S 83S. Published 2013 May 1. doi:10.3945/an.112.003483
33. Mazidi M, Rezaie P, Kengne AP, Mobarhan MG, Ferns GA. Gut microbiome and metabolic syndrome. *Diabetes Metab Syndr*. 2016;10(2 Suppl 1):S150 S157. doi:10.1016/j.dsx.2016.01.024
34. Verma D, Garg PK, Dubey AK. Insights into the human oral microbiome. *Arch Microbiol*. 2018;200(4):525 540. doi:10.1007/s00203-018-1505-3
35. Sun S, Wei H, Zhu R, *et al*. Biology of the Tongue Coating and Its Value in Disease Diagnosis. *Complement Med Res*. 2018;25(3):191 197. doi:10.1159/000479024
36. Dominik Nischwitz. *It's All In Your Mouth. Biological Dentistry And The Surprising Impact Of Oral Health On Whole Body Wellness*. 2020. Chelsea Green Publishing.
37. Monje M. Myelin Plasticity and Nervous System Function. *Annu Rev Neurosci*. 2018;41:61 76. doi:10.1146/annurev-neuro-080317-061853
38. Duhamel G, Prevost VH, Cayre M, *et al*. Validating the sensitivity of inhomogeneous magnetization transfer (ihMT) MRI to myelin with fluorescence microscopy. *Neuroimage*. 2019;199:289 303. doi:10.1016/j.neuroimage.2019.05.061

39. Wang SS, Zhang Z, Zhu TB, Chu SF, He WB, Chen NH. Myelin injury in the central nervous system and Alzheimer's disease. *Brain Res Bull*. 2018;140: 162 168. doi:10.1016/j.brainresbull.2018.05.003
40. Allen DR, Huang MU, Morris NB, *et al*. Impaired Thermoregulatory Function during Dynamic Exercise in Multiple Sclerosis. *Med Sci Sports Exerc*. 2019;51(3):395 404. doi:10.1249/MSS.0000000000001821
41. Hachim MY, Elemam NM, Maghazachi AA. The Beneficial and Debilitating Effects of Environmental and Microbial Toxins, Drugs, Organic Solvents and Heavy Metals on the Onset and Progression of Multiple Sclerosis. *Toxins* (Basel). 2019;11(3):147. Published 2019 Mar 5. doi:10.3390/toxins11030147 Form
42. Hal A Huggins. *Solving the MS mystery: help, hope and recovery*. 2002. Dragon Slayer Publication.
43. Andrew Hall Cutler. *Amalgam illness. Diagnosis and treatment*. 2017. noamalgam.com
44. Epstein SS. *Unreasonable risk. How to avoid cancer from cosmetics and personal care products*. 2001. Published by Environmental Toxicology, Chicago Illinois.
45. Alroughani R, Boyko A. Pediatric multiple sclerosis: a review. *BMC Neurol*. 2018;18(1):27. Published 2018 Mar 9. doi:10.1186/s12883-018-1026-3
46. Whitehouse CR, Boullata J, McCauley LA. The potential toxicity of artificial sweeteners. *AAOHN J*. 2008;56(6):251 261. doi:10.3928/08910162-20080601-02
47. Ochoa-Repáraz J, Kirby TO, Kasper LH. The Gut Microbiome and Multiple Sclerosis. *Cold Spring Harb Perspect Med*. 2018;8(6):a029017. Published 2018 Jun 1. doi:10.1101/cshperspect.a029017
48. StrattonCW,WheldonDB(2006) Multiple sclerosis: an infectious syndrome involving Chlamydophila pneumoniae. *TRENDS in Microbiology* Vol.14 No.11
49. Alan MacDonald. *Migrating worm in the brain can cause MS*. https://vimeo.com/166688480 lecture, college of American pathologists.
50. Enig MG. *Know Your Fats: The Complete Primer for Understanding the Nutrition of Fats, Oils, and Cholesterol*. Bethesda Press, Silver Spring, MD, 2000.
51. Ravnskov U. *The Cholesterol Myths. Exposing the fallacy that saturated fat and cholesterol cause heart disease*. 2000. NewTrends Publishing.
52. Corning B, Copland AP, Frye JW. The Esophageal Microbiome in Health and Disease. *Curr Gastroenterol Rep*. 2018;20(8):39. Published 2018 Aug 1. doi:10.1007/s11894-018-0642-9
53. Zhou Q, Melton DA. Pancreas regeneration [published correction appears in *Nature*. 2018 Aug;560(7720):E34]. *Nature*. 2018;557(7705):351 358. doi:10.1038/s41586-018-0088-0
54. Khan MN, Raza SS, Hussain AK, Nadeem MD, Ullah F. Pancreatic Duct Stones. *J Ayub Med Coll Abbottabad*. 2017;29(1):154 156.
55. Johnson CD, Besselink MG, Carter R. Acute pancreatitis. *BMJ*. 2014;349: g4859. Published 2014 Aug 12. doi:10.1136/bmj.g4859
56. Ertz-Archambault N, Keim P, Von Hoff D. Microbiome and pancreatic cancer: A comprehensive topic review of literature. *World J Gastroenterol*. 2017;23(10): 1899 1908. doi:10.3748/wjg.v23.i10.1899
57. Masterjohn C. On the trail of the elusive x factor: a sixty-two-year-old mystery finally solved. *Wise Traditions*. 2007;8(1).
58. Campbell-McBride N. *GAPS Stories. Personal Accounts of improvement and recovery through the GAPS Nutritional protocol*. 2012. Medinform Publishing.
59. Quagliariello A, Del Chierico F, Russo A, *et al*. Gut Microbiota Profiling and

Gut-Brain Crosstalk in Children Affected by Pediatric Acute-Onset Neuropsychiatric Syndrome and Pediatric Autoimmune Neuropsychiatric Disorders Associated With Streptococcal Infections. *Front Microbiol.* 2018;9:675. Published 2018 Apr 6. doi:10.3389/fmicb.2018.00675

60. Marti H. The Discovery of Helminth Life Cycles. *Adv Parasitol.* 2019;103:1 10. doi:10.1016/bs.apar.2019.02.001
61. Sures, B., Siddall, R. and Taraschewski, H. Certain parasites, particularly intestinal acanthocephalans and cestodes of fish, can accumulate heavy metals at concentrations that are orders of magnitude higher than those in the host tissues or the environment. *Parasit Today*, 1999 Jan;15(1):16–21.
62. Garzón M, Pereira-da-Silva L, Seixas J, *et al.* Association of enteric parasitic infections with intestinal inflammation and permeability in asymptomatic infants of São Tomé Island. *Pathog Glob Health.* 2017;111(3):116 127. doi:10.1080/20477724.2017.1299831
63. Yasuda K, Nakanishi K. Host responses to intestinal nematodes. *Int Immunol.* 2018;30(3):93 102. doi:10.1093/intimm/dxy002
64. Rendon A, Schäkel K. Psoriasis Pathogenesis and Treatment. *Int J Mol Sci.* 2019;20(6):1475. Published 2019 Mar 23. doi:10.3390/ijms20061475
65. Campbell-McBride N. *GAPS Stories. Personal Accounts of improvement and recovery through the GAPS Nutritional protocol.* 2012. Medinform Publishing.
66. Quigley EMM. The Spectrum of Small Intestinal Bacterial Overgrowth (SIBO). *Curr Gastroenterol Rep.* 2019;21(1):3. Published 2019 Jan 15. doi:10.1007/s11894-019-0671-z
67. Wüthrich B, Schmid A, Walther B, Sieber R. Milk consumption does not lead to mucus production or occurrence of asthma. *J Am Coll Nutr.* 2005;24(6 Suppl): 547S 55S. doi:10.1080/07315724.2005.10719503
68. Rawls M, Ellis AK. The microbiome of the nose. *Ann Allergy Asthma Immunol.* 2019;122(1):17 24. doi:10.1016/j.anai.2018.05.009
69. Cheli R, Ciancamerla G. Die durch Medikamente verusachte Gastritis [Drug-induced gastritis]. *Gastroenterol Fortbildungskurse Prax.* 1973;4:59 65.
70. Dominik Nischwitz. *It's All In Your Mouth. Biological Dentistry And The Surprising Impact Of Oral Health On Whole Body Wellness.* 2020. Chelsea Green Publishing.
71. Howden CW, Hunt RH. Spontaneous hypochlorhydria in man: possible causes and consequences. *Dig Dis.* 1986;4(1):26 32. doi:10.1159/000171134
72. Noto JM, Peek RM Jr. The gastric microbiome, its interaction with Helicobacter pylori, and its potential role in the progression to stomach cancer. *PLoS Pathog.* 2017;13(10):e1006573. Published 2017 Oct 5. doi:10.1371/journal.ppat.1006573
73. Castaño-Rodríguez N, Goh KL, Fock KM, Mitchell HM, Kaakoush NO. Dysbiosis of the microbiome in gastric carcinogenesis. *Sci Rep.* 2017;7(1): 15957. Published 2017 Nov 21. doi:10.1038/s41598-017-16289-2
74. Camilleri M, Chedid V, Ford AC, *et al.* Gastroparesis. *Nat Rev Dis Primers.* 2018;4(1):41. Published 2018 Nov 1. doi:10.1038/s41572-018-0038-z
75. Wilkinson JM, Cozine EW, Loftus CG. Gas, Bloating, and Belching: Approach to Evaluation and Management. *Am Fam Physician.* 2019;99(5):301 309.
76. Ritchie WP Jr. Alkaline reflux gastritis. Late results on a controlled trial of diagnosis and treatment. Ann Surg. 1986;203(5):537 544. doi:10.1097/ 00000658-198605000-00014
77. Bhandari S, Jha P, Thakur A, Kar A, Gerdes H, Venkatesan T. Cyclic vomiting syndrome: epidemiology, diagnosis, and treatment. *Clin Auton Res.* 2018; 28(2):203 209. doi:10.1007/s10286-018-0506-2

78. Mort RL, Jackson IJ, Patton EE. The melanocyte lineage in development and disease [published correction appears in *Development*. 2015 Apr 1;142(7):1387]. *Development*. 2015;142(4):620 632. doi:10.1242/dev.106567
79. Ezzedine K, Eleftheriadou V, Whitton M, van Geel N. Vitiligo. *Lancet*. 2015;386(9988):74 84. doi:10.1016/S0140-6736(14)60763-7
80. Grunnet I, Howitz J, Reymann F, Schwartz M. Vitiligo and pernicious anemia. *Arch Dermatol*. 1970;101(1):82 85.
81. Andreas NJ, Kampmann B, Mehring Le-Doare K. Human breast milk: A review on its composition and bioactivity. *Early Hum Dev*. 2015;91(11):629 635. doi:10.1016/j.earlhumdev.2015.08.013
82. Quigley M, Embleton ND, McGuire W. Formula versus donor breast milk for feeding preterm or low birth weight infants. *Cochrane Database Syst Rev*. 2018;6(6):CD002971. Published 2018 Jun 20. doi:10.1002/14651858.CD002971.pub4

Index